Global Health: Changing Health Technology

Global Health: Changing Health Technology

Editor: Tandy Rocco

AMERICAN
MEDICAL PUBLISHERS
www.americanmedicalpublishers.com

AMERICAN
MEDICAL PUBLISHERS
www.americanmedicalpublishers.com

Cataloging-in-Publication Data

Global health : changing health technology / edited by Tandy Rocco.
p. cm.
Includes bibliographical references and index.
ISBN 979-8-88740-135-5
1. World health. 2. Public health. 3. Medical technology. 4. Medical geography.
5. Medical innovations. 6. Biomedical engineering. I. Rocco, Tandy.
RA441 .G56 2023
362.1--dc23

American Medical Publishers,
41 Flatbush Avenue,
1st Floor, New York,
NY 11217, USA

ISBN 979-8-88740-135-5 (Hardback)

Contents

Preface

Global health is an area of study, research, and practice that focuses on improving health and achieving equity in health for all people around the world. The objectives of global health include improving worldwide health, reducing disparities, and protecting global threats that overlook national borders. It consists of various perspectives that emphasize the factors and administration of health in international contexts. Medicine, epidemiology, demography, economics, and other social sciences such as sociology, development studies, psychology, anthropology, cultural studies and law, can help in recognizing the determinants of health in societies. Technology plays a major role in the advancement of healthcare and medicine. Digital technologies such as artificial intelligence (AI), virtual reality (VR), healthcare trackers, wearables, sensors, telehealth, and telemedicine, etc. are now being used increasingly to make the healthcare systems cheaper, faster, and more effective in managing diseases. The topics included in this book on global health and health technology are of utmost significance and will provide incredible insights to the readers. It will help the readers in keeping pace with the rapid changes in this field.

The information contained in this book is the result of intensive hard work done by researchers in this field. All due efforts have been made to make this book serve as a complete guiding source for students and researchers. The topics in this book have been comprehensively explained to help readers understand the growing trends in the field.

I would like to thank the entire group of writers who made sincere efforts in this book and my family who supported me in my efforts of working on this book. I take this opportunity to thank all those who have been a guiding force throughout my life.

Editor

1

3-Dimensional Facial Analysis—Facing Precision Public Health

Gareth Baynam[1,2,3,4,5,6,7], Alicia Bauskis[3], Nicholas Pachter[1,4,8], Lyn Schofield[1,9], Hedwig Verhoef[10], Richard L. Palmer[11], Stefanie Kung[11], Petra Helmholz[11], Michael Ridout[11], Caroline E. Walker[3], Anne Hawkins[1], Jack Goldblatt[1,4], Tarun S. Weeramanthri[12], Hugh J. S. Dawkins[3,8,9,13] and Caron M. Molster[3]*

[1] Genetic Services of Western Australia, Department of Health, Government of Western Australia, Perth, WA, Australia, [2] Western Australian Register of Developmental Anomalies, Perth, WA, Australia, [3] Office of Population Health Genomics, Public Health Division, Department of Health, Government of Western Australia, Perth, WA, Australia, [4] School of Paediatrics and Child Health, University of Western Australia, Perth, WA, Australia, [5] Institute for Immunology and Infectious Diseases, Murdoch University, Perth, WA, Australia, [6] Telethon Kids Institute, Perth, WA, Australia, [7] Spatial Sciences, Department of Science and Engineering, Curtin University, Perth, WA, Australia, [8] School of Pathology and Laboratory Medicine, University of Western Australia, Perth, WA, Australia, [9] Centre for Comparative Genomics, Murdoch University, Perth, WA, Australia, [10] Cooperative Research Centre for Spatial Information, Perth, WA, Australia, [11] School of Spatial Sciences, Curtin University, Perth, WA, Australia, [12] Public Health Division, Department of Health, Government of Western Australia, Perth, WA, Australia, [13] Centre for Population Health Research, Curtin Health Innovation Research Institute, Curtin University of Technology, Perth, WA, Australia

Correspondence:
Gareth Baynam
gareth.baynam@health.wa.gov.au

Precision public health is a new field driven by technological advances that enable more precise descriptions and analyses of individuals and population groups, with a view to improving the overall health of populations. This promises to lead to more precise clinical and public health practices, across the continuum of prevention, screening, diagnosis, and treatment. A phenotype is the set of observable characteristics of an individual resulting from the interaction of a genotype with the environment. Precision (deep) phenotyping applies innovative technologies to exhaustively and more precisely examine the discrete components of a phenotype and goes beyond the information usually included in medical charts. This form of phenotyping is a critical component of more precise diagnostic capability and 3-dimensional facial analysis (3DFA) is a key technological enabler in this domain. In this paper, we examine the potential of 3DFA as a public health tool, by viewing it against the 10 essential public health services of the "public health wheel," developed by the US Centers for Disease Control. This provides an illustrative framework to gage current and emergent applications of genomic technologies for implementing precision public health.

Keywords: public health, 3D facial scan, rare diseases, spatial information, genomics and genetics, developmental disabilities

INTRODUCTION

Rare diseases (RD) are increasingly recognized nationally (1) and globally as a public health priority (2, 3). While individually, RD have a low prevalence, it is estimated that the combined prevalence is between 6 and 8% of the population (2, 4). Most RD have a genetic association and are often severely debilitating, impair physical and mental abilities, and shorten life expectancy (5). These characteristics present clinical and public health challenges. These include the need for early and accurate diagnosis and for identifying emerging technologies to enhance the delivery of clinical and public health practices for affected individuals (1).

The RD community has collectively nominated timely accurate diagnosis and earlier intervention with improved therapeutic options as key issues (6). This context and this challenge also provide opportunities for innovation and creating new knowledge. One such opportunity for improved diagnosis and treatment is through the clarity that can be achieved with detailed analysis and representation of the phenotype of genetic and rare disorders. Broadly, a phenotype is the set of observable characteristics of an individual resulting from the interaction of a genotype with the environment; in medicine, it is used to describe some deviation from normal morphology, physiology, or behavior. Greater phenotypic clarity is being advanced through imaging, the use of standards for phenotypic description, and their combination. This "precision" or "deep" phenotyping affords medicine and science a unique opportunity to generate biological insights.

An emerging deep phenotyping application is 3-dimensional facial analysis (3DFA). In the RD domain, 3DFA has been investigated and is increasingly being implemented, primarily for diagnostic purposes (7–9). 3DFA is also being applied to monitor existing and novel therapies, an area in which it has a nascent role (10, 11). 3DFA involves the investigation of deeply precise 3D facial data that can be acquired with various facial imaging technologies and applied to deliver scientific insights. The technological innovations enabling 3DFA include advances in imaging hardware, analytical techniques, and the combination with other, e.g., text-based, advances.

Approaches such as 3DFA, and other forms of deep phenotyping, mean that RD are providing a fruitful domain for precision approaches to medicine and public health. This is highlighted by a series of targeted precision initiatives in multiple countries, including in the United States, programs based at the National Institutes of Health at the Centers for Mendelian Genetics and the Undiagnosed Diseases Program and Network (12, 13); in Japan, via its Agency for Medical Research and Development under its rare and intractable diseases pillar; and in Western Australia (WA), through a coordinated suite of initiatives being implemented under the *WA Rare Diseases Strategic Framework 2015–2018* (1, 9).

PRECISION TECHNOLOGIES IN PUBLIC HEALTH

Precision public health has been defined as "the application and combination of new and existing technologies, which more precisely describe and analyze individuals and their environment over the life course, in order to tailor preventive interventions for at-risk groups and improve the overall health of the population." Thus, precision public health complements and extends precision medicine's focus by recognizing that precise interventions are needed at both the individual and population levels.

Herein, we outline the state of play of current and emergent 3DFA applications, specifically within a precision public health paradigm, and using congenital and rare disorders as an exemplar. As an illustrative framework, we use the 10 essential public health services of "the public health wheel" (14). This framework operationalizes the three core functions of public health, namely, assessment, policy-making, and assurance.

MONITOR HEALTH STATUS TO IDENTIFY AND SOLVE COMMUNITY HEALTH PROBLEMS

Congenital anomalies are an important class of mainly RD accounting for 12–15% of people with RD and are also known as birth defects (15). The causes of these conditions can be divided into genetic (e.g., monogenic disorders), multifactorial (e.g., cleft palate), and environmental exposures [e.g., fetal alcohol syndrome (FAS)]. Congenital anomalies accounted for 732,000 disability-adjusted life years lost, in 2010, in Western Europe alone (16).

A considerable proportion of congenital anomalies are associated with facial dysmorphology (17), either through the presence of congenital anomalies in known syndromes with well-documented facial dysmorphology (e.g., cardiac anomalies in Noonan syndrome), or in the recurrent co-coding of individual congenital anomalies and facial dysmorphism in individuals (17). Furthermore, hundreds of disorders (18), which are collectively and variably described as "dysmorphic syndromes" or "developmental disorders," have characteristic facies. In these instances, 3DFA has potential to contribute to the improved speed and accuracy of diagnosis for a sizeable proportion of the general population. This will contribute to more accurate epidemiological data, including more precise estimates of the incidence, prevalence, and burden of congenital disorders.

DIAGNOSE AND INVESTIGATE HEALTH PROBLEMS AND HEALTH HAZARDS IN THE COMMUNITY

3-Dimensional facial analysis is being developed for deeply precise diagnostic applications across a broad range of typically rare conditions with well-established facial dysmorphic patterns (8), see **Figures 1** and **2**. Additionally, it is increasingly and objectively unlocking hitherto undetected, or underappreciated,

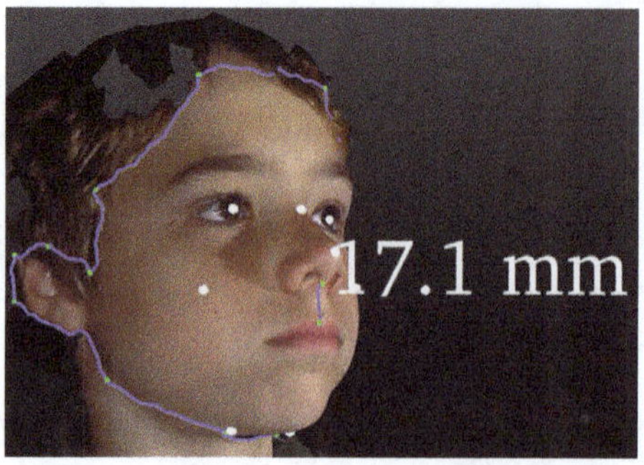

FIGURE 1 | Some functionality of 3DFA. The purple line around the facial periphery demonstrates a cropping and facial segmentation tool. White dots are automated land marking. The vertical purple line demonstrates an application of the measuring tool, in this case showing a 17.1 mm philtral length.

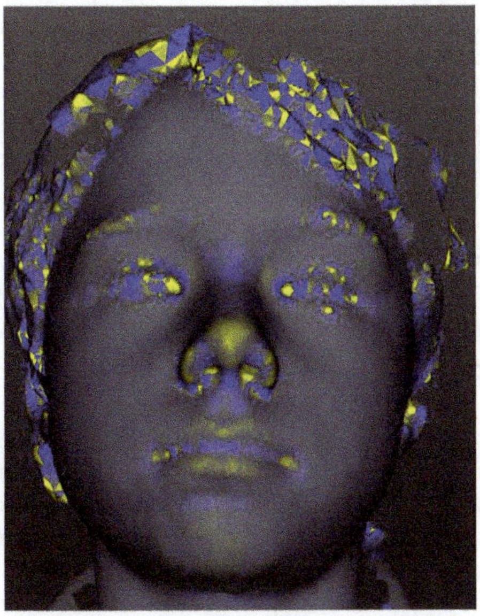

FIGURE 2 | The tool has modular analysis components. This figure demonstrates one such module, curvature analysis, which is demonstrated in a yellow-blue color scale.

facial diagnostic signatures (7). For example, speech delay is common in rare conditions, and in one study of kindergarten children, approximately 7% had language-specific impairments (19). A potential 3DFA application is using facial signatures as early predictors of language delay, either in those from the general population or in those at high familial risk, e.g., siblings of children with autism. The presence of a group of rare disorders, characterized by severe speech impairment and with overlapping facial features, collectively called Angelman-like syndromes (20), supports the possibility of using facial signatures to predict speech delay. There are also numerous other rare disorders that are associated with variable degrees of speech delay, e.g., Cornelia de Lange syndrome and biologically related disorders (21), that have characteristic, and overlapping facial phenotypes. It is likely that other children, with or without known syndromes, will have facial signatures that are indicative of speech delay that may offer a novel way for early screening for language delay to target early intervention.

INFORM, EDUCATE, AND EMPOWER PEOPLE ABOUT HEALTH ISSUES

We all have a face. It is our unique expression of who we are, it reflects our life experiences and communicates our emotions to the world. From birth, our faces are a window to our being and our portal of interaction with our world. Our faces speak of the community from whence we came, and of the communities to which we belong, the ultimate expression of our connection as individuals. Our face is a canvas for the arts, a window for education, a living record of the diversity of the environment and our origins. Our face is also a biological billboard that advertises our physical and mental wellness, our aging, and our disease. We commonly say, "you look ill," "you look well," "you look in pain," and we can, for instance, readily recognize a child with Down's syndrome by their facial features. Objectively documenting and harnessing these facial clues that underlie common parlance and innate recognition capacities, can be used to inform, educate, and empower people for health.

A person who has a 3D image taken of their face can almost immediately see the computer-generated image. This recognizable and relatable image enables patients and their families to gain a new perspective of their health, or the health of a relative. Within WA, the technology has recently been used with primary school students who participated in a project to support equitable innovation for Aboriginal health. As the parameters of normal facial contours vary with ethnicity, it is important to compile reference scans for different ethnic groups. The children involved in this project were delighted to be able to view and manipulate their 3D facial images. "They especially loved being able to turn their faces upside down to look up their noses!" (22).

MOBILIZE COMMUNITY PARTNERSHIPS AND ACTION TO IDENTIFY AND SOLVE HEALTH PROBLEMS

Projects focusing on the delivery of novel ways to diagnose and monitor rare disorders have been undertaken with the key support of patient advocacy organizations in Australia (e.g., Rare Voices Australia, Fabry Australia, Mucopolysachharide and Related Diseases Society Australia, Short Statured People's Association of Australia) and internationally (e.g., International MPS Network, Costello Syndrome Family Association, CFC International). Similarly, projects focused on equitable health innovation to address RD have been developed and delivered in partnership with Aboriginal leaders, health workers, and communities. These projects have been important to the development of interest in and application of 3DFA.

The desire to address RD, together with the multifarious and crosscutting aspects of faces described above, has provided a unique vehicle for mobilizing community partnerships to engage in the identification and solution of health problems. A 2015 event organized as part of an ongoing platform for harmonizing translational research across premier hospitals, research institutes, government, and the community is an illustrative case (23). The "Faces of WA" event coalesced cross-sector interest in 3DFA applications from across science, arts, research, education, and data analytics communities.

DEVELOP POLICIES AND PLANS THAT SUPPORT INDIVIDUAL AND COMMUNITY HEALTH EFFORTS

In 2015, WA released the state-wide *WA Rare Diseases Strategic Framework 2015–2018* (1), which includes, but is not limited, to the following objectives: build on existing services for RD diagnosis and screening; identify emerging technologies to enhance the delivery of health care for RD, including to rural and remote areas; engage with people living with RD, their carers and families; promote active participation of people living with RD with their health care; build epidemiology and health system evidence for RD by improving diagnosis and disease classification; and strengthen clinical and translational research in RD. The implementation of 3DFA contributes to most of these objectives.

An example of a disease-specific policy in WA is the *Fetal Alcohol Spectrum Disorders (FASD) Model of Care* (24). FASD has been prioritized as a public health issue in Australia and other countries, and a cohesive, multilevel, and community-focused suite of approaches is required to address this preventable disorder group. The *FASD Model of Care* identifies health care and public health prevention strategies as the most important means of reducing FASD. The implementation and use of 3DFA has the potential to address several of these recommendations, including but not limited to screening and early diagnosis. FAS is part of the of FASD continuum for which characteristic facial features are obligate for diagnosis. These facial characteristics are known to vary by ethnicity (25, 26), and there is a paucity of data on the Australian Aboriginal population. A pragmatic, but potentially imprecise, approach using African-American facial standards has been implemented for FAS diagnosis. Should these be unfit for purpose, epidemiological, and diagnostic data may be inaccurate with implications for targeted health and prevention strategies. Potentially, the ethnic variation of Aboriginal facial features could be more objectively addressed with the precision of currently available 3D approaches.

ENFORCE LAWS AND REGULATIONS THAT PROTECT HEALTH AND ENSURE SAFETY

Clinicians and public health practitioners advocate for, review, evaluate, revise, educate, and enforce compliance with laws and regulations. This must include new and existing laws and regulations related to the use of genomic and other technologies, and the information generated from their use (27).

The genetic and genomic information about individuals, and that obtained from 3DFA, forms part of and expands the individual's health information. It may also provide information about the individual's relatives, which may be of interest to them, especially where prevention or treatment is available. Health professionals may inform the individual of how the genetic information relates to their relatives; however, confidentiality requirements prevent the disclosure of this information to the relatives, without the consent of the individual, except in specific circumstances outlined in relevant legislation and regulations. Internationally and variably, legislation has been enacted to regulate the collection, use, and disclosure of health information. In Australia, the 2006 amendments to *the Privacy Act 1988* allow for health practitioners to use or disclose an individual's genetic information, without their consent, where there is a reasonable belief that doing so is necessary to lessen or prevent a serious threat to the life, health, or safety of their relatives. Irrespective of jurisdictional differences in legislation and its implementation, the principle remains that new phenotypic technologies that reveal indications of familial disease may have implications for life insurance, employment, and reproductive choices, so they need to conform with legislated codes for privacy protection, disclosure, and data sharing.

LINK PEOPLE TO NEEDED PERSONAL HEALTH SERVICES AND ASSURE THE PROVISION OF HEALTH CARE WHEN OTHERWISE UNAVAILABLE

Linking people to needed services includes developing mechanisms to assure the provision of such services to marginalized and underserved populations. In relation to RD, three such population groups in WA are people living with long-standing undiagnosed conditions, those living in rural and remote areas, and Aboriginal Australians. Improved diagnostic services utilizing new genomic technologies and 3DFA are enabling more equitable access to services for these populations.

At the level of state-wide clinical practice, 3DFA has been implemented in services that improve population access to RD diagnostics. The Rare and Undiagnosed Diseases Diagnostic service at Genetic Services of WA (9) integrates genomic diagnostics into a state-wide clinical service that includes outreach clinics. The Undiagnosed Diseases Program Western Australia is a cross-disciplinary service provided within the local children's hospital but also accessible to children across the state. These complementary programs aim to find diagnoses for those with long-standing, undiagnosed conditions.

Given the (increasing) transportability and reducing cost of 3D facial imaging systems, 3DFA is being implemented in remote outreach clinics by initially using a model of periodic deployment of a portable camera. Permanent placement of scanners in key regional locations is planned for the future. This is to facilitate point-of-care diagnostics, treatment, and monitoring and to enhance referral, i.e., by pairing submission of 3D images with text-based referrals and consultation processes.

ASSURE COMPETENT PUBLIC AND PERSONAL HEALTH-CARE WORKFORCE

Facial gestalt is key to diagnosis for numerous genetic conditions (e.g., Velocardiofacial syndrome, Williams syndrome, Noonan syndrome) and non-genetic conditions [e.g., fetal valproate syndrome (FAS)]. Through the creation of tools that objectively determine facial patterns and unlock knowledge, diagnostic ability and workforce competency can be improved. The increasingly transportable nature of the approach also suits capacity building in remote regions; training in 3DFA could contribute to workforce development. Coupled with the non-invasive nature of 3DFA, this increasing portability, and the very nature of faces, it also provides a unique opportunity to engage with this new technology as a bridge to deeper engagement with other (e.g., genomic) technologies.

EVALUATE EFFECTIVENESS, ACCESSIBILITY, AND QUALITY OF PERSONAL AND POPULATION-BASED HEALTH SERVICES

The value of clarifying a diagnosis is undeniable (28). Improved diagnostic certainty through the precision of 3DFA provides novel opportunities to evaluate health care, for instance, in assessing the diagnostic programs for rare genetic diseases through direct and objective comparison of facial phenotypic and molecular diagnostic approaches. Additionally, by improving certainty of the diagnosis of RD, one could more accurately assess interventions targeted to the reduction of the burden of these conditions. Given the marked disparity between the proportion of the population with RD and their combined health system costs, supporting the need for early diagnosis and intervention has the potential to drive cost savings across the health system (29).

3-Dimensional facial analysis is being used to monitor the effectiveness of drug therapy, which provides new avenues to assess drug response for both localized facial anomaly (10) and systemic disease (11). An example of 3DFA's use to monitor drug response was an application in mucopolysaccharidosis type I (MPS I). This lysosomal storage disease is caused by the body's inability to produce a specific enzyme, it expresses a pattern of progressive facial dysmorphology and it is treatable by drug therapy. 3DFA was used to monitor a child with MPS I undergoing treatment to demonstrate that the rate at which facial dysmorphology was advancing was reduced (11). 3DFA has also been used to monitor a child receiving a treatment (rapamycin) for a craniofacial anomaly. This child had extensive facial malformations and monitoring of their facial features using 3DFA showed a progressive improvement in their condition (10). In addition to observing treatment and disease progression in a standard clinical setting, 3DFA may also have a monitoring role in clinical trials.

RESEARCH FOR NEW INSIGHTS AND INNOVATIVE SOLUTIONS TO HEALTH PROBLEMS

Rare diseases are a hot bed for technological innovation and recurrently discoveries in RD have delivered innovations for common diseases (30). While 3DFA is yielding translational insights into innovations for diagnosis, treatment, and monitoring in the RD domain, it is also particularly suited to examining the overlap between rare and more common diseases. Notably, population level studies demonstrated that common genetic variations (polymorphisms) were associated with discrete patterns of facial variation. Notably, these facial signatures recapitulated the characteristic facies of the respective genetic syndrome due to rare genetic variation (pathogenic mutations). This highlights further evidence of the overlap between common and rare phenotypes with implications for possible reciprocal (rare-common) insights.

An example of a common disease that is poised for 3D facial translational research is obstructive sleep apnea (OSA). Through determining the facial signatures of OSA, 3DFA can be used as a complementary tool for OSA screening and classification. Again reflecting the potential for joint insights into rare and common diseases, OSA is a condition seen in RD, where it regularly has an earlier onset than in the general population (e.g., MPS syndromes).

A further promising area is face-to-text conversion. Conversion of a 3D facial image to standardized text-based descriptive terms known as human phenotype ontology (HPO) is an ideal way to achieve this. These standardized terms can be used computationally (i.e., are machine readable) and can then be used for report generation and for integration with text-based diagnostics. Face-to-text conversion has been performed for a limited subset of facial HPO terms (31). It needs to be extended to the full set and be further validated by human experts.

CONCLUSION

3-Dimensional facial analysis is a prototypical precision public health tool that delivers non-invasive, non-irradiating, transportable, and community engaging deep phenotyping. It enables multisector applications that can be increasingly implemented across the spectrum of public health. It can be applied to individuals as well as for single RD. Finally, insights generated in RD could be investigated in more common diseases.

AUTHOR CONTRIBUTIONS

GB, HD, CM, and AB contributed equally to the coordination of content and drafting the manuscript. GB, NP, JG, and AH contributed expert content to the clinical genomics components. TW, HD, CM, CW, and AB contributed to the expert content on public health genomics. HV, LS, RP, SK, PH, and MR contributed to the informatics and 3 dimensional facial scanning content. GB, HD, JG, TW, and CW are chief investigators of the Australian National Health and Medical Research Council APP1055319, and LS is employed on this grant.

FUNDING

The authors acknowledge their involvement in the International Rare Disease Research Consortium (IRDiRC) and the support from The Western Australian Government Department of Health as part of its commitment to the goals of the IRDiRC. The authors gratefully acknowledge the combined financial support-in-part from the RD-Connect-European Union Seventh Framework Programme (HEALTH. 2012.2. 1.1-1-C) under grant agreement number 305444; RD Connect: an integrated platform connecting databases, registries, biobanks, and clinical bioinformatics for rare disease research; and from the Australian National Health and Medical Research Council APP1055319 under the NHMRC–European Union Collaborative Research Grants scheme. GB acknowledges the WA Department of Health Raine Clinical Research Fellowship.

REFERENCES

1. Office of Population Health Genomics. *WA Rare Diseases Strategic Framework 2015-2018*. Perth, Australia: Public Health Division, Department of Health Western Australia (2015).
2. European Organisation for Rare Diseases. *Rare Diseases: Understanding this Public Health Priority*. Paris, France: EURORDIS (2005).
3. Valdez R, Ouyang L, Bolen J. Public health and rare diseases: oxymoron no more. *Prev Chronic Dis* (2016) 13:E05. doi:10.5888/pcd13.150491
4. Aymé S, Rodwell C. *Report on the State of the Art of Rare Disease Activities in Europe*. Paris: European Union Committee of Experts on Rare Disease, European Union. (2013).
5. Schieppati A, Henter J-I, Daina E, Aperia A. Why rare diseases are an important medical and social issue. *Lancet* (2008) 371(9629):2039–41. doi:10.1016/S0140-6736(08)60872-7
6. Molster C, Youngs L, Hammond E, Dawkins H. National rare diseases coordinating committee, and national rare diseases working group (2012). Key outcomes from stakeholder workshops at a symposium to inform the development of an Australian national plan for rare diseases. *Orphanet J Rare Dis* (2012) 7:50. doi:10.1186/1750-1172-7-50
7. Hammond P, Suttie M, Hennekam R, Allanson J, Shore E, Kaplan F. The face signature of fibrodysplasia ossificans progressiva. *Am J Med Genet A* (2012) 158A(6):1368–80. doi:10.1002/ajmg.a.35346
8. Baynam G, Walters M, Claes P, Kung S, LeSouef P, Dawkins H, et al. The facial evolution: looking backward and moving forward. *Hum Mutat* (2013) 34(1):14–22. doi:10.1002/humu.22219
9. Baynam G, Pachter N, McKenzie F, Townshend S, Slee J, Kiraly-Borri C, et al. The rare and undiagnosed diseases diagnostic service – application of massively parallel sequencing in a state-wide clinical service. *Orphanet J Rare Dis* (2016) 11(1):77. doi:10.1186/s13023-016-0462-7
10. Baynam GS, Walters M, Dawkins H, Bellgard M, Halbert AR, Claes P. Objective monitoring of mTOR inhibitor therapy by three-dimensional facial analysis. *Twin Res Hum Genet* (2013) 16(4):840–4. doi:10.1017/thg.2013.49
11. Kung S, Walters M, Claes P, LeSouef P, Goldblatt J, Martin A, et al. Monitoring of therapy for mucopolysaccharidosis type I using dysmorphometric facial phenotypic signatures. *JIMD Rep* (2015) 22:99–106. doi:10.1007/8904_2015_417
12. Taruscio D, Groft SC, Cederroth H, Melegh B, Lasko P, Kosaki K, et al. Undiagnosed diseases network international (UDNI): white paper for global actions to meet patient needs. *Mol Genet Metab* (2015) 116(4):223–5. doi:10.1016/j.ymgme.2015.11.003
13. National Institutes of Health. *NIH-Wide Strategic Plan: Turning Discovery into Health*. Bethesda, MD: Department of Health and Human Services (2016).
14. Centers for Disease Control and Prevention. *The Public Health System and the 10 Essential Public Health Services*. (2016). Available from: http://www.cdc.gov/nphpsp/essentialservices.html
15. European Surveillance of Congential Anomalies. *Congenital Anomalies Are a Major Cause of Mainly Rare Diseases*. Italy: EUROCAT, European Commission (2012).
16. Murray CJ, Vos T, Lozano R, Naghavi M, Flaxman AD, Michaud C, et al. Disability-adjusted life years (DALYs) for 291 diseases and injuries in 21 regions, 1990-2010: a systematic analysis for the Global Burden of Disease study 2010. *Lancet* (2012) 380(9859):2197–223. doi:10.1016/S0140-6736(12)61689-4
17. Department of Health Western Australian. *Western Australian Register of Developmental Anomalies*. (2016). Available from: http://www.kemh.health.wa.gov.au/services/register_developmental_anomalies/
18. Possum. *Pictures of Standard Syndromes and Undiagnosed Malformations*. (2016). Available from: http://www.possum.net.au/
19. Tomblin JB, Records NL, Buckwalter P, Zhang X, Smith E, O'Brien M. Prevalence of specific language impairment in kindergarten children. *J Speech Lang Hear Res* (1997) 40(6):1245–60. doi:10.1044/jslhr.4006.1245
20. Tan WH, Bird LM, Thibert RL, Williams CA. If not Angelman, what is it? A review of Angelman-like syndromes. *Am J Med Genet A* (2014) 164A(4):975–92. doi:10.1002/ajmg.a.36416
21. Deardorff MA, Noon SE, Krantz ID. Cornelia de Lange syndrome. In: Pagon RA, Adam MP, Ardinger HH, Wallace SE, Amemiya A, Bean LJH, et al., editors. *GeneReviews*. Seattle, WA: University of Washington (1993).
22. Department of Health Western Australia. *The face value of rare disease project*. Healthview Magazine. (2016). p. 15.
23. Western Australian Health Translation Network. *Faces of Western Australia*. (2015). Available from: http://www.scienceontheswan.com.au/?pgid=627
24. Department of Health Western Australia. *Fetal Alcohol Spectrum Disorder Model of Care*. Perth, Australia: Health Networks Branch, Department of Health Western Australia (2010).
25. Suttie M, Foroud T, Wetherill L, Jacobson JL, Molteno CD, Meintjes EM, et al. Facial dysmorphism across the fetal alcohol spectrum. *Pediatrics* (2013) 131(3):e779–88. doi:10.1542/peds.2012-1371
26. Fetal Alcohol Syndrome Diagnostic and Prevention Network. *Lip-Philtum Guides*. (2016). Available from: https://depts.washington.edu/fasdpn/htmls/lip-philtrum-guides.htm
27. McWalter K, Gaviglio A. Introduction to the special issue: public health genetics and genomics. *J Genet Couns* (2015) 24(3):375–80. doi:10.1007/s10897-015-9825-9
28. Sorensen G. *White Paper: Diagnosis, Misdiagnosis, and the Value of Knowing*. USA: Siemens Medical Solutions (2014).
29. Walker CE, Mahede T, Davis G, Miller LJ, Girschik J, Brameld K, et al. The collective impact of rare diseases in Western Australia: an estimate using a population-based cohort. *Genet Med* (2016) 143:1–7. doi:10.1038/gim.2016.143
30. Gahl W. The battlefield of rare diseases: where uncommon insights are common. *Sci Transl Med* (2012) 4(154):154ed157. doi:10.1126/scitranslmed.3004980
31. Claes P, Liberton DK, Daniels K, Rosana KM, Quillen EE, Pearson LN, et al. Modeling 3D facial shape from DNA. *PLoS Genet* (2014) 10(3):e1004224. doi:10.1371/journal.pgen.1004224

2

Bergenin Activates SIRT1 as a Novel Therapeutic Agent for Osteogenesis of Bone Mesenchymal Stem Cells

Weiduo Hou[1,2†], Chenyi Ye[1,2†], Mo Chen[3], Weixu Li[1,2], Xiang Gao[1,2], Rongxin He[1,2], Qiang Zheng[1,2*] and Wei Zhang[1,2*]*

[1] Department of Orthopedics, Second Affiliated Hospital, School of Medicine, Zhejiang University, Hangzhou, China, [2] Research institute of Orthopaedics, Zhejiang University, Hangzhou, China, [3] Department of Rheumatology, Second Affiliated Hospital, School of Medicine, Zhejiang University, Hangzhou, China

***Correspondence:**
Wei Zhang
zhangweilook@zju.edu.cn
Qiang Zheng
2100057@zju.edu.cn
Weixu Li
zrlwx@zju.edu.cn

†These authors have contributed equally to this work.

Bone mesenchymal stem cells (BMSCs) are important candidates for bone regeneration. The role of Bergenin, a C-glucoside of 4-O-methyl gallic acid obtained from the species, Bergenia, in BMSC osteogenesis has not yet been elucidated. We therefore investigated the effects of Bergenin on the osteogenesis of BMSCs and found that Bergenin enhanced osteoblast-specific markers and downregulated the adipocyte-specific markers *in vitro*. Furthermore, using a rat calvarial defect model, we found that Bergenin significantly improved bone healing, as determined by imaging and histological analyses. Moreover, it also upregulated SIRT1 expression. A SIRT1 inhibitor (EX 527) decreased the enhanced bone mineral formation caused by Bergenin. Taken together, these findings show that Bergenin accelerated the osteogenic differentiation of BMSCs, at least partly through the activation of SIRT1.

Keywords: Bergenin, bone mesenchymal stem cells, osteogenesis, SIRT1, bone regeneration

INTRODUCTION

In clinical practice, approximately 5–10% of fractures result in delayed healing or nonunions, followed by morbidities and functional limitations (Dozza et al., 2018). Bone-marrow-derived mesenchymal stem cells (BMSCs) have the potential to differentiate into bone tissue, making them attractive candidates for bone regeneration (Walmsley et al., 2016). Accordingly, it is essential to identify therapeutic strategies to enhance BMSC osteogenesis.

Bergenin is a colorless, crystallin isocoumarin primarily obtained from the species, Bergenia. It is a C-glucoside of 4-O-methyl gallic acid (Barai et al., 2018) and has been reported to engage in antioxidant, anti-inflammatory, antiarthritic, immunomodulatory, antinarcotic, wound-healing, antidiabetic, and *in vitro* neuroprotective activities. Barai et al. (2018) reported that Bergenin might prevent neurodegenerative disorders. Bergenin inhibited methylglyoxal-induced oxidative stress and inflammation-induced cytokine expression in MC3T3-E1 cells (Lee and Choi, 2018). Wang et al. (2017) reported that Bergenin ameliorated experimental colitis in mice by enhancing expression of SIRT1 to inhibit NF-κB-mediated macrophage activation. Based on the promising beneficial role of SIRT 1 on osteogenesis and bone metabolism (Feng et al., 2016; Deng et al., 2017; Zainabadi et al., 2017; Qu et al., 2018; Zhang et al., 2018; Wang et al., 2019), it is of great interest to explore the possible impact of Bergenin on osteogenesis.

To date, the pharmacological actions of Bergenin during osteogenesis have not yet been elucidated. We hypothesized that Bergenin may promote the osteogenic differentiation of BMSCs through the activation of SIRT1. The results of our study showed that Bergenin enhanced the osteogenic differentiation of BMSCs both *in vitro* and *in vivo*.

MATERIALS AND METHODS

Cells and Reagents

Human BMSCs, as previously reported (Zhang et al., 2015), were purchased from Cyagen Biosciences (from multiple healthy adult donators aged 18–45 years, HUXMA-01001, Guangzhou, China). These cells can differentiate into osteoblasts, adipoblasts, and chondrocytes under specific induction conditions. Adherent cells were trypsinized and passaged after reaching 80% confluence (2–3 days after seeding). Cells from passages 3–5 were used in subsequent experiments. As previously reported (Wang et al., 2017), Bergenin (purity > 99%) was purchased from JingZhu Biological Technology (Nanjing, China). EX 527, a SIRT1 inhibitor, was prepared by Selleck Chemicals (Houston, TX, USA). This study was carried out in accordance with the principles of the Basel Declaration and recommendations of Zhejiang University. The protocol was approved by the Animal Ethics Committee of Zhejiang University.

Cytotoxicity Assay

To evaluate the impact of Bergenin on the viability of BMSCs, CCK-8 (Dojindo, Kumanoto, Japan) assay and 3-(4, 5-dimethylthiazolyl-2)-2,5-diphenyltetrazolium bromide (MTT) assay (Beyotime, Shanghai, China) were applied. The cells (5000/well) were seeded into 96-well plates and allowed to adhere for 24 h. After that, cells were treated with different concentrates of Bergenin. After the treatment for 1, 5, and 7 days, the medium was removed, and the cells were treated with 10% CCK-8 solution or 0.5 mg/ml MTT solution in 100 μl of low-glucose Dulbecco's Modified Eagle's Medium without fetal bovine serum for 3 h at 37°C. Absorbance at 450 nm, which was directly proportional to cell proliferation, was measured by a microplate reader (ELX808; BioTek, Winooski, VT, USA).

Osteogenic Differentiation and Adipogenic Differentiation Protocol of BMSCs

BMSCs ($3 \times 10^4/cm^2$) were cultured in complete growth medium (HUXMA-90011, Cyagen Biosciences) and incubated at 37°C under 5% CO_2. For osteogenic differentiation, the cells were subsequently cultured in osteogenic induction medium (HUXMA-90021; Cyagen Biosciences). For adipogenic differentiation of BMSCs, cells were induced in adipogenic induction medium (HUXMA-90031; Cyagen Biosciences). The cells were maintained by the addition of fresh osteogenic induction medium every 2–3 days.

Measurement of Alkaline Phosphatase (ALP) Activity

According to a previous study (Zhou et al., 2015a), we first lysed the cells with RIPA lysis buffer (Beyotime, Shanghai, China) to measure the ALP activity of cells. Then, ALP activity was measured using a *p*-nitrophenyl phosphate colorimetric determination (Sigma-Aldrich, Shanghai, China). All tests were performed according to the manufacturer's protocols. The ALP activity was also measured in blood samples taken at the time of animal sacrifice.

Alizarin Red (ARS) and Oil Red O Staining

After the induction of osteogenic differentiation, mineral deposition was assessed by ARS (Cyagen Biosciences). Cells were fixed in 4% paraformaldehyde (Sangon Biotech, Shanghai, China) for 15 min at room temperature and then washed with distilled water twice. A 1% solution of Alizarin Red was added and incubated for 10 min at room temperature; this was followed by rinsing with distilled water. Photographs of images were then taken using an inverted microscope (Leica, Wetzlar, Germany).

After the induction of adipogenic differentiation, fat droplet was assessed by Oil Red O staining kit (Cyagen Biosciences). Cells were fixed in 4% paraformaldehyde (Sangon Biotech, Shanghai, China) for 15 min at room temperature and then washed with distilled water twice. An Oil Red O staining was added and incubated for 30 min at room temperature; this was followed by rinsing with distilled water. Photographs of images were then taken using an inverted microscope (Leica, Wetzlar, Germany).

Immunofluorescence

Cells ($3 \times 10^4/cm^2$) were cultured in induction medium in a 12-well plate, and runt-related transcription factor 2 (RUNX2) and SIRT1 were detected using a fluorescence microscope (EU5888; Leica) after 3 days' induction. Briefly, the cells were fixed in 4% paraformaldehyde for 15 min at room temperature after treatment. They were then blocked for 30 min in 0.01% Triton X-100 and 5% bovine serum albumin. Fixed cells were washed and incubated overnight with anti-RUNX2 (#12556S; 1:400; Cell Signaling Technology, Shanghai, China) and SIRT1 (#8469S; 1:100; Cell Signaling Technology). Cells were then incubated with a fluorescence-conjugated secondary antibody (ab150077 or ab150075, Abcam, Shanghai, China) for 120 min at room temperature, and nuclei were stained with 4',6-diamidino-2-phenylindole (DAPI; Sigma-Aldrich, Shanghai, China) for 5 min; they were then observed using an inverted fluorescence microscope (Leica).

Quantitative Real-Time Polymerase Chain Reaction

Total cellular RNA was isolated using RNAiso reagent (Takara Bio, Kusatsu, Japan) and reverse-transcribed into cDNA in a reaction volume of 20 μl with Prime Script RT Master Mix (Takara Bio) according to our previous study (Zhang et al., 2018). After that, 1 μl of cDNA was used as the template for the quantitative real-time polymerase chain reaction (qPCR). All gene transcripts were quantified by PCR using the Power SYBR® Green PCR Master Mix (Takara Bio) on the ABI StepOnePlus

System (Applied Biosystems, Warrington, UK). According to the manufacturer's instructions, the cycle conditions of PCR were as follows: 95°C for 30 s, 40 cycles of 95°C for 5 s, and 60°C for 30 s. The relative target gene expression levels were calculated using the 2–ΔΔCt method. The mRNA of the target genes and the housekeeping gene (GAPDH) were quantified in separate tubes. All primers were synthesized by Sangon Biotech. Primers used are followed: GAPDH, Forward: CGGACCAATACGACCAAATCCG; Reverse: AGCC ACATCGCTCAGACACC; ALP, Forward: TTGACCTCCTCGG AAGACACTCTG; Reverse: CGCCTGGTAGTTGTTGTGAGCA TAG;RUNX2, Forward: ACTTCCTGTGCTCGGTGCT; Reverse: GACGGTTATGGTCAAGGTGAA; COL1A, Forward: GAGA GCATGACCGATGGATT; Reverse: CCTTCTTGAGGTTGCC AGTC; PPARγ, Forward: GGGATCAGCTCCGTGGATCT; Reverse: TGCACTTTGGTACTCTTGAAGTT; SIRT1 Forward: TAGCCTTGTCAGATAAGGAAGGA; Reverse: ACAGCTTCA CAGTCAACTTTGT.

Western Blot Analysis

Cells were lysed in RIPA lysis buffer (Beyotime) with a proteasome inhibitor (Beyotime). Total proteins were separated by 10% sodium dodecyl sulfate-polyacrylamide gel electrophoresis and then transferred to a polyvinylidene fluoride membrane (Millipore, Shanghai, China). After blocking in 5% nonfat milk for 2 h, the membranes were incubated overnight at 4°C with antibodies specific for glyceraldehyde 3-phosphate dehydrogenase (A00227-1; 1:8,000; Boster Biological Technology, Wuhan, China), RUNX2 (#12556S; 1:1,000; Cell Signaling Technology), PPARγ (#2435S; 1:1,000; Cell Signaling Technology), or SIRT1(#8469S; 1:1,000; Cell Signaling Technology). Horseradish-peroxidase-conjugated goat anti-rabbit IgG (BA1056; 1:5000; Boster Biological Technology) was used as a secondary antibody for 2 h at room temperature. The immunoreactive bands were detected using an enhanced chemiluminescent detection reagent (Millipore, Shanghai, China). Signal intensity was measured using a Bio-Rad XRS chemiluminescence detection system (Bio-Rad, Hercules, CA, USA).

In Vivo Evaluation of Rats

The accelerated bone-forming ability of Bergenin was assessed in a calvarial defect model in Sprague–Dawley rats (Aghaloo et al., 2007; Sun et al., 2014). All experiments were conducted in accordance with the Animal Care and Use Committee guidelines of Zhejiang province and the Institutional Animal Care and Use Committee of Zhejiang University. Three-month-old male (approximately 200 g) Sprague–Dawley rats were obtained from the Academy of Medical Sciences of Zhejiang province. According to our previous studies (Ye et al., 2018; Zhang et al., 2018), rats were anesthetized with 0.3% sodium pentobarbital (Sigma-Aldrich) intraperitoneally at 30 mg/kg body weight. A trephine drill was utilized under constant irrigation to create a 4-mm, critically sized defect in the parietal bone. Care was taken to avoid injury to the underlying dura mater. All rats received the above surgical procedures. The rats were divided randomly into two groups: a control group (sham) and an experimental (Bergenin) group (n = 6/group). To conduct effective statistical analysis, sample size ≥ 4/group is required. In this study, n = 6/group was set, which was consistent with our previous study (Chen et al., 2017) and other published studies (Chen et al., 2017; Deng et al., 2018; Wang et al., 2018). As reported in previous studies (Gao et al., 2015; Yun et al., 2015; Wang et al., 2017), the Bergenin group was intraperitoneally treated with Bergenin in phosphate-buffered saline (PBS) at 50 mg/kg body weight weekly after surgery, throughout the 8 weeks; the sham group was treated with an equal volume of PBS.

The rats were sacrificed in a CO_2 chamber at 8 weeks after surgery. The cranium was collected for radiographic and histological analyses, and the serum was assessed for ALP activity.

Microcomputed Tomography Evaluation

To evaluate callus formation and bridging bone formation at bone defect sites 8 weeks postoperatively, the craniums were scanned using a μCT-100 imaging system (Scanco Medical, Brüttisellen, Switzerland) with X-ray energy settings of 70 kVp, 1,024 reconstruction matrix, 14.8-μm slice thickness, and an exposure time of 300 ms. According to previous studies (Shinozaki et al., 2014; Toda et al., 2014), after three-dimensional (3D) reconstruction using the manufacturer's software was conducted, a square region of interest (ROI) centered on the area of the defects was selected for further qualitative and quantitative analyzes. The bone volume fraction (bone volume/total volume, BV/TV) was calculated by 3D standard microstructural analysis.

Histological Evaluation

Samples were fixed with 4% paraformaldehyde for 24–48 h at room temperature and decalcified using 10% EDTA (Sigma-Aldrich) with a solution change once weekly for more than 8 weeks at 4°C before embedding in paraffin. Serial sections with a thickness of 5 μm were cut and mounted onto polylysine-coated slides. Consistent with previous studies (Shinozaki et al., 2014; Toda et al., 2014), the cross section of the central area of the defects was serially cut at 5 μm thick for further histological evaluation. Hematoxylin and eosin and Masson staining were performed separately on consecutive tissue sections, as described in our previous study (Zhang et al., 2016).

Statistical Analysis

Statistical analysis was performed using SPSS statistical software for Windows, version 19.0 (IBM, Armonk, NY, USA). All experiments were performed in at least triplicate, and the data are presented as the mean ± standard deviation. Statistical significance was determined using a two-tailed Student's t test when comparing two groups and by a one-way analysis of variance followed by Bonferroni's *post hoc* test when comparing more than two groups. A value of $P \leq 0.05$ was considered to represent a statistically significant difference.

RESULTS

Bergenin had no Adverse Effect on the Viability of BMSCs

To determine the cytotoxic potential of Bergenin, its effects on BMSC viability were evaluated by the CCK-8 and MTT assay. No significant cytotoxic effect was observed between groups treated with and without Bergenin (**Figure 1**).

Bergenin Upregulated the Levels of Osteo-Specific Markers Under Osteogenic Conditions

ALP activity is an important marker for the osteogenesis of BMSCs. After treatments using 1–100 μM Bergenin, the ALP activity of the experimental group was increased on days 3 and 5 after the induction of osteogenic differentiation, compared with that of the control group (**Figure 2A**).

To assess the role of Bergenin in the osteogenic differentiation of BMSCs, the levels of osteo-specific genes and proteins, including ALP, RUNX2, and COL1A1, were determined. The qPCR analysis revealed that the ALP, RUNX2, and COL1A1 mRNA levels were significantly increased on days 3 and 5 after the induction of osteogenic differentiation in BMSCs in the presence versus the absence of Bergenin (1 or 100 μM) ($P < 0.05$; **Figure 2B–E**).

Western blot analysis revealed that RUNX2 protein expression was increased by 10–100 μM Bergenin treatment on day 3 after the induction of osteogenic differentiation. Moreover, on day 5, there was a higher level of RUNX2 protein expression in BMSCs treated with certain doses of Bergenin, when compared with those from the control group (**Figure 2F–K**). Moreover, Alizarin Red staining showed significantly more calcium deposits in the 1–100 μM Bergenin treatment group (**Figure 2L**). Using immunofluorescence analysis, we also found higher levels of Runx2 and COL1A1 due to Bergenin on day 3 (10 or 100 μM) (**Figure 2M**).

Bergenin Downregulated the Levels of Adipo-Specific Markers Under Adipogenic Conditions

PPARγ is a master regulator of adipogenic differentiation of BMSCs. Western blot analysis revealed that PPARγ protein expression was decreased by 1–100 μM Bergenin treatment on days 3 and 5 after the induction of osteogenic differentiation (**Figure 3A** and **B**). Furthermore, oil Red O staining found significantly less fat droplet in the 1–100 μM Bergenin treatment group (**Figure 3C**).

Bergenin Activated SIRT1 Expression

Based on the vital beneficial role of SIRT1 on osteogenesis (Feng et al., 2016; Deng et al., 2017; Zainabadi et al., 2017; Qu et al., 2018; Zhang et al., 2018; Wang et al., 2019) and the results of previous studies (Wang et al., 2017), we measured the SIRT1 mRNA and protein levels. The results of qPCR and Western blot analyses indicated lower expression of SIRT1 in the control group, compared with certain dose of the Bergenin-treated group (**Figure 2D** and **E**). Moreover, using immunofluorescence analysis, we also found increased levels of SIRT1 due to Bergenin on day 3 after the induction of osteogenic differentiation (10 or 100 μM) (**Figure 2H**).

Accelerated Osteogenic Differentiation of BMSCs Due to the Presence of Bergenin was Partially Impaired by a SIRT1-Specific Inhibitor (EX 527)

To confirm the role of SIRT1, we investigated the effect of its specific inhibitor (EX 527) on the osteogenic differentiation of BMSCs. According to previous studies, EX-527 is the most specific and potent SIRT1 inhibitor (Li et al., 2011; Sasca et al., 2014; Nikseresht et al., 2018). EX-527 (10 μM) was added to osteogenic induction medium (Li et al., 2011); after 3 days, the expression of osteo-specific markers was determined. **Figure 4A** and **B** shows that lower levels of RUNX2 were found in the Bergenin + inhibitor-treated cells compared with cells treated with Bergenin alone. Blocking SIRT1 also decreased the levels of mineralization (**Figure 4C**). In a similar manner, the downregulation of SIRT1 by EX-527 inhibited the expression of osteo-specific genes (*ALP*, *RUNX2*, and *COL1A1*) (**Figure 4D**).

Bergenin Accelerated Bone Formation in a Calvarial Defect Model in Rats

To assess the *in vivo* effect of Bergenin on osteogenesis, a rat calvarial defect model was used. The morphology of new bone formation was characterized using microcomputed tomography (micro-CT)

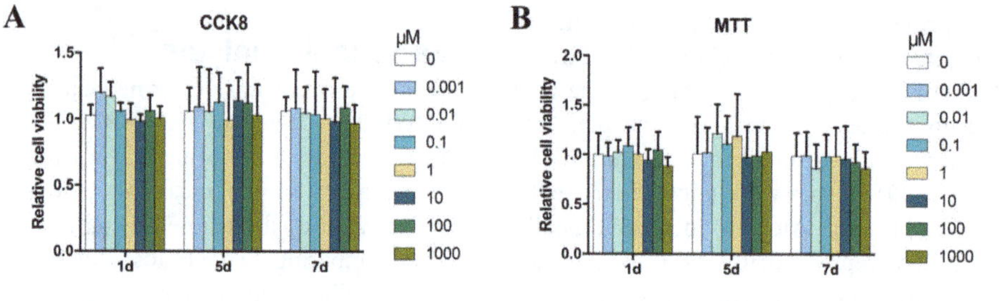

FIGURE 1 | Effects of Bergenin on cell activity in human bone marrow mesenchymal stem cells (BMSCs). **(A)** The effects of Bergenin on BMSC viability were detected using Cell Counting Kit-8. **(B)** The effects of Bergenin on BMSC viability were detected using MTT assay. Data are expressed as the mean ± standard deviation (SD), $n = 3$. *$P < 0.05$ vs. BMSCs without Bergenin.

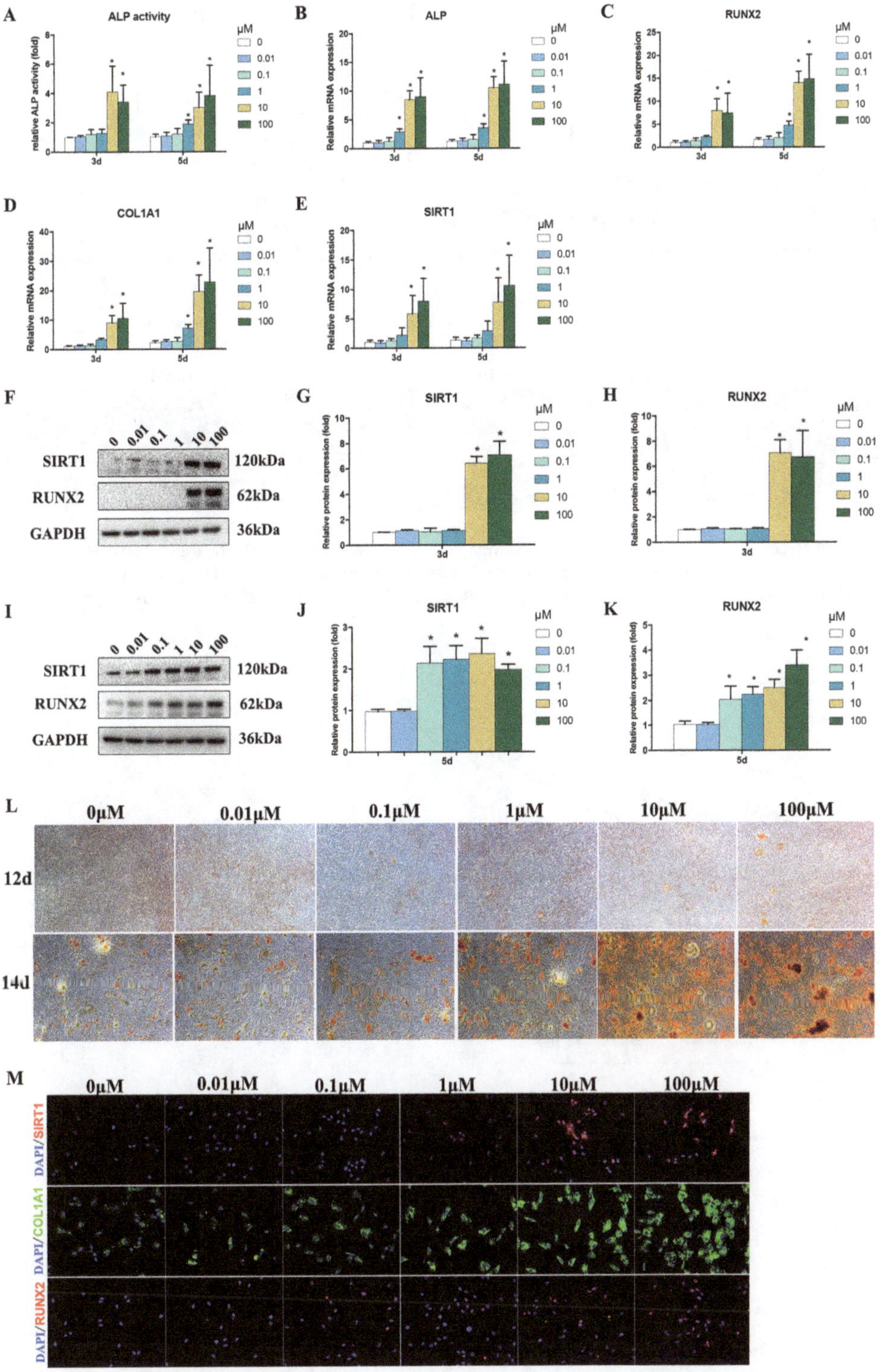

FIGURE 2 | Effects of Bergenin on osteogenesis of bone marrow mesenchymal stem cells (BMSCs). **(A)** The effects of Bergenin on alkaline phosphatase activity at days 3 and 5 during the osteogenic differentiation of BMSCs. **(B–E)** mRNA expression of RUNX2, ALP, and COL1A1 was determined by quantitative reverse transcription polymerase chain reaction at day 3 and day 5 during osteogenic differentiation. mRNA expression levels were normalized to GAPDH. **(F–K)** The expression of RUNX2 and SIRT1 protein was determined by Western blot analysis after osteogenic differentiation at days 3 and 5. Protein expression levels were normalized to glyceraldehyde-3-phosphate dehydrogenase. Data are expressed as the mean ± standard deviation (SD) of three independent experiments, and one of three independent experiments is shown. Data are expressed as the mean ± SD, $n = 3$. $^{*}P < 0.05$ vs. BMSCs treated with osteogenic induction medium alone. **(L)** Alizarin red staining at days 12 and 14 of osteogenic differentiation. Magnification ×40. **(M)** Immunofluorescence staining showing that the protein levels of RUNX2, COL1A1, and SIRT1 are upregulated by the addition of Bergenin (10 or 100 μM) at day 3 of osteogenic differentiation. COL1A1 is stained green. RUNX2 and SIRT1 are stained red. Nuclei are stained with 4′,6-diamidino-2-phenylindole (blue). Magnification ×200.

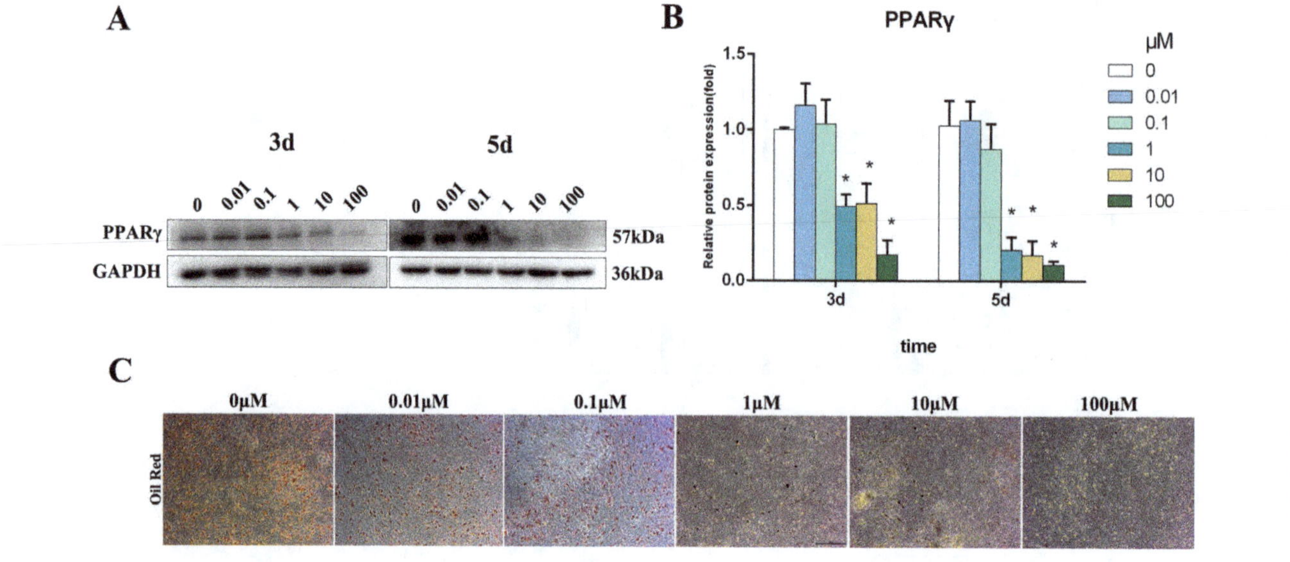

FIGURE 3 | Effects of Bergenin on adipogenesis of bone marrow mesenchymal stem cells (BMSCs). **(A and B)** The expression of PPARγ protein was determined by Western blot analysis after adipogenic differentiation at days 3 and 5. Protein expression levels were normalized to glyceraldehyde-3-phosphate dehydrogenase. *$P < 0.05$ vs. BMSCs treated with osteogenic induction medium alone. **(C)** Oil Red O staining at days 14 of adipogenic differentiation. Magnification ×40.

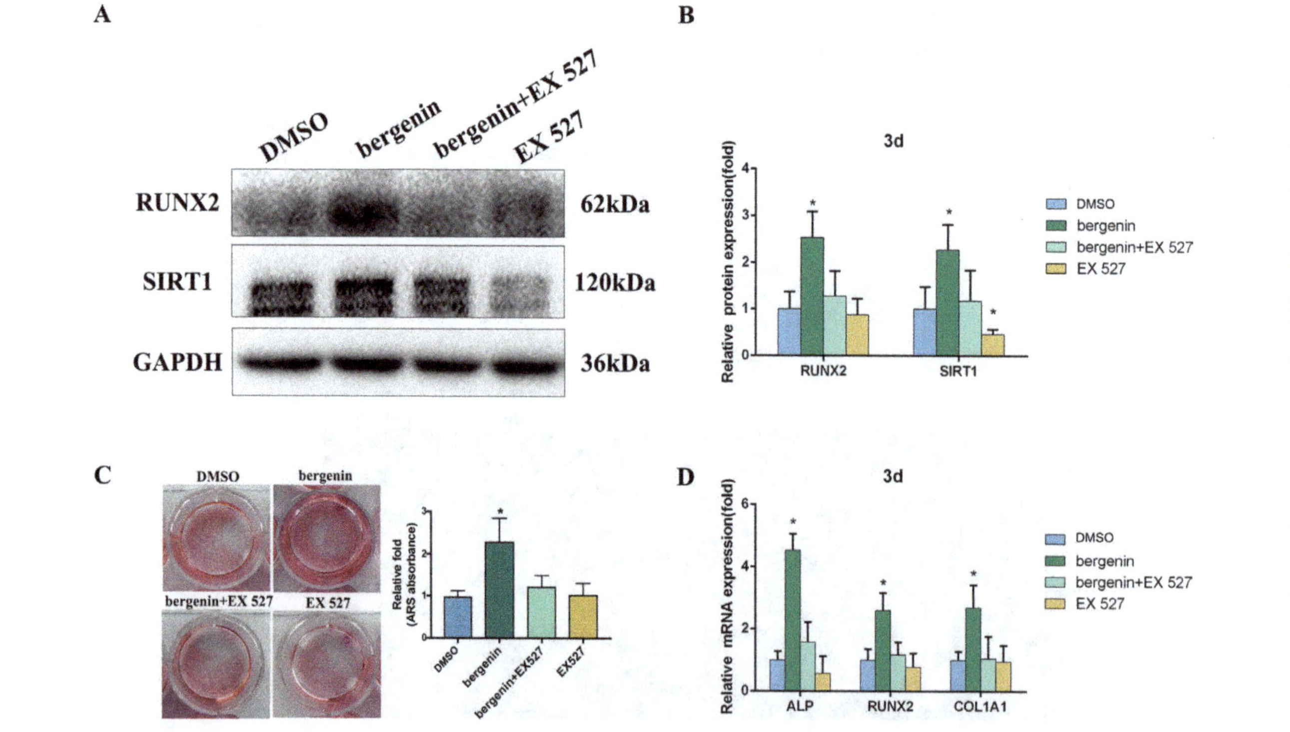

FIGURE 4 | Effects of a SIRT1-specific inhibitor (EX 527) on the enhanced expression of an osteoblast-specific gene of bone marrow mesenchymal stem cells by Bergenin. **(A and B)** The expression of RUNX2 and SIRT1 in blank, control + EX 527, Bergenin (10 μM), and Bergenin (10 μM) + EX 527 groups was determined by Western blot analysis. EX 527 (10 μM) was applied for 1 h, followed by culture in osteogenic induction medium with Bergenin for 3 days. Protein expression levels were normalized to glyceraldehyde-3-phosphate dehydrogenase. Data are expressed as the mean ± standard deviation (SD) of three independent experiments, and one of three independent experiments is shown. Data are expressed as the mean ± SD. *$P < 0.05$ vs. group with osteogenic induction medium alone. **(C)** Alizarin red staining and quantification of mineralization at day 12 of osteogenic differentiation. **(D)** The mRNA expression of RUNX2, ALP, and COL1A1 in blank, control + EX 527, Bergenin (10 μM), and Bergenin (10 μM) + EX 527 groups was determined by quantitative reverse transcription polymerase chain reaction. EX 527 (10 μM) was applied for 1 h, followed by culture in osteogenic induction medium with Bergenin for 3 days. mRNA expression levels were normalized to GAPDH. *$P < 0.05$ vs. BMSCs treated with osteogenic induction medium alone.

analysis. Representative images are shown in **Figure 5A**. Micro-CT revealed that the Bergenin group showed increased bone formation in the calvarial defect compared with the sham group at 8 weeks after surgery. Quantification of the mineralized areas also showed a significant increase in mineralization tissues in the Bergenin group (**Figure 5B**). Additionally, higher levels of ALP activity were detected in the serum of the Bergenin group (**Figure 5C**).

Representative histological photographs of each group, including hematoxylin and eosin and Masson's trichrome staining, are shown in **Figure 5D** and E. In the Bergenin group, a thick callus consisting of newly formed woven bone tissue was observed in the defect area, with a narrower distance between bone defects, compared with the control animals.

DISCUSSION

To the best of our knowledge, this is the first demonstration that the SIRT1 agonist Bergenin effectively promoted both the *in vitro* and *in vivo* osteogenesis. First, it promoted the osteo-specific markers and mineralization forming of BMSCs and inhibited the adipogenesis *in vitro*. It also enhanced bone formation in a bone defect model and upregulated the expression of SIRT1. Moreover, blocking the activation of SIRT1 decreased the enhanced osteogenesis of BMSCs due to the presence of Bergenin. Taken together, these findings indicated that Bergenin accelerated the osteogenic differentiation of BMSCs, at least partly through upregulation of SIRT1.

Bone defects and nonunions occur frequently in clinical settings. Bergenin is one of the plant-derived chemical constituents in traditional medicine and engages in multiple biological activities. Importantly, previous studies have reported that it can affect bone metabolism. Nazir et al. (2007) reported that it showed antiarthritic activity through the possible modulation of the Th1/Th2 cytokine balance. Kwang et al. revealed that Bergenin had protective effects on methylglyoxal-induced cytotoxicity in MC3T3-E1 osteoblasts (Suh et al., 2018). Pretreatment with Bergenin before methylglyoxal exposure reduced mitochondrial dysfunction,

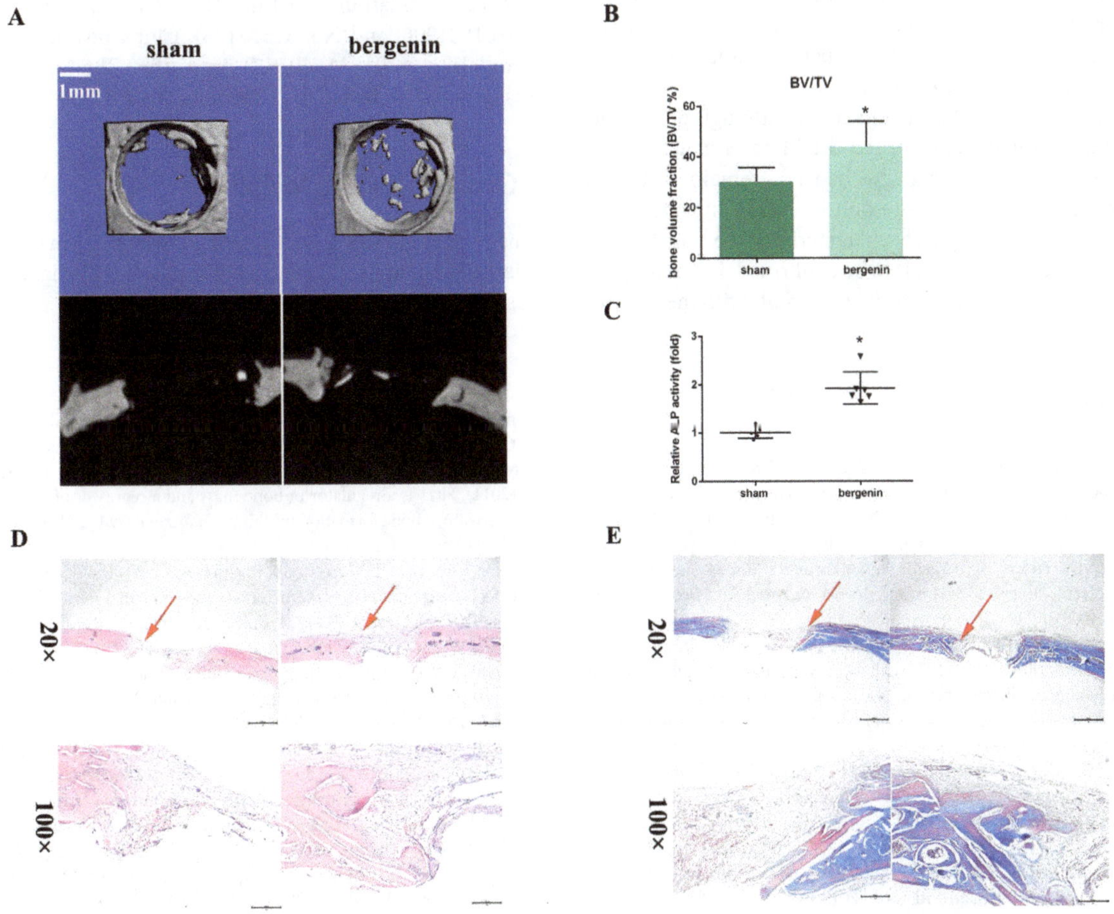

FIGURE 5 | Bergenin accelerated bone formation in a calvarial defect model in rats. **(A)** Microcomputed tomography analysis for bone healing. **(B)** Bone volume was analyzed by microcomputed tomography. Data are expressed as the mean ± standard deviation (SD). Reactions were performed in triplicate. $^*P < 0.05$ vs. bone defects with PBS (sham group). **(C)** ALP activity in serum, $^*P < 0.05$ vs. bone defects with PBS (sham group). **(D)** Histologic analysis for bone healing. HE, hematoxylin and eosin staining; Magnification ×40 (bar = 500 μm) and ×100 (bar = 200 μm). **(E)** Masson, Masson's trichrome staining. Magnification ×40 (bar = 500 μm) and ×100 (bar = 200 μm).

indicating that Bergenin may prevent the development of diabetic osteopathy (Lee and Choi, 2018). In our study, we found that Bergenin upregulated the levels of osteo-specific markers (ALP, RUNX2, and COL1A1) and accelerated the mineralization of BMSCs *in vitro*. Moreover, increased bone formation was found after Bergenin treatment *in vivo*. Of note, numerous studies have demonstrated that fat-induction factors inhibit osteogenesis, and, conversely, bone-induction factors hinder adipogenesis (Chen et al., 2016a; Chen et al., 2016b). Likewise, in our study, we found that Bergenin could inhibit the levels of adipo-specific marker (PPARγ) and suppress the lipid droplet formation.

Increasing evidence has demonstrated that SIRT1 can promote bone formation (Cohen-Kfir et al., 2011; Chen et al., 2014; Qu et al., 2016). Tseng et al. (2011) reported that resveratrol promoted the osteogenesis of human mesenchymal stem cells by upregulating RUNX2 gene expression *via* the SIRT1/FOXO3A axis. Moreover, SIRT1 also inhibits adipogenesis (Zhou et al., 2015b). A previous study indicated that Bergenin could improve the expression of SIRT1 by inhibiting inflammation (Wang et al., 2017). Consistent with these results, we also found that Bergenin acted as an activator of SIRT1. Bergenin upregulated protein and mRNA expression of SIRT1 in a dose-independent manner. Furthermore, the accelerated osteogenic differentiation of BMSCs due to the presence of Bergenin was partially impaired by the addition of a SIRT1-specific inhibitor (EX 527).

Our study has several limitations. First, although our results indicated that Bergenin upregulated SIRT1 to enhance BMSC osteogenesis, the underlying mechanism remains unclear. Second, as the long-term dose–response relationship and safety of Bergenin were not adequately characterized, the translational relevance of these findings needs to be confirmed. In addition, in this study, we did not compare the *in vivo* results with the positive control group, which absolutely causes osteogenesis, by classic drugs or gold standard clinically. Future studies are required.

CONCLUSION

Based on our data, we found that Bergenin enhanced the osteogenic differentiation of BMSCs, partly through activation of SIRT1. Bergenin may therefore be a novel therapeutic agent for the treatment of bone defects.

AUTHOR CONTRIBUTIONS

WZ and QZ contributed to the design and funding sources to this study. WZ, WH, and MC drafted the manuscript. WL, XG, RH, and CY did all the *in vitro* and *in vivo* parts of the study. All authors have contributed significantly and read and approved the final manuscript.

FUNDING

This study was supported by a grant from the National Natural Science Foundation of China (No. 81802221, No. 81672147, No. 81501906, and No. 81572124), China postdoctoral science foundation (2018M640567) and the Zhejiang Provincial postdoctoral preferred foundation (zj20180131).

ACKNOWLEDGMENTS

This work was also supported by a grant from China postdoctoral science foundation (2018M640567) and the Zhejiang Provincial postdoctoral preferred foundation (zj20180131).

REFERENCES

Aghaloo, T. L., Amantea, C. M., Cowan, C. M., Richardson, J. A., Wu, B. M., Parhami, F., et al. (2007). Oxysterols enhance osteoblast differentiation *in vitro* and bone healing *in vivo*. *J. Orthop. Res.* 25 (11), 1488–1497. doi: 10.1002/jor.20437

Barai, P., Raval, N., Acharya, S., Borisa, A., Bhatt, H., and Acharya, N. (2018). Neuroprotective effects of bergenin in Alzheimer's disease: investigation through molecular docking, *in vitro* and *in vivo* studies. *Behav. Brain Res.* 356, 18–40. doi: 10.1016/j.bbr.2018.08.010

Chen, E. E. M., Zhang, W., Ye, C. C. Y., Gao, X., Jiang, L. L. J., Zhao, T. T. F., et al. (2017). Knockdown of SIRT7 enhances the osteogenic differentiation of human bone marrow mesenchymal stem cells partly *via* activation of the Wnt/beta-catenin signaling pathway. *Cell Death Dis.* 8 (9), e3042. doi: 10.1038/cddis.2017.429

Chen, H., Liu, X., Chen, H., Cao, J., Zhang, L., Hu, X., et al. (2014). Role of SIRT1 and AMPK in mesenchymal stem cells differentiation. *Ageing Res. Rev.* 13, 55–64. doi: 10.1016/j.arr.2013.12.002

Chen, Q., Shou, P., Zheng, C., Jiang, M., Cao, G., Yang, Q., et al. (2016a). Fate decision of mesenchymal stem cells: adipocytes or osteoblasts? *Cell Death Differ.* 23 (7), 1128–1139. doi: 10.1038/cdd.2015.168

Chen, Y., Liu, X., Liu, R., Gong, Y., Wang, M., Huang, Q., et al. (2017). Zero-order controlled release of BMP2-derived peptide P24 from the chitosan scaffold by chemical grafting modification technique for promotion of osteogenesis *in vitro* and enhancement of bone repair *in vivo*. *Theranostics* 7 (5), 1072–1087. doi: 10.7150/thno.18193

Chen, Y. H., Chung, C. C., Liu, Y. C., Yeh, S. P., Hsu, J. L., Hung, M. C., et al. (2016b). Enhancer of zeste homolog 2 and histone deacetylase 9c regulate age-dependent mesenchymal stem cell differentiation into osteoblasts and adipocytes. *Stem Cells* 34 (8), 2183–2193. doi: 10.1002/stem.2400

Cohen-Kfir, E., Artsi, H., Levin, A., Abramowitz, E., Bajayo, A., Gurt, I., et al. (2011). Sirt1 is a regulator of bone mass and a repressor of Sost encoding for sclerostin, a bone formation inhibitor. *Endocrinology* 152 (12), 4514–4524. doi: 10.1210/en.2011-1128

Deng, Y., Guo, T., Li, J., Guo, L., Gu, P., and Fan, X. (2018). Repair of calvarial bone defect using Jarid1a-knockdown bone mesenchymal stem cells in rats. *Tissue Eng. Part A* 24 (9-10), 711–718. doi: 10.1089/ten.tea.2017.0168

Deng, Z., Wang, Z., Jin, J., Wang, Y., Bao, N., Gao, Q., et al. (2017). SIRT1 protects osteoblasts against particle-induced inflammatory responses and apoptosis in aseptic prosthesis loosening. *Acta. Biomater.* 49, 541–554. doi: 10.1016/j.actbio.2016.11.051

Dozza, B., Salamanna, F., Baleani, M., Giavaresi, G., Parrilli, A., Zani, L., et al. (2018). Nonunion fracture healing: evaluation of effectiveness of demineralized bone matrix and mesenchymal stem cells in a novel sheep bone nonunion model. *J. Tissue. Eng. Regen. Med.* 12 (9), 1972–1985. doi: 10.1002/term.2732

Feng, G., Zheng, K., Song, D., Xu, K., Huang, D., Zhang, Y., et al. (2016). SIRT1 was involved in TNF-alpha-promoted osteogenic differentiation of human DPSCs through Wnt/beta-catenin signal. *In Vitro Cell Dev. Biol. Anim.* 52 (10), 1001–1011. doi: 10.1007/s11626-016-0070-9

Gao, X. J., Guo, M. Y., Zhang, Z. C., Wang, T. C., Cao, Y. G., and Zhang, N. S. (2015). Bergenin plays an anti-inflammatory role *via the* modulation of MAPK and NF-kappaB signaling pathways in a mouse model of LPS-induced mastitis. *Inflammation* 38 (3), 1142–1150. doi: 10.1007/s10753-014-0079-8

Lee, K. H., and Choi, E. M. (2018). Effects of bergenin on methylglyoxal-induced damage in osteoblastic MC3T3-E1 cells. *J. Appl. Toxicol.* 38 (4), 585–593. doi: 10.1002/jat.3565

Li, Y., He, X., Li, Y., He, J., Anderstam, B., Andersson, G., et al. (2011). Nicotinamide phosphoribosyltransferase (Nampt) affects the lineage fate determination of mesenchymal stem cells: a possible cause for reduced osteogenesis and increased adipogenesis in older individuals. *J. Bone Miner. Res.* 26 (11), 2656–2664. doi: 10.1002/jbmr.480

Nazir, N., Koul, S., Qurishi, M. A., Taneja, S. C., Ahmad, S. F., Bani, S., et al. (2007). Immunomodulatory effect of bergenin and norbergenin against adjuvant-induced arthritis—a flow cytometric study. *J .Ethnopharmacol.* 112 (2), 401–405. doi: 10.1016/j.jep.2007.02.023

Nikseresht, S., Khodagholi, F., and Ahmadiani, A. (2018). Protective effects of ex-527 on cerebral ischemia–reperfusion injury through necroptosis signaling pathway attenuation. *J. Cell Physiol.* 234, 1816–1826. doi: 10.1002/jcp.27055

Qu, B., Gong, K., Yang, H., Li, Y., Jiang, T., Zeng, Z., et al. (2018). SIRT1 suppresses high glucose and palmitate-induced osteoclast differentiation *via* deacetylating p66Shc. *Mol. Cell Endocrinol.* 474, 97–104. doi: 10.1016/j.mce.2018.02.015

Qu, B., Ma, Y., Yan, M., Gong, K., Liang, F., Deng, S., et al. (2016). Sirtuin1 promotes osteogenic differentiation through downregulation of peroxisome proliferator-activated receptor gamma in MC3T3-E1 cells. *Biochem. Biophys. Res. Commun.* 478 (1), 439–445. doi: 10.1016/j.bbrc.2016.06.154

Sasca, D., Hahnel, P. S., Szybinski, J., Khawaja, K., Kriege, O., Pante, S. V., et al. (2014). SIRT1 prevents genotoxic stress-induced p53 activation in acute myeloid leukemia. *Blood* 124 (1), 121–133. doi: 10.1182/blood-2013-11-538819

Shinozaki, Y., Toda, M., Ohno, J., Kawaguchi, M., Kido, H., and Fukushima, T. (2014). Evaluation of bone formation guided by DNA/protamine complex with FGF-2 in an adult rat calvarial defect model. *J. Biomed. Mater. Res. B Appl. Biomater.* 102 (8), 1669–1676. doi: 10.1002/jbm.b.33143

Suh, K. S., Chon, S., and Choi, E. M. (2018). Bergenin increases osteogenic differentiation and prevents methylglyoxal-induced cytotoxicity in MC3T3-E1 osteoblasts. *Cytotechnology* 70 (1), 215–224. doi: 10.1007/s10616-017-0135-y

Sun, H., Wu, Y., Fu, D., Liu, Y., and Huang, C. (2014). SIRT6 regulates osteogenic differentiation of rat bone marrow mesenchymal stem cells partially *via* suppressing the nuclear factor-kappaB signaling pathway. *Stem Cells* 32 (7), 1943–1955. doi: 10.1002/stem.1671

Toda, M., Ohno, J., Shinozaki, Y., Ozaki, M., and Fukushima, T. (2014). Osteogenic potential for replacing cells in rat cranial defects implanted with a DNA/protamine complex paste. *Bone* 67, 237–245. doi: 10.1016/j.bone.2014.07.018

Tseng, P. C., Hou, S. M., Chen, R. J., Peng, H. W., Hsieh, C. F., Kuo, M. L., et al. (2011). Resveratrol promotes osteogenesis of human mesenchymal stem cells by upregulating RUNX2 gene expression *via the* SIRT1/FOXO3A axis. *J. Bone Miner. Res.* 26 (10), 2552–2563. doi: 10.1002/jbmr.460

Walmsley, G. G., Ransom, R. C., Zielins, E. R., Leavitt, T., Flacco, J. S., Hu, M. S., et al. (2016). Stem cells in bone regeneration. *Stem Cell Rev.* 12 (5), 524–529. doi: 10.1007/s12015-016-9665-5

Wang, H., Hu, Z., Wu, J., Mei, Y., Zhang, Q., Zhang, H., et al. (2019). Sirt1 promotes osteogenic differentiation and increases alveolar bone mass *via* Bmi1 activation in mice. *J. Bone Miner. Res.*, e3677. doi: 10.1002/jbmr.3677

Wang, K., Li, Y. F., Lv, Q., Li, X. M., Dai, Y., and Wei, Z. F. (2017). Bergenin, acting as an agonist of PPARgamma, ameliorates experimental colitis in mice through improving expression of SIRT1, and therefore inhibiting NF-kappaB-mediated macrophage activation. *Front. Pharmacol.* 8, 981. doi: 10.3389/fphar.2017.00981

Wang, X., Zeng, D., Weng, W., Huang, Q., Zhang, X., Wen, J., et al. (2018). Alendronate delivery on amino modified mesoporous bioactive glass scaffolds to enhance bone regeneration in osteoporosis rats. *Artif. Cells Nanomed. Biotechnol.* 46 (sup2), 171–181. doi: 10.1080/21691401.2018.1453825

Ye, C., Chen, M., Chen, E., Li, W., Wang, S., Ding, Q., et al. (2018). Knockdown of FOXA2 enhances the osteogenic differentiation of bone marrow-derived mesenchymal stem cells partly *via* activation of the ERK signalling pathway. *Cell Death Dis.* 9 (8), 836. doi: 10.1038/s41419-018-0857-6

Yun, J., Lee, Y., Yun, K., and Oh, S. (2015). Bergenin decreases the morphine-induced physical dependence *via* antioxidative activity in mice. *Arch. Pharm. Res.* 38 (6), 1248–1254. doi: 10.1007/s12272-014-0534-y

Zainabadi, K., Liu, C. J., and Guarente, L. (2017). SIRT1 is a positive regulator of the master osteoblast transcription factor, RUNX2. *PLoS One* 12 (5), e0178520. doi: 10.1371/journal.pone.0178520

Zhang, L., Bao, D., Li, P., Lu, Z., Pang, L., Chen, Z., et al. (2018). Particle-induced SIRT1 downregulation promotes osteoclastogenesis and osteolysis through ER stress regulation. *Biomed. Pharmacother.* 104, 300–306. doi: 10.1016/j.biopha.2018.05.030

Zhang, W., Chen, E., Chen, M., Ye, C., Qi, Y., Ding, Q., et al. (2018). IGFBP7 regulates the osteogenic differentiation of bone marrow-derived mesenchymal stem cells *via* Wnt/beta-catenin signaling pathway. *FASEB J.* 32 (4), 2280–2291. doi: 10.1096/fj.201700998RR

Zhang, W., Xue, D., Hu, D., Xie, T., Tao, Y., Zhu, T., et al. (2015). Secreted klotho protein attenuates osteogenic differentiation of human bone marrow mesenchymal stem cells *in vitro via* inactivation of the FGFR1/ERK signaling pathway. *Growth Factors.* 33 (5-6), 356–365. doi: 10.3109/08977194.2015.1108313

Zhang, W., Xue, D., Yin, H., Wang, S., Li, C., Chen, E., et al. (2016). Overexpression of HSPA1A enhances the osteogenic differentiation of bone marrow mesenchymal stem cells *via* activation of the Wnt/beta-catenin signaling pathway. *Sci. Rep.* 6, 27622. doi: 10.1038/srep27622

Zhou, W., Liu, Z., Yao, J., Chi, F., Dong, K., Yue, X., et al. (2015a). The effects of exenatide microsphere on serum BGP and ALP levels in ZDF rats after implantation. *Clin. Implant. Dent. Relat. Res.* 17 (4), 765–770. doi: 10.1111/cid.12184

Zhou, Y., Zhou, Z., Zhang, W., Hu, X., Wei, H., Peng, J., and Jiang, S. (2015b). SIRT1 inhibits adipogenesis and promotes myogenic differentiation in C3H10T1/2 pluripotent cells by regulating Wnt signaling. *Cell Biosci.* 5, 61. doi: 10.1186/s13578-015-0055-5

3

Optimizing Patient Risk Stratification for Colonoscopy Screening and Surveillance of Colorectal Cancer: The Role for Linked Data

David B. Preen[1], Iris Lansdorp-Vogelaar[2], Hooi C. Ee[3], Cameron Platell[4], Dayna R. Cenin[1,2], Lakkhina Troeung[1], Max Bulsara[1,5] and Peter O'Leary[6]*

[1] *Centre for Health Services Research, School of Population and Global Health, The University of Western Australia, Perth, WA, Australia,* [2] *Department of Public Health, Erasmus University Medical Centre, Rotterdam, Netherlands,* [3] *Department of Gastroenterology, Sir Charles Gairdner Hospital, Nedlands, WA, Australia,* [4] *Colorectal Cancer Research Unit, The University of Western Australia, Perth, WA, Australia,* [5] *Institute for Health Research, University of Notre Dame, Fremantle, WA, Australia,* [6] *Faculty of Health Sciences, Curtin University, Perth, WA, Australia*

Keywords: colorectal cancer, colonoscopy, screening, clinical guidelines, adenoma, risk stratification

***Correspondence:**
David B. Preen
david.preen@uwa.edu.au

INTRODUCTION

Colorectal cancer (CRC) is the third most common cancer worldwide, with an estimated 1.4 million new cases and almost 700,000 related deaths globally each year (1). In Australia, CRC is the second most commonly reported cancer and second most common cause of cancer-related death (2). Moreover, Australia has the fourth highest incidence of CRC for men and fifth highest for women internationally (3, 4). Incidence rates of CRC have at least doubled in many countries since the mid-1970s (5–7), although trends vary across countries with stabilizing or declining rates in more recent years reported in Western Europe and the United States (US), respectively. This trend is reversed for high-income nations that have recently made the transition from low-income economies (8, 9).

In the majority of cases, CRC develops from non-malignant precursor adenomatous colonic polyps (adenomas) (10), with the overall adenoma burden dependent on the number, size, villosity, dysplasia grade, and location of adenomas in the colon. Importantly, the average interval from adenoma appearance to development of CRC is >10 years (11), and the removal of adenomas reduces CRC incidence and mortality (12, 13). This affords an excellent opportunity for early detection through screening and regular colonoscopic surveillance, and the condition meets the World Health Organization criteria for diseases suited to screening (14). Patients with prior adenoma are therefore recommended to undergo regular surveillance colonoscopy (15). Increased surveillance, in addition to advances in surgical and adjuvant therapy (16), has been shown to reduce CRC incidence and increase median 5-year survival for CRC from 55.0% in the early 1980s to 65.3% by 2005 (16).

Lifetime prevalence of adenoma is 40–50% (17), however, the majority of adenomas never develop into malignant neoplasms and only 4–5% of the population eventually develop CRC (18). Consequently, simply identifying the presence of adenomas does not represent the most efficient approach for making informed recommendations for the need and timing of follow-up colonoscopic surveillance and the overall adenoma burden and specific adenoma characteristics should be factored into clinical decision making (12, 13).

USE OF COLONOSCOPY FOR CRC DETECTION

Although some population-based screening programs exist employing fecal occult blood testing (FOBT), colonoscopy remains the "gold-standard" for detection of CRC and precursor adenomas

(19). However, others have suggested that colonoscopy is overused as a primary screening and surveillance tool leading to sizable increases in the rates of colonoscopy in many countries (20–22).

In Australia, rising usage of colonoscopy has been seen for over two decades, with Medicare claims for the procedure increasing by 250% in the last 10 years (23). This increase has occurred simultaneously with increased capacity within the private hospital sector (24). Given the current trajectory, and when considered with population aging and the promotion of earlier screening, it is estimated that over 1 million colonoscopies will be performed annually by 2020 in Australia (population 24 million) (25). Similar relative trends have been reported elsewhere, with greater absolute increases, in countries such as the US (26). Such demand is not sustainable for most health systems, both in terms of provider capacity and health-care costs, estimated to be in the multiple billions of dollars annually in western nations (27). Furthermore, if projected increases in demand are realized, access to this service will be compromised, especially in public health systems. Already in Australia waiting times for colonoscopy exceeding 250 days are not uncommon (28, 29).

RISK STRATIFICATION APPROACHES TO CRC DETECTION AND PREVENTION

Researchers, including our team, have previously called for greater consideration of personalized risk stratification approaches to primary screening for CRC (30); however, less consideration has been given to the potential benefits of such approaches for ongoing surveillance. Targeting colonoscopy to patients who stand to benefit most (i.e., those at higher risk of CRC) through robust risk stratification would reduce the burden of colonoscopies to both patients and the health system, while maintaining the preventive benefits of surveillance colonoscopy. Such targeting could reduce burden for lower-risk patients, who are less likely to benefit and reduce waiting times for high-risk patients who require more regular surveillance. In addition, as most adenoma patients face a lifetime of burdensome colonoscopies with its associated bowel preparation and procedural risks, targeting surveillance to high-risk patients would also likely increase compliance with recommended follow-up colonoscopy intervals, which is often poor; only 36% of patients comply with clinical guideline recommended intervals for surveillance colonoscopy in Australia (31). Moreover, with increasing incidence in CRC seen in younger age groups (32, 33), especially those under eligibility age thresholds for FOBT programs (34), and differential surveillance colonoscopy compliance based on patient insurance status (35), risk stratification holds additional benefits for particular patient groups.

The literature on risk stratification for CRC prevention primarily incorporates factors such as family history and sociodemographics (age, sex, and socioeconomic status) with some models also incorporating genetic variants associated with CRC susceptibility (36). Where surveillance colonoscopy is considered, adenoma number, size, villosity, and dysplasia grade at the most recent investigation are the more common determinants for recommending future surveillance intervals, whereas other factors including proximal or distal adenoma location, and the total adenoma burden over time are often overlooked as risk factors for future CRC.

INCORPORATING DATA FROM MULTIPLE PRIOR COLONOSCOPIES

The cumulative burden of prior colorectal adenoma has almost exclusively been omitted from risk stratification approaches for surveillance colonoscopy, often due to unavailability of data. Most research in this area has only incorporated data from the most recent colonoscopy. However, it is likely that the risk of adenoma recurrence or development of CRC is modified by prior adenoma and/or changes in adenoma characteristics over time. Therefore, risk increases are likely conditional on adenoma characteristics from multiple earlier examinations rather than just the most recent investigation.

To date, there has been little published work which has considered longitudinal colonoscopy history for risk prediction of CRC. Estimates from a relatively small study ($n < 3{,}000$) of Dutch patients investigated predictive ability of baseline colonoscopy on adenoma burden for up to two subsequent colonoscopies (37). The authors reported that optimizing timing of colonoscopy surveillance by incorporating multiple risk factors could result in 20% fewer surveillance colonoscopies being required annually, while maintaining the same level of effectiveness in terms of cancer detection and life-years gained (37). Three other studies have reported on rates of advanced adenoma or CRC incorporating up to two surveillance colonoscopies (38–40), although, as commented by the US Multi-Society Task Force on Colorectal Cancer (41), all have important limitations possibly resulting in selection bias. Despite these weaknesses, findings were consistent across these studies suggesting that accounting for longitudinal colonoscopy history could provide important information for CRC risk prediction. While these results are encouraging, there is currently a complete lack of findings in the literature beyond the second surveillance colonoscopy. Consequently, the extent to which adenoma burden over a patient's life mediates future CRC risk is largely unknown.

Due to the lack of empirical data in this area, recommended intervals for follow-up colonoscopy in most national clinical guidelines, such as those in the US, UK, Australia, and Europe (15, 41–43), are almost exclusively based on results of the latest examination alone. Consequently, existing international guidelines are arguably a compromise that may not accurately define optimal intervals for repeat surveillance in patients with detected adenomas over multiple prior colonoscopies.

In Australia, clinical guidelines advocate that a risk assessment combining the results at baseline and at least one repeat surveillance examination may be a superior tool for CRC prediction than reliance on findings at the latest examination (15). However, there is no guidance provided on how to use that information other than a general statement that endoscopists should be encouraged to consider previous colonoscopy findings. The authors of the Australian Clinical Guidelines for Colonoscopy Surveillance recognize this limitation and recommend further research to determine CRC risk after a series of surveillance examinations, stratified by risk parameters of the baseline adenomas (15). This has also been highlighted as an important area in an Australian gap analysis (44).

OPPORTUNITIES IN THE CURRENT DATA ENVIRONMENT

The emergence of whole-population data linkage systems in many countries has afforded the opportunity to combine comprehensive data from a range of health service data collections for large samples over decades. Such linkage systems provide a powerful resource for conducting longitudinal research on large or even entire populations and have benefits for minimizing, if not overcoming, limitations due to sample size, selection bias, response or recall bias, loss-to-follow-up, and ascertainment of accurate health service exposure and outcome measures. The use of such data has become commonplace in health research (45), and linkage of whole-population non-consented service data for research purposes is an accepted ethical approach (46).

Data from such linkage systems could also lay the foundation for more robust risk stratification of populations, incorporating a wide range of sociodemographic, clinical, and genetic factors depending on the data available to be linked. Linkage systems, such as the Western Australian Data Linkage System (47), use widely accepted probabilistic-matching techniques and already have capacity to link decades of cancer registry, inpatient, pathology, and mortality data, combined with the ability to genealogically link patients at the individual-level to derive familial history of disease and "genetic" risk factors. Such data provide a unique platform to investigate different risk stratification models for CRC detection through colonoscopy surveillance. Moreover, due to the extensive observation periods that can be investigated, these systems provide the opportunity to incorporate data based on findings over multiple surveillance colonoscopies, which have been omitted from the literature to date but are likely an important component for precision targeting of ongoing surveillance windows. Additional linkage to National Bowel Cancer Screening Program records and large cohort studies, which may provide information on a range of health behaviors not routinely captured in administrative data such as smoking, alcohol consumption, diet, and physical activity would further enhance the ability to precisely stratify CRC risk and tailor appropriate follow-up intervals. The lack of such behavioral risk factor information, rarely captured in administrative data, is a potential limitation and arguably does not allow all risk factors to be considered in risk stratification models. However, available administrative data do allow targeting of factors most relevant to guideline-based decision making in this area. Furthermore, the approach proposed in this paper would still provide an advance on existing risk-stratification models as a result of accounting for the cumulative burden of prior colorectal adenoma which has been omitted from risk stratification approaches to CRC screening and surveillance to date.

In addition, when combined with the availability of tools such as MISCAN-Colon, a well-established microsimulation model for CRC (48, 49), evaluation of the cost-effectiveness of different risk stratification models for informing timing of ongoing follow-up colonoscopy for CRC is possible. Such work can also be tailored to jurisdictional-specific settings and precedents exist for the adaption of the MISCAN-Colon model to local settings, such as the Australian-specific variant of MISCAN-Colon (50).

CONCLUSION

Whole-population data linkage systems are uniquely placed to allow robust longitudinal investigation to develop risk stratification models for CRC surveillance. Systems would require the capacity to link data collections comprising demographic, cancer registry, hospital inpatient, pathology, mortality, and genealogical factors over multiple decades at the whole-of-population level. The ability to link additional behavioral risk factor data (e.g., smoking, alcohol consumption, and dietary intake) from sources such as large cohort studies would also add value. The linking of such data collections would allow relevant risk factors to be accounted for in risk stratification models, including the incorporation of complete colonoscopy history and adenoma burden over time, which represents a potentially important modifying factor for cancer risk but is currently not included in risk modeling for recurrent adenoma of CRC.

In addition to providing greater precision with patient risk profiling, estimates can be used in cost-effectiveness analyses to determine optimal colonoscopy surveillance intervals for patients at different levels of cancer risk. This could reduce costs to the health system without a reduction in the number of CRCs that surveillance colonoscopy prevents. Such information also has capacity to support rational decisions concerning the best strategy for repeat surveillance via colonoscopy for patients at both low and high risk for CRC and reduce excessive delays for surveillance colonoscopy, especially for high-risk patients. Moreover, it creates an evidence-base for recommendations that would be immediately implementable in clinical practice with the potential to influence national colonoscopy surveillance guidelines.

AUTHOR CONTRIBUTIONS

DP was the lead investigator for the project to which this opinion piece relates and was responsible for concept development, undertaking the relevant literature critique and drafting the initial manuscript. IL-V provided direct health economics and colorectal cancer screening expert input and was involved (along with DP) with developing the overall concept. PO and DC provided genetic and risk stratification for cancer screening input. HE and CP provided colorectal clinical and surgical input. MB and LT provided methodological expertise. All the authors were involved with developing the manuscript and provided detailed feedback and commentary on all iterations of the draft paper.

FUNDING

This paper arises from a project grant funded by the Australian National Health and Medical Research Council (NHMRC) (APP1123495).

REFERENCES

1. International Agency for Research on Cancer. *Colorecatal Cancer: Estimated Incidence, Mortality and Prevalence Worldwide in 2012.* World Health Organisation (2016). Available from: http://globocan.iarc.fr/Pages/fact_sheets_cancer.aspx
2. Australasian Association of Cancer Registries. *Cancer in Australia: An Overview*. Cancer Series 2012; no. 74. Cat. no. CAN 70.
3. Ferlay J, Soerjomataram I, Dikshit R, Eser S, Mathers C, Rebelo M, et al. Cancer estimated incidence, mortality and prevalence worldwide: sources, method and major patterns in GLOBOCAN 2012. *Int J Cancer* (2015) 136(5):E359–86. doi:10.1002/ijc.29210
4. National Cancer Insitute. *Age-Adjusted Colorectal Cancer Incidence and Mortality Rates for 2008 for 32 Countries 2015.* (2017). Available from: http://healthcaredelivery.cancer.gov/icsn/colorectal/mortality.html
5. American Cancer Society. *Cancer Facts & Figures for African Americans 2005–2016.* (2016). Available from: http://www.cancer.org/docroot/STT/stt_0.asp
6. Boyle P, Ferlay J. Mortality and survival in breast and colorectal cancer. *Nat Clin Pract Oncol* (2008) 2(9):424–5. doi:10.1038/ncponc0288
7. National Institutes of Health. *What You Need To Know About Cancer of the Colon and Rectum*. Maryland: US Department of Health and Human Services & National Institutes of Health (2006).
8. Boyle P, Langman JS. ABC of colorectal cancer: epidemiology. *BMJ* (2000) 321(7264):805–8. doi:10.1136/bmj.321.7264.805
9. World Cancer Research Fund and American Institute for Cancer Research. *Food, Nutrition, Physical Activity, and the Prevention of Cancer: A Global Perspective.* Washington, DC: American Institute for Cancer Research (2007).
10. Morson BC. The evolution of colorectal carcinoma. *Clin Radiol* (1984) 35(6):425–31. doi:10.1016/S0009-9260(84)80033-1
11. Winawer SJ, Fletcher RH, Miller L, Godlee F, Stolar MH, Mulrow CD, et al. Colorectal cancer screening: clinical guidelines and rationale. *Gastroenterology* (1997) 112(2):594–642. doi:10.1053/gast.1997.v112.agast970594
12. Martínez M, Baron JA, Lieberman DA, Schatzkin A, Lanza E, Winawer SJ, et al. A pooled analysis of advanced colorectal neoplasia diagnoses after colonoscopic polypectomy. *Gastroenterology* (2009) 136(3):832–41. doi:10.1053/j.gastro.2008.12.007
13. van Heijningen E, Lansdorp-Vogelaar I, Kuipers EJ, Dekker E, Lesterhuis W, Ter Borg F, et al. Features of adenoma and colonoscopy associated with recurrent colorectal neoplasia based on a large community-based study. *Gastroenterology* (2013) 144(7):1410–8. doi:10.1053/j.gastro.2013.03.002
14. Wilson J, Junger G. Principles and practice of screening for disease. *Public Health Paper No 34*. Geneva: World Health Organization (1968).
15. Cancer Council Australia Colonoscopy Surveillance Working Party. *Clinical Practice Guidelines for Surveillance Colonoscopy in Adenoma Follow-Up; Following Curative Resection of Colorectal Cancer; and for Cancer Surveillance in Inflammatory Bowel Disease.* Sydney: Cancer Council Australia (2011).
16. Howlader N, Noone AM, Krapcho M, Garshell J, Miller D, Altekruse SF, et al. *SEER Cancer Statistics Review, 1975-2013.* Bethesda, MD: National Cancer Institute (2016). Available from: http://seer.cancer.gov/csr/1975_2012/
17. Rex D, CB W, Hofstad B, editors. *Colon Polyps: Prevalence, Incidence and Growth Rates.* Oxford: Blackwell (2003).
18. *ACIM (Australian Cancer Incidence and Mortality) Books: Colorectal (Bowel) Cancer.* Australian Institute of Health and Welfare (2017). Available from: http://www.aihw.gov.au/acim-books/
19. Smith GA, O'Dwyer PJ. Sensitivity of double contrast barium enema and colonoscopy for the detection of colorectal neoplasms. *Surg Endosc* (2001) 15:649–52. doi:10.1007/s004640000372
20. Bian J, Bennett C, Cooper G, D'Alfonso A, Fisher D, Lipscomb J, et al. Assessing colorectal cancer screening adherence of Medicare fee-for-service beneficiaries age 76 to 95 years. *J Oncol Pract* (2016) 12(6):e670–80. doi:10.1200/JOP.2015.009118
21. Johnson MR, Grubber J, Grambow SC, Maciejewski ML, Dunn-Thomas T, Provenzale D, et al. Physician non-adherence to colonoscopy interval guidelines in the veterans affairs healthcare system. *Gastroenterology* (2015) 149(4):938–51. doi:10.1053/j.gastro.2015.06.026
22. Kruse GR, Khan SM, Zaslavsky AM, Ayanian JZ, Sequist TD. Overuse of colonoscopy for colorectal cancer screening and surveillance. *J Gen Intern Med* (2015) 30(3):277–83. doi:10.1007/s11606-014-3015-6
23. National Bowel Cancer Screening Program Working Group. *Improving Colonoscopy Services in Australia.* Canberra: Australian Government Department of Health and Ageing (2009).
24. *Review of MBS Colonoscopy Items.* Department of Health and Ageing (2011). Available from: http://www.health.gov.au/internet/main/publishing.nsf/Content/Colonoscopy_Review
25. Pignone MP, Flitcroft KL, Howard K, Trevena LJ, Salkeld GP, St John DJB. Costs and cost-effectiveness of full implementation of a biennial faecal occult blood test screening program for bowel cancer in Australia. *Med J Aust* (2011) 194(4):180–5.
26. Klabunde CN, Cronin KA, Breen N, Waldron WR, Ambs AH, Nadel MR. Trends in colorectal cancer test use among vulnerable populations in the United States. *Cancer Epidemiol Biomarkers Prev.* (2011) 20(8):1611–21. doi:10.1158/1055-9965.EPI-11-0220
27. Ladabaum U, Song K. Projected national impact of colorectal cancer screening on clinical and economic outcomes and health services demand. *Gastroenterology* (2005) 129(4):1151–62. doi:10.1053/j.gastro.2005.07.059
28. Viiala CH, Tang KW, Lawrence IC, Murray K, Olynyk JK. Waiting times for colonoscopy and colorectal cancer diagnosis. *Med J Aust* (2007) 186(6):282–5.
29. Miles J. QLD health complaints commissioner demands open waiting lists. *Courier Mail* (2012).
30. Cenin D, O'Leary P, Lansdorp-Vogelaar I, Preen D, Jenkins M, Moses E. Integrating personalised genomics into risk stratification models of population screening for colorectal cancer. *ANZ J Public Health* (2016) 41(1):3–4. doi:10.1111/1753-6405.12587
31. Bampton PA, Sandford JJ, Young GP. Applying evidence-based guidelines improves use of colonoscopy resources in patients with a moderate risk of colorectal neoplasia. *Med J Aust* (2002) 176(4):155–7.
32. Siegel RL, Jemal A, Ward EM. Increase in incidence of colorectal Cancer among young men and women in the United States. *Cancer Epidemiol Biomarkers Prev* (2009) 18(6):1695–8. doi:10.1158/1055-9965.EPI-09-0186
33. Troeung L, Sodhi-Berry N, Martini A, Malacova E, Ee H, O'Leary P, et al. Increasing incidence of colorectal cancer in adolescents and young adults aged 15-39 years in western australia 1982-2007: examination of colonoscopy history. *Front Public Health* (2017) 5:179. doi:10.3389/fpubh.2017.00179
34. Australian Institute of Health and Welfare. *National Bowel Cancer Screening Program: Monitoring Report 2013–14.* Canberra: Australian Institute of Health and Welfare (2015). Report No.: Cat No: Can 92.
35. Gimeno García AZ. Factors influencing colorectal cancer screening participation. *Gastroenterol Res Pract* (2012). doi:10.1155/2012/483417
36. Win AK, Macinnis RJ, Hopper JL, Jenkins MA. Risk prediction models for colorectal cancer: a review. *Cancer Epidemiol Biomarkers Prev* (2012) 21(3):398–410. doi:10.1158/1055-9965.EPI-11-0771
37. van der Meulen M, van Hees F, Korfage I, van Heijningen E, van Ballegooijen M, de Koning HJ, et al. *Surveillance after Polypectomy – Towards Successful Implementation of Guidelines.* Netherlands: The Netherlands Organisation for Health Research and Development (2015).
38. Laiyemo AO, Pinsky PF, Marcus PM, Lanza E, Cross AJ, Schatzkin A, et al. Utilization and yield of surveillance colonoscopy in the continued follow-up study of the Polyp Prevention Trial. *Clin Gastroenterol Hepatol* (2009) 7:562–7. doi:10.1016/j.cgh.2008.12.009
39. Pinsky PF, Schoen RE, Weissfeld JL, Church T, Yokochi LA, Doria-Rose VP, et al. The yield of surveillance colonoscopy by adenoma history and time to examination. *Clin Gastroenterol Hepatol* (2009) 7:86–92. doi:10.1016/j.cgh.2008.07.014
40. Robertson DJ, Burke CA, Welch G, Haile RW, Sandler RS, Greenburg R, et al. Using the results of a baseline and a surveillance colonoscopy to predict recurrent adenomas with high-risk characteristics. *Ann Intern Med* (2009) 151:103–9. doi:10.7326/0003-4819-151-2-200907210-00007
41. Lieberman DA, Rex DK, Winawer SJ, Giardiello FM, Johnson DA, Levin TR. Guidelines for colonoscopy surveillance after screening and polypectomy: update by the US Multi-Society Task Force on Colorectal Cancer. *Gastroenterology* (2012) 143(3):844–57. doi:10.1053/j.gastro.2012.06.001

42. Cairns S, Scholefield J, Steele R. British Society of Gastroenterology: guidelines for colorectal cancer screening and surveillance. *Gut* (2010) 59:666–90. doi:10.1136/gut.2009.179804
43. Dekker E, van Leerdam ME, Hazewinkel Y, Sanduleanu S, Vasen HF, Lansdorp-Vogelaar I, et al. *Dutch Guideline Colonoscopy Surveillance.* Rotterdam: Dutch Association of Gastroenterology Liver Physicians (2013).
44. Dear R, Barratt AL, Evans A, Simes J, Newsom J, Kent D, et al. Identifying and prioritising gaps in colorectal cancer trials research in Australia. *Med J Aust* (2012) 197(9):507–11. doi:10.5694/mja12.10623
45. Brook EL, Rosman DL, Holman CDJ. Public good through data linkage: measuring research outputs from the Western Australia Data Linkage System. *ANZ J Public Health* (2008) 32(1):19–23. doi:10.1111/j.1753-6405.2008.0010160.x
46. Kelman CW, Bass AJ, Holman CDJ. Research use of linked health data: a best practice protocol. *ANZ J Public Health* (2002) 26(3):251–5. doi:10.1111/j.1467-842X.2002.tb00682.x
47. *Western Australian Data Linkage System (WADLS).* Western Australia: Department of Health (2016). Available from: http://www.datalinkage-wa.org.au/
48. Lansdorp-Vogelaar I, Kuntz KM, Knudsen AB, van Ballegooijen M, Zauber AG, Jemal A. Contribution of screening and survival differences to racial disparities in colorectal cancer rates. *Cancer Epidemiol Biomarker Prev* (2012) 21(5):728–36. doi:10.1158/1055-9965.EPI-12-0023
49. Loeve F, Boer R, van Oortmarssen GJ, van Ballegooijen M, Habbema JD. The MISCAN-COLON simulation model for the evaluation of colorectal cancer screening. *Comput Biomed Res* (1999) 32(1):13–33. doi:10.1006/cbmr.1998.1498
50. Cenin D, St John J, Slevin T, Ledger MJ, Lansdorp-Vogelaar I. Optimising the expansion of the National Bowel Cancer Screening Program. *Med J Aust* (2014) 201(8):456–61. doi:10.5694/mja13.00112

4

Community-Level Pharmaceutical Interventions to Reduce the Risks of Polypharmacy in the Elderly

***Orenzio Soler*[1]* *and Jorge Otávio Maia Barreto*[2]**

[1] School of Pharmacy, Health Science Institute, Federal University of Pará, Belém, Brazil,

[2] Fiocruz School of Government, Fiocruz Brasília, Osvaldo Cruz Foundation, Brasília, Brazil

Correspondence:
Orenzio Soler
orenziosoler@ufpa.br

Background: Patients over 65 years of age taking multiple medications face several risks, and pharmaceutical interventions can be useful to improve quality of care and reduce those risks. However, there is still no consensus on the effectiveness of these interventions aimed at promoting changes in clinical, epidemiological, economic, and humanistic outcomes for various service delivery, organizational, financial, and implementation-based interventions. The objective of this overview of systematic reviews was to summarize evidence on the effectiveness of community-level pharmaceutical interventions to reduce the risks associated with polypharmacy in the population over 65 years of age.

Method: This overview used a previously described protocol to search for systematic review articles, with and without meta-analysis, and economic evaluations, without any language or time restrictions, including articles published up to May 2018. The following databases were searched: the Cochrane Library, Epistemonikos, Health Evidence, Health Systems Evidence, Virtual Health Library, and Google Scholar. The basic search terms used were "elderly," "polypharmacy," and "pharmaceutical interventions." The findings for outcomes of interest were categorized using a taxonomy for health policies and systems. Equity-related questions were also investigated. The studies were evaluated for methodological quality and produced a narrative synthesis.

Results: A total of 642 records were retrieved: 50 from Health Evidence, 197 from Epistemonikos, 194 from Cochrane, 116 from Health Systems Evidence, and 85 from the Virtual Health Library. Of these, 16 articles were selected: 1 overview of systematic reviews, 12 systematic reviews, and 3 economic evaluations. There is evidence of improvement in clinical, epidemiological, humanistic, and economic outcomes for various types of community-level pharmaceutical interventions, but differences in observed outcomes may be due to study designs, primary study sample sizes, risk of bias, difficulty in aggregating data, heterogeneity of indicators and quality of evidence included in the systematic reviews that were assessed. It is necessary to optimize the methodological designs of future primary and secondary studies.

Conclusion: Community-level pharmaceutical interventions can improve various clinical, epidemiological, humanistic and economic outcomes and potentially reduce risks associated with polypharmacy in the elderly population.

Keywords: elderly, polypharmacy, pharmaceutical interventions, overview, systematic review

INTRODUCTION

It is estimated that 21% of the world's population will be over 65 years of age by the year 2050. The elderly have complex health needs as they often have multiple comorbidities. An estimated 30% of elderly persons are prescribed 5 to 12 medications (United Nations, 2017). The elderly not only use more medications but also experience physiological changes, i.e., pharmacokinetic and pharmacodynamic changes, that increase the risk of adverse events. Between 10 and 30% of hospitalizations in this population are consequences of drug-related complications, which are potentially avoidable through adequate management (World Health Organization, 2015). The provision of care to this population represents one of the greatest challenges for health systems worldwide.

Community-level care for the elderly can be provided in various types of facilities, including community pharmacies. The terminology used to describe care units for the elderly differs around the world: hospices, long-term care facilities, nursing homes, skilled nursing facilities, and assisted living facilities (Pinto and Von-Simson, 2012). These types of facilities vary with regard to their infrastructure, the profile of the professionals employed, and the type of care offered (partial or full and/or individual or collective).

Elderly persons, particularly those residing in nursing homes, are susceptible to polypharmacy. Polypharmacy is defined as the prescription of multiple drugs to an individual (Duerden et al., 2013). The negative consequences of polypharmacy include prescription errors (PE), potentially inappropriate prescription (PIP), and potentially inappropriate medication (PIM), which can lead to drug-related problems (DRP) and/or drug-related negative outcomes (DNO) such as adverse drug events (ADEs) and/or adverse drug reactions (ADRs). The prevalence of polypharmacy in the elderly is high, although it varies widely depending on the definitions used, the facility type and the geographical location (Santos et al., 2007; Brasil Ministério da Saúde, 2014; Leelakanok et al., 2017).

The differences between "adequate polypharmacy" and "inadequate polypharmacy" are now recognized. "Adequate polypharmacy" occurs when multiple drugs are prescribed to an individual with multiple morbidities, in an evidence-based manner; i.e., the combination of prescribed medications will ensure a good quality of life, improve longevity, and minimize drug toxicity. "Inadequate polypharmacy" occurs when multiple medications are inappropriately prescribed, beyond the clinical needs; that is, when the intended benefit with the drug is not achieved, leading to unnecessary risks and negative health outcomes (Duerden et al., 2013).

Improving the quality of medication prescribing for the elderly also involves reducing the irrational use of medications, leading to better health outcomes. To address this challenge, frameworks for the evaluation of key factors related to the occurrence of inappropriate prescriptions as well as interventions to improve this professional conduct have been developed.

According to the Canadian Agency for Drugs and Technologies in Health (CADTH), there are several types of interventions targeted at various levels and components of health systems (Higgins and Green, 2011):

- Professional: (i) Interventions targeted at professionals to improve their prescribing practices; (ii) Interventions targeted at consumers to improve the use of medications.
- Organizational: Interventions that involve a change in the structure or delivery of health care.
- Financial: Interventions that focus on professional reimbursement, incentives, and penalties.
- Regulatory: Interventions that aim to change the provision of health services through regulatory frameworks.

These interventions require health professionals to analyze the pharmacotherapeutic strategy established for a patient. This is a continuous process that identifies and solves DRP and/or DNO based on need, efficacy and safety, with the goal of increasing effectiveness and decreasing the risks of pharmacotherapy. Examples include therapeutic strategy-related interventions, interventions related to the quantity of drugs and health education interventions (Brasil Ministério da Saúde, 2014). It is hypothesized, although there is no consensus, that professional, organizational, regulatory and financial interventions targeted at prescribers and consumers can be effective for improving the prescription and rational use of medications.

Goal

This overview investigated the available evidence on the effects of community-level pharmaceutical interventions to reduce the risks associated with polypharmacy in the elderly population over 65 years of age.

METHODS

Search Strategy

This overview covered studies published in the following databases: Cochrane Library, Epistemonikos, Health Evidence, Health Systems Evidence, Virtual Health Library (Portuguese acronym: BVS), and Google Scholar. There was no language or time restriction, including articles published up to May 2018. Systematic reviews, with or without meta-analysis, and economic evaluations were included. The search strategy included medical subject headings (MeSH) and health sciences descriptors (DeCS), using the keywords "Elderly," "Polypharmacy," and "Pharmaceutical intervention." The search was adapted to the various electronic databases. Details of the search strategies are provided in **Supplementary Material 1**.

This study addressed the following question: Which community-level pharmaceutical interventions reduce the risks associated with polypharmacy in the elderly population over 65 years of age? In accordance with the PICO guidelines (Santos et al., 2007), studies with the following characteristics were included: Population (P): Individuals over 65 years of age; Intervention (I): Pharmaceutical interventions (pharmaceutical care); Control (C): No pharmaceutical intervention or any other intervention; and Outcome (O): Clinical, epidemiological, humanistic, and economic outcomes.

Studies focused on other age groups, such as adolescents and adults aged between 18 and 64 years, were excluded, along with studies that addressed interventions at other levels of care. The interventions of interest were those focused on identifying and solving problems related to polypharmacy, pharmaceutical care and reduction of the risks of medication use, at the community level.

Review Process

Data Selection, Categorization, and Extraction

The identification and selection of studies followed the Cochrane Collaboration methods for systematic reviews (Higgins and Green, 2011). The retrieved studies were imported into the Rayyan QCRI (Ouzzani et al., 2016) online platform, and the references from the included and excluded studies were imported into the Mendeley reference manager (Mendeley et al., 2017). The titles and abstracts of the retrieved studies were independently selected by two reviewers (OS; JB). All disagreements were resolved by consensus among the reviewers. The selection process was documented and is presented in the flowchart adapted from the Preferred Reporting Items for Systematic Reviews and Meta-Analyzes (PRISMA) guidelines (Moher et al., 2009) (**Figure 1**).

For the categorization of pharmaceutical interventions, the taxonomy proposed by the CADTH (Canadian Agency for Drugs Technologies in Health., 2018) and the Cochrane Effective Practice and Organization of Care (EPOC) taxonomy (Khalil et al., 2017) were used to classify interventions as professional, organizational, financial, regulatory or multifaceted. The outcomes of these interventions were compared to the outcomes of interventions by other professionals, outcomes with no pharmaceutical intervention or outcomes with any other community-level intervention. As outcome criterion, clinical and humanistic outcomes, including access to services (output), as well as epidemiological and economic outcomes were used. Other definitions and concepts are available in **Supplementary Material 2**.

An extraction form was used to collect the data of interest: article title, authors, journal, year of publication, last year of research, objectives, methods, statistics, risk of bias, main results, gaps, limitations, recommendations, equity analysis, quality assessment, conflicts of interest, and unanswered questions.

Excluded Articles

In total, 642 records were retrieved: 50 from Health Evidence, 197 from Epistemonikos, 194 from Cochrane, 116 from Health Systems Evidence, and 85 from the Virtual Health Library, with no articles retrieved from Google Scholar. Of these, 117 duplicates were removed, leaving 525 records. The titles and abstracts of the eligible studies were independently assessed by two reviewers (OS; JB). During the screening, 472 articles were excluded due to inadequacies regarding outcomes, target population, design and/or type of study and type of publication. A total of 53 articles were preselected based on the inclusion criteria. After reading the full text of the articles, 27 were excluded because of the scenarios, intervention types and outcomes. In the end, 16 articles were selected for this overview. The list of excluded articles is available in **Supplementary Material 3**.

Data Synthesis

A narrative-descriptive synthesis was prepared. This synthesis describes the interventions and evidence found, including the main findings relevant to the aims of this overview.

Quality Assessment of Included Studies

The quality assessment was performed independently for each study by two reviewers (OS; JB), and the results were compared. Disagreements were resolved by consensus. We used A MeaSurement Tool to Assess systematic Reviews (AMSTAR) (Shea et al., 2007) and the checklist for Assessment of Economic Evaluation Studies (AEES) (Silva et al., 2014) to evaluate the quality of systematic reviews. Individual evaluations are available in **Supplementary Materials 4, 5**.

Equity Considerations

Equity aspects were considered for the included studies, in particular, design approaches and reporting of issues related to health inequities. We used the PROGRESS framework (National Collaborating Centre for Methods and Tools, 2015), which includes place of residence, race/ethnicity/culture/language, occupation, sex/gender, religion, education level, socioeconomic status, and social capital. The PROGRESS framework was used to identify whether there were approaches and/or issues related to inequities in the outcomes of interest, in order to develop research and/or adapt research evidence and inform the design of new interventions (O'Neill et al., 2014).

The protocol of this overview was previously registered in PROSPERO (Booth, 2013) under number CRD42018093788/2018 (Soler and Barreto, 2018).

RESULTS

Profile and Characteristics of the Reviews

Sixteen articles met the inclusion criteria. The included studies were published between 2007 and 2017. They included 1 overview of systematic reviews, 12 systematic reviews, and 3 economic evaluations. The countries where the primary studies in these reviews were conducted include high-, middle-, and low-income countries. The characteristics of the included studies are

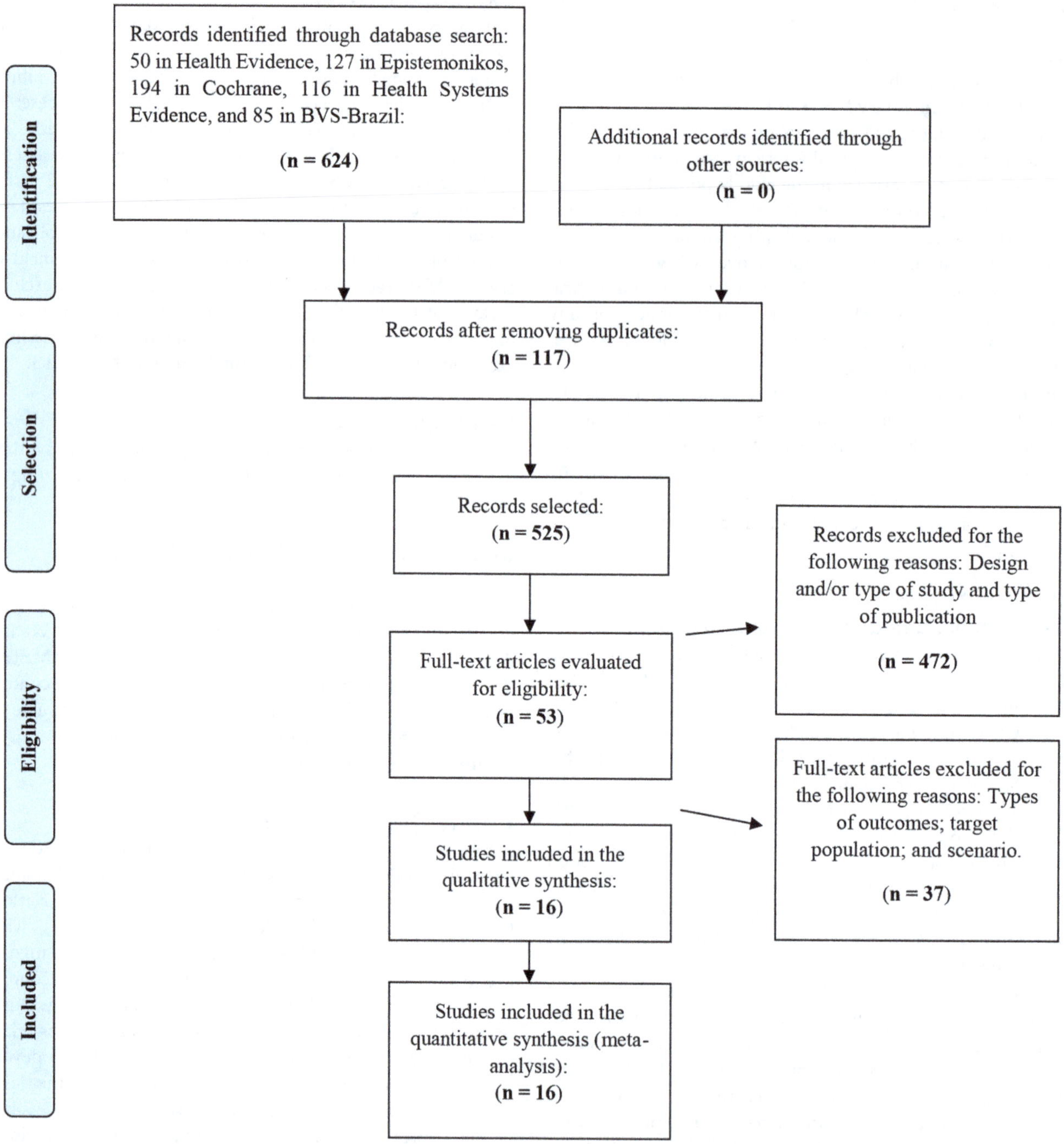

FIGURE 1 | Flowchart of the selection process of the articles included in the review. Adapted from Moher et al. (2009). Complementary information: www.prisma-statement.org.

provided in **Supplementary Material 6** and the distribution of studies by country and continent in **Supplementary Material 7**.

Categories of Interventions and Outcomes

The categorization of interventions and outcomes based on the adopted frameworks is shown in **Tables 1**, **2**. Clinical, epidemiological and humanistic outcomes, including access to services, were categorized for professional, organizational, financial, regulatory, and multifaceted interventions.

Methodological Quality of Included Studies

The systematic reviews were graded based on the AMSTAR criteria, with scores varying from low to high quality (**Supplementary Material 4**). The economic evaluation

TABLE 1 | Map of evidence on interventions for clinical outcomes.

Interventions			Clinical outcomes						
			Polypharmacy: medication errors		Adherence	Drug-related problems			
			Reduction of potentially inappropriate prescriptions (PIP)	**Improvement of use of appropriate and safe medications**	**Improvement of adherence**	**Reduction of adverse drug events**	**Reduction of adverse drug reactions**	**Reduction of drug-drug interactions**	**Reduction of drug-related negative health Outcomes**
Professional interventions	Targeted at prescribers	Clinical case analysis and/or evaluation	(Kaur et al., 2009; Alldred et al., 2013; Olaniyan et al., 2015)	(Kaur et al., 2009; Alldred et al., 2013; Olaniyan et al., 2015)	(Kaur et al., 2009; Alldred et al., 2013; Olaniyan et al., 2015)	*	*	*	*
		Review of drug use	(Hajjar et al., 2007; Kaur et al., 2009; Mathumalar et al., 2011; Patterson et al., 2012; Cooper et al., 2015; Jórdan-Sánchez et al., 2015; Olaniyan et al., 2015; Khalil et al., 2017)	(Hajjar et al., 2007; Kaur et al., 2009; Mathumalar et al., 2011; Patterson et al., 2012; Cooper et al., 2015; Jórdan-Sánchez et al., 2015; Olaniyan et al., 2015; Khalil et al., 2017)	(Hajjar et al., 2007; Kaur et al., 2009; Mathumalar et al., 2011; Patterson et al., 2012; Cooper et al., 2015; Jórdan-Sánchez et al., 2015; Olaniyan et al., 2015; Khalil et al., 2017)	(Hajjar et al., 2007)	(Hajjar et al., 2007)	(Hajjar et al., 2007)	(Hajjar et al., 2007)
		Educational interventions for prescribers	(Hajjar et al., 2007; Kaur et al., 2009; Mathumalar et al., 2011; Olaniyan et al., 2015)	(Hajjar et al., 2007; Kaur et al., 2009; Mathumalar et al., 2011; Olaniyan et al., 2015)	(Hajjar et al., 2007; Kaur et al., 2009; Mathumalar et al., 2011; Olaniyan et al., 2015)	*	*	*	*
	Targeted at users and caregivers	Educational interventions for users and/or caregivers	(Kaur et al., 2009; Mathumalar et al., 2011; Olaniyan et al., 2015)	(Kaur et al., 2009; Mathumalar et al., 2011; Olaniyan et al., 2015)	(Kaur et al., 2009; Mathumalar et al., 2011; Olaniyan et al., 2015)	*	*	*	*
Organizational interventions	Use of information and communication technology	Active search for user data and information	(Olaniyan et al., 2015)	(Olaniyan et al., 2015)	(Olaniyan et al., 2015)	*	*	*	*
		Drug information services	(Kaur et al., 2009)	(Kaur et al., 2009)	(Kaur et al., 2009)	*	*	*	*
		Clinical decision-making support systems	(Kaur et al., 2009; Mathumalar et al., 2011; Cooper et al., 2015)	(Kaur et al., 2009; Mathumalar et al., 2011; Cooper et al., 2015)	(Kaur et al., 2009; Mathumalar et al., 2011; Cooper et al., 2015)	*	*	*	*
		Use of risk screening tools	(Patterson et al., 2012; Olaniyan et al., 2015)	(Patterson et al., 2012; Olaniyan et al., 2015)	(Patterson et al., 2012; Olaniyan et al., 2015)	*	*	*	*

(Continued)

TABLE 1 | Continued

Interventions		Clinical outcomes						
		Polypharmacy: medication errors		Adherence	Drug-related problems			
		Reduction of potentially inappropriate prescriptions (PIP)	Improvement of use of appropriate and safe medications	Improvement of adherence	Reduction of adverse drug events	Reduction of adverse drug reactions	Reduction of drug-drug interactions	Reduction of drug-related negative health Outcomes
	Provision of pharmaceutical care services	(Mathumalar et al., 2011; Patterson et al., 2012; Lee et al., 2013; Sáez-Benito et al., 2013; Cooper et al., 2015; Olaniyan et al., 2015; Babar et al., 2017)	(Mathumalar et al., 2011; Patterson et al., 2012; Lee et al., 2013; Sáez-Benito et al., 2013; Cooper et al., 2015; Olaniyan et al., 2015; Babar et al., 2017)	(Mathumalar et al., 2011; Patterson et al., 2012; Lee et al., 2013; Sáez-Benito et al., 2013; Cooper et al., 2015; Olaniyan et al., 2015; Babar et al., 2017)	(Lee et al., 2013)	(Lee et al., 2013)	(Lee et al., 2013)	(Lee et al., 2013)
	Technical management of medications	(Olaniyan et al., 2015)	(Olaniyan et al., 2015)	(Olaniyan et al., 2015)	*	*	*	*
	Financial interventions: incentive programs to change prescribing practices	*	*	*	*	*	*	*
Governmental Interventions	Regulatory interventions: governmental policies regulating prescriptions	(Kaur et al., 2009)	(Kaur et al., 2009)	(Kaur et al., 2009)	*	*	*	*
Multifaceted interventions		(Hajjar et al., 2007; Alldred et al., 2013; Lee et al., 2013; Cooper et al., 2015; Olaniyan et al., 2015)	(Hajjar et al., 2007; Alldred et al., 2013; Lee et al., 2013; Cooper et al., 2015; Olaniyan et al., 2015)	(Hajjar et al., 2007; Alldred et al., 2013; Lee et al., 2013; Cooper et al., 2015; Olaniyan et al., 2015)	Sáez-Benito et al., 2013	Sáez-Benito et al., 2013	Sáez-Benito et al., 2013	Sáez-Benito et al., 2013

*The references in parentheses indicate the studies that presented evidence for each intervention/outcome studied. *Not studied and/or no evidence.*
community-level pharmaceutical interventions to reduce the risks of polypharmacy in the elderly: overview of systematic reviews and economic evaluations.

TABLE 2 | Map of evidence on interventions for access to services, epidemiological, humanistic, and economic outcomes.

Interventions			Access to services (output)					Epidemiological outcomes		Humanistic outcomes		Economic outcomes
			Reduction of outpatient visits	Reduction of house visits	Reduction of visits to urgent and emergency services	Reduction of hospitalizations	Reduction of hospitalization time	Reduction of morbidity	Reduction of mortality	Improvement of health status relative to clinical outcomes and surrogate outcomes	Improvement of health-related quality of life HRQoL	Reduction of medication costs
Professional interventions	Targeted at prescribers	Clinical case analysis and/or evaluation	*	*	*	*	*	(Hajjar et al., 2007)	(Hajjar et al., 2007)	*	*	*
		Review of drug use	*	*	*	*	*	(Hajjar et al., 2007)	(Hajjar et al., 2007)	*	*	*
		Educational interventions for prescribers	*	*	*	*	*	(Hajjar et al., 2007)	(Hajjar et al., 2007)	*	*	*
	Targeted at users	Educational interventions for users and/or caregivers (uniprofessional and/or multiprofessional)	*	*	*	*	*	(Hajjar et al., 2007)	(Hajjar et al., 2007)	*	*	*
Organizationa interventions	Use of information and communication technology	Active search for user data and information	*	*	*	*	*	*	*	*	*	*
		Drug information services	*	*	*	*	*	*	*	*	*	*
		Clinical decision-making support systems	*	*	*	*	*	*	*	*	*	*
		Use of risk screening tools	*	*	*	*	*	*	*	*	*	*
	Provision of pharmaceutical care services		*	*	*	(Lee et al., 2013; Babar et al., 2017)	*	*	*	(Lee et al., 2013)	(Lee et al., 2013; Jórdan-Sánchez et al., 2015)	(Bojke et al., 2010; Jórdan-Sánchez et al., 2015)
	Technical management of medications (medication logistics)		*	*	*	*	*	*	*	*	(Bojke et al., 2010; Desborougha et al., 2011)	*
Financial interventions-incentive programs to change prescribing practices			*	*	*	*	*	*	*	*	*	*
Governmental interventions: regulatory interventions - governmental policies that regulate prescriptions			*	*	*	*	*	*	*	*	*	*
Multifaceted interventions			*	*	*	*	*	*	*	*	*	*

*The references in parentheses indicate the studies that presented evidence for each intervention/outcome studied. *Not studied and/or no evidence.*
Community-level pharmaceutical interventions to reduce the risks of polypharmacy in the elderly: overview of systematic reviews and economic evaluations.

studies were considered of high quality based on the AEES criteria (**Supplementary Material 5**).

The level of noncompliance with the AMSTAR criteria may be related to the year of publication of the article, as earlier studies tended to have lower scores. The least frequently met AMSTAR criteria, in ascending order, were list of studies (included and excluded), methods for aggregating study results, evaluation, and documentation of scientific quality of included studies, evaluation of probability of publication bias, the inclusion of gray literature, and declaration of conflicts of interest.

Reported Results

Synthesis of Evidence on Interventions for Clinical Outcomes

The results presented in **Table 1** show the effects of various categories of interventions (professional, organizational, governmental, and multifaceted) on clinical outcomes related to polypharmacy and medication errors, adherence, and drug-related problems. The reported outcomes include reduced prescription of potentially inappropriate medicines, improved use of appropriate and safe medications, improved adherence, and reduced adverse drug events, adverse drug reactions, drug-drug interactions, and drug-related negative health outcomes.

Professional Interventions:

Review of drug use

Hajjar et al. (2007), Kaur et al. (2009), Mathumalar et al. (2011), Patterson et al. (2012), Cooper et al. (2015), Jórdan-Sánchez et al. (2015), Olaniyan et al. (2015), Khalil et al. (2017), presented evidence regarding the reduction of polypharmacy, medication errors, prescription of potentially inappropriate medications; improvement of the use of appropriate and safe medications; and improvement of adherence. Hajjar et al. (2007) also found evidence for clinical outcomes related to reduction of drug-related problems, adverse drug events, adverse drug reactions, drug-drug interactions, and drug-related negative health outcomes.

Clinical Case Analysis and/or Evaluation

Kaur et al. (2009), Alldred et al. (2013), Olaniyan et al. (2015), and have published evidence on clinical outcomes related to the reduction of polypharmacy, medication errors, and prescription of potentially inappropriate medications; improvement of the use of appropriate and safe medications; and improvement of adherence.

Educational Interventions Targeted at Prescribers

Kaur et al. (2009), Hajjar et al. (2007), Olaniyan et al. (2015), and Mathumalar et al. (2011) provided evidence for clinical outcomes related to the reduction of polypharmacy, medication errors and prescription of potentially inappropriate medications; improvement of the use of appropriate and safe medications; and improvement of adherence.

Educational Interventions Targeted at Users and/or Caregivers

Kaur et al. (2009), Olaniyan et al. (2015), and Mathumalar et al. (2011), and presented evidence for clinical outcomes related to the reduction polypharmacy, medication errors, and prescription of potentially inappropriate medications; improvement of the use of appropriate and safe medications; and improvement of adherence.

Organizational Interventions

Use of Information and/or Communication Technology for Active Search of Data and User Information

Olaniyan et al. (2015) presented evidence for clinical outcomes related to the reduction of polypharmacy, medication errors and prescription of potentially inappropriate medications; improvement of the use of appropriate and safe medications; and improvement of adherence.

Use of Information and/or Communication Technology for Drug Information Services

Kaur et al. (2009) presented evidence for clinical outcomes related to the reduction of polypharmacy, medication errors, and prescription of potentially inappropriate medications; improvement of the use of appropriate and safe medications; and improvement of adherence.

Use of Information and/or Communication Technology for Clinical Decision-Making Support Systems

Kaur et al. (2009), Mathumalar et al. (2011), and Cooper et al. (2015) presented evidence for clinical outcomes related to the reduction of polypharmacy, medication errors, and prescription of potentially inappropriate medications; improvement of the use of appropriate and safe medications; and improvement of adherence.

Use of Information and/or Communication Technology for Risk Screening Tools

Patterson et al. (2012) and Olaniyan et al. (2015) presented evidence for clinical outcomes related to the reduction of polypharmacy, medication errors, and prescription of potentially inappropriate medications; improvement of the use of appropriate and safe medications; and improvement of adherence.

Provision of Pharmaceutical Care Services

Mathumalar et al. (2011), Patterson et al. (2012), Lee et al. (2013), Sáez-Benito et al. (2013), Cooper et al. (2015), Olaniyan et al. (2015), and Babar et al. (2017) presented evidence for clinical outcomes related to the reduction of polypharmacy, medication errors, and prescription of potentially inappropriate medications; improvement of the use of appropriate and safe medications; and improvement of adherence. Lee et al. (2013) also found data on clinical outcomes regarding the reduction of drug-related problems, adverse drug events, adverse drug reactions, drug-drug interactions, and drug-related negative health outcomes.

Technical Management of Medications and/or Medication Logistics

Olaniyan et al. (2015) presented evidence for clinical outcomes related to the reduction of polypharmacy, medication errors, and prescription of potentially inappropriate medications; improvement of the use of appropriate and safe medications; and improvement of adherence.

Governmental Interventions: Regulation of Prescribing Practices

Kaur et al. (2009) presented evidence for clinical outcomes related to the reduction of polypharmacy, medication errors, and prescription of potentially inappropriate medications; improvement of the use of appropriate and safe medications; and improvement of adherence.

Financial Interventions: Incentive Programs to Change Prescribing Practices

Among the evaluated articles, no article specifically addressed this type of intervention, although there is evidence that such interventions can be effective in improving prescribing quality. It should be noted, however, that the CADTH has published evidence on interventions related to the improvement of prescribing quality using financial interventions (Higgins and Green, 2011).

Multifaceted Interventions

Hajjar et al. (2007), Alldred et al. (2013), Lee et al. (2013), Cooper et al. (2015), and Olaniyan et al. (2015), and presented evidence for clinical outcomes related to the reduction of polypharmacy, medication errors, and prescription of potentially inappropriate medications; improvement of the use of appropriate and safe medications; and improvement of adherence. Lee et al. (2013) also found data on clinical outcomes related to the reduction of drug-related problems, adverse drug events, adverse drug reactions, drug-drug interactions, and drug-related negative health outcomes.

Synthesis of Evidence on Epidemiological, Humanistic, and Economic Outcomes and Access to Services

The **Table 2** shows the effects of different interventions (professional, organizational, governmental, financial, and multifaceted) on different outcomes: access to services (reduction of outpatient visits, home visits, visits to emergency and emergency services, hospitalizations hospital, time of hospital stay), epidemiological (morbidity and mortality), humanistic (improvement of health status, improvement of health-related quality of life), and economic (reduction of drug costs).

Professional Interventions:

Clinical Case Analysis and/or Evaluation

Hajjar et al. (2007) have presented evidence on epidemiological outcomes including reduction of morbidity and mortality.

Review of Drug Use

Hajjar et al. (2007) have presented evidence on epidemiological outcomes including reduction of morbidity and mortality.

Educational Interventions Targeted at Prescribers

Hajjar et al. (2007) have presented evidence on epidemiological outcomes including reduction of morbidity and mortality.

Educational Interventions Targeted at Users

Hajjar et al. (2007) have presented evidence on epidemiological outcomes including reduction of morbidity and mortality.

Organizational Interventions:

Provision of Pharmaceutical Care Services

Lee et al. (2013) and Babar et al. (2017) presented evidence on the improvement of access to services (output) and reduced hospital admissions. Lee et al. (2013) also found evidence for humanistic outcomes related such improved health status in terms of both clinical and surrogate outcomes. Jórdan-Sánchez et al. (2015) found evidence for improvement of health-related quality of life (HRQoL). Bojke et al. (2010) and Jórdan-Sánchez et al. (2015) found evidence on the reduction of drug costs. There is evidence that, on average, pharmaceutical care is economically viable and cost-effective, with an 80% probability reported by Bojke et al. (2010).

Equity Considerations in Included Studies

With regard to equity, we found that the criteria described in the studies were limited to place of residence in high-, middle-, and low-income countries. There was no mention of whether individuals lived in urban or rural areas, their race/ethnicity/culture/language or their sex/gender (**Table 3**). Thus, in general, the included studies did not address equity and did not include subgroup analyses to identify socioeconomic differences.

DISCUSSION AND CONCLUSION

This study aimed to provide an overview of systematic reviews and economic evaluations that addressed community-level pharmaceutical interventions to reduce the risks associated with polypharmacy in the elderly over 65 years. The elderly constitute the age group most at risk of polypharmacy and most susceptible to adverse events. For this population group, care at the community level represents one of the greatest challenges for health systems, especially for universal healthcare systems.

Polypharmacy refers to the prescription of both adequate and inadequate medications. Prescriptions must be made in a way that explicitly considers the overall effects of the total drug regimen and should be based on strong evidence to ensure rational use of medications.

Pharmaceutical care is an important part of universal healthcare systems in regard to ensuring rational use of drugs. Services provided at the points of care that include pharmaceutical care, whether delivered individually or collectively, are particularly important.

TABLE 3 | PROGRESS framework.

Article	EQUITY: approaches and issues related to equity							
	P	R	O	G	R	E	S	S
Khalil et al., 2017	(+)	*	(–)	♀♂	(–)	(–)	(–)	–
Babar et al., 2017	(+)	(–)	(–)	♀♂	(–)	(–)	(–)	–
Loh et al., 2016	(+)	(–)	(–)	♀♂	(–)	(–)	(–)	–
Cooper et al., 2015	(+)	(–)	(–)	♀♂	(–)	(–)	(–)	–
Jokanovic et al., 2015	(+)	(–)	(–)	♀♂	(–)	(–)	(–)	–
Jórdan-Sánchez et al., 2015	(+)	(–)	(–)	♀	(–)	**	***	****
Olaniyan et al., 2015	(+)	(–)	(–)	♀♂	(–)	(–)	(–)	–
Alldred et al., 2013	(+)	(–)	(–)	♀♂	(–)	(–)	(–)	–
Lee et al., 2013	(+)	(–)	(–)	♀♂	(–)	(–)	(–)	–
Sáez-Benito et al., 2013	(–)	(–)	(–)	♀♂	(–)	(–)	(–)	–
Patterson et al., 2012	(+)	*	(–)	♀♂	(–)	(–)	(–)	–
Desborougha et al., 2011	(+)	(–)	(–)	♀♂	(–)	(–)	*****	–
Mathumalar et al., 2011	(+)	(–)	(–)	♀♂	(–)	(–)	(–)	–
Bojke et al., 2010	(+)	(–)	(–)	♀♂	(–)	(–)	(–)	–
Kaur et al., 2009	(–)	(–)	(–)	♀♂	(–)	(–)	(–)	–
Hajjar et al., 2007	(–)	(–)	(–)	♀♂	(–)	(–)	(–)	–

P, Place of residence; R, Race/ethnicity/culture/language; O, Occupation; G, Sex/gender; R, Religion; E, Education level; S, Socioeconomic status; S, Social capital.
(+), High-, middle- and low-income countries, with no information about whether individuals live in urban or rural areas.
(–), No information.
♂, male; ♀, female.
, White and non-white; **, Lack of formal education; *, Mobility problem; ****, Living with a partner; *****, Own house.*
Source: Pharmaceutical interventions at the community level to reduce risks of polypharmacy in the elderly: an overview of systematic reviews and economic assessments.

LIMITATIONS

This overview used systematic methods and a rigorous approach to identify and provide an up-to-date global synthesis of community-level pharmaceutical interventions that reduce the risks associated with polypharmacy in the elderly over 65 years of age.

A limitation of this study was that the results found did not allow a comparison between the studies, the quality of the evidence presented and the ethical conflicts. It is possible that potentially eligible systematic reviews might have been missed because they used different synonyms of the key descriptors.

The authors of the selected systematic reviews often warned readers to be cautious in the interpretation of the results, especially in view of the difficulty of aggregating data and the heterogeneity of the studies in terms of the variety, types, intensity and multiplicity of indicators and the use of narrative synthesis, as a meta-analysis was not possible.

IMPLICATIONS FOR PROFESSIONAL PRACTICE

The categories of interventions included in this overview (professional, organizational, regulatory, financial, and multifaceted) demonstrated the benefits of pharmaceutical care for improving outcomes in the elderly over 65 years of age. There is evidence that an adequate system for managing, prescribing, monitoring, and evaluating the use of medications is effective in reducing polypharmacy and improving adherence to medications, while decreasing drug costs, medication errors, drug-related problems, adverse drug reactions, drug-drug interactions, drug-related negative health outcomes, and hospital admissions. Such systems also improve access to services, the use of safe and adequate medications and health-related quality of life.

Implications for Research

In terms of implications for research, there is a substantial number of international studies showing that community-level interventions that reduce the risks associated with polypharmacy are complex and varied; there is no single path. However, authors of the systematic reviews selected in this overview highlight issues that remain unanswered, namely:

- Is there a difference between the socioeconomic and cultural profile of the elderly in terms of equity and clinical, humanistic, epidemiological, and economic outcomes?
- What types and/or models of pharmaceutical interventions provide monetary gains when compared to other intervention models?
- Is there a good cost-effectiveness and/or cost-utility ratio (life years gained, disability days avoided, QALY or DALY) in the long term for pharmaceutical care users?
- Are there psychological effects on patients receiving pharmaceutical care in terms of clinical, humanistic, epidemiological, and economic outcomes?
- Is there a positive impact of pharmaceutical care on the cognitive function and functional capacity of elderly patients?
- Which indicators are more specific and sensitive in measuring pharmaceutical interventions and their correlation with clinical, humanistic, epidemiological, and economic outcomes?
- Do multifaceted strategies for pharmaceutical care have a synergistic effect on clinical, humanistic, epidemiological, and economic outcomes?
- What is the minimum time (time scale) and/or frequency (daily, weekly, monthly) of pharmaceutical care provided to elderly patients necessary to be effective and/or efficient?
- Are the positive effects on clinical, humanistic, epidemiological, and economic outcomes persistent in the long-term?

There is a need for further investigation of the effect of various types of pharmaceutical interventions (professional, organizational, regulatory, financial, and multifaceted) on the improvement of pharmaceutical care in the elderly over 65 years of age.

Implications for Policies and Programs

As for the implications for policies and programs, pharmaceutical care stands out from an economic perspective as it is an efficient intervention to optimize prescribed medications and improve the quality of life in elderly persons taking multiple medications.

Results from a cost-utility analysis suggest that pharmaceutical care is cost-effective.

There is evidence—with 80% probability—that pharmaceutical care is economically viable and profitable. This supports its incorporation into pharmaceutical assistance programs and/or policies, especially in universal healthcare systems based on access, quality and rational and sustainable use of medications at all levels of health care.

We know how important it is to ensure the establishment and implementation of evidence-based policies. Thus, we reiterate that, in universal and sustainable healthcare systems, pharmaceutical assistance and/or pharmaceutical care must be based on evidence of the efficacy and safety of the drugs, the effectiveness of the medications and the efficiency of the treatments.

Finally, we recommend that pharmaceutical professionals committed to efficient health policies should be included in multidisciplinary care teams to ensure that the elderly have access to high-quality and safe pharmacotherapy and a better quality of life.

AUTHOR CONTRIBUTIONS

OS defined the research questions and prepared the research protocol in conjunction with JB. OS designed the study and conducted the bibliographic searches and the analyses. JB refined the research question in the original draft and contributed to the study design by helping with the literature review and article review. The authors read and approved the final version of the manuscript.

FUNDING

DIREB 017 FIO 16—Project: Support for the Improvement of technology management in SUS through a platform for translation, exchange, and social appropriation of knowledge. Coordinator: JB. The content of the review is the sole responsibility of the individual authors and does not reflect the opinions of Fiocruz-Brasília or the Brazilian Ministry of Health.

ACKNOWLEDGMENTS

The authors thank the Oswaldo Cruz Foundation, Regional Unit of Brasília, Fiocruz School of Government, the Graduate Program in Public Health Policies, and the Ministry of Health of Brazil.

REFERENCES

Alldred, D. P., Raynor, D. K., Hughes, C., Barber, N., Chen, T. F., and Spoor, P. (2013). Interventions to optimise prescribing for older people in care homes (Review). *Cochrane. Database Syst. Rev.* 2:CD009095. doi: 10.1002/14651858.CD009095.pub2

Babar, Z. D., Kousar, R., Murtaza, G., Azhar, S., Khan, S. A., and Curley, L. (2017). Randomized controlled trials covering pharmaceutical care and medicines management: a systematic review of literature. *Res. Soc. Admin. Pharm.* 1:19. doi: 10.1016/j.sapharm.2017.06.008

Bojke, C., Sculpher, M., Campion, P., Chrystyn, H., Coulton, S., Cross, B., et al. (2010). Cost-effectiveness of shared Pharmaceutical care for older patients: RESPECT trial findings. *Br. J. Gen. Pract.* 60:e20-27. doi: 10.3399/bjgp09X482312

Booth, A. (2013). PROSPERO's progress and activities 2012/13. *Syst. Rev.* 2:111. doi: 10.1186/2046-4053-2-111

Brasil Ministério da Saúde. (2014). *Serviços farmacêuticos na atenção básica à saúde. Secretaria de Ciência, Tecnologia e Insumos Estratégicos.* Departamento de Assistência Farmacêutica e Insumos Estratégicos. - Brasília: Ministério da Saúde, 108 p.: il. - (Cuidado farmacêutico na atenção básica; caderno 1).

Canadian Agency for Drugs and Technologies in Health (2018). *CADTH Evidence Drive. Search Rx for Change Database. CADTH publishes. Canadian Copyright.* Available online at: https://www.cadth.ca/resources/rx-for-change/database/ (accessed August 12, 2018).

Cooper, J. A., Cadogan, C. A., Patterson, S. M., Kerse, N., Bradley, M. C., Ryan, C., et al. (2015). Interventions to improve the appropriate use of polypharmacy in older people: a Cochrane systematic review. *BMJ Open* 5:e009235. doi: 10.1136/bmjopen-2015-009235

Desborougha, J. A., Sachb, T., Bhattacharya, D., Holland, R. C., and Wright, D. J. (2011). A cost-consequences analysis of an adherence focused pharmacist-led medication review servisse. *Int. J. Pharmacy Pract.* 20, 41–49. doi: 10.1111/j.2042-7174.2011.00161.x

Duerden, M., Avery, T., and Payne, R. (2013). *Polypharmacy and Medicines Optimization. Making it Safe and Sound.* London: The King's Fund; First published by The King's Fund Charity Registration Number: 1126980.

Hajjar, E. R., Cafiero, A. C., and Hanlon, J. T. (2007). Polypharmacy in elderly patients. *Am. J . Geriatr. Pharmacother.* 5, 341–355. doi: 10.1016/j.amjopharm.2007.12.002

Higgins, J. P. T., and Green, S. (2011). *Cochrane Handbook for Systematic Reviews of Interventions.* Vol. 1 *de Wiley Cochrane Series.* London: John Wiley & Sons.

Jokanovic, N., Tan, E. C. K., Dooley, M. J., Kirkpatrick, C. M., and Bell, J. S. (2015). Prevalence and factors associated with polypharmacy in long-term care facilities: a systematic review. *JAMDA* 16:535.e11.

Jódan-Sánchez, F., Malet-Larrea, A., Martín, J., García-Mochón, L., López del Amo, M., Martínez-Martínez, F., et al. (2015). Cost-utility analysis of a medication review with follow-up service for older adults with polypharmacy in community pharmacies in spain: the conSIGUE Program. *PharmacoEconomics* 33, 599–610. doi: 10.1007/s40273-015-0270-2

Kaur, S., Mitchell, G., Vitetta, L., and Roberts, M. S. (2009). Interventions that can reduce inappropriate prescribing in the elderly - a systematic review. *Drugs Aging.* 26, 1013–1028. doi: 10.2165/11318890-000000000-00000

Khalil, H., Bell, B., Chambers, H., Sheikh, A., and Avery, A. J. (2017). Professional, structural and organizational interventions in primary care for reducing medication errors. *Cochrane Database Syst. Rev.* 10:CD003942. doi: 10.1002/14651858.CD003942.pub3

Lee, J. K., Slack, M. K., Martin, J., Ehrman, C., and Chisholm-Burns, M. (2013). Geriatric Patient Care by U.S. Pharmacists in healthcare teams: systematic review and meta-analyses. *J. Am. Geriatr. Soc.* 61, 1119–1127. doi: 10.1111/jgs.12323

Leelakanok, N., Holcombe, A. L., Lund, B. C., Gu, X., and Schweizer, M. L. (2017). Association between polypharmacy and death: a systematic review and meta-analysis. *J. Am. Pharmac. Assoc.* 57, 729–38.e10. doi: 10.1016/j.japh.2017.06.002

Loh, Z., Cheen, M., and Wee, H. (2016). Humanistic and economic outcomes of pharmacist-provided medication review in the community-dwelling elderly: a systematic review and meta-analysis. *J. Clin. Pharmacy Therapeut.* 41, 621–633. doi: 10.1111/jcpt.12453

Mathumalar, L., Shonella, S., Dean, F. B., Bottle, A., and Azeem, M. (2011). Interventions to optimise prescribing in care homes: systematic review. *Age Ageing* 40, 150–162. doi: 10.1093/ageing/afq161

Mendeley, J. A., Thomson, M., and Coyne, R. P. (2017). *How and When to Reference*. Available online at https://www.howandwhentoreference.com (accessed July 7, 2018).

Moher, D., Liberati, A., Tetzlaff, J., and Altman, D. G. (2009). The PRISMA Group. Preferred reporting items for systematic reviews and meta-analyses: the PRISMA statement. *PLoS Med.* 6:e1000097. doi: 10.1371/journal.pmed.1000097

National Collaborating Centre for Methods and Tools (2015). *PROGRESS Framework: Applying An Equity Lens to Interventions*. Hamilton, ON: McMaster University.

Olaniyan, J. O., Ghaleb, M., Dhillon, S., and Robinson, P. (2015). Safety of medication use in primary care. *Int. J. Pharmacy Pract.* 23, 3–20. doi: 10.1111/ijpp.12120

O'Neill, J., Tabish, H., Welch, V., Petticrew, M., Pottie, K., Clarke, M., et al. (2014). Applying an equity lens to interventions: using, PROGRESS ensures consideration of socially stratifying factors to illuminate inequities in health. *J. Clin. Epidemiol.* 67, 56–64. doi: 10.1016/j.jclinepi.2013.08.005

Ouzzani, M., Hammady, H., Fedorowicz, Z., and Elmagarmid, A. (2016). Rayyan — a web and mobile app for systematic reviews. *Syst. Rev.* 5:210. doi: 10.1186/s13643-016-0384-4

Patterson, S. M., Hughes, C., Kerse, N., Cardwell, C. R., and Bradley, M. C. (2012). Interventions to improve the appropriate use of polypharmacy for older people. *Cochr. Database Syst. Rev.* 5:CD008165. doi: 10.1002/14651858.CD008165.pub2

Pinto, S. P. L. C., and Von-Simson, O. R. M. (2012). Instituições de longa permanência para idosos no Brasil: sumário da legislação. *Rev. Brasil. Geriatr. Gerontol.* 15, 169–174. doi: 10.1590/S1809-98232012000100018

Sáez-Benito, L., Fernandez-Llimos, F., Feletto, E., Gastelurrutia, M. A., Martinez-Martinez, F., and Benrimo, S. (2013). Evidence of the clinical effectiveness of cognitive pharmaceutical services for aged patients. *Age Ageing* 42, 442–449. doi: 10.1093/ageing/aft045

Santos, C. M. C., Pimenta, C. A. M., and Nobre, M. C. (2007). A estratégia PICO para a construção da pergunta de pesquisa e busca de evidências. *Rev. Latino-Am. Enfermagem* 15, 508–511. doi: 10.1590/S0104-11692007000300023

Shea, B. J., Grimshaw, J. M., Wells, G. A., Boers, M., Andersson, N., Hamel, C., et al. (2007). Development of AMSTAR: a measurement tool to assess the methodological quality of systematic reviews. *BMC Med. Res. Methodol.* 7:10. doi: 10.1186/1471-2288-7-10

Silva, E. M., Galvão, T. F., Pereira, M. G., and Silva, M. T. (2014). Estudos de avaliação econômica de tecnologias em saúde: roteiro para análise crítica. *Rev. Panam. Salud. Publica.* 35, 219–227.

Soler, O., and Barreto, J. (2018). *Pharmaceutical Interventions in Community Level to Reduce Risks of Polypharmacy in the Elderly: An Overview of Systematic Reviews and Economic Evaluations*. York, UK: PROSPERO: International prospective register of systematic reviews. Available online at: http://www.crd.york.ac.uk/PROSPERO/display_record.php?ID=CRD42018093788

United Nations, Department of Economic and Social Affairs, Population Division (2017). *World Population Prospects: The 2017 Revision, Key Findings and Advance Tables*. Working Paper No. ESA/P/WP/248.

World Health Organization (2015). *World Report on Ageing and Health*. Geneva: World Health Organization, 246.

5

Administrative Data Linkage in Brazil: Potentials for Health Technology Assessment

M Sanni Ali[1,2,3], Maria Yury Ichihara[3,4], Luciane Cruz Lopes[5], George C.G. Barbosa[3], Robespierre Pita[3], Roberto Perez Carreiro[3], Djanilson Barbosa dos Santos[6], Dandara Ramos[3], Nivea Bispo[3], Fabiana Raynal[7], Vania Canuto[7], Bethania de Araujo Almeida[3], Rosemeire L. Fiaccone[3,4,8], Marcos E. Barreto[3,9,10], Liam Smeeth[1,3†] and Mauricio L. Barreto[3,4†]*

[1] Faculty of Epidemiology and Population Health, Department of Non-communicable Disease Epidemiology, London School of Hygiene and Tropical Medicine, London, United Kingdom, [2] Nuffield Department of Orthopaedics, Rheumatology and Musculoskeletal Sciences (NDORMS), Center for Statistics in Medicine (CSM), University of Oxford, Oxford, United Kingdom, [3] Centre for Data and Knowledge Integration for Health (CIDACS), Instituto Gonçalo Muniz, Fundação Osvaldo Cruz, Salvador, Brazil, [4] Institute of Public Health, Federal University of Bahia (UFBA), Salvador, Brazil, [5] University of Sorocaba–UNISO, São Paulo, Brazil, [6] Centro de Ciências da Saúde, Federal University of Recôncavo of Bahia (UFRB), Salvador, Brazil, [7] Department of Management and Incorporation of Health Technology, Ministry of Health (DGITS/MS), Brasília, Brazil, [8] Department of Statistics, Federal University of Bahia (UFBA), Salvador, Brazil, [9] Department of Computing, Federal University of Bahia (UFBA), Salvador, Brazil, [10] Institute of Health Informatics, University College London, London, United Kingdom

***Correspondence:**
M Sanni Ali
sanni.ali@lshtm.ac.uk

Health technology assessment (HTA) is the systematic evaluation of the properties and impacts of health technologies and interventions. In this article, we presented a discussion of HTA and its evolution in Brazil, as well as a description of secondary data sources available in Brazil with potential applications to generate evidence for HTA and policy decisions. Furthermore, we highlighted record linkage, ongoing record linkage initiatives in Brazil, and the main linkage tools developed and/or used in Brazilian data. Finally, we discussed the challenges and opportunities of using secondary data for research in the Brazilian context. In conclusion, we emphasized the availability of high quality data and an open, modern attitude toward the use of data for research and policy. This is supported by a rigorous but enabling legal framework that will allow the conduct of large-scale observational studies to evaluate clinical, economical, and social impacts of health technologies and social policies.

Keywords: administrative data, Brazil, data linkage, epidemiological studies, health technology assessment, record linkage

INTRODUCTION

Health technology assessment (HTA), also known as healthcare technology assessment or medical technology assessment, is the systematic evaluation of the properties, intended and unintended effects and/or impacts of health technologies and interventions (Batarrita, 1999; Banta, 2009). It is an investigative process that evaluates the clinical (effectiveness and safety), economical (cost or cost-effectiveness), ethical, and social consequences of using new or existing technologies in health with the main goal of improving "value for money" in health care (Banta, 2009; Kristensen et al., 2009). Health technologies can be any intervention in health with the aim of promoting health and prevent, diagnose, or treat disease, examples include: drugs, devices, procedures, and the organizational, educational, informational, and support systems within which health care is delivered to the population (Banta, 2009). HTAs are useful to a wide range of decision makers in healthcare: government policy makers, insurance companies, and other payers, industries, planners, administrators, clinicians, and patients. Although the goal of HTA is to support policy decision and not sole knowledge generation, it must be carried out with integrity and using solid scientific methods to yield valid results (Banta, 2009).

In the mid-1980s, a new constitution in Brazil ruled that health is a right of all citizens and a duty of the State. This was the starting point for the building up of the Brazilian unified national health system [Sistema Único de Saúde (SUS), literally the "Single Health System"]. Since that moment, the Brazilian government showed strong interest in HTA, particularly after organizing and leading, in collaboration with Pan American Health Organization/World Health Organization (PAHO/WHO), on a HTA conference in Brasilia, Brazil (Banta, 2009; Guimarães, 2014). The discussions involved the political aspects of HTAs, including the questionable effectiveness of technologies used in health, cost and cost-effectiveness, and the process of technology transfer. In the years from 2000 to 2008, substantial actions were taken in HTA: (1) Several seminars and consultations were held. (2) Key institutional changes were made at the Ministry of Health (MoH), including the formation of the Department of Science and Technology (DST); the Secretariat of Science, Technology and Strategic Inputs (SSTSI); and the Commission for the Incorporation of Technologies (the Commission). Later, the DST joined the International Network of Agencies in HTA. (3) Policies were developed by the federal government to encourage HTA and its application for clinical, management, and policy decisions. The SSTSI was then given the mandate for policy implementation in relation to pharmaceuticals within the SUS. At the same time, a process flow for incorporating technologies under the auspices of SUS and Supplementary Health System (SHS) was established, which was later redefined. Furthermore, the SSTSI was assigned to oversight the Commission; to evaluate and recommend the incorporation, alteration, or exclusion of products for the SUS and SHS procedure lists; to propose the revision of therapeutic guidelines; and to order and carry out HTA-specific studies. (4) Several academic institutions, such as the Federal University of Rio de Janeiro and the State University of Sao Paulo, developed HTA research initiative and the Brazilian Network for HTA (REBRATS), coordinated by MoH, was established by the adhesion of HTA groups scattered throughout universities, medical schools, and teaching hospitals (Banta, 2009; Guimarães, 2014).

In December 2011, the National Committee for Health Technology Incorporation into SUS (CONITEC) was created by the Brazilian Government through a Federal Law (12.401/2011) and regulated by Presidential Decree (7.646 from December 21, 2011). Aiming to provide greater agility, transparency, and efficiency to the health technologies, incorporation or disinvestment processes, CONITEC has set a new milestone to health management with innovative precepts in HTA in Brazil. With the objective of providing administrative, technical, and scientific support to CONITEC, the Executive Secretariat of CONITEC was created, which is in charge of the Department of Management and Incorporation of Health Technologies (DGITS) of the SSTSI of the MoH. The actions developed by DGITS, assisted by a network of national institutions (hospitals and universities), which are partners of CONITEC, have been successful in promoting public consultations, making decisions about claims, and acquiring health technology products and services (Guimarães, 2014). Currently, most of the HTA procedures within the REBRATS realm make predominant use of secondary sources of information, especially studies in the field of meta-analyses and other publications, for the incorporation of technologies (Guimarães, 2014).

Brazil has a long tradition of keeping records of health-related information for administrative purposes owing to the establishment of SUS, its informatics department (DATASUS), and the substantial progress made toward Universal Health Coverage (UHC) (Paim et al., 2011). Despite the efforts made by the MoH to harmonize the recording of information, a great disparity exists among various health institutions related to data collection processes. In addition, individual data collected by different health services (for example, hospital and mortality registries) lack unique key identifiers for individuals, hence, combining these data sources is not a trivial task. These factors, in addition to the technological infrastructure and skilled human resource constraints, have limited the use of routinely collected data to generate evidence to support clinical and policy decisions and to answer important epidemiological questions.

However, in the past decade, several big data and record linkage initiatives, different record linkage software packages (for example, Reclink, Atylmo, and CIDACS-RL) (Camargo and Coeli, 2000; Pita et al., 2018), and international collaborations on research and capacity building have emerged. The use of record linkage technology to integrate data that are not available in a single data set by supplementing information from other data sources and/or validate information collected in one data source has made the conduct of health outcomes research possible in the Brazilian setting (Camargo and Coeli, 2000; Pinto et al., 2017). The HTA field in Brazil will benefit from such institutional and technological advances in data processing and analysis to produce evidence on the (cost-)effectiveness and safety of health technologies, as well as their impact of social, economic, and health policies. Hence, the objective of this manuscript was to review the main health care and socioeconomic databases, recent advances in the use of big data and data linkage tools; and to highlight the potentials and challenges of using secondary data and data linkage for health outcomes and policy research, as well as HTA.

This manuscript is organized as follows: the section *Databases Used in Health Outcomes/Policy Research in Brazil* describes the major databases used in health outcomes/policy research in Brazil, the section *Data Linkage* introduces important concepts in data linkage, the section *Data Linkage Initiatives in Brazil* describes major initiatives in creation of data centers and development of data linkage in Brazil, the section *Record Linkage Tools Developed and/or Used in Brazil* summarizes record linkage algorithms developed/used in Brazilian databases, the section *Challenges and Opportunities* highlights major challenges in the use of secondary data for health research in Brazil, and the section *Conclusion* concludes the manuscript.

DATABASES USED IN HEALTH OUTCOMES/POLICY RESEARCH IN BRAZIL

In Brazil, the main databases storing health-related information are generated from SUS (de Mello Jorge et al., 2010; Paim et al., 2011; Souza et al., 2016). These databases can be classified into: (1) epidemiological (such as the Live Births Information System/SINASC; the Mortality Information System/SIM; the Information System for Notifiable Diseases/SINAN), which are used for surveillance, evaluation, and research to address public health questions; (2) administrative (such as the Outpatient Information System/SIA-SUS and the Hospital Information System/SIH-SUS), which are used for accounting and control of the production of the services provided; and (3) clinical, which are used to store clinical data on patients for future reference (Souza et al., 2016).

In addition, other government sectors also generate and manage data on demographic and socio-economic characteristics of the Brazilian population. For example, the Ministry of Social Development maintains an electronic database ("Cadastro Único," CadUnico) for provision of social services, such as the Conditional Cash Transfer Program (BFP) and the Housing Program (MCMV). These databases, in combination with others, have been used to study social determinants of health and evaluations of social policies on health (Rasella et al., 2013; Nunes et al., 2016; Machado et al., 2018). **Table 1** summarizes some details about the main databases publicly available from SUS and other governmental sources in Brazil.

TABLE 1 | Databases From the Brazilian Public Health System (SUS) and Other Government Sources.

Abbreviation	Year	Registers
CadUnico	2003	Individuals and their socio-economic characteristic applying for social benefits.
BFP	2003	Individuals receiving BF payments.
SINASC	1990	All births in Brazil including the type of pregnancy and delivery.
SIM	1975	All deaths in Brazil including ICD-10 cause of death.
SINAN	1993	Diseases of compulsory notification using ICD-10 codes.
SIH-SUS	1993	Patient admissions in the network of public hospitals under SUS.
SIA-SUS	1995	Outpatient visits by SUS.
APAC-SIA	1996	High-cost ambulatory procedures and high-cost medicines.
RHC	1967	Cancer patients in (public or private) hospitals responsible for oncology care.
RCBP	1967	Cancer patients in centers located mostly in major cities.
SISMAMA	2004	Information about breast and gynaecological cancer screening.
SI-PNI	1973	Dispensed immunobiologicals.
SIAB-SUS	1998	Home visits, and medical and nursing care performed in households and health unit
SISLAB-GAL	2008	Laboratory test including cases of Compulsory Notification.
NOTIVISA	2008	Spontaneous reports of suspected cases of Adverse Drug Events.
SNGPC	2007	Dispensing movement data (inputs and outputs) of the drugs subject to special control and antimicrobials.
SINITOX	1980	Cases of intoxication and poisoning.
PFPB	2004	Medication dispensation in the FPB Program.

Cadastro Único

Large social inequalities and poverty are major historical characteristics of Latin America and Brazil, in particular (Bértola and Williamson, 2017). To reduce poverty and inequalities, Brazil has implemented several social protection policies including the Conditional Cash Transfer Program—"Bolsa Familia Program," the housing program "Minha Casa Minha Vida," and the access to water program "Cisterns," among others. In 2003, the Brazilian government created the unified registration for social programs, Cadastro Único (CadUnico), to facilitate implementation and to support decisions related to applications for any of the available social protection programs (Mostafa and Silva, 2007). CadUnico is an electronic database comprising individual records of 114 million people (57% of the Brazilian population, until 2015). It has information on the household characteristics and individual members, who applied to any of the 20 social benefits (from 2004 onward) and those who received any social benefit (since 2001), including detailed demographic, economic, and social conditions of the household (Mostafa and Silva, 2007; Rodrigues, 2017). It is continuous for new applicants, and those already registered have to update the information every 2 years. For those who had their benefits turned down but want to reapply and those who are already receiving a benefit, the information update is mandatory. The extensive coverage of this social registry, the availability of individually identified data, and the possibility of linking them to other health care databases, such as SIM/SINASC/SINAN, allow for designing individual level longitudinal studies to evaluate the impact of social protection programs on health outcomes (such as diseases, hospitalizations, and deaths) (Paim et al., 2011, Rasella et al., 2013; Nunes et al., 2016; Machado et al., 2016a) and has inspired the development of the 100 Million Brazilian Cohort (Pinto et al., 2017; Pita et al., 2018).

Bolsa Família Program

The Brazilian government introduced the largest conditional cash transfer program in the developing world called "Bolsa Família Program" in 2003 as a merger of the pre-reform cash transfers (Lindert et al., 2007). The aim was to reduce current poverty and inequality, by providing a minimum level of income for extremely poor families and to break the inter-generational transmission of poverty by conditioning these transfers on beneficiary compliance with human capital requirements. The conditionalities include: 1) children aged 7 to 17 years have to attend a minimum of 85% schooling days; 2) children up to 7 years of age must complete vaccination and growth monitoring; and 3) beneficiary families with pregnant women, nursing mothers, or children younger than 7 years should follow a health and nutrition agenda (pre- and post-natal care, vaccination, and health and nutrition surveillance). It is implied that making the benefits conditional on "positive" behaviors can further increase the chances of breaking out of the poverty cycle through increased education or improved health. The program also seeks to help empower BFP beneficiaries by linking them to other complementary services, such as health and education (Lindert et al., 2007; Paes-Sousa et al., 2011).

BFP targets were identified through geographic and household assessment methods based on per capita household income. Geographic targeting is applied at federal and municipal levels where as family eligibility is determined based on household registry data that was collected locally and transmitted to the central database, the CadUnico (Lindert et al., 2007). The cash transfers are intended for poor and extremely poor households, with additional payments when a household include children up to 17 years of age (up to two payments per family), or pregnant women (up to nine monthly payments) or lactating women (up to six monthly payments). The original income ceilings for eligibility to the BFP program were set at a fixed monthly per capita household income of R $100 (US $48) for poor families and R $50 (US $25) for extremely poor families. To account for increases in the cost of living, the thresholds were increased in 2006 to R$120 (US $57) for poor families and R$60 (US $29) for extremely poor families (Machado et al., 2018). Additional adjustments were made in 2009 (R$140 for poor and R$70 for extremely poor families) and in 2014 (R$154 for poor and R$77 for extremely poor families). BFP covers 23% of the Brazilian population with the benefits ranging from $18 to a maximum of $175 per month. The mother, when present, must receive the monthly payment on behalf of the whole family (Paiva et al., 2013).

The BFP has attracted significant attention both in Brazil and beyond. As such, several studies have been conducted to evaluate the impact of this program on several health-related outcomes, such as poverty reduction (Soares et al., 2006), inequalities (Soares et al., 2006), crime (Chioda et al., 2016; Machado et al., 2018), leprosy incidence (Nery et al., 2014), and child mortality and hospital admissions (Rasella et al., 2013). Information recorded for each household include date of start of the benefit, period of receipt, and amount of monthly cash transferred (Ministro da Cidadania, 2017). This database, in combination with CadUnico, provides socio-economic information for nearly half of the Brazilian population in the lower income category.

SINASC

The Live Births Information System (Sistema de Informação Sobre Nascidos Vivos [SINASC]), created in 1990 by the MoH, contains vital information on live births in Brazil with the most significant characteristics about the newborn, the mother, the pregnancy, and the delivery. The system includes consolidated data since 1994 and operates with a standardized model of the birth certificate (the Declaration of Live Birth, DNV, a "declaração de nascido vivo"), a legal document completed by the health provider who assisted the delivery and then collected by health secretariat (Frias et al., 2014).

SINASC includes information on place of delivery (hospital or home), the mother who gave birth (including name, age, place of residence, marital status, education, number of children, and number of previous live and still births), the pregnancy (number of prenatal appointments, length of gestation, type of pregnancy: singleton or twin, type of delivery); and the newborn (gestational age, birth weight, sex, ethnicity, the presence and type of birth anomalies for live and stillbirths, and 1- and 5-min APGAR score for live births) (da Saúde, 2011). SINASC uses the International Classification of Disease Version 10 (ICD-10) for coding congenital defects (do Nascimento et al., 2018).

Data must be uploaded by SUS's local level manager, the Municipal Health Secretariat, who are also responsible for processing, consolidating, evaluating, and analyzing these data to support decision-making at local level. Data completeness and coverage are very high, with more than 90% completeness for most variables at country level and capturing 97% of Brazilian registered births (Pedraza, 2012; Oliveira et al., 2015). However, this coverage is heterogeneous within the country, with large variations among the states and some with low percentages particularly those located in the North and Northeast regions. In addition, under-registration of births is still common in some regions of the country and inconsistency of records in variables, such as mother's education, race, and number of prior childbirths, is still high in North and Northeast regions (Oliveira et al., 2015; Hunter and Sugiyama, 2018). SINASC, in combination with SIM (the Mortality Information System) and SIH (the Hospital Information System), has been used to study the impacts, burden, and/patterns of diseases (Paixao et al., 2018), pregnancy-related hospitalizations (Moura et al., 2018), impact of socio-economic inequalities on prenatal consultation (Mallmann et al., 2018), factors affecting neonatal mortality (Kropiwiec et al., 2017; Paixao et al., 2018), the use of ICD-10 coding system on congenital disease ascertainment (do Nascimento et al., 2018). SINASC and SIM/SIH also provide data that are used as parameters in the HTA studies.

SIM

The Mortality Information System (Sistema de Informação sobre Mortalidade [SIM]) was the first subsystem of health information created in 1975 and managed by MoH, containing records of all deaths in Brazil, including fetal deaths. These records are based on the standard death certificate (called the Declaration of Death; DO, "declaração de óbito"), a required legal document, and fetal death certificate collected by the state health secretariat, which contributes to the improvement in the registration of data (Oliveira et al., 2015). Information recorded include: name, date of birth, date of death, sex, ethnicity, educational level, marital status, occupation, place of death, type of health service where death occurred (hospital, another type of health unit, home, or elsewhere), ICD-10 code causes of death (main and secondary) and comorbidities (up to two) (Victora and Barros, 2001). The correct coding of the cause of death, according to ICD-10, is of great importance for the good quality of SIM data. Like SINASC, the coverage in SIM is heterogeneous within the country, with large variations among the states and some with low percentages particularly those located in the North and Northeast regions (Victora and Barros, 2001).

SIM, with SIH/SINASC, has been used in linkage studies (Kropiwiec et al., 2017; Paixao et al., 2018), characterization of trends and regional patterns in (cause-specific) maternal and infant mortality (Victora and Barros, 2001), trends and disparities in cancer mortality (Alves et al., 2009; Girianelli et al., 2014; Braga et al., 2017; Prado da Fonseca et al., 2018), among others. SIM has good coverage and quality, and death characterization. However, delays in data processing, under-reporting of deaths, high numbers of ill-defined cause of death, variation of the quality and coverage in different geographical areas, as well as incorrect filling of death certificates, are some of the limitations (Victora and Barros, 2001; Santos et al., 2008).

SINAN

The Notifiable Diseases Information System [Sistema de Informação de Agravos de Notificação (SINAN)] was implemented gradually and disorderly from 1993. In 1998, it became mandatory to feed the system with data on diseases of compulsory notification, such as tuberculosis, leprosy, human immunodeficeincy virus/acquired immune deficiency syndrome (HIV-AIDS), leishmaniasis, dengue, and Zika. There is a national list of these diseases; however, some states could also include their own specific health problems or outbreaks. Information on disease, using ICD-10 code, is collected through forms filled by health professionals who attend patients with suspected diseases. There are three documents: 1) Individual Notification Form (FIN), filled at the hospital when there is a suspicion of obligatory notifiable disease, outbreak, or new/unknown diseases. This form is followed by: 2) Negative Notification, when there is no disease confirmation; 3) Individual Investigation Form (FII) on identification of the source of infection and transmission mechanism. Each disease record includes different variables, but all include: name, sex, date of birth, place of residence, years of education, date of onset, and clinical aspects of the disease such as symptoms, laboratory tests, disease severity, and sometimes the outcome of the treatment (Paixao et al., 2018). SINAN facilitates the study determinants of obligatory notifiable diseases; indicates the risks of diseases; and facilitates standardization of procedures, investigations, and forms for notifiable diseases. However, there is under-reporting especially of patients from private practices, delay in data processing and correction, and long and complicated information flow (Laguardia et al., 2004).

SINAN, linked to SIM and/or SINASC, has been used to evaluate maternal and child health outcomes (Paixao et al., 2018), incidence and prevalence studies (Tanaka et al., 2017), tuberculosis (Oliveira et al., 2012a; Saraceni et al., 2018), and HIV studies after linkage with other administrative databases SISCEL (Laboratory Tests Control Systems) and SICLOM (Medication Logistics Control System) administrative databases made available in 2000 and 2006, respectively (Saraceni et al., 2018). SICLOM database covers all people living with HIV and receiving ART (antiretroviral therapy), both in public and private health care sectors. SISCEL database, on the other hand, covers only those people living with HIV who had CD4 and viral load tests conducted in public laboratories (Saraceni et al., 2018).

SIH

The Hospital Information System [Sistema de Informações Hospitalares (SIH)] is the national administrative database established in 1991 and comprises information on patient admissions in the network of public hospitals under SUS and private hospitals contracted by the SUS. It has information on over 75% of the country's hospitalizations that are covered/funded by the SUS. Hospitalizations in SUS require completion of a standard form (authorization for hospitalization) that captures patients' personal data, symptoms, and ICD-10 codes of the initial diagnosis. This form and other information recorded by the SIH-SUS on diagnoses, treatment, test results, and billing are standardized throughout Brazil. The resulting data are checked and validated by local health authorities and subsequently transmitted to regional and national levels (Coelho et al., 2016).

Variables recorded include: sex, age, number of hospitalizations, the total amount and value of reimbursed hospital services, days and average length of stay, mortality, among others (Melione and Jorge, 2008; Coelho et al., 2016). SIH has high agility, good morbidity information; it is regularly submitted to audit and payment review; and also allows for monitoring of surveillance epidemiology. However, it mainly covers the public health system which accounts for about 70% of the total admissions and it is constantly changing (Medeiros et al., 2005; Melione and Jorge, 2008; Coelho et al., 2016; Machado et al., 2016a). Although it was created with an administrative purpose, it has been frequently used to monitor population health states and observational studies of adverse drug events (Martins et al., 2018) and health care costs (Quarti Machado Rosa et al., 2018).

SIA-SUS

The Outpatient/Ambulatory Information System of SUS [Sistema de Informações Ambulatoriais do Sistema Único de Saúde (SIA-SUS)] was implemented throughout the country in 1995 and records outpatient visits through the Ambulatory Production bulletin (BPA). Data processing occurs in a decentralized way in which each state and municipality, duly qualified, can register, program, process, and pay for the production of its health facilities under its management. For the generation of information, SIA uses some basic systems, such as the SUS Procedure Chart Management System (SIGTAP), capture application, such as magnetic ambulatory production bulletin, and authorization of magnetic ambulatory procedures. Both capture applications allow recording of basic-, medium-, and high-complexity care procedures. SIA is widely used for HTA studies, since it provides, in addition to the quantitative procedure performed in the SUS, the cost of these procedures for SUS (Machado et al., 2016b).

APAC-SIA

The System of High Complexity Procedures Authorization (APAC-SIA) is a SIA sub-system, established in 1996, constituted by individual registers of high-cost ambulatory procedures and high-cost medicines for specific diseases such as biologics (Brito et al., 2005; Peres et al., 2016; Machado et al., 2016b). Access to high-cost medicines is *via* SUS's Specialized Component of Pharmaceutical Service through a form that comprises useful clinical information of the patient (Machado et al., 2016b). This database contains information on name, national health card number, age, sex, mother's name, address, main procedure code and name, amount of procedures, brief description of diagnosis, ICD-10 code, concomitant diseases, and health care professional number and register code.

The High Complexity Oncology Procedures Authorizations (APAC-ONCO) database contains additional information, including diagnosis date, primary cancer site; histopathology description and final diagnosis; ICD-10 topography; lymph node invasion (yes/no); metastasis locations; tumor, node, metastasis (TNM) stage; and stage by different system. It also records information on previous treatment and current treatment (surgery, chemotherapy, or radiotherapy), including description and start date, scheme, planned duration, and irradiated areas. APAC-ONCO has been used in cancer studies after linkage with other databases, such as SIM (Machado et al., 2016b; Peres et al., 2016), SIH, the breast cancer screening information system (SISMAMA) (Peres et al., 2016), and the hospital-based cancer registry (RCBP) (Peres et al., 2016).

Cancer Information Systems

The cancer registry is a service for collecting, storing, analyzing, interpreting, and systematically disseminating cancer data and includes: 1) The Hospital Cancer Registry (RHC) for recording information about cancer patients seen in a particular hospital (public or private) responsible for oncology care. RHC has administrative purposes, such as estimation of future demand, equipment needs, and human resources. It is considered highly representative of the baseline population and is useful to determine diagnosis efficiency, stage at diagnosis, and treatment. 2) The Population-Based Cancer Registry (RCBP) which was established in 1967 with 26 centers located mostly in major cities. It monitors the frequency of new cancer cases between regions and over time by collecting diagnoses from different sources (clinicians and pathologists) or the death data (when the main cause is cancer). Both registries record socio-demographic information about the patient (age, education level, marital status and place of residence), family history of cancer, source and year of referral, date of diagnosis, diagnosis and previous cancer treatment, characteristics of the tumor (synchronous tumor and laterality), date of first appointment and initiation of the treatment, type of treatment received, stage at diagnosis and tumor evolution after the treatment, and cost of diagnosis and treatment (Ferreira et al., 2017).

The National Cancer Institute (INCA) branch of the MoH in partnership with DATASUS has also implemented the Information System for the Control of Breast Cancer (SISMAMA), an online tool that register information about breast and gynaecological cancer screening. In Brazil, mammograms are encouraged by SUS targeting the female population older than 50 years and has been performed every 2 years, or annually in the case of altered clinical examinations (Cecilio et al., 2015). Women presenting with familial history are encouraged to undergo annual screening of the breasts (Lima-Costa and Matos, 2007). It is estimated that 50% of Brazilian women older than 50 years have had at least one mammography in their life (Lima-Costa and Matos, 2007; Anderson et al., 2011). SISMAMA was conceived as a management tool that capture, organize, and make available data about the population tested; test results (mammograms and ultrasounds, and breast cytopathology and histopathology); follow-up of abnormal cases; the quality of the services; as well as other essential information generated in the course of providing screening tests (Passman et al., 2011). Data collection begins in the primary care setting, typically with a physician's order for a screening or diagnostic mammogram. Mammography results are classified using the Breast Imaging Reporting and Data System (BI-RADS) developed by the American College of Radiology (ACR). SISMAMA has been used in several studies after linkage with SIM, SIA-APAC, and SIH-SUS (Freire et al., 2015; Peres et al., 2016; Tomazelli et al., 2018a; Tomazelli et al., 2018b).

SI-PNI

The National Immunization Program Information System [Sistema de Informação do Programa Nacional de Imunização (SI-PNI)] contains records on dispensed immunobiologicals. It was developed by PNI in partnership with DATASUS and is comprise several subsystems: 1) the Information System of the Immunization Program Assessment (SI-API) which provides data on vaccination coverage (routine and campaigns), dropout rate, immunization control bulletins. API can be used by the federal, state, regional, and municipal levels; 2) the Immunobiological Inventory and Distribution Information System (SI-EDI) which controls the supply and distribution of immunobiologicals at the state and federal levels; 3) the Information System of adverse events following vaccination (SI-EAPV), which allows the vigilance of adverse events after administration of the vaccine; 4) the Information System of the Instrument Evaluation Program (SI-PAIS) and the Information System of the Evaluation Program of the Supervision Instrument in Vaccine Room (SI-PAISSV), which contribute for standard evaluation profile and fast delivery of tabulated results; 5) the Information System for the Assessment of Immunobiologicals Used (SI-AIU), which evaluates the lost and utilized doses; 6) the Information System of the Reference Center for Special Immunobiological (SI-CRIE) which informs adverse events and utilization of special immunobiologicals (da Nóbrega et al., 2010).

SI-PNI enables quantitative analysis of vaccination coverage by vaccine type, doses given, and dropout rate throughout the country by age group, time, and geographical area (Assis Moura et al., 2018). Within SI-PNI, it is also possible to perform monthly follow-up of vaccination activities regarding the quantity of distributed and applied doses, coverage, and adverse events post-vaccination (EAPV). SI-PNI uses single identifying number shown on the "National Health Card" [Cart ao Nacional de Sa ude (CNS)], hence, the vaccinated and their origins can be identified, allowing to find unvaccinated ones and give them a dose. Linkage to different national databases enables conduct of observational studies on vaccine effectiveness (Domingues and Teixeira, 2013; Sato, 2015). In addition, SI-PNI can be used as parameter to assess and modeling economics evaluation of new vaccines.

SIAB

The Basic Health Care Information System [Sistema de Informação da Atenção Básica (SIAB)] was created in 1998 by DATASUS, in conjunction with the co-ordination of community health/health care Secretariat (COSAC/SAS). It assists monitoring and evaluation of activities carried out by the community health agents

(ACS), aggregating and processing the data from the home visits, as well as the medical and nursing care performed in households and health unit (Da Silva and Laprega, 2005; Frias et al., 2012). Data are collected using the forms for enrolment, and follow-up of families is served by the family health teams and community health agents. It contains data on socio-economic characteristics; health (morbidity); residences of households and their individuals; and medical follow-up data on priority groups such as pregnant women, diabetics, hypertensives, and leprosy patients having tuberculosis, and children younger than 2 years (the mother's name and address, age of the child, date of death, and cause of death). In addition, medical and nursing consultations, request for additional examinations, referrals, as well as notification of some diseases, for example, pneumonia in children younger than 5 years are recorded.

SISLAB

Brazil has a national network of public laboratories, the National System of Public Health Laboratories [Sistema Nacional de Laboratórios de Saúde Pública (SISLAB)]. The laboratories are organized hierarchically (national, regional, state, and municipal level) by the degree of complexity of activities, in accordance with the principles of SUS, related to health surveillance including epidemiological surveillance, surveillance in environmental health, sanitary surveillance, and medical assistance (da Saúde, 2004). In 2008, the MoH, aiming to improve laboratory information through the General Coordination of Public Health Laboratories (CGLAB) and DATASUS, elaborated the Laboratory Environment Management System [Gerenciador de Ambiente Laboratorial (GAL)]. GAL is a free software with its own communication patterns, distributed, robust and flexible architecture, and multi-platforms (Jesus et al., 2013; Júnior et al., 2017). The national module of the GAL manages, monitors, and concentrates the results of the laboratory tests informed by the State Modules of the following six areas: Medical Biology, Environmental and Worker Health, Animal, Quality Control, Management, and Quality and Biotechnology. Therefore, GAL is a computerized system applied to the examinations and tests of samples of human, animal, and environmental origins, following the protocols of the MoH.

GAL sends laboratory test results from suspected or confirmed cases of Compulsory Notifications (flu, tuberculosis, leishmaniasis, dengue, zika, yellow fever, pertussis, and meningitis, among others) to the SINAN. It also contains data on viral hepatitis markers, serological diagnosis of HIV, tumor markers, diagnosis of zoonosis and related biological factors, analysis of water quality in health facilities and environmental health surveillance service (Jesus et al., 2013; Júnior et al., 2017). The SISLAB-GAL data contribute decisively to surveillance in Brazil, but its integration with other social-economic information (for example, data from CadUnico) and health care data (for example, SIM/SIH) would allow to conduct several epidemiological studies.

NOTIVISA

The National Notification System for Health Surveillance [Sistema de Notificações em Vigilância Sanitária (NOTIVISA)], created in 2008, is an online computerized information system of the National Sanitary Surveillance Agency (ANVISA) that receives spontaneous reports of suspected cases of Adverse Drug Events. It covers the Brazilian territory and is considered the largest and most important repository of Adverse Drug Events data from the National Pharmacovigilance System (SINAF) of the country (de Vigilância Sanitária, 2008). NOTIVISA allows the obtaining and circulation of information on health problems to users, sudden or undesirable effect, and/or malfunctions related to health products marketed in Brazil. The NOTIVISA system has enabled adoption of adequate measures of control, safety alerts, besides providing information to update the existing legislation and/or to propose new legislation as well as sanitary recommendations for the adoption of measures that ensure the protection and health promotion of the population (Branco et al., 2015).

Data from NOTIVISA have been used in studies to investigate the occurrence of reports related to health products in the post-marketing phase, such as the occurrence of Adverse Events and Technical Complaints related to the use of a vascular catheter (Oliveira and Rodas, 2017), to describe the adverse events related to healthcare products that resulted in death in Brazil (Maia et al., 2018).

SNGPC

The National System for Management of Controlled Products [Sistema Nacional de Gerenciamento de Produtos Controlados (SNGPC)], implemented in late 2007 and early 2008, is a sanitary surveillance information system that captures dispensing movement data (inputs and outputs) of the drugs subject to the special control as well as antimicrobials and updates in pharmacies and private drug stores in the country. The SNGPC main objectives include: to monitor the dispensation of drugs and narcotics, and psychotropic substances and their precursors; to optimize the book keeping process; to allow monitoring of prescription habits and consumption of controlled substances in a given region to propose control policies; to collect data that allow the generation of up-to-date and reliable information for the National Health Surveillance Service (SNVS) for decision making; and to streamline the actions of health surveillance (de Vigilância Sanitária, 2010)

The data feeding the system comes from the prescription of qualified medical professionals, retained at the time of dispensing the drug in the pharmaceutical establishment, and invoices for the purchase of medicines suppliers. The main operational actors of the SNGPC are the pharmacists in charge of the pharmacies and drug stores, and SNVS health surveillance professionals. SNGPC has been used in studies to examine the consumption of appetite suppressant drugs (Mota et al., 2014), the consumption of psychotropic anorectic drugs (Martins et al., 2012), and the frequency as well as distribution of the consumption of benzodiazepine anxiolytics in private pharmacies and drug stores (Azevedo et al., 2016).

PFPB

The Popular Pharmacy Program [Programa Farmácia Popular do Brasil (PFPB)] was created in 2004, within the scope of the SUS, to expand access to medicines for the most common diseases among citizens. One of the objectives of the program was to favor low-income people by making treatment feasible in the face of the high price of medicines. It also supports the population of the private health network as an alternative, since they have access to medicines with prices more affordable. PFPB was also aimed to contribute to the reduction of the expenses generated by the purchase of medicines and minimize the expenses of the SUS with hospitalizations that are caused by the abandonment of the treatment (Inocencio and De Vivo, 2011).

The PFPB developed two axes of action: the own network of public Popular Pharmacies (rede Própria) and accredited private retail pharmacies of PFPB (PFPB-E, "Aqui Tem Farmácia Popular" or ATFP). Popular Pharmacies, operating since 2004, have a list of 112 medicines which are dispensed at cost representing a reduction of up to 90% of the market value. The PFPB-E, considered as an expansion of PFPB in partnership with pharmacies and drugstores of the private network, was created with the objective of expanding the coverage of pharmaceutical assistance and promoting the integrity of health care (Coelho Filho et al., 2004). In this modality, the MoH subsidizes 90% of the reference value for diseases, such as dyslipidemia, Parkinson's, glaucoma, osteoporosis, rhinitis, contraceptives, and geriatric diapers. As of 2011, with the creation of "Health Without Price" ("Saúde Não tem Preço"), the two axes of action started to count on free medicines for asthma, diabetes and hypertension. It has the potential for linkage since it contains tax number (Cadastro de Pessoas Físicas [CPF]) of individual patients (Coelho Filho et al., 2004).

SINITOX

The National Toxic-Pharmacological Information System [Sistema Nacional de Informações Tóxico-Farmacológicas (SINITOX)] was created in 1980 and is linked to FIOCRUZ. It is responsible for the collection, compilation, analysis, and dissemination of cases of intoxication and poisoning registered by the National Network of Information and Assistance Centers Toxicological—RENACIAT. RENACIAT is currently composed of 36 units located in 19 states and the federal district which provide information and guidance on the diagnosis, prognosis, treatment and prevention of intoxications, as well as on the toxicity of chemical and biological substances and the risks they cause to health (Bortoletto and Bochner, 1999).

The differences in structure, setup, and content of all these different databases can lead to significant challenges in use of these data for HTA and decision-making. In addition, there are considerable challenges regarding the lack of governance. Most often, there are poor or no standards for collaboration; there is a lack of incentives for data sharing; and there are issues with regard to patient consent, privacy, and data security that may severely hamper access to such data. As a result, the costs for data protection would be very high to comply with relevant regulation (Annemans, 2017).

Despite the availability of all these SUS and related databases, there are still key challenges in the use of secondary data for HTA, pharmacovigilance, and supporting decision-making. Data linkage is one of the available approaches that can be used to mitigate lack of integration and standardization observed in such databases. Record linkage can help generate useful and high quality data sets to conduct research, and support formulation and evaluation of public policy. However, linking these databases is not a trivial task mainly due to the lack of common key identifiers amongst all the databases, as well other technical issues related to data quality, standardization, availability, and volume (number of records). **Table 2** summarizes some attributes encountered in most of these databases, which are potential candidates for linkage purposes.

DATA LINKAGE

Data linkage, also called record linkage, is the process of combining records about the same individual or entity from two or more different data sources (Winkler, 2006; Jurczyk et al., 2008a) or the process of identifying duplicate records in the same data set (Jurczyk et al., 2008a). In principle, record linkage problem consists of developing a classifier that categorizes record pairs as "linked" or "non-linked" with reasonable accuracy (Jurczyk et al., 2008a). It enables the aggregation of data not available in a single data set thereby supplementing information on an individual with information from other data sources, validating information collected in one data source, or to de-duplicate records within a single data source (Winkler, 2006; Jurczyk et al., 2008a). Record linkage also has additional applications, such as building longitudinal profile of individuals and case-identification in capture-recapture studies (Sayers et al., 2015).

There are two main types of linkage algorithms: deterministic and probabilistic. Deterministic linkage methods vary from a one-step procedure using a single unique identifier or a set of several attributes (called "exact" deterministic linkage) to step-wise algorithmic linkages involving a series of progressively less restrictive steps to allow variation between record attributes (called "iterative" deterministic linkage). A record pair is classified as "linked" if it meets the criteria or parameters at any step; otherwise is classified as "non-linked" (Dusetzina et al., 2014). Probabilistic linkage methods, on the other hand, takes advantage of differences in the discriminatory power of each attribute and apply calculation of similarity scores, as well as decision rules, to classify record pairs as linked, potentially linked (treated as dubious records in most linkage tools) and non-linked (Newcombe et al., 1959; Fellegi and Sunter, 1969; Dusetzina et al., 2014). It can also

TABLE 2 | Potential Linkeage Attributs amongst SUS databases.

Attribute	Meaning	Databases
Name	Full Name	CadUnico, BFP, SIM, SINAN, SINASC, SIH-SUS, SIA-SUS (APAC-SIA), SISMAMA, SIAB, SISLAB-GAL
Mother's name	Full Name	CadUnico, BFP, SIM, SINAN, SINASC, SIH-SUS, SIA-SUS (APAC-SIA), SISMAMA, SIAB, SISLAB-GAL
Data of birth	Date, Month, Year	CadUnico, BFP, SIM, SINAN, SINASC, SIH-SUS, SIA-SUS (APAC-SIA), SISMAMA, SIAB, SISLAB-GAL
Municipality Codo	7 Digit Numeric	CadUnico, BFP, SIM, SINAN, SINASC, SIH-SUS, SIA-SUS (APAC-SIA), SISMAMA, SIAB, SISLAB-GAL
Sex	Male/Female	CadUnico, BFP, SIM, SINAN, SINASC, SIH-SUS, SIA-SUS (APAC-SIA), SISMAMA, SIAB, SISLAB-GAL

deal with some inconsistencies between records with missing data, i.e., it has the capacity to link records with errors in the linking fields (Dusetzina et al., 2014).

Since its introduction by Newcombe (Newcombe et al., 1959) and mathematical formalization by Fellegi and Sunter (Fellegi and Sunter, 1969), several variations of record linkage and computerized tools have emerged to meet different requirements and challenges, such as accuracy, speed, and scalability. Many of these tools have a general purpose, allowing a combination of existing configurations and methodologies (Camargo and Coeli, 2000; Elfeky et al., 2002; Christen et al., 2004; Christen, 2008; Schnell et al., 2009; Pita et al., 2018). While most of these methods are probabilistic, some of them apply a combination of deterministic and probabilistic linkages (called "hybrid" methods) (Pita et al., 2018). In general, a successful linkage processing involves several main steps: pre-processing, blocking and indexing, field comparison, weight vector classification, and accuracy assessment (Christen, 2008) as depicted in **Figure 1**.

The pre-processing step involves data cleansing and standardization whereby incomplete and incorrectly formatted data is converted into well-defined, consistent form (Christen et al., 2004; Christen, 2008). Specific approaches to deal with missing data can be applied at this step to i) remove missing fields or entire records or ii) impute missing values based on standard or calculated values. Pre-processing may also involve anonymization using different privacy-preserving techniques, such as Bloom filters (Inan et al., 2008; Pita et al., 2018), to protect sensitive data from disclosure and unauthorized use.

Executing a linkage routine between data sets A and B will result in a number of field comparisons defined by the product $|A| * |B|$. In a big data context, these numbers make pairwise comparisons impractical and lead to a number of infrastructure, data processing, and data analysis challenges (Peek et al., 2014; Harron et al., 2017). To circumvent scalability challenges over big data sets, different approaches have been used in the literature, such as parallelism/distribution and blocking (or indexing) strategies, as well as their combinations (Christen, 2008; Pita et al., 2018). Other initiatives have also proposed the use of cluster-based platforms, multi-processors or graphics processing units (GPUs) (Boratto et al., 2018; Pita et al., 2018). Blocking and indexing step generates pairs of candidate records pertaining to the same comparison blocks (Christen, 2012). These methods drastically decrease the number of candidate record pairs to a feasible number thereby speeding up the linkage performance over big data sets while still maintaining linkage accuracy. Several indexing techniques used in linkage solutions are well described in the literature (Christen, 2012).

The field comparison step involves using several functions to measure the similarity of attributes for each record pair. The choice of the functions is dependent on the content of the field: string comparison functions are used for names and addresses whereas numerical comparison functions are used for fields, such as date, age, and numerical values (Christen, 2012). Once a vector of numerical similarity values is calculated for each record pair, the candidate record pairs are classified as linked (i.e., candidate pairs that are linked deterministically or probabilistically by the linkage software), non-linked or possibly linked, based on one or more cutoff (threshold) points, in the weight vector classification step as shown in **Figure 2**.

During the final step—accuracy assessment—evaluates the linkage algorithm and the quality of the linkage (i.e., it estimates rates of linkage errors: missed matches and false matches).Linkage accuracy is often assessed using a gold standard dataset where the true match status of each pair of records is known. Comparing the probabilistically linked dataset to the gold-standard dataset will identify true matches, true non-matches, false matches, and missed matches. Hence, measures of linkage quality such as sensitivity, positive predictive value, and F-measure can be easily derived. When gold standard dataset is not available,alternative approaches such as sensitivity analysis, comparison of characteristics of linked and non-linked data, and identification of implausible matches could be used to quantify the rate of linkage errors (Christen, 2008)

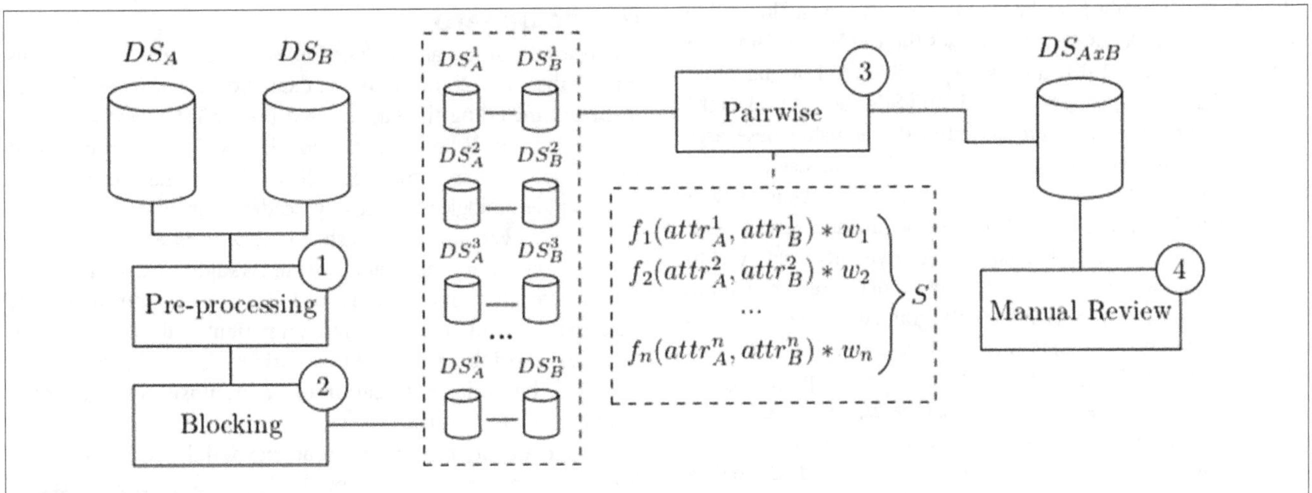

FIGURE 1 | Common flowchart of a data linkage tool: Raw data are pre-processed (1) and split into smaller blocks (2). Pairwise comparison is performed among records within similar blocks using functions that produce a similarity measure for each attribute. A weighted vector is then used to average each individual similarity measure into a single score S (3). Manual review the dataset generated after the pairwise comparison is optionally performed (4). Data source A (DS_A), data source B (DS_B), number of blocks (n), attributes (attr), weights (w), score (S), and linked data DS_{AxB}.

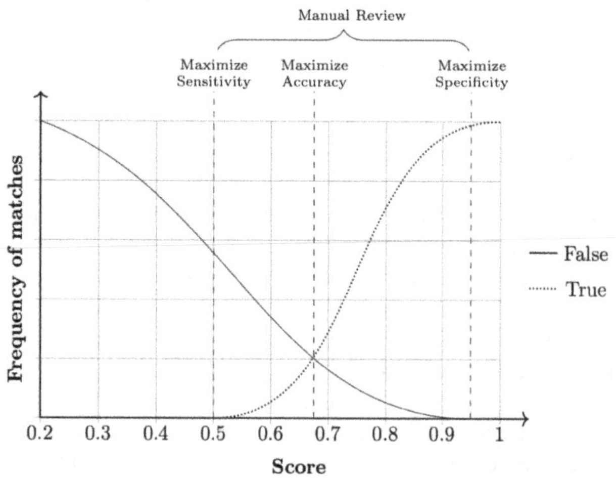

FIGURE 2 | Example of a frequency analysis of a data set produced by the linkage pipeline. Three cut-off points can be chosen according to specific needs. Any pair in between sensitivity and specificity cutoffs is considered a dubious match and thus passed for manual review. When manual review is not possible, a common approach is to choose a cut-off point that averages sensitivity and specificity, maximizing accuracy.

DATA LINKAGE INITIATIVES IN BRAZIL

In the last decade, the use of big data for research in Brazil has increased substantially due to several factors: data access, creation of research groups and data centers, development of efficient record linkage tools, and international research collaborations, among others. In this section, we describe three data centers specialized in the use of big data as well as development of record linkage tools:

CIDACS

The Centre for Data and Knowledge Integration for Health [Centro de Integração de Dados e Conhecimentos para Saúde (CIDACS)] is a data linkage center managed by the Oswaldo Cruz Foundation (FIOCRUZ),′ officially launched in December 2016 and located in Salvador, State of Bahia, Brazil. It houses the 100 Million Brazilian Cohort (Pita et al., 2018) and is responsible for housing other large databases, such as SINAN, SIM, and SINASC, as well as the development of other new and innovative studies using these large databases. An agreement signed between the Ministry of Social Development (MoSD), FIOCRUZ, UFBA, and the University of Brasilia (UnB); the MoSD permitted the acquisition, after ethical approvals, of a copy of CadUnico and BF payments from 2004 to 2015. Negotiations with the MoH, in particular, the Department for Health Information (DATASUS) granted CIDACS copies of SINASC, SINAN and SIM from 2000 to 2015. Copies of SIH, SISVAN, and "Minha Casa Minha Vida" (housing program) are also available, whereas access to other databases, such as "Cisterns" (Wells), is in negotiation at the time of writing this paper.

The center operates with a strong governance; an advanced data platform comprising the computational infrastructure needed for receipt, storage, curation, and integration of large databases, and extraction of data sets for specific analysis; and a physical structure carefully designed to give full physical protection for the data when handling non-anonymized data sets as well as to manage access and analysis of de-identified or anonymized data sets. All standard operation procedures (SOPs) for data manipulation, cleaning, linkage, and for meta-data production are being defined according to international standards. In the past few years, CIDACS has developed algorithms for data anonymization and data linkage including the two linkage algorithms ("AtyImo," a tool used in less safe environments where the identifier information must be masked or anonymized, and "CIDACS-RL," which is used under extremely safe environments without masking). Linkage using both tools were already validated and, for the optimum threshold (best trade-off of sensitivity and specificity), the accuracy of both algorithms is above 90% (Pita et al., 2018).

Minas Gerais

The research group at the Federal University of Minas Gerais had also made significant achievement in record linkage. In partnership with the MoH's team, the team has been working on the National Health Database Centered on Individual: a 15-year cohort of individual-level historical data, preserving patient privacy, integrating SIH, SIA, SIM, SINASC, and SINAN (Guerra et al., 2018). It will allow researchers to generate real-world evidence using clinical, pharmacological, and pharmacoeconomic studies.

The group has also developed a parallel deduplication algorithm, called FER-APARDA, using probabilistic record linkage, as well as PAREIA (Santos et al., 2007; dos Santos Filho, 2008). PAREIA's crucial contributions are two-fold: 1) the proposed blocking scheme uses predicates from fields or portions of them, making a junction of disjunctions to prevent input errors to separate true matches from the right blocks. 2) The use of high-performance computing techniques and programming languages to guarantee its suitability to big data scenarios. This initiative has enabled several scientific investigations, such as the study of a criminal network by identifying distinct offenders on a graph-based police event database (dos Santos Fraga, 2009).

Rio de Janero

The research group at the State University of Rio de Janeiro has made substantial contribution on data science and record linkage in Brazil, including the largely used probabilistic record linkage tool based on Fellegi-Sunter model, RecLink (Camargo and Coeli, 2000; Camargo and Coeli, 2006). Reclink has been used in many epidemiological studies by academic institutions and the MoH which were mostly published in *Reports in Public Health*,[1] a scientific repository maintained by the Oswaldo Cruz Foundation. They have also employed record linkage on administrative databases to study mortality rate on patients submitted to high complex cardiology procedures (Migowski et al., 2011) and to assess the under notification of tuberculosis cases in Brazil (Oliveira et al., 2012b).

Main contributions of this group, beyond the reported linked databases, comprise the use of the Expectation Maximization (EM) algorithm to predict the best settings for model tuning (Junger, 2006), the use of phonetic code in blocking step (Coeli

[1] https://scielosp.org/grid/csp/

and Camargo, 2002), and the rule-based matching. Recent work on the development of an open source version, the OpenRecLink (de Camargo and Coeli, 2015) has provided a multi-platform solution suitable to international users. Additional efforts have been made to define a cut-off point on probabilistic record linkage results (Verzinhasse Peres et al., 2014) and building a data warehouse for the integration of three Brazilian health information systems concerned with the production of ambulatory and hospital procedures for cancer care, and cancer mortality: SIH-SUS, APAC-ONCO, and SIM (Freire et al., 2015).

RECORD LINKAGE TOOLS DEVELOPED AND/OR USED IN BRAZIL

In the past decade, the use of secondary data for research in Brazil has grown substantially. This is due to several factors: availability of large data sources, development of efficient linkage tools, legislation in Brazil favoring the used of secondary data for Brazil, the need to evaluate several public policies, and international collaborations, among others.

RecLink

RecLink (RecLinkIII) is an open source C++ based probabilistic linkage algorithm specifically developed for the Portuguese language phonetics (Camargo and Coeli, 2000). Its flexible Graphical User Interface (GUI) allows the user to customize the tool and read different data sets easily. The interface is also used to define the behavior of the tool, such as the pre-processing steps, blocking and matching parameters (Camargo and Coeli, 2006). RecLink uses a custom format for input, which means the original data sets first have to be converted to standard formats to be linked. It has functions related to the standardization of common fields, including manipulation of names (case sensitive conversions, preposition and accent removal in names, and removal of commas and punctuation marks), standardization of date formats, and correct classification of missing values. Standardization of character attributes, such as date of birth and sex, is performed using the dBASE database manager, whereas a Soundex code developed for this purpose is used for strings, such as names and municipality (Camargo and Coeli, 2000; Camargo and Coeli, 2006).

RecLink performs record linkage in two steps: 1) blocking step, which separates the two data sets to be linked into smaller data sets according to the configuration provided by the user and 2) matching weight calculation and pairwise comparison of records that belong to the same block (Camargo and Coeli, 2000). The blocking stage can be conducted in one-step procedure using a single attribute, such as municipality(Paixao et al., 2018) or multi-step procedure using different combinations of attributes (Capuani et al., 2014). The Levenshtein string comparator is used to compare names; it is defined as the minimum number of insertions, deletions, or substitutions necessary to change one string into another (the values varying between 1, perfect similarity and 0, total disagreement). RecLink uses three different weight systems that can be selected by the user: 1) the pure and simple comparison, which only classifies records as matches if their attributes are strictly identical; 2) the character sequence comparison, which evaluates each pair of attributes from both records and returns how many different characters they have; and 3) the fuzzy comparison, which returns a normalized score consisting of the size of the longest common sequence of characters divided by the size of the longest attribute. The default m-probabilities and u-probabilities of 0.9 and 0.1, respectively, are often used (Oliveira et al., 2012a; Paixao et al., 2018).

RecLink is the most popular linkage tool in Brazil that has been used in several population linkage-based studies (Oliveira et al., 2012a; Capuani et al., 2014; Paixao et al., 2018). It also has several functions for other applications, such as de-duplication, standard query language (SQL) exporting, and frequency tables calculation. The software is available for free use and licensed under GPL (Camargo and Coeli, 2000; Camargo and Coeli, 2006).

Python Linkage Algorithm

Python linkage algorithm (PLA) is a Python based deterministic algorithm developed for passive data collection with cohorts of HIV-infected patients at FIOCRUZ Rio de Janeiro. The tool aims to maximize accuracy and to minimize the need for clerical (manual) review in data linkage (Pacheco et al., 2008b). It was primarily implemented to assist in retrieval of information on the vital status of people living with HIV/AIDS (PLWHA) who are lost to follow-up in two large urban HIV/AIDS cohorts: Rio de Janeiro cohort database (Schechter et al., 1994) and TB-HIV in Rio (THRio) (Pacheco et al., 2011). The Rio de Janeiro cohort database was originally designed to validate the WHO-HIV staging system in a developing country, whereas the THRio cohort was designed to assess the impact of implementing isoniazid prophylactic therapy among HIV-positive patients with indications for prophylaxis in Rio de Janeiro (Pacheco et al., 2011; Saraceni et al., 2014). PLA has also been adapted to cross-reference PLWHA public databases to both tuberculosis and AIDS cohort databases (Pacheco et al., 2008a; Grinsztejn et al., 2013).

The algorithm has a hierarchical structure and correlates records using exact comparisons. It allows for specific errors in names and dates, measured by means of phonetic codes and a string similarity score based on a recursive longer common substring algorithm, implemented in the "difflib" library from Python, which helps dealing with specific differences between sequences and dates. PLA runs both in a fully automated procedure (PLA-FAP) and in association with clerical/manual review of records that are not classified as true matches or non-matches (PLA-MR). Patient name, mother name, and date of birth are used as matching fields with parameter estimates obtained with the Expectation–Maximization algorithm. Date of birth is allowed to have only one digit mistake in any position or the common swap between day and month (only if they were exactly the same but swapped) (Pacheco et al., 2008b). The Levenshtein distance string comparator measure is used to compare the field name and mother name (Fonseca et al., 2010). The algorithm uses score values chosen empirically during its development using different data sources (Pacheco et al., 2008b).

The combination of these measurements and score values determine several levels of inclusion and exclusion, called automatic codes, which depends on how much information is available or missing. Records with complete information are treated independently from records with missing information. Whenever a pair of records is neither automatically included nor automatically excluded by the criteria, this pair is kept in the final merged database, marked as an unresolved pair for possible further manual review. The algorithm is hierarchical in the sense that lower codes mean more similar records hence perfect matches, but codes used for records with full information, even if higher, are more robust than codes for missing records. The algorithm is not "greedy": the same record in the test database linked with a lower code (exact match) to one record could also be linked to another one with a higher code (poor match). This feature is useful in dealing with databases with one-to-many relations, for example in the case of tuberculosis surveillance databases (Pacheco et al., 2008b; Fonseca et al., 2010).

PLA has been validated using several cohorts Pacheco et al. (2008b); Pacheco et al. (2011); Saraceni et al. (2014); de Paula et al. (2018) and has comparable accuracy to RecLink, which intrinsically require manual review, and outperformed RecLink significantly in the presence of incomplete data without manual inspection (sensitivity: 98.4% for PLA versus 94.6% RecLink, $p < 0.05$) Pacheco et al. (2008a, 2008b, 2009, 2011); Grinsztejn et al. (2013).

Atylmo

Atylmo was developed by UFBA and CIDACS between 2013 and 2016 to support a joint Brazil–UK project aimed at developing large population-based cohorts. It was written in Python, freely available on Github, and runs distributed over Spark (Pinto et al., 2017; Pita et al., 2018) or in parallel over CUDA over hybrid (multicore+multi-GPU) architectures. It implements a pipeline comprising data pre-processing (cleansing, standardization, blocking, and anonymization), pairwise comparison and matching decision, and accuracy assessment (Pita et al., 2018).

Data pre-processing in Atylmo is responsible to clean and standardize names, filling null/missing fields with default values, and remove duplicate records. Blocking is based on different predicates built with five linking attributes (name, mother name, date of birth, sex, and municipality). In an effort to reduce errors due to typos or missing values that could lead records being inserted in wrong blocks, Atylmo uses a predicate of attributes in its blocking stage. Anonymization is based on Bloom filters, which guarantee privacy-preserving requisites related to sensitive (identifiable) data, allowing Atylmo to run within less protected environments, if needed. A Bloom filter is a 128-bit vector in which bigrams (pair of characters) are represented as 0 or 1 depending on some hash functions. It is useful to reduce the effort during pairwise comparison; instead of comparing strings directly, one can compare binary vectors using the Sørensen's Dice similarity function (Pita et al., 2018). Dice is defined as: Dice = (2 h)/(a + b), where h is the total of 1's at the same positions in both filters, and a and b are the total of 1's in the first and second filters, respectively. A Dice = 1 means filters are completely equal, decreasing to 0 (zero) depending on existing differences. The current implementation normalizes Dice indices between 0 and 10.000. Dice costs less to compute than other editing distance functions, improving Atylmo's speed (Pita et al., 2018).

Atylmo implements a two-round linkage step in which a mixture of deterministic and probabilistic methods can be used together to generate high accurate data marts (domain specific data). The weights of each attribute are determined by the amount of bits they occupy in the Bloom, meaning that important attributes, such as name will have a larger bloom length over less important attributes. In the hybrid approach, categorical attributes are matched exactly whereas names and dates (both more prone to errors) are probabilistically classified as: exact (Dice = 10,000), strong (10,000 ≥ Dice ≥ 9,000), weak (9,000 > Dice ≥ 8,000), and unpaired (8,000 ≤ Dice). This approach results in some flexibility in the combinations of exact and approximate comparisons. As a result, three output data sets are produced: true positive (TP) pairs, true negative (TN) pairs, and "dubious records" [false positive (FP) and false negative (FN) matches]. This classification is based on upper and lower cutoff points representing boundaries for TP and TN matches, respectively. Further analysis of the cutoff points is performed to retrieve more true (positive and negative) pairs and an iterative second round analysis of dubious pairs, shifting these points in each iteration, is conducted to retrieve additional records into these two groups (Pinto et al., 2017; Pita et al., 2018).

Finally, accuracy assessment can be performed manually based on gold standards (when existent) to certify small data marts or automatically based on supervised machine learning methods (Pita et al., 2017) in big data marts. Supervised methods use the same data produced during the accuracy assessment of previous linkage to fit a model that can be later used to classify new records. Atylmo, in comparison to previous linkage tools freely available, has reasonably better accuracy and shorter execution time with a major advantage to scale upward to huge databases (Pita et al., 2018). The current version of Atylmo based on the NVIDIA's CUDA library is able to probabilistically link databases of up 80 million records in around 60 s over multiple GPU architectures (Boratto et al., 2018).

CIDACS-RL

CIDACS-RL, created at CIDACS in Salvador, is a Java-based search engine indexing linkage tool. It was developed to mitigate accuracy and scalability challenges in linking huge administrative electronic health and socioeconomic data sets, in the order of millions of records, stored within the center. To achieve this, instead of using usual blocking strategies, CIDACS-RL uses indexing, query and scoring modules provided by Apache Lucene (Białecki et al., 2012) and inverted index and term frequency-inverse document frequency (TF-IDF) to reduce the number of comparisons. The TF-IDF weight is composed by the normalized TF (the number of times a word appears in a document divided by the total number of words in that document) and the IDF (computed as the logarithm of the total number of documents divided by the number of documents where the specific term appears).

Within the CIDACS environment, all data sets are submitted to data cleansing and quality assurance processes after entering data linkage step. Those processes guarantee that linkage attributes are standardized and cleansed. Similarly to other methods, CIDACS-RL performs record linkage in two steps. If two databases A and B were to be linked and $|\cdot|$ denotes the number of records in a given database, assuming $|A| > |B|$ (i.e., A is the largest database: the indexing module take as input the linkage attributes from data set A (larger data set) and builds an index A_i (Białecki et al., 2012). A challenging issue in linking huge data sets is to reduce the number of pairwise comparisons, therefore, CIDACS-RL uses the query module as a blocking stage. Hence, instead of comparing each record of data set B with every record of data set A, CIDACS-RL query a small subset of similar records from A_i and apply comparison functions on them.

As Apache Lucene provides different query types, CIDACS-RL uses a mixture of queries functions (exact, semi-exact or fuzzy) to overcome different errors expected to exist in data linkage attributes (Białecki et al., 2012). Exact query takes each linkage attribute as a parameter and returns only records in which every attribute is equal to those used for querying. Semi-exact query is a modification of exact query composed of an arrangement of n1 linkage attributes, hence, enabling retrieval of candidate pairs where only one attribute is different between the query record and result pairs. Unlike exact and semi-exact queries, fuzzy query allows differences on any number of attributes. Each query function (exact, semi-exact or fuzzy) takes each record in data set B to query in A_i and returns a set of similar records based on TF-IDF.

Since some attributes may have semantic meaning which the TF-IDF does not account for, CIDACS-RL relies on a custom scoring function tailored for Brazilian data sources to compare record pairs. This function is based on different metrics and approaches, depending on the type of attribute. CIDACS-RL supports four kinds of attributes: string, categorical, date, and IBGE municipality code. The IBGE code is a seven-digit numeric code where the first two digits represent one of Brazil's 27 states, the following four digits represent one of 5,570 municipalities and the last digit is used for verification purposes. Next, each record in data set B which was used as source for the query is compared with all records retrieved from A_i and returns the most similar record based on the custom scoring function. The function returns all pairs matched along with the score obtained; if any record with a score greater than the threshold is found on exact or semi-exact queries, the pair is added to the resulting set and fuzzy query is not executed.

FRIL

Fine-grained Records Integration and linkage Tool (FRIL) is a Java based tool providing a set of highly customizable functions. Data integration (or reconciliation) is supported through different merging and splitting functions. It uses searching methods to determine which pairs of records will be compared from both data sets to be linked. FRIL has two different search methods: nested loop join and sorted neighborhood. Nested loop method performs "all to all" comparison, which is the same as no blocking. Sorted neighborhood defines a window limit in a way that records outside the window are not compared, reducing the number of comparisons (Jurczyk et al., 2008a; Jurczyk et al., 2008b).

To compare record pairs, FRIL implements four types of distance functions: edit distance, soundex, Q-gram and equality. All distances are normalized between 0 (total disagreement) and 1 (total agreement). Edit distance consists of the number of changes needed to make both attributes equal. Soundex transforms the attributes to a new form that takes the word sound into account, which can be useful when dealing with attributes, such as names and addresses, which are informed using speech. Equality just assigns 1 if the attribute is equal and 0 otherwise (Jurczyk et al., 2008a; Jurczyk et al., 2008b). Regarding the decision process, FRIL allows for matching weights to be assigned to each attribute by the user. The matching weights are then used to compute a normalized weighted average that is the similarity score for the pair. Similarity score is used to make a decision classifying the pair as match, non-match, or uncertain, according to thresholds defined by the user (Jurczyk et al., 2008a). Uncertain pairs can be later manually labeled as matches or non-matches, if needed. FRIL has been used in Brazilian databases and comparative studies of linkage algorithms, however, the performance in huge data sets was sub-optimal compared others, such as AtyImo (Pita et al., 2018).

Febrl

Freely extensible biomedical record linkage (Febrl) is a Python-based data linkage pipeline, implementing data cleansing, de-duplication, and pairwise comparison. Its modular architecture contains a handful of functions that can be used in the linkage process. The tool has a graphical interface (GUI) that can be used to customize settings according to the data sets and desired results. Febrl is organized in two main parts: pre-processing and the linkage itself. There is also a data exploration functionality that can be used to visualize the data and make sure it was loaded correctly (Christen et al., 2004; Christen, 2008).

Febrl supports several text-based data set formats: columnar text files, CSV, and SQL databases. Pre-processing comprises data cleaning and standardization through different standard functions for names, dates, and addresses. There is also an implementation of Hidden Markov Models (HMM) for name and address segmentation. For example, a single attribute name can be split into first name and second name. The HMMs can also be applied to addresses to extract multiple attributes (such as ZIP code, house number, city name, and state) from a single one. Febrl also has functions for date standardization, which are useful when two data sets have different date formats (Christen et al., 2004; Christen, 2008).

Pairwise comparison includes blocking methods and multiple functions to compare attributes. Febrl contains seven blocking implementations. They aim to reduce the amount of comparisons, and thus reducing the computational cost of the linkage. Febrl allows for each attribute to be compared using a different comparison function. Hence, it is possible to explore different strategies to find the one that better fits the set of attributes in the given data set; the tool has more than 20 different comparison functions. When comparing two records, each comparison function returns a score for attribute pair. On top of the score produced by each comparison function, it is necessary to use a definitive classifier, for weight vector classification, that generates a single score for the pair. The classification process can be supervised or unsupervised. After the classification step, it is also possible to customize the output of the system. This option allows the user to specify if the output will be one-to-one or one-to-many comparison (Christen, 2008). Similarly, comparative studies on data linkage tools in huge Brazilian databases showed slightly sub-optimal performance compared to RecLink and AtyImo (Pita et al., 2018). **Table 3** compares the five recording linkage tools using different attributes.

TABLE 3 | Comparative analysis of existing linkage tools.

Feature	RecLink	PLA	Atylmo	CIDACS-RL	FRIL	Febrl
Deterministic	Pure Comparison	Exact Comparison	Hybrid approach	Exact query	Equality function	Exact comparison functions
Probabilistic	Character Sequence and fuzzy	Automatic codes	Fully probabilistic	Semi-exact and fuzzy queries	Edit distance, soundex and Q-gram	Approximate comparison functions
Blocking	One step (single attribute) and multi-step predicates)	No	Predicates	TF-IDF indexing	Nested loop join and Sorted neighbourhood	Block, Ssorted and fuzzy (bigram)
Anonymization	No	No	Bloom Fliter	No	No	No
Manual review of Dubious records	No	PLA-MR	Second round with adjusted cut-offs	Yes	Yes	Yes
Automated review of dubious records	No	PLA-FAP	Machine learning-based	No	Yes (expectation maximization)	Expected
Open source, freely available	Yes(GPL)	No	Yes	No	Yes	Yes

CHALLENGES AND OPPORTUNITIES

Linked administrative data sets hold the potential to change the research landscape in the HTA arena, since linkage constitutes a valuable tool for combining individual-level information (biological, behavioral, socio-economical, clinical, and environmental) from different sources. This combined information can be used for population-based research applications with implications for public health, as well supporting public policy decision making.

Administrative data differ substantially from data generated by the academic community. Government data is collected in a logical format over time and refers to the totality of populations or specific groups; academic data is limited in scope, generally collected over a defined period for specific purposes. The use of linked administrative data for research, compared to those of primary data, often has several challenges and limitations. However, it can have several advantages: 1) large sample size, enabling statistical power for stratified analysis, making possible to explore epidemiological questions in different sub-populations; 2) it can help rebuild the prospective characteristic of the data, allowing for longitudinal studies at relatively lower cost with retrospective data; 3) it can also help answer questions that require detailed data on hard-to-reach populations, such as children; and 4) it can also help generate evidence with a high level of external validity and applicability for policy making as it captures the real-world setting. In the area of HTA, administrative data holds the potential to contribute to the development of high-quality and powerful research that furnishes scientific evidence for use by policy makers.

Brazil has made substantial effort to improve the quality of the data collected as part of service delivery. Although huge variation exists between regions and states, most data sets contain incomplete, inconsistent, inaccurate data that vary in content, format, and structure. This has substantial impact on data pre-processing requirements, quality of linked data, and internal validity of research findings from the data (Harron et al., 2017). Although considerable proportion of missing values in non-mandatory variables in a specific data set can be expected, for example education and occupation, key variables are more likely to be complete. In addition, similar variables are recorded in different data sets: a missing variable in one data set can be recorded in another data set; hence, in some circumstances, the linkage process can recover this missing variable.

Importantly, due to lack of unique key identifiers, all linkage tools used in Brazilian data including RecLink, AtyImo, and CIDACS-RL, rely on names, sex, date of birth, and municipality as linkage attributes (Camargo and Coeli, 2000; Pita et al., 2018). Brazilian names are often recorded in different ways, for example, an individual with five names might have only the first and last name recorded in one data set but all the five names recorded in the other data set (Harron et al., 2017; Paixao et al., 2018). In addition, there are misspellings, abbreviations, and punctuation marks with names and municipalities, and different date formats with date of birth which require a time-consuming data cleansing and sometimes sophisticated techniques for standardization. The level of data cleansing performed should take into account preserving the discriminative power of individual identifiers and the ability to distinguish one record from another (Harron et al., 2017). To minimize errors and improve comparison of record pairs, RecLink (Camargo and Coeli, 2000; Camargo and Coeli, 2006) and CIDAS-RL use string comparators and phonetic coding adapted to Brazilian names, whereas AtyImo uses a predicate of attributes in its blocking stage and Bloom filters (Pita et al., 2018).

The availability of huge volumes of data also provides opportunities to explore the effect of interventions or policies on frequent as well as rare health outcomes and in sub-populations including vulnerable groups (e.g., children, woman, ethnic minorities). At the same time, storage, processing, and analysis of such huge data has proved challenging for research institutions despite recent technological advances. The 100 Million Brazilian Cohort, an electronic database comprising individual records of approximately 114 million people (57% of the Brazilian population) is one example. The extensive coverage in the social registry: CadUnico, the availability of individually identified data, and the possibility to link to other health care data sets made it possible to design individual level longitudinal studies to evaluate the impact of BFP and other social protection programs on health and health-related outcomes.

CIDACS, the data center located in Salvador, needed to utilize sophisticated infrastructures for storage and processing of data, yet it took several days to link some data sets. Again, the lack of unique key identifiers in the databases to be linked required the use of techniques (for example, the use of predicates and Bloom filters in AtyImo or search engine indexing and scoring in CIDACS-RL) to reduce computation time at both blocking and comparison steps of the linkage process. Freely available linkage software, such as FRIL, Febril, or RecLink, crashed when attempting to run the linkage to build the 100 Million Brazilian Cohort, even on high-speed computers, prompting the need for developing efficient linkage tools: AtyImo and CIDACS-RL. Furthermore, the large size of the linked data may pose analytic challenges for standard statistical packages, such as SPSS and R, to run advanced statistical methods, for example propensity score matching.

Providing access to and usage of administrative data sets containing personal identifiable information for linkage purposes also presents a range of privacy challenges, mainly with regard to ethical and legal issues in the effort to protect personal data. Processing, linkage, and analysis of data should be conducted in accordance with the principles and criteria designed to ensure individuals' privacy, data security, and the ethical use of data containing personal information. This could vary from country to country or from center to center. For example, CIDACS's big data platform utilizes: 1) a combination of physical and virtual environments including the separation of data curation, linkage and analysis, 2) a hierarchical data access policy ensuring that only a specified number of individuals possess the highest level of access to all data elements for treatment purposes, and 3) privacy-preserving linkage tool, for example, AtyImo uses hash functions to anonymize relevant fields before the record linkage stage (Pinto et al., 2017; Pita et al., 2018). The hash functions, in addition to anonymization, help to speed up the linkage process (Pita et al., 2018) despite complicating the process of assessing the similarity between identifiers on different records (Harron et al., 2017). On the other hand, CIDACS-RL uses safe heaven to protect privacy while processing and linking data sets.

In the center's access and analysis environment, researchers have exclusive permission to access anonymized linked data sets *via* the coded data variables relevant to their field of study, after obtaining approval from the institutional review board. Access to data sets can be in person at the data center or through a Virtual Private Network (VPN), in accordance with sound information security practices. These includes: 1) submission of detailed research project accompanied by favorable ethical opinion and filled forms for the data plan provided by CIDACS to support the linkage and extraction of variables contained in the available databases, which should be restricted to those necessary to answer the questions in the proposed study. Detailed descriptions of the processes to be applied and the analyses to be conducted on the data are also desirable to avoid methodological biases. 2) Signature of the "Terms of Responsibility" related to the access and use of data.

Administrative data are generally collected by government departments or agencies for specific purposes, which contain personal information that may be confidential and/or sensitive, such as data collected for the execution of social programs or health service delivery. The use of these data for secondary use in restricted research requires a case-by-case analysis taking into account the balance between risks and benefits to individuals and the predominant public interest. Linking of records between different data sources, administrative or non-governmental, requires individualized data for the application of record linkage techniques, in the absence of unique identifier in the different data sources. As a result, access, processing, and analysis of data containing personal information for the purpose of research and the generation of evidence for decision making in public health policy require legal basis, physical and virtual security arrangements, exclusive use for a purpose previously specified, appropriate credentials for access, and favorable ethical opinion of the proposed study (Harron et al., 2017).

In Brazil, the Law on Access to Information (LAI) provides guidelines for the organs and entities of the federal public administration to adjust their information management policies by promoting the necessary adjustments to the registration, processing and archiving of documents and information. However, LAI does not address the use of information collected or stored by government for use in research because it is more focused on public transparency. A general law for the protection and processing of personal data including data for research purposes, the Personal Data Protection Bill, processed by the Chamber of Deputies since 2012 was recently sanctioned presidential. The General law on the Protection of Personal Data (Law 13709/2018) determines the rights of citizens to their personal data and the criteria that public and private agents will have to obey in dealing with them. It requires the regulator to request privacy risk reports to make sure that personal data are being safely processed, stored, and accessed. Hence, the law might present challenges for governance and management of the entire life cycle of the data requiring investments in computer infrastructure and specialized personnel, and adherence to good information security practices, to maintain the privacy and confidentiality of personal data. The law, which will come into force in February 2020, is the first Brazilian law on the subject and will establish specific norms for the treatment of personal information for public health research.

CONCLUSION

Brazil has high quality of health care records, growing number of linkage centers, and an open, modern attitude toward use of data for research and policy including HTA, supported by a rigorous but enabling legal framework. Despite the technical, infrastructural, and legal challenges with the use of huge secondary data for research, data linkage creates a unique opportunity to conduct large-scale observational studies to generate evidence on the impact of health technologies and health/social policies.

AUTHOR CONTRIBUTIONS

LS, MSA, and MLB contributed to the conception and design of the study. MSA wrote the first draft of the manuscript with substantial contributions by other authors on the different sections of the manuscript. All authors have read and revised the manuscript critically for important intellectual content, and approved the final version of the manuscript.

FUNDING

This work is part of the The 100 Million Brazilian Cohort project funded by the Wellcome Trust, Grant code: 202912/B/16/Z.

REFERENCES

Alves, C. M. M., Guerra, M. R., and Bastos, R. R. (2009). Tendência de mortalidade por câncer de colo de útero para o estado de minas gerais, brasil, 1980-2005. *Cad. Saude Publica* 25, 1693–1700. doi: 10.1590/S0102-311X2009000800005

Anderson, B. O., Cazap, E., El Saghir, N. S., Yip, C.-H., Khaled, H. M., Otero, I. V., et al. (2011). Optimisation of breast cancer management in low-resource and middle-resource countries: executive summary of the breast health global initiative consensus, 2010. *Lancet Oncol.* 12, 387–398. doi: 10.1016/S1470-2045(11)70031-6

Annemans, L. (2017). The use of real world data throughout an innovative medicine's lifecycle.

Assis Moura, A. D., Leite Braga, A. V., Borges Carneiro, A. K., da Silva Alves, E. C., Marques Bastos, C. M., Nunes, I. H., et al. (2018). Rapid monitoring of vaccination to prevent measles in Ceara State, Brazil, 2015. *Epidemiol. Serv. Saude* 27, e2016380. doi: 10.5123/S1679-49742018000200017

Azevedo, Â. J. P. d., Araújo, A. A. d., and Ferreira, M. Â. F. (2016). Consumo de ansiolíticos benzodiazepínicos: uma correlação entre dados do sngpc e indicadores sociodemográficos nas capitais brasileiras. *Cien. Saude Colet.* 21, 83–90. doi: 10.1590/1413-81232015211.15532014

Banta, D. (2009). What is technology assessment? *Int. J. Technol. Assess. Health Care* 25, 7–9. doi: 10.1017/S0266462309090333

Batarrita, J. A. (1999). International network of agencies for health technology assessment (inahta) or the need for collaboration in the evaluation of health technologies. *Med. Clin.* 112, 86–89.

Bértola, L., and Williamson, J. (2017). *Has Latin American Inequality Changed Direction?: Looking Over the Long Run.* (AG, Switzerland: Springer Nature). doi: 10.1007/978-3-319-44621-9

Białecki, A., Muir, R., and Ingersoll, G. (2012). "Apache lucene 4," in *SIGIR 2012 workshop on open source information retrieval*, vol. 17. Portland, OR USA.

Boratto, M., Alonso, P., Pinto, C., Melo, P., Barreto, M., and Denaxas, S. (2018). Exploring hybrid parallel systems for probabilistic record linkage. *J. Supercomput.* 75, 1137–1149. doi: 10.1007/s11227-018-2328-3

Bortoletto, M. É., and Bochner, R. (1999). Drug impact on human poisoning in Brazil. *Cad. Saude Publica* 15, 859–869. doi: 10.1590/S0102-311X1999000400020

Braga, S. F. M., de Souza, M. C., and Cherchiglia, M. L. (2017). Time trends for prostate cancer mortality in Brazil and its geographic regions: an age–period–cohort analysis. *Cancer Epidemiol.* 50, 53–59. doi: 10.1016/j.canep.2017.07.016

Branco, N. M. C., Lopes, R. G., Silva, M. F., and Romão, C. M. C. A. P. (2015). Notivisa e os laboratórios de saúde pública: a interface da informação em vigilância sanitária. *Vigil. Sanit. Debate: Sociedade, Ciência & Tecnologia* 3, 130–134. doi: 10.3395/2317-269x.00242

Brito, C., Portela, M. C., and Vasconcellos, M. T. L. d. (2005). Public care for breast cancer women in the state of Rio de Janeiro, Brazil. *Rev. Saúde Pública* 39, 874–881. doi: 10.1590/S0034-89102005000600002

Camargo, K. R. d., and Coeli, C. M. (2000). Reclink: aplicativo para o relacionamento de bases de dados, implementando o método probabilistic record linkage. *Cad. Saude Publica* 16, 439–447. doi: 10.1590/S0102-311X2000000200014

Camargo, K. R. d. Jr., and Coeli, C. M. (2006). Reclink 3: nova versão do programa que implementa a técnica de associação probabilística de registros (probabilistic record linkage). *Cad. Saúde Colet. (Rio J.)* 14, 399 404. doi: 10.1590/S0102-311X2000000200014

Capuani, L., Bierrenbach, A. L., Abreu, F., Takecian, P. L., Ferreira, J. E., and Sabino, E. C. (2014). Accuracy of a probabilistic record-linkage methodology used to track blood donors in the mortality information system database. *Cad. Saude Publica* 30, 1623–1632. doi: 10.1590/0102-311X00024914

Cecilio, A. P., Takakura, E. T., Jumes, J. J., dos Santos, J. W., Herrera, A. C., Victorino, V. J., et al. (2015). Breast cancer in Brazil: epidemiology and treatment challenges. *Breast Cancer* 7, 43. doi: 10.2147/BCTT.S50361

Chioda, L., De Mello, J. M., and Soares, R. R. (2016). Spillovers from conditional cash transfer programs: Bolsa família and crime in urban Brazil. *Econ. Educ. Rev.* 54, 306–320. doi: 10.1016/j.econedurev.2015.04.005

Christen, P. (2008). "Febrl-: an open source data cleaning, deduplication and record linkage system with a graphical user interface," in *Proceedings of the 14th ACM SIGKDD international conference on Knowledge discovery and data mining* (Las Vegas, Nevada, USA: ACM), 1065–1068. doi: 10.1145/1401890.1402020

Christen, P. (2012). A survey of indexing techniques for scalable record linkage and deduplication. *IEEE Trans. Knowl. Data Eng.* 24, 1537–1555. doi: 10.1109/TKDE.2011.127

Christen, P., Churches, T., Hegland, M., and Springer. (2004). "Febrl–a parallel open source data linkage system," in *Pacific-Asia Conference on Knowledge Discovery and Data Mining* vol. 3056. Lecture Notes in Computer Science. (Berlin, Heidelberg: Springer).

Coelho, G. E., Leal, P. L., de Paula Cerroni, M., Simplicio, A. C. R., and Siqueira, J. B., Jr. (2016). Sensitivity of the dengue surveillance system in Brazil for detecting hospitalized cases. *PLoS Negl. Trop. Dis.* 10, e0004705. doi: 10.1371/journal.pntd.0004705

Coelho Filho, J. M., Marcopito, L. F., and Castelo, A. (2004). Perfil de utilização de medicamentos por idosos em área urbana do nordeste do brasil. *Rev. Saúde Pública* 38, 557–564. doi: 10.1590/S0034-89102004000400012

Coeli, C. M., and Camargo., K. R. d. (2002). Evaluation of different blocking strategies in probabilistic record linkage. *Rev. Bras. Epidemiol.* 5, 185–196. doi: 10.1590/S1415-790X2002000200006

da Nóbrega, A. A., da Silva Teixeira, A. M., and Lanzieri, T. M. (2010). Avaliação do sistema de informação do programa de imunizações (si-api).

da Saúde, M. (2011). Manual de instruções para o preenchimento da declaração de nascido vivo.

da Saúde, M. (2004). Portaria gm/ms n.2031, de 23 de setembro de 2004. dispõe sobre a organização do sistema nacional de laboratórios de saúde pública.

Da Silva, A., and Laprega, M. (2005). Critical evaluation of the primary care information system (siab) and its implementation in ribeirão preto, São Paulo, Brazil. *Cad. Saude Publica* 21, 1821. doi: 10.1590/S0102-311X2005000600031

de Camargo, K. R., and Coeli, C. M. (2015). Going open source: some lessons learned from the development of openreclink rumo ao software aberto: algumas lições aprendidas com o desenvolvimento do openreclink. *Cad. Saude Publica* 31, 257–263. doi: 10.1590/0102-311X00041214

de Mello Jorge, M. H. P., Laurenti, R., and Gotlieb, S. L. D. (2010). Avaliação dos sistemas de informção em saúde no brasil. *Cad. Saúde Colet.* 18, 07–18.

de Paula, A. A., Pires, D. F., Alves Filho, P., de Lemos, K. R. V., Barçante, E., and Pacheco, A. G. (2018). A comparison of accuracy and computational feasibility of two record linkage algorithms in retrieving vital status information from HIV/AIDS patients registered in Brazilian public databases. *Int. J. Med. Inform.* 114, 45–51. doi: 10.1016/j.ijmedinf.2018.03.005

de Vigilância Sanitária, A. N. (2008). Diretrizes para o gerenciamento do risco em farmacovigilância.

de Vigilância Sanitária, A. N. (2010). Sistema nacional de gerenciamento de produtos controlados – sngpc.

do Nascimento, R. L., Castilla, E. E., Dutra, M. d. G., and Orioli, I. M. (2018). Icd-10 impact on ascertainment and accuracy of oral cleft cases as recorded by the Brazilian national live birth information system. *Am. J. Med. Genet. A* 176, 907–914. doi: 10.1002/ajmg.a.38634

Domingues, C. M. A. S., and Teixeira, A. M. d. S. (2013). Vaccination coverage and impact on vaccine-preventable diseases in Brazil between 1982 and 2012: National immunization program progress and challenges. *Epidemiol. Serv. Saúde* 22, 9–27. doi: 10.5123/S1679-49742013000100002

dos Santos Filho, W. (2008). Algoritmo paralelo e eficiente para o problema de pareamento de dados.

dos Santos Fraga, W. (2009). *Caracterização Das Redes De Infratores Extraídas De Ocorrências Policiais E Identificação De Pessoas-Chave.* Master's thesis, Federal University of Minas Gerais, http://www.bibliotecadigital.ufmg.br/dspace/handle/1843/SLSS-7XGF9B.

Dusetzina, S. B., Tyree, S., Meyer, A.-M., Meyer, A., Green, L., and Carpenter, W. R. (2014). An overview of record linkage methods.

Elfeky, M. G., Verykios, V. S., and Elmagarmid, A. K. (2002). "Tailor: a record linkage toolbox," in *Proceedings 18th International Conference on Data Engineering* (Washington, DC, USA: IEEE Computer Society), 17–28. doi: 10.1109/ICDE.2002.994694

Fellegi, I. P., and Sunter, A. B. (1969). A theory for record linkage. *J. Am. Stat. Assoc.* 64, 1183–1210. doi: 10.1080/01621459.1969.10501049

Ferreira, N. A. S., de Carvalho, S. M. F., Valenti, V. E., Bezerra, I. M. P., Batista, H. M. T., de Abreu, L. C., et al. (2017). Treatment delays among women with breast cancer in a low socio-economic status region in Brazil. *BMC Womens Health* 17, 13. doi: 10.1186/s12905-016-0359-6

Fonseca, M. G. P., Coeli, C. M., Lucena, F. d. F. d. A., Veloso, V. G., and Carvalho, M. S. (2010). Accuracy of a probabilistic record linkage strategy applied to identify deaths among cases reported to the Brazilian aids surveillance database. *Cad. Saude Publica* 26, 1431–1438. doi: 10.1590/S0102-311X2010000700022

Freire, S. M., Souza, R. C. d., and Almeida, R. T. d. (2015). Integrating Brazilian health information systems in order to support the building of data warehouses. *Res. Biomed. Eng.* 31, 196–207. doi: 10.1590/2446-4740.0666

Frias, P. G. d., Cavalcanti, M. d. R. B. A., Mullachery, P. H., Damacena, G. N., and Szwarcwald, C. L. (2012). An evaluation of the registration of deaths of infants aged less than one year in the basic care information system (siab). *Rev. Bras. Saúde Mater. Infant.* 12, 15–25. doi: 10.1590/S1519-38292012000100002

Frias, P. G. d., Szwarcwald, C. L., and Lira, P. I. C. d. (2014). Evaluation of information systems on live births and mortality in Brazil in the 2000s. *Cad. Saude Publica* 30, 2068–2280. doi: 10.1590/0102-311X00196113

Girianelli, V., Gamarra, C., and Azevedo e Silva, G. (2014). Os grandes contrastes na mortalidade por câncer do colo uterino e de mama no brasil. *Rev. Saude Publica* 48, 459–467. doi: 10.1590/S0034-8910.2014048005214

Grinsztejn, B., Luz, P. M., Pacheco, A. G., Santos, D. V., Velasque, L., Moreira, R. I., et al. (2013). Changing mortality profile among HIV-infected patients in Rio de Janeiro, Brazil: shifting from aids to non-aids related conditions in the haart era. *PLoS One* 8, e59768. doi: 10.1371/journal.pone.0059768

Guerra, A. A., Jr., Pereira, R. G., Gurgel, E. I., Cherchiglia, M., Dias, L. V., Ávila, J., et al. (2018). Building the national database of health centred on the individual: administrative and epidemiological record linkage-Brazil, 2000-2015. *Int. J. Pop. Data Sci.* 3 (1), 446. doi: 10.23889/ijpds.v3i1.446

Guimarães, R. (2014). Technological incorporation in the unified health system (sus): the problem and ensuing challenges. *Cien. Saude Colet.* 19, 4899–4908. doi: 10.1590/1413-812320141912.04642014

Harron, K., Dibben, C., Boyd, J., Hjern, A., Azimaee, M., Barreto, M. L., et al. (2017). Challenges in administrative data linkage for research. *Big Data Soc.* 4, 2053951717745678. doi: 10.1177/2053951717745678

Hunter, W., and Sugiyama, N. B. (2018). Making the newest citizens: achieving universal birth registration in contemporary Brazil. *J. Dev. Stud.* 54, 397–412. doi: 10.1080/00220388.2017.1316378

Inan, A., Kantarcioglu, M., Bertino, E., and Scannapieco, M. (2008). "A hybrid approach to private record linkage," in *Data Engineering, 2008. ICDE 2008. IEEE 24th International Conference on* (Washington, DC, USA: IEEE Computer Society), 496–505. doi: 10.1109/ICDE.2008.4497458

Inocencio, M., and De Vivo, B. (2011). Acesso a medicamentos: análise das estratégias do estado para o desenvolvimento do programa farmácia popular. *Cad. Gest. Publica Cid.* 16, 201–221. doi: 10.12660/cgpc.v16n59.3700

Jesus, R. d., Guimarães, R. P., Bergamo, R., Santos, L. C. F. d., Matta, A. S. D. d., Júnior, P., et al. (2013). Laboratory environment management system: account of an experience with a transformational tool for laboratory management and health surveillance. *Epidemiol. Serv. Saúde* 22, 525–529. doi: 10.5123/S1679-49742013000300018

Junger, W. L. (2006). Estimação de parâmetros em relacionamento probabilístico de bancos de dados: uma aplicação do algoritmo em para o reclink. *Cad. Saúde Colet. (Rio J.)* 14, 225–232.

Júnior, P., Matta, A. S. D. d., Jesus, R. d., Guimarães, R. P., Souza, L. R. d. O., Brant, J. L., et al. (2017). Laboratory environment management system-gal: assessment of a tool for sentinel surveillance of influenza-like illness, Brazil, 2011-2012. *Epidemiol. Serv. Saúde* 26, 339–348. doi: 10.5123/S1679-49742017000200011

Jurczyk, P., Lu, J. J., Xiong, L., Cragan, J. D., and Correa, A. (2008a). Fine-grained record integration and linkage tool. *Birth Defects Res. Part A Clin. Mol. Teratol.* 82, 822–829. doi: 10.1002/bdra.20521

Jurczyk, P., Lu, J. J., Xiong, L., Cragan, J. D., and Correa, A. (2008b). "Fril: a tool for comparative record linkage," in *AMIA annual symposium proceedings*, vol. 2008. (Bethesda, Md: American Medical Informatics Association), 1, 440.

Kristensen, F. B., Mäkelä, M., Neikter, S. A., Rehnqvist, N., Håheim, L. L., Mørland, B., et al. (2009). European network for health technology assessment, eunethta: planning, development, and implementation of a sustainable european network for health technology assessment. *Int. J. Technol. Assess. Health Care* 25, 107–116. doi: 10.1017/S0266462309990754

Kropiwiec, M. V., Franco, S. C., and Amaral, A. R. d. (2017). Factors associated with infant mortality in a Brazilian city with high human development index. *Rev. Paul. Pediatr.* 35, 391–398. doi: 10.1590/1984-0462/;2017;35;4;00006

Laguardia, J., Domingues, C. M. A., Carvalho, C., Lauerman, C. R., Macário, E., and Glatt, R. (2004). Information system for notifiable diseases (sinan): challenges in developing a national health information system. *Epidemiol. Serv. Saúde* 13, 135–146.

Lima-Costa, M. F., and Matos, D. L. (2007). Prevalence and factors associated with mammograms in the 50-69-year age group: a study based on the Brazilian national household sample survey (pnad-2003). *Cad. Saude Publica* 23, 1665–1673. doi: 10.1590/S0102-311X2007000700018

Lindert, K., Linder, A., Hobbs, J., and De la Brière, B. (2007). *The nuts and bolts of Brazil's Bolsa Família Program: implementing conditional cash transfers in a decentralized context.* Tech. rep., Social Protection Discussion Paper.

Machado, D. B., Rodrigues, L. C., Rasella, D., Barreto, M. L., and Araya, R. (2018). Conditional cash transfer programme: Impact on homicide rates and hospitalisations from violence in Brazil. *PLoS One* 13, e0208925. doi: 10.1371/journal.pone.0208925

Machado, J. P., Martins, M., and Leite, I. d. C. (2016a). Quality of hospital databases in Brazil: some elements. *Rev. Bras. Epidemiol.* 19, 567–581. doi: 10.1590/1980-5497201600030008

Machado, M. A. d. Á., Moura, C. S. d., Ferré, F., Bernatsky, S., Rahme, E., and Acurcio, F. d. A. (2016b). Treatment persistence in patients with rheumatoid arthritis and ankylosing spondylitis. *Rev. Saúde Pública* 50, 50. doi: 10.1590/S1518-8787.2016050006265

Maia, C. S., Freitas, D. R. C. d., Gallo, L. G., and Araújo, W. N. d. (2018). Registry of adverse events related to health care that results in deaths in Brazil, 2014-2016. *Epidemiol. Serv. Saúde* 27, e2017320. doi: 10.5123/S1679-49742018000200004

Mallmann, M. B., Boing, A. F., Tomasi, Y. T., Anjos, J. C. d., and Boing, A. C. (2018). Evolution of socioeconomic inequalities in conducting prenatal consultations among Brazilian parturient women: analysis of the period 2000-2015. *Epidemiol. Serv. Saúde* 27, e2018022. doi: 10.5123/S1679-49742018000400014

Martins, A. C., Giordani, F., Guaraldo, L., Tognoni, G., and Rozenfeld, S. (2018). Adverse drug events identified in hospitalized patients in Brazil by international classification of diseases (icd-10) code listings. *Cad. Saude Publica* 34, e00222417. doi: 10.1590/0102-311x00222417

Martins, E. L. M., Amaral, M. d. P. H. d., Ferreira, M. B. C., Mendonça, A. É. d., Pereira, M. C. S., Pereira, D. C., et al. (2012). Prescriptions for anorectic psychotropic drugs in the municipality of juiz de fora, minas gerais, Brazil. *Cien. Saude Colet.* 17, 3331–3342. doi: 10.1590/S1413-81232012001200018

Medeiros, K. R. d., Machado, H. d. O. P., Albuquerque, P. C. d., and Gurgel, G. D., Jr. (2005). The health information system as a human resources policy tool: an important mechanism for the detection of labor force needs in the unified health system. *Cien. Saude Colet.* 10, 433–440. doi: 10.1590/S1413-81232005000200021

Melione, L. P. R., and Jorge, M. H. P. d. M. (2008). Data reliability of hospital admissions due to external causes in a public hospital in São José Dos Campos, São Paulo, Brazil. *Rev. Bras. Epidemiol.* 11, 379–392. doi: 10.1590/S1415-790X2008000300005

Migowski, A., Chaves, R. B. M., Coeli, C. M., Ribeiro, A. L. P., Tura, B. R., Kuschnir, M. C. C., et al. (2011). Acurácia do relacionamento probabilístico na avaliação da alta complexidade em cardiologia. *Rev. Saúde Pública* 45, 269–275. doi: 10.1590/S0034-89102011005000012

Ministro da Cidadania. (2017). Bolsa família e cadastro Único no seu município. Available at: http://mds.gov.br/assuntos/bolsa-familia/ (Accessed March 12, 2017).

Mostafa, J., and Silva, K. d. (2007). *Brazil's single registry experience: A tool for pro-poor social policies.* Ministry of Social Development and Fight Against Hunger. Available at: http://www.cashdividend.net/wp-content/uploads/2013/06/Brazils-Single-Registry.pdf

Mota, D. M., Oliveira, M. G. d., Bovi, R. F., Silva, S. F., Cunha, J. A. F., and Divino, J. A. (2014). Are there irrationalities in the consumption of anti-obesity drugsin Brazil? a pharmaco-econometric analysis of panel datasets. *Cien. Saude Colet.* 19, 1389–1400. doi: 10.1590/1413-81232014195.17242013

Moura, B. L. A., Alencar, G. P., Silva, Z. P. d., and Almeida, M. F. d. (2018). Hospitalizations due to complications of pregnancy and maternal and perinatal outcomes in a cohort of pregnant women in the Brazilian unified national health system in São Paulo, Brazil. *Cad. Saude Publica* 34, e00188016. doi: 10.1590/0102-311x00188016

Nery, J. S., Pereira, S. M., Rasella, D., Penna, M. L. F., Aquino, R., Rodrigues, L. C., et al. (2014). Effect of the Brazilian conditional cash transfer and primary health care programs on the new case detection rate of leprosy. *PLoS Negl. Trop. Dis.* 8, e3357. doi: 10.1371/journal.pntd.0003357

Newcombe, H. B., Kennedy, J. M., Axford, S., and James, A. P. (1959). Automatic linkage of vital records. *Science* 130, 954–959. doi: 10.1126/science.130.3381.954

Nunes, E. C., Rosa, R. d. S., and Bordin, R. (2016). Hospitalizations for cholecystitis and cholelithiasis in the state of Rio Grande do Sul, Brazil. *Arq. Bras. Cir. Dig. (São Paulo)* 29, 77–80. doi: 10.1590/0102-6720201600020003

Oliveira, C. G. d., and Rodas, A. C. D. (2017). Postmarketing surveillance in Brazil: vascular catheters–an overview of notifications of adverse events and technical complaints. *Cien. Saude Colet.* 22, 3247–3257. doi: 10.1590/1413-812320172210.17612017

Oliveira, G. P. d., Pinheiro, R. S., Coeli, C. M., Barreira, D., and Codenotti, S. B. (2012a). Mortality information system for identifying underreported cases of tuberculosis in Brazil. *Rev. Bras. Epidemiol.* 15, 468–477. doi: 10.1590/S1415-790X2012000300003

Oliveira, G. P. d., Pinheiro, R. S., Coeli, C. M., Barreira, D., and Codenotti, S. B. (2012b). Uso do sistema de informação sobre mortalidade para identificar subnotificação de casos de tuberculose no brasil. *Rev. Bras. Epidemiol.* 15, 468–477. doi: 10.1590/S1415-790X2012000300003

Oliveira, M. M. d., Andrade, S. S. C. d. A., Dimech, G. S., Oliveira, J. C. G. d., Malta, D. C., Neto, R., et al. (2015). Avaliação do sistema de informações sobre nascidos vivos. brasil, 2006 a 2010. *Epidemiol. Serv. Saúde*, 24, 629–640. doi: 10.5123/S1679-49742015000400005

Pacheco, A. G., Durovni, B., Cavalcante, S. C., Lauria, L., Moore, R. D., Moulton, L. H., et al. (2008a). Aids-related tuberculosis in Rio de Janeiro, Brazil. *PLoS One* 3, e3132. doi: 10.1371/journal.pone.0003132

Pacheco, A. G., Saraceni, V., Tuboi, S. H., Lauria, L. M., Moulton, L. H., Faulhaber, J. C., et al. (2011). Estimating the extent of underreporting of mortality among HIV-infected individuals in Rio de Janeiro, Brazil. *AIDS Res. Hum. Retroviruses* 27, 25–28. doi: 10.1089/aid.2010.0089

Pacheco, A. G., Saraceni, V., Tuboi, S. H., Moulton, L. H., Chaisson, R. E., Cavalcante, S. C., et al. (2008b). Validation of a hierarchical deterministic record-linkage algorithm using data from 2 different cohorts of human immunodeficiency virus-infected persons and mortality databases in Brazil. *Am. J. Epidemiol.* 168, 1326–1332. doi: 10.1093/aje/kwn249

Pacheco, A. G., Tuboi, S. H., May, S. B., Moreira, L. F., Ramadas, L., Nunes, E. P., et al. (2009). Temporal changes in causes of death among HIV-infected patients in the haart era in Rio de Janeiro, Brazil. *J. Acquir. Immune Defic. Syndr.* 51, 624. doi: 10.1097/QAI.0b013e3181a4ecf5

Paes-Sousa, R., Santos, L. M. P., and Miazaki, É. S. (2011). Effects of a conditional cash transfer programme on child nutrition in Brazil. *Bull. World Health Organ.* 89, 496–503. doi: 10.2471/BLT.10.084202

Paim, J., Travassos, C., Almeida, C., Bahia, L., and Macinko, J. (2011). The Brazilian health system: history, advances, and challenges. *Lancet* 377, 1778–1797. doi: 10.1016/S0140-6736(11)60054-8

Paiva, L. H., Falcão, T., and Bartholo, L. (2013). Do bolsa-família ao brasil sem miséria in *Programa Bolsa Família: uma década de inclusão e cidadania*. Eds. T. Campello and M. C., Neri (IPEA: Brasília), 25–46.

Paixao, E. S., Harron, K., Campbell, O., Teixeira, M. G., Maria da Conceição, N. C., Barreto, M. L., et al. (2018). Dengue in pregnancy and maternal mortality: a cohort analysis using routine data. *Sci. Rep.* 8, 9938. doi: 10.1038/s41598-018-28387-w

Passman, L. J., Farias, A. M. R. O., Tomazelli, J. G., de Abreu, D. M. F., Dias, M. B. K., de Assis, M., et al. (2011). Sismama—implementation of an information system for breast cancer early detection programs in Brazil. *Breast* 20, S35–S39. doi: 10.1016/j.breast.2011.02.001

Pedraza, D. F. (2012). Qualidade do sistema de informações sobre nascidos vivos (sinasc): análise crítica da literatura. *Cien. Saude Colet.* 17, 2729–2737. doi: 10.1590/S1413-81232012001000021

Peek, N., Holmes, J., and Sun, J. (2014). Technical challenges for big data in biomedicine and health: data sources, infrastructure, and analytics. *Yearb. Med. Inform.* 9, 42. doi: 10.15265/IY-2014-0018

Peres, S. V., Latorre, M. d. R. D. d., Tanaka, L. F., Michels, F. A. S., Teixeira, M. L. P., Coeli, C. M., et al. (2016). Quality and completeness improvement of the population-based cancer registry of são paulo: linkage technique use. *Rev. Bras. Epidemiol.* 19, 753–765. doi: 10.1590/1980-5497201600040006

Pinto, C., Dantas, R., Sena, S., Reis, S., Fiaccone, R., Amorim, L., et al. (2017). Accuracy of probabilistic linkage: The Brazilian 100 million cohort. *Proc. Int. Conf. Biomed. Health Informat.* Available at: http://discovery.ucl.ac.uk/1542411/3/Denaxas_Barreto_BHI2017Final.pdf

Pita, R., Mendonça, E., Reis, S., Barreto, M., and Denaxas, S. (2017). "A machine learning trainable model to assess the accuracy of probabilistic record linkage," in *International Conference on Big Data Analytics and Knowledge Discovery* (Regensburg, Germany: Springer, Cham), 214–227. doi: 10.1007/978-3-319-64283-3_16

Pita, R., Pinto, C., Sena, S., Fiaccone, R., Amorim, L., Reis, S., et al. (2018). On the accuracy and scalability of probabilistic data linkage over the Brazilian 114 million cohort. *IEEE J. Biomed. Health Inform*, 346–353. doi: 10.1109/JBHI.2018.2796941

Prado da Fonseca, E., Cristina do Amaral, R., Carlos Pereira, A., Martins Rocha, C., and Tennant, M. (2018). Geographical variation in oral and oropharynx cancer mortality in Brazil: a Bayesian approach. *Int. J. Environ. Res. Public Health* 15, 2641. doi: 10.3390/ijerph15122641

Quarti Machado Rosa, M., dos Santos Rosa, R., Correia, M. G., Araujo, D. V., Bahia, L. R., and Toscano, C. M. (2018). Disease and economic burden of hospitalizations attributable to diabetes mellitus and its complications: a nationwide study in Brazil. *Int. J. Environ. Res. Public Health* 15, 294. doi: 10.3390/ijerph15020294

Rasella, D., Aquino, R., Santos, C. A., Paes-Sousa, R., and Barreto, M. L. (2013). Effect of a conditional cash transfer programme on childhood mortality: a nationwide analysis of Brazilian municipalities. *Lancet* 382, 57–64. doi: 10.1016/S0140-6736(13)60715-1

Rodrigues, M. P. C. (2017). Compliance with labor standards: measuring the effectiveness of policies against child labor and modern slavery in Brazil.

Santos, I. S., Menezes, A., Mota, D. M., Albernaz, E. P., Barros, A. J., Matijasevich, A., et al. (2008). Infant mortality in three population-based cohorts in southern Brazil: trends and differentials. *Cad. Saude Publica* 24, s451–s460. doi: 10.1590/S0102-311X2008001500011

Santos, W., Teixeira, T., Machado, C., Meira, W., Jr., Ferreira, R., Guedes, D. et al. (2007). "A scalable parallel deduplication algorithm," in *Computer Architecture and High Performance Computing, 2007. SBAC-PAD 2007. 19th International Symposium on* (Gramado, RS, Brazil: IEEE), 79–86. doi: 10.1109/SBAC-PAD.2007.32

Saraceni, V., Benzaken, A. S., Pereira, G. F. M., Andrade, K. B., Oliveira, P. B., Arakaki-Sanchez, D., et al. (2018). Tuberculosis burden on aids in Brazil: a study using linked databases. *PLoS One* 13, e0207859. doi: 10.1371/journal.pone.0207859

Saraceni, V., Cohn, S., Cavalcante, S. C., Pacheco, A. G., Moulton, L. H., Chaisson, R. E., et al. (2014). Prevalent tuberculosis (tb) at HIV diagnosis in Rio de Janeiro, Brazil: the TB/HIV in Rio (thrio) cohort. *J. Acquir. Immune Defic. Syndr.* 67, 98. doi: 10.1097/QAI.0000000000000247

Sato, A. P. S. (2015). National immunization program: computerized system as a tool for new challenges. *Rev. Saúde Pública* 49, 39. doi: 10.1590/S0034-8910.2015049005925

Sayers, A., Ben-Shlomo, Y., Blom, A. W., and Steele, F. (2015). Probabilistic record linkage. *Int. J. Epidemiol.* 45, 954–964. doi: 10.1093/ije/dyv322

Schechter, M., Zajdenverg, R., Machado, L. L., Pinto, M. E., Lima, L., and Perez, M. A. (1994). Predicting cd4 counts in HIV-infected Brazilian individuals: a model based on the world health organization staging system. *J. Acquir. Immune Defic. Syndr.* 7, 163–168.

Schnell, R., Bachteler, T., and Reiher, J. (2009). Privacy-preserving record linkage using bloom filters. *BMC Med. Inform. Decis. Mak.* 9, 41. doi: 10.1186/1472-6947-9-41

Soares, F. V., Soares, S. S. D., Medeiros, M., Osório, R. G., et al. (2006). *Cash transfer programmes in Brazil: impacts on inequality and poverty.* Working Papers 21, International Policy Centre for Inclusive Growth.

Souza, A. M. d. F. M., de Oliveira, S. B., and Daher, E. P. (2016). Mapping the hospital billing process: The case of the a federal hospital in Rio de Janeiro. *Procedia Comput. Sci.* 100, 671–676. doi: 10.1016/j.procs.2016.09.210

Tanaka, L. F., Latorre, M. d. R. D., Gutierrez, E. B., Heumann, C., Herbinger, K.-H., and Froeschl, G. (2017). Trends in the incidence of aids-defining and non-aids-defining cancers in people living with aids: a population-based study from Sao Paulo, Brazil. *Int. J. STD AIDS* 28, 1190–1198. doi: 10.1177/0956462417692924

Tomazelli, J. G., Girianelli, V. R., and Silva, G. A. (2018a). Estratégias usadas no relacionamento entre sistemas de informações em saúde para seguimento das mulheres com mamografias suspeitas no sistema único de saúde. *Rev. Bras. Epidemiol.* 21, e180015. doi: 10.1590/1980-549720180015

Tomazelli, J. G., Girianelli, V. R., and Silva, G. A. (2018b). Women screened for breast cancer: follow-up through health information systems, Brazil, 2010-2012. *Epidemiol. Serv. Saúde*, 27, e2017445. doi: 10.5123/S1679-49742018000300005

Verzinhasse Peres, S., Dias de Oliveira Latorre, M. d. R., Silva Michels, F. A., Fiengo Tanaka, L., Medina Coeli, C., and Furquim de Almeida, M. (2014). Determinação de um ponto de corte para a identificação de pares verdadeiros pelo método probabilístico de linkage de base de dados. *Cad. Saúde Colet.* 22, 428–436. doi: 10.1590/1414-462X201400040017

Victora, C. G., and Barros, F. C. (2001). Infant mortality due to perinatal causes in Brazil: trends, regional patterns and possible interventions. *Sao Paulo Med. J.* 119, 33–42. doi: 10.1590/S1516-31802001000100009

Winkler, W. E. (2006). Overview of record linkage and current research directions. In *Bureau of the Census* (Citeseer). doi: 10.1002/9780470057339.var022.

ABBREVIATIONS

ACR	American College of Radiology
ACS	Agentes comunitários de saúde ("The community health agents")
Anvisa	Agência Nacional de Vigilância Sanitária ("National Agency for Health Surveillance")
APAC-ONCO	Autorizações de Procedimentos de Alta Complexidade Oncológica ("The High Complexity Oncology Procedures Authorizations for Oncology")
APGAR	Appearance, Pulse, Grimace, Activity, and Respiration
ATFP	Aqui Tem Farmácia Popular (accredited private retail pharmacies)
AUC	Area under (receiver operating characteristic) curve
BFP	Bolsa Familia Program ("the Conditional Cash Transfer Program")
BPAI	Boletim de Produção Ambulatorial Individualizado ("Individual Outpatient Production Periodicals")
BPA	Boletim de Produção Ambulatorial ("The Ambulatory Production bulletin")
BI-RADS	Breast Imaging Reporting and Data System
CadUnico	Cadastro Unico
CGLAB	Coordenação Geral de Laboratórios de Saúde Pública ("The General Coordination of Public Health Laboratories")
CIs	Confidence intervals
CIDACS	Centro de Integração de Dados e Conhecimentos para Saúde ("the Centre for Data and Knowledge Integration for Health")
CIDACS-RL	CIDACS record linkage
CNS	Cartão Nacional de Saúde ("National Health Card")
CONITEC-SUS	Comissão Nacional de Incorporação de Tecnologias no Sistema Único de Saúde ("The National Committee for Health Technology Incorporation into SUS")
COSAC/SACS	Coordenação de Saúde da Communidade/ Secretaria de Assistência à Saúde ("co-ordination of community health/health care Secretariat")
CPF	Cadastro de Pessoas Físicas ("Individual Taxpayer Registry number")
DATASUS	Departamento de Informática do Sistema, Único de Saúde ("Department for Health Information")
DO	a declaração de, óbito (" The Declaration of Death")
DGITS	Departamento de Gestão e Incorporação de Tecnologias em Saúde ("The Department of Management and Incorporation of Health Technologies")
DNV	Declaração de Nascido Vivo ("the declaration of live birth")
DSA	Data set A
DSB	Data set B
DSAXB	Data set A and B linked

DST	Departamento de Ciência e Tecnologia - Decit ("The Department of Science and Technology ")
EM	Expectation Maximization
Febrl	Freely extensible biomedical record linkage
FII	Ficha Individual de Investigação ("Individual Investigation Form ")
FIN	Ficha Individual de Notificação ("Individual Notification Form")
FIOCRUZ	Fundação Oswaldo Cruz ("The Oswaldo Cruz Foundation")
FRIL	Fine-grained Records Integration and linkage Tool
GAL	Gerenciador de Ambiente Laboratorial ("the Laboratory Environment Management System"
GPUs	Graphics Processing Units
GUI	Graphical User Interface
HMMs	Hidden Markov Models; IBGE, Instituto Brasileiro de Geografia e Estatística ("Brazilian Institute of Geography and Statistics") Instituto Nacional de Câncer
ICD	International Classification of Diseases
LAI	The Law on Access to Information
MCMV	Minha Casa Minha Vida (the Housing Program)
MoH	Ministry of Health; NOTIVISA, Sistema de Notificações em Vigilância Sanitária ("The National Notification System for Health Surveillance")
PAHO/WHO	Pan American Health Organization/World Health Organization (PAHO/WHO)
PFPB	Programa Farmácia Popular do Brasil ("The Brazilian Popular Pharmacy Program")
PLA	Python linkage algorithm
PLA-FAP	Python linkage algorithm—fully automated procedure
PLA-MR	Python linkage algorithm—manual review
PLWHA	People living with HIV/AIDS
PNI	do Programa Nacional de Imunização ("The National Immunization Program")
PPV	Positive predictive value
RAM	Random-access memory
RCBP	Registros de Câncer de Base Populacional ("The Population-Based Cancer Registry")
REBRATS	Rede Brasileira de Avaliação de Tecnologias em Saúde ("the Brazilian Network for HTA")
RENACIAT	Rede Nacional de Centros de Informação e Atenção Toxicológical ("the National Network of Information Centers and Toxicological Attention")
RHC	de Registro Hospitalar de Câncer ("The Hospital Cancer Registry")
ROC	Receiver operating characteristic
SIAB	Sistema de Informação da Atenção Básica ("The Basic Health Care Information System")
SI-AIU	Sistema de Informação de Apuração dos Immunobiológicos Utilizados ("the Immunization Program Evaluation System")
SI-API	Sistema de Informação de Avaliação do Programa de Immunização ("the Immunization Program Evaluation Information System")
SI-CRIE	Sistema de Informação do Centro de Referência para Immunobiológicos Especiais ("the Information System of the Reference Center Ffor Special Immunobiologicals")
SI-EAPV	Sistema de Informação de Eventos Adversos Pós Vacinais ("the Information System of adverse events following vaccinations")
SI-EDI	Sistema de Informação de Estoque e Distribuição de Immunobiológicos ("the Immunobiological Inventory and Distribution Information System")

6

Outcome Measures Used in Ocular Gene Therapy Trials: A Scoping Review of Current Practice

Jasleen K. Jolly[1,2,3]*, Holly Bridge*[2] *and Robert E. MacLaren*[1,3]*

[1] *Nuffield Laboratory of Ophthalmology, Nuffield Department of Clinical Neurosciences, University of Oxford, Oxford, United Kingdom,* [2] *Wellcome Integrative Neuroimaging Centre, Nuffield Department of Clinical Neurosciences, University of Oxford, Oxford, United Kingdom,* [3] *Oxford Eye Hospital, Oxford University Hospitals NHS Foundation Trust, Oxford, United Kingdom*

***Correspondence:**
Robert E. MacLaren
enquiries@eye.ox.ac.uk

Multiple gene therapy trials are occurring for a variety of ophthalmic diseases around the world. The safety of gene therapy in the eye has been established, and the next step is to reliably assess efficacy. This is primarily done through the use of imaging techniques and visual function measures. Standardized visual function assessments, however, were originally developed for a clinical setting and may not be suitable for detecting and quantifying therapeutic changes. This scoping review takes a comprehensive look at current practice in terms of the outcome measures defined at trial registration. These were compared to the outcome measures reported in the literature. All published trials reported the pre-registered primary outcome measure. A range of additional secondary outcomes were reported that were not originally planned. Gaps in gene therapy assessment exist and further discussion are required to find a way forward, particularly as more conditions progress to phase 2 and 3 trials. Several factors impacting on trial design and outcome measure choice are discussed.

Keywords: clinical trial, gene therapy, genetic eye disease, outcome measure, retinal imaging, vision, visual function

INTRODUCTION

The eye presents the perfect organ for gene therapy. It is an immune privileged site, which is protected by the blood retinal barrier. The target cells, such as photoreceptors and retinal pigment epithelium are frequently non-dividing, meaning any intervention is likely to last for life. The different structures in the eye can be visualized due to the optical clarity inherent in the eyeball or can be imaged with well-documented techniques (Zysk et al., 2007; Fleckenstein et al., 2014). The structures in the eye can be targeted by various surgical procedures. Finally, many disease processes have a degree of symmetry. This means that, when treating one eye, the other eye can act as a control for comparison. For these reasons, ocular gene therapy is being trialed as an experimental treatment for an increasing number of conditions. There are established techniques to measure both structural and functional changes, with work ongoing in this field to evaluate the different diseases being treated. The success of gene therapy can be determined by the pattern of change seen in visual function measurement. Since visual function is the major marker for success of gene therapy, it is critical to establish guidelines for best practice.

Gene therapy can follow several different strategies. Most commonly, it is the supplementation of a defective gene with a working copy in affected target cells, as happens in achromatopsia and choroideremia. However, in some cases, such as with neovascular age-related macular degeneration, the gene expression may introduce a factor to help dampen the disease response. The mode of action is less important than the disease being investigated in determining the appropriate measures to use for trial monitoring. The Monaciano Symposium identified the measurement of treatment outcome as an area requiring priority review in order to aid the robustness of clinical interventional trials (Thompson et al., 2015). It calls for the investigation into appropriate outcome measures for each disease to measure structure and function without adding an unreasonable burden on the patient. They propose a standardization of testing protocols and data analysis. The reproducibility and reliability of tests should also be pre-defined.

With the increase in the number of trials using ocular gene therapy, the importance of adequate outcome measures is gathering interest. The success of gene therapy relies on three key aspects. The viral vector is developed over several years and optimized in animal models before reaching human trials (Koilkonda et al., 2014; Patrício et al., 2017). Much work has been conducted on optimizing the delivery of the therapeutic vector (Salvetti et al., 2017; Xue et al., 2017). Another component required for success of clinical trials is the adequate measurement of therapeutic impact. This requires a combination of the evaluation of ocular structure *via* imaging, and measurement of visual function. Standardized clinical visual function measures were largely developed for use in a clinical setting rather than for the assessment of novel interventions and may not always be adequate for measurement of a therapeutic effect. For example, the 100-hue test for color vision has wide normative ranges, making interpretation of longitudinal data difficult (Kinnear and Sahraie, 2002). The relationship of the outcome measures to disease progression, and therefore, the therapeutic window should also be better understood to interpret clinical trial findings. In addition, disease features such as visual field loss may make the conduct the test difficult.

A systematic review of gene therapy for retinal disease has been registered on the PROSPERO database (CRD42017056500) by London City University, but not yet completed. This specifies visual outcome as the outcome measure for assessing the success of trials, but the type of vision measure being looked at is not detailed, demonstrating the importance of providing further guidance on this topic. Additionally, as bilateral gene therapy will become more common, there will no longer be a control eye to provide a comparison as is done in many phase 1 trials, making vision outcome even more critical (MacLaren, 2016). Visual function is a combination of many aspects of vision, including detail, color, contrast, speed of vision, and night vision. The objective of this paper is to review the outcome measures listed and published for registered gene therapy trials in order to establish current practice, and to consider the scope for development of relevant outcome measures.

METHOD

All clinical interventional trials must be registered on a publically available database. The databases on Clinicaltrials.gov (RRID: SCR_002309), EU clinical trials register (RRID SCR_005956), and the NIH clinical trials register were searched for all registrations by the end of October 2018, using the following search terms: gene therapy, subretinal injection, intravitreal injection, STX eye trial, Nightstar, Applied genetic, MeiraGTx, Hemera, Oxford Biomedica, Sanofi, Spark, ProQR, GenSight, and Genzyme.

Duplicate records were omitted from analysis. Natural history studies or studies specifically for long-term follow up of patients in a previous trial were also excluded in order to focus on the primary interventional trials. We then searched for any results from studies with a registered start date of greater than 12 months before October 2018. This was done *via* PubMed, study group websites, and Scopus. Searches were conducted using the investigator details and registered study name. Publications for the same study were grouped together and analyzed as an integrated dataset, with discrepancies between the primary outcome measure on the clinical trials record *versus* the final publications being noted.

RESULTS

Listed Outcome Measures

We identified 50 unique clinical trials on the registers for 17 ophthalmic indications (**Supplementary Figure**). Lebers congential amaurosis, Leber hereditory optic neuritis, and choroideremia are the only conditions currently in phase 3 trials. Outcome measures were analyzed according to clinical trial phase and were separated into four categories: safety, validated tests, novel test methods, and non-specific (**Supplementary Table**).

Visual acuity was included in almost all studies as either a primary or a secondary measure. Various forms of perimetry also featured highly in the outcome measures list. Out of the 50 trials, 16 used broad descriptors which did not make clear what data were being collected or how it was going to be used. This included descriptors such as visual function or specifying imaging techniques with no details of the aspect of the images to be examined. One did not specify any outcome measures.

Published Trials

One trial marked as completed has not yet been published (NCT00001735). Eighteen trials have associated results in the peer-reviewed literature. **Table 1** details the correlation between the trial register record and the outcomes reported in the peer-reviewed papers. Where primary and secondary outcomes were explicitly stated in the paper, these were recorded if also reported in the results. Anything not reported in the results or supplemental sections was not counted. In reports where primary or secondary was not made clear, all measures reported were recorded, and primary *versus* secondary was inferred from emphasis and context.

There was 100% compliance with reporting on the pre-specified primary outcome measures. Sixteen trials pre-specified one or more secondary outcome measure. These were met in full by 68% (11) trials. Five trials did not meet all of the

TABLE 1 | Comparison of clinical trial record and published outcomes in ocular gene therapy trials.

Study ID (clinicaltrials.gov), disease and gene therapy delivery method	Phase; full/prelim	Pre-specified primary outcome	Reported primary outcome	Pre-specified secondary outcome	Reported secondary outcome
NCT01024998 Neovascular AMD AAV intravitreal (Heier et al., 2017)	I; full	Adverse events, maximum tolerated dose	Adverse events, change in VA and vector DNA concentration in biological samples	Decreased retinal thickness	Transgene expression in aqueous fluid and OCT thickness
NCT01494805 Neovascular AMD AAV subretinal (Rakoczy et al., 2015; Constable et al., 2017)	I/II; both	Adverse events and laboratory measures	Adverse events and laboratory measures	VA, foveal thickness, and CNV lesion	VA, retinal thickness, and standard injection retreatments
NCT01301443 Neovascular AMD lentivirus subretinal (Campochiaro et al., 2017)	I; full	Adverse events	Adverse events, change in VA, ocular inflammation, IOP, laboratory measures	OCT intraretinal fluid	Transgene expression, OCT macular thickening, lesion measures on fluorescein angiography, VA
NCT01461213 Choroideremia AAV subretinal (MacLaren et al., 2014; Edwards et al., 2016)	I/II; prelim	VA	VA	Microperimetry, OCT, and AF	Microperimetry threshold, OCT thickness, AF area
NCT02553135 Choroideremia AAV subretinal (Lam et al., 2019)	II; full	Adverse events	VA, adverse events	Macular autofluorescence, microperimetry	Microperimetry, contrast sensitivity, color vision, autofluorescence area, OCT ellipsoid zone and choroidal thickness assessments, safety
NCT02671539 Choroideremia AAV subretinal (Fischer et al., 2018)	II; full	VA	VA	Adverse events, autofluorescence, microperimetry, contrast sensitivity, color vision	Microperimetry, autofluorescence area, OCT ellipsoid zone and choroidal thickness, safety
NCT02077361 Choroideremia AAV subretinal (Dimopoulos et al., 2018)	I/II; full	Adverse events	Safety including adverse events	Microperimetry, Goldmann visual field, multifocal ERG, FST, OCT, photos, and autofluorescence	VA, autofluorescence area, OCT ellipsoid zone, microperimetry, quality of life questionnaire
NCT01482195 MERTK AAV subretinal (Ghazi et al., 2016)	I; full	Adverse events and laboratory measures	Safety measures	VA and FST	VA, FST, OCT thickness
NCT01267422 LHON AAV intravitreal (Wan et al., 2016)	Not given; prelim	VA, laboratory measures	VA, laboratory measures	IOP, neutralizing antibody assay, OCT RNFL thickness, computerized visual field mean deviation and visual field index, VEP, ERG, liver, and kidney function	Visual field index and mean deviation, VEP, OCT RNFL thickness, and blood tests
NCT02161380 LHON AAV intravitreal (Feuer et al., 2016)	I; prelim	Toxicity	Loss of VA	None	OCT RNFL thickness, pattern ERG, and adverse events
NCT01496040 LCA AAV subretinal (Le Meur et al., 2018)	I/II; full	Biodistribution in urine and nasal samples	Adverse events and biodsitribution	ERG, questionnaire, distance VA, near VA, color vision, pupillometry, microperimetry, and dark adaptation	Chorioretinal imaging, OCT thickness, undefined questionnaire, distance VA, nystagmus measures, visual field, microperimetry, fMRI, ERG, pupillometry, and mobility test
NCT00749957 LCA AAV subretinal (Weleber et al., 2016)	I/II; full	Adverse events	Adverse events	Static perimetry and VA	VA, static perimetry hill of vision, kinetic perimetry hill of vision, ERG, OCT, photography, and quality of life questionnaire
NCT00481546 LCA AAV subretinal (Hauswirth et al., 2008; A. V. Cideciyan et al., 2008; Artur V. Cideciyan et al., 2009; Jacobson et al., 2012; Artur V. Cideciyan et al., 2015)	I; both	Toxicity, symptoms, and, adverse events	Laboratory measures, symptoms, and adverse events	Visual function	VA, FST, dark adaptation kinetics, chromatic stimuli sensitivity, kinetic perimetry, OCT thickness, fixation analysis, pupillary light reflex, mobility testing, eye movements, and fMRI

(Continued)

TABLE 1 | Continued

Study ID (clinicaltrials.gov), disease and gene therapy delivery method	Phase; full/prelim	Pre-specified primary outcome	Reported primary outcome	Pre-specified secondary outcome	Reported secondary outcome
NCT00516477 LCA AAV subretinal (Maguire et al., 2008, Maguire et al., 2009; Ashtari et al., 2011; Testa et al., 2013)	I; both	Safety and tolerability	Adverse events	Change in visual function psychophysical and objective measures	Pupillary light reflex, nystagmus testing, kinetic perimetry, microperimetry, OCT, AF, FST, ERG, mobility testing, and fMRI
NCT01208389 LCA 2nd eyes (Bennett et al., 2016)	I/II; prelim	Adverse events	Adverse events	VA, VF, pupillary light response, mobility testing, FST, and contrast sensitivity	FST, kinetic perimetry, VA, pupillary light reflex, mobility, and fMRI
NCT00643747 LCA AAV subretinal (J W B Bainbridge et al., 2008; James W.B. Bainbridge et al., 2015; Ripamonti et al., 2015)	I/II; both	Inflammation	Adverse events	Visual function	Laboratory measures, VA, kinetic perimetry, microperimetry, dark-adapted perimetry, mobility, contrast sensitivity, color vision, spectral sensitivity, retinal imaging, and ERG
NCT00999609 LCA AAV subretinal (Russell et al., 2017)	3; full	Multi-luminance mobility testing bilateral	Multi-luminance mobility testing bilateral	FST, multi-luminance mobility testing monocular, and VA	FST, multi-luminance mobility testing monocular, VA, kinetic perimetry, Humphrey static visual fields, contrast sensitivity, and pupil light reflex
NCT02317887 XLRS AAV intravitreal (Cukras et al., 2018)	1; full	Adverse events, retinal structure, ocular structure	Adverse events, inflammation	Visual function, OCT, ERG, AAV antibodies	VA, microperimetry, ERG, OCT macular thickness, AAV antibodies

References provided in brackets. AF, fundus autofluorescence; AMD, age-related macular degeneration; ERG, electroretinogram; FST, full-field stimulus threshold; IOP, intraocular pressure; OCT, ocular coherence tomography; RNFL, retinal nerve fiber layer; VA, visual acuity; VEP, visual evoked potential.

outcome measures but did meet some of them. In addition, 83% (15/18) trials reported additional outcome measures, including a range of features, such as retinal imaging, aspects of visual function, and fMRI imaging. **Figure 1A** demonstrates the number of additional secondary outcomes carried out in the published literature but not originally included in the register as a histogram. **Figure 1B** shows the array of the visual function tests reported. VA was the most commonly used assessment of visual function. Perimetry was also commonly used but could take several different forms; each of which is targeting different areas of the visual field. Mobility testing is not standardized and appears in almost half the published trials. Electroretinograms are measured in a similar number of trials but are standardized due to ISCEV standards. The tests listed in low number of trials are generally non-standardized exploratory techniques such as fixation analysis and dark-adapted perimetry.

DISCUSSION

Adverse events are a key part of phase 1 trials as would be expected. Visual acuity is also a frequent factor in determining treatment effects and is reported in 94% of trials. It is a widely accepted measure, both clinically and by medical regulatory authorities. VA has been reported to have higher variability in low vision patients so strategies to optimize VA measurements in patients with disease need to be better established (Kiser et al., 2005).

Even within trials for the same disease, visual outcome measures used differ across sites, making direct comparison difficult. This is especially problematic due to the small numbers of patients involved in these highly specialized trials. The ideal way forward would be to conduct formal natural history studies and additional validation studies of novel outcome measures where existing measures are not sufficient or appropriate. The length of natural history studies should be determined by the nature of the disease being investigated. Fast progressing conditions will require a shorter follow-up period of 1 or 2 years. Slower progressive conditions should ideally have a longer follow-up period. An initial audit of imaging and functional data collected in the clinical environment can provide guidance on the speed of progression as a starting point such as conducted by Jolly et al., 2016 and 2017 in choroideremia (Jolly et al., 2016, Jolly et al., 2017). Combining structural and functional data will be helpful in better understanding the disease process as well as treatment impact in both natural history trials as well as in final outcome measures chosen.

Outcome measures should ideally be based on the biology of the disease and related to measurement of the therapeutic target within the eye, in order to maximize the chance of measuring a real therapeutic effect. This may change in end-stage disease *versus* trials designed for early disease states. The balance of structural *versus* functional measures is likely to change in late stage *versus* early stage disease. If the novel outcome measures are established in the disease prior to the interventional trials, the data can be submitted to the regulatory authorities in

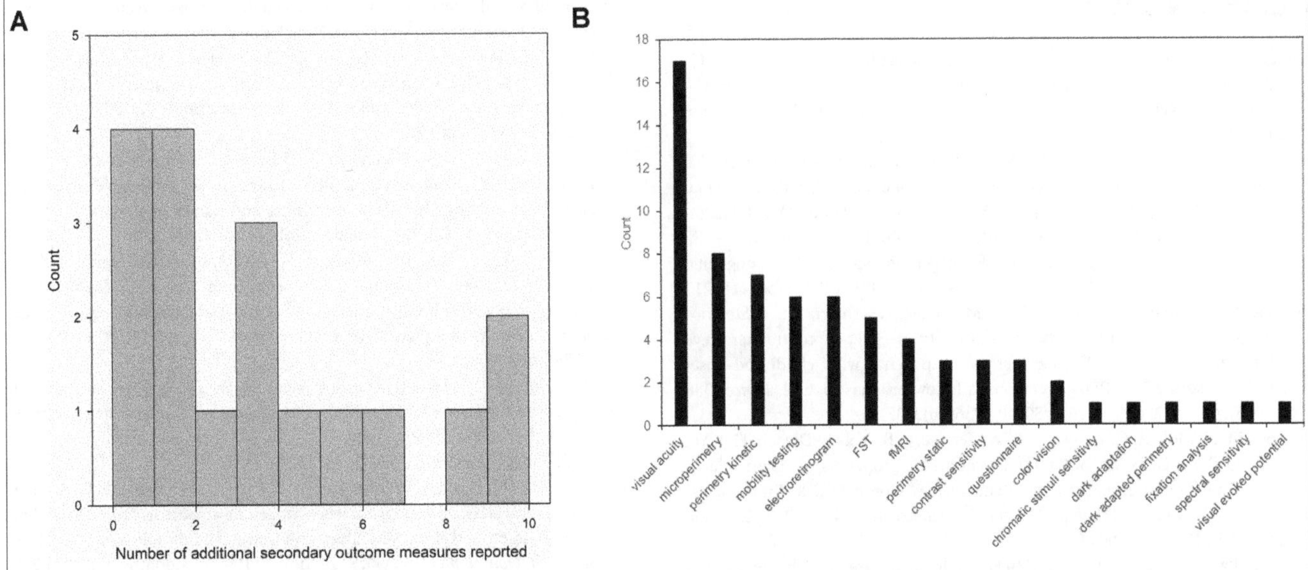

FIGURE 1 | (A) Histogram to show the number of additional outcome measures reported by 79% of trials with peer-reviewed publications. **(B)** Range of visual function tests currently used as secondary outcome measures in reported ocular gene therapy trials from **Table 1**.

advance of the interventional trials. This would increase the acceptability of these measures. Outcome measures should be based on an understanding of the underlying disease process as well as the impact of the gene therapy as determined by the expected impact of the viral vector and cells likely to be transfected. A significant advantage of this approach would be the likelihood of reaching the final outcome more quickly due to the use of targeted and sensitive markers of disease.

Patient quality of life is highly dependent on their perception of the world. Subjective assessment using validated instruments can provide insights into visual perception from the patients' perspective and can be considered as part of the battery of outcome measures (De Boer et al., 2004). Defining success based on clinical (such as repeatability) and patient (such as improvement required for greater quality of life) factors will make a stronger case for the success of therapy, particularly for phase 2 and 3 trials (Mcglothlin and Lewis, 2014). Although questionnaire results may be considered biased due to the patients motivation, the subjective feedback can provide very powerful evidence for the real world impact of any therapy in a way that clinical measures are unable to achieve. Many funding bodies in the United Kingdom encourage the use of patient and participant involvement in research as the insights they can provide can have an influence on guiding researchers to improved clinical trial design, as well as impact when reporting results (Boote et al., 2011).

Despite visual function being highlighted as an important factor in the success of gene therapy trials, little progress has been made on developing a coherent approach worldwide (Thompson et al., 2015). Other fields have highlighted similar issues for gene therapy (Lähteenvuo and Ylä-Herttuala, 2017). As more diseases are targeted by a gene therapy approach, and trials progress to phases 2 and 3, this will become ever more important. Cataract formation is a side effect of the invasive vector delivery techniques (Gupta et al., 2007; Hasler et al., 2015). Moreover, patients are followed up over long periods of time, increasing the chance of age-related cataract formation. Thus, it is necessary to account for the effect of cataract on visual function measures to ensure that any deficits do not interfere with determining the impact of gene therapy. Otherwise, results may be skewed in a negative way masking the therapeutic effect. Greater investment is needed in exploring disease parameters in more detail in order to complete gene therapy trials in an effective, timely, and cost-effective manner. This review provides an important starting point for clinical trial design.

AUTHOR CONTRIBUTIONS

JJ and RM contributed conception and design of the study. JJ performed the data analysis and wrote the first draft of the manuscript. HB and RM contributed to manuscript revision, read and approved the submitted version.

FUNDING

This study is funded by the National Institute for Health Research (NIHR) [Clinical Doctoral Research Fellowship CA-CDRF-2016-02-002 for Jasleen K Jolly]. The views expressed are those of the authors and not necessarily those of the NHS, the NIHR or the Department of Health and Social Care. The sponsor and funding organization had no role in the design or conduct of this research.

REFERENCES

Ashtari, M., Cyckowski, L. L., Monroe, J. F., Marshall, K. A., Chung, D. C., Auricchio, A., et al. (2011). The human visual cortex responds to gene therapy—mediated recovery of retinal function. *J. Clin. Invest.* 121 (6), 2160–2168. doi: 10.1172/JCI57377

Bainbridge, J. W. B., Smith, A. J., Barker, S. S., Robbie, S., Henderson, R., Balaggan, K., et al. (2008). Effect of gene therapy on visual function in leber's congenital amaurosis. *N. Engl. J. Med.* 358 (21), 2231–2239. doi: 10.1056/NEJMoa0802268

Bainbridge, J. W. B., Mehat, M. S., Sundaram, V., Robbie, S. J., Barker, S. E., Ripamonti, C., et al. (2015). Long-term effect of gene therapy on Leber's congenital amaurosis. *N. Engl. J. Med.* 372 (20), 1887–1897. doi: 10.1056/NEJMoa1414221

Bennett, J., Wellman, J., Marshall, K. A., McCague, S., Ashtari, M., DiStefano-Pappas, J., et al. (2016). Safety and durability of effect of contralateral-eye administration of AAV2 gene therapy in patients with childhood-onset blindness caused by RPE65 mutations: a follow-on phase 1 trial. *Lancet* 388 (10045), 661–672. doi: 10.1016/S0140-6736(16)30371-3

De Boer, M. R., Moll, A. C., de Vet, H. C. W., Terwee, C. B., Völker-Dieben, H. J. M., and van Rens, G. H. M. B. (2004). Psychometric properties of vision-related quality of life questionnaires: a systematic review." Ophthalmic & Physiological Optics. *J. Br. Coll. Ophthalmic Opticians (Optometrists)* 24 (4), 257–273. doi: 10.1111/j.1475-1313.2004.00187.x

Boote, J., Baird, W., and Sutton, A. (2011). Public involvement in the design and conduct of clinical trials: a narrative review of case examples. *Trials* 12 (S1), A82. doi: 10.1186/1745-6215-12-S1-A82

Campochiaro, P. A., Lauer, A. K., Sohn, E. H., Mir, T. A., Naylor, S., Anderton, M. C., et al. (2017). Lentiviral vector gene transfer of endostatin/angiostatin for macular degeneration (GEM) study. *Hum. Gene Ther.* 28 (1), 99–111. doi: 10.1089/hum.2016.117

Cideciyan, A. V., Aleman, T. S., Boye, S. L., Schwartz, S. B., Kaushal, S., Roman, A. J., et al. (2008). Human gene therapy for RPE65 isomerase deficiency activates the retinoid cycle of vision but with slow rod kinetics. *Proc. Natl. Acad. Sci.* 105 (39), 15112–15117. doi: 10.1073/pnas.0807027105

Cideciyan, A. V., Aguirre, G. K., Jacobson, S. G., Butt, O. H., Schwartz, S. B., Swider, M., et al. (2015). Pseudo-fovea formation after gene therapy for RPE65-LCA. *Invest. Ophthalmol. Visual Sci.* 56 (1), 526–537. doi: 10.1167/iovs.14-15895

Cideciyan, A. V., Hauswirth, W. W., Aleman, T. S., Kaushal, S., Schwartz, S. B., Boye, S. L., et al. (2009). Human RPE65 Gene Therapy for Leber congenital amaurosis: persistence of early visual improvements and safety at 1 year. *Hum. Gene Ther.* 20 (9), 999–1004. doi: 10.1089/hum.2009.086

Constable, I. J., Lai, C. M., Magno, A. L., French, M. A., Barone, S. B., Schwartz, S. D., et al. (2017). Gene therapy in neovascular age-related macular degeneration: three-year follow-up of a phase 1 randomized dose escalation trial. *Am. J. Ophthalmol.* 177, 150–158. doi: 10.1016/j.ajo.2017.02.018

Cukras, C., Wiley, H. E., Jeffrey, B. G., Sen, H. N., Turriff, A., Zeng, Y., et al. (2018). Retinal AAV8-RS1 gene therapy for X-linked retinoschisis: initial findings from a phase I/IIa trial by intravitreal delivery. *Mol. Ther.* 26 (9), 2282–2294. doi: 10.1016/j.ymthe.2018.05.025

Dimopoulos, I. S., Hoang, S. C., Radziwon, A., Binczyk, N. M., Seabra, M. C., MacLaren, R. E., et al. (2018). Two-year results after AAV2-mediated gene therapy for choroideremia: the Alberta experience. *Am. J. Ophthalmol.* 193, 130–142. doi: 10.1016/j.ajo.2018.06.011

Edwards, T. L., Jolly, J. K., Groppe, M., Barnard, A. R., Cottriall, C. L., Tolmachova, T., et al. (2016). Visual acuity after retinal gene therapy for choroideremia. *N. Engl. J. Med.* 374 (20), 1996–1998. doi: 10.1056/NEJMc1509501

Feuer, W. J., Schiffman, J. C., Davis, J. L., Porciatti, V., Gonzalez, P., Koilkonda, R. D., et al. (2016). Gene therapy for Leber hereditary optic neuropathy: initial results. *Ophthalmology* 123 (3), 558–570. doi: 10.1016/j.ophtha.2015.10.025

Fischer, M. D., Ochakovski, G. A., Beier, B., Seitz, I. P., Vaheb, Y., Kortuem, C., et al. (2018). Changes in retinal sensitivity after gene therapy in choroideremia. *Retina (Philadelphia, Pa.).* doi: 10.1097/IAE.0000000000002360

Fleckenstein, M., Issa, P. C., and Holz, F. G. (2014). "Fundus Autofluorescence Imaging in Retinal Dystrophies," in *Inherited chorioretinal dystrophies: a textbook and atlas.* Eds. Bernard Puech, Jean-Jacques De Laey, and Graham E Holder (Berlin, Heidelberg. Springer Berlin Heidelberg), 41–59. doi: 10.1007/978-3-540-69466-3_6

Ghazi, N. G., Abboud, E. B., Nowilaty, S. R., Alkuraya, H., Alhommadi, A., Cai, H., et al. (2016). Treatment of retinitis pigmentosa due to MERTK mutations by ocular subretinal injection of adeno-associated virus gene vector: results of a phase I trial. *Hum. Genet.* 135 (3), 327–343. doi: 10.1007/s00439-016-1637-y

Gupta, O. P. I., Weichel, E. D., Regillo, C. D., Fineman, M. S., Kaiser, R. S., Ho, A. C., et al. (2007). Postoperative complications associated with 25-gauge pars plana vitrectomy. *Ophthalmic Surg. Lasers Imaging* 38 (4), 270–275. doi: 10.3928/15428877-2007-07

Hasler, P. W., Bloch, S. B., Villumsen, J., Fuchs, J., Lund-Andersen, H., and Larsen, M. (2015). Safety study of 38 503 intravitreal ranibizumab injections performed mainly by physicians in training and nurses in a hospital setting. *Acta Ophthalmol.* 93 (2), 122–125. doi: 10.1111/aos.12589

Hauswirth, W. W., Aleman, T. S., Kaushal, S., Cideciyan, A. V., Schwartz, S. B., Wang, L., et al. (2008). Treatment of leber congenital amaurosis due to RPE65 mutations by ocular subretinal injection of adeno-associated virus gene vector: short-term results of a phase I trial. *Hum. Gene Ther.* 19 (10), 979–990. doi: 10.1089/hum.2008.107

Heier, J. S., Kherani, S., Desai, S., Dugel, P., Kaushal, S., Cheng, S. H., et al. (2017). Intravitreous injection of AAV2-SFLT01 in patients with advanced neovascular age-related macular degeneration: a phase 1, open-label trial. *Lancet* 390 (10089), 50–61. doi: 10.1016/S0140-6736(17)30979-0

Jacobson, S. G., Cideciyan, A. V., Ratnakaram, R., Heon, E., Schwartz, S. B., Roman, A. J., et al. (2012). Gene therapy for leber congenital amaurosis caused by RPE65 mutations: safety and efficacy in fifteen children and adults followed up to three years. *Arch. Ophthalmol.* 130 (1), 9–24. doi: 10.1001/archophthalmol.2011.298

Jolly, J. K., Edwards, T. L., Moules, J., Groppe, M., Downes, S. M., and MacLaren, R. E. (2016). A qualitative and quantitative assessment of fundus autofluorescence patterns in patients with choroideremia. *Invest. Opthalmol. Visual Sci.* 57 (10), 4498. doi: 10.1167/iovs.15-18362

Jolly, J. K., Xue, K., Edwards, T. L., Groppe, M., and MacLaren, R. E. (2017). Characterizing the natural history of visual function in choroideremia using microperimetry and multimodal retinal imaging. *Invest. Ophthalmol. Visual Sci.* 58 (12), 5575–5583. doi: 10.1167/iovs.17-22486

Kinnear, P. R., and Sahraie, A. (2002). New Farnsworth-Munsell 100 hue test norms of normal observers for each year of age 5–22 and for age decades 30–70. *Br. J. Ophthalmol.* 86, 1408–1411. doi: 10.1136/bjo.86.12.1408

Kiser, A. K., Mladenovich, D., Eshraghi, F., Bourdeau, D., and Dagnelie, G. (2005). Reliability and consistency of visual acuity and contrast sensitivity measures in advanced eye disease. *Optom. Vision Sci.* 82 (11), 946–954. doi: 10.1097/01.opx.0000187863.12609.7b

Koilkonda, R. D., Yu, H., Chou, T.-H., Feuer, W. J., Ruggeri, M., Porciatti, V., et al. (2014). Safety and effects of the vector for the leber hereditary optic neuropathy gene therapy clinical trial. *JAMA Ophthalmol.* 132 (4), 409. doi: 10.1001/jamaophthalmol.2013.7630

Lähteenvuo, J., and Ylä-Herttuala, S. (2017). Advances and challenges in cardiovascular gene therapy. *Hum. Gene Ther.* 28 (11), 1024–1032. doi: 10.1089/hum.2017.129

Lam, B. L., Davis, J. L., Gregori, N. Z., MacLaren, R. E., Girach, A., Verriotto, J. D., et al. (2019). Choroideremia gene therapy phase 2 clinical trial: 24-month results. *Am. J. Ophthalmol.* 197, 65–73. doi: 10.1016/j.ajo.2018.09.012

MacLaren, R. E. (2016). Benefits of gene therapy for both eyes. *Lancet* 388 (10045), 635–636. doi: 10.1016/S0140-6736(16)30783-8

MacLaren, R. E., Groppe, M., Barnard, A. R., Cottriall, C. L., Tolmachova, T., Seymour, L., et al. (2014). Retinal gene therapy in patients with choroideremia: initial findings from a phase 1/2 clinical trial. *Lancet* 383 (9923), 1129–1137. doi: 10.1016/S0140-6736(13)62117-0

Maguire, A. M., Simonelli, F., Pierce, E. A., Pugh, E. N., Mingozzi, F., Bennicelli, J. L., et al. (2008). Safety and efficacy of gene transfer for leber's congenital amaurosis. *N. Engl. J. Med.* 358 (21), 2240–2248. doi: 10.1056/NEJMoa0802315

Maguire, A. M., High, K. A., Auricchio, A., Wright, J. F., Pierce, E. A., Testa, F., et al. (2009). Age-dependent effects of RPE65 gene therapy for leber's congenital amaurosis: a phase 1 dose-escalation trial. *Lancet* 374 (9701), 1597–1605. doi: 10.1016/S0140-6736(09)61836-5

Mcglothlin, A. E., and Lewis, R. J. (2014). Minimal clinically important difference defining what really matters to patients. *JAMA* 312 (13), 1342–1343. doi: 10.1001/jama.2014.13128

Meur, G. L., Lebranchu, P., Billaud, F., Adjali, O., Schmitt, S., Bézieau, S., et al. (2018). Safety and long-term efficacy of AAV4 gene therapy in patients with RPE65 leber congenital amaurosis. *Mol. Ther.* 26 (1), 256–268. doi: 10.1016/j.ymthe.2017.09.014

Patrício, M. I., Barnard, A. R., Orlans, H. O., McClements, M. E., and MacLaren, R. E. (2017). Inclusion of the Woodchuck hepatitis virus posttranscriptional regulatory element enhances AAV2-driven transduction of mouse and human retina. *Mol. Ther. - Nucleic Acids* 6, 198–208. doi: 10.1016/j.omtn.2016.12.006

Rakoczy, E. P., Lai, C. M., Magno, A. L., Wikstrom, M. E., French, M. A., Pierce, C. M., et al. (2015). Gene Therapy with recombinant adeno-associated vectors for neovascular age-related macular degeneration: 1 year follow-up of a phase 1 randomised clinical trial. *Lancet* 386 (10011), 2395–2403. doi: 10.1016/S0140-6736(15)00345-1

Ripamonti, C., Henning, G. B., Robbie, S. J., Sundaram, V., van den Born, L. I., Casteels, I., et al. (2015). Spectral sensitivity measurements reveal partial success in restoring missing rod function with gene therapy. *J. Vision* 15 (20), 1–16. doi: 10.1167/15.15.20

Russell, S., Bennett, J., Wellman, J. A., Chung, D. C., Yu, Z. F., Tillman, A., et al. (2017). Efficacy and safety of voretigene neparvovec (AAV2-HRPE65v2) in patients with RPE65-mediated inherited retinal dystrophy: a randomised, controlled, open-label, phase 3 trial. *Lancet* 390 (10097), 849–860. doi: 10.1016/S0140-6736(17)31868-8

Salvetti, A. P., Patrício, M. I., Barnard, A. R., Orlans, H. O., Hickey, D. G., and MacLaren, R. E. (2017). Impact of vital dyes on cell viability and transduction efficiency of AAV vectors used in retinal gene therapy surgery: an in vitro and *in vivo* analysis. *Transl. Vision Sci. Technol.* 6 (4), 4. doi: 10.1167/tvst.6.4.4

Testa, F., Maguire, A. M., Rossi, S., Pierce, E. A., Melillo, P., Marshall, K., et al. (2013). Three-year follow-up after unilateral subretinal delivery of adeno-associated virus in patients with leber congenital amaurosis type 2. *Ophthalmology* 120 (6), 1283–1291. doi: 10.1016/j.ophtha.2012.11.048

Thompson, D. A., Ali, R. R., Banin, E., Branham, K. E., Flannery, J. G., Gamm, D. M., et al. (2015). Advancing therapeutic strategies for inherited retinal degeneration: recommendations from the monaciano symposium. *Invest. Ophthalmol. Visual Sci.* 56 (2), 918–931. doi: 10.1167/iovs.14-16049

Wan, X., Pei, H., Zhao, M. J., Yang, S., Hu, W. K., He, H., et al. (2016). Efficacy and safety of RAAV2-ND4 treatment for leberâ (Tm) s hereditary optic neuropathy. *Sci. Rep.* 6, 2–11. doi: 10.1038/srep21587

Weleber, R. G., Pennesi, M. E., Wilson, D. J., Kaushal, S., Erker, L. R., Jensen, L., et al. (2016). Results at 2 years after gene therapy for RPE65-deficient leber congenital amaurosis and severe early-childhood-onset retinal dystrophy. *Ophthalmology* 123 (7), 1606–1620. doi: 10.1016/j.ophtha.2016.03.003

Xue, K., Groppe, M., Salvetti, A. P., and MacLaren, R. E. (2017). Technique of retinal gene therapy: delivery of viral vector into the subretinal space. *Eye* 31 (9), 1308–1316. doi: 10.1038/eye.2017.158

Zysk, A. M., Nguyen, F. T., Oldenburg, A. L., Marks, D. L., and Boppart, S. A. (2007). Optical coherence tomography: a review of clinical development from bench to bedside. *J. Biomed. Opt.* 12 (5), 51403. doi: 10.1117/1.2793736

7

Variation in Population Vulnerability to Heat Wave in Western Australia

Jianguo Xiao[1], Tony Spicer[1], Le Jian[1,2], Grace Yajuan Yun[1], Changying Shao[1], John Nairn[3], Robert J. B. Fawcett[4], Andrew Robertson[1] and Tarun Stephen Weeramanthri[1]*

[1] Public Health Division, Department of Health, Government of Western Australia, Perth, WA, Australia, [2] School of Public Health, Curtin University, Perth, WA, Australia, [3] Australian Bureau of Meteorology, Adelaide, SA, Australia, [4] Australian Bureau of Meteorology, Melbourne, VIC, Australia

***Correspondence:**
Jianguo Xiao
jianguo.xiao@health.wa.gov.au

Heat waves (HWs) have killed more people in Australia than all other natural hazards combined. Climate change is expected to increase the frequency, duration, and intensity of HWs and leads to a doubling of heat-related deaths over the next 40 years. Despite being a significant public health issue, HWs do not attract the same level of attention from researchers, policy makers, and emergency management agencies compared to other natural hazards. The purpose of the study was to identify risk factors that might lead to population vulnerability to HW in Western Australia (WA). HW vulnerability and resilience among the population of the state of WA were investigated by using time series analysis. The health impacts of HWs were assessed by comparing the associations between hospital emergency department (ED) presentations, hospital admissions and mortality data, and intensities of HW. Risk factors including age, gender, socioeconomic status (SES), remoteness, and geographical locations were examined to determine whether certain population groups were more at risk of adverse health impacts due to extreme heat. We found that hospital admissions due to heat-related conditions and kidney diseases, and overall ED attendances, were sensitive indicators of HW. Children aged 14 years or less and those aged 60 years or over were identified as the most vulnerable populations to HWs as shown in ED attendance data. Females had more ED attendances and hospital admissions due to kidney diseases; while males had more heat-related hospital admissions than females. There were significant dose–response relationships between HW intensity and SES, remoteness, and health service usage. The more disadvantaged and remotely located the population, the higher the health service usage during HWs. Our study also found that some population groups and locations were resilient to extreme heat. We produced a mapping tool, which indicated geographic areas throughout WA with various vulnerability and resilience levels to HW. The findings from this study will allow local government, community service organizations, and agencies in health, housing, and education to better identify and understand the degree of vulnerability to HW throughout the state, better target preparatory strategies, and allocate limited resources to those most in need.

Keywords: heat wave, vulnerability, socioeconomic status, geographical variation, morbidity, mortality, Western Australia

INTRODUCTION

A heat wave (HW) is a prolonged period of excessively hot weather. Heat waves have caused more deaths in Australia since European settlement than all other natural hazards combined, and are predicted to increase in frequency, duration, and intensity, with a doubling of the number of HW-related deaths in the next 40 years (1, 2). Currently, there is no standardized definition for HW internationally or among different jurisdictions in Australia. A recent study conducted in Western Australia (WA) found that the excess heat factor (EHF) metric was the best HW indicator among the three metrics examined to predict greatest health service demand (3). That study's outcomes were only based on Perth's metropolitan population, which required new studies to test the validity of EHF for the whole of WA.

Heat waves typically affect large geographical areas over the course of three or more days. Many jurisdictions, including WA, have created extreme heat emergency management plans to respond to HW events. With large populations and limited resources, many jurisdictions lack the precision to target the most at risk populations with appropriate public health interventions, and many HW plans are based on assumptions and research from other states and countries. There has been little verification of whether a particular population group is at higher risk or even resilient to HWs, although acclimatization, individual susceptibility, and community and geographical characteristics all affect heat-related effects on mortality and morbidity (2, 4–7). Past epidemiological studies have established consistently identifiable vulnerable groups to extreme heat. Young children and the elderly are commonly identified at high risk of morbidity and mortality during the period of HWs (8–11), whereas people with renal, respiratory, and cardiovascular conditions are susceptible to heat due to hyperthermia and dehydration (12–14). However, there have only been a limited number of studies examining the geographical variation and effects of socioeconomic status (SES) on people's response to HW.

Western Australia is the largest state in Australia with varying geographic features and climates that range from temperate areas in the south to tropical areas in the north. Seventy-eight percent of the population is based in the Perth metropolitan area with the remaining 22% scattered throughout regional and remote areas. To improve preparedness and response arrangements for HWs, there is a need to determine which populations are at higher risk of heat exposure and what are the risk factors related to it. Our study aims to characterize the relationship between HW intensity and health service demand of different population groups in different regions of WA. By identifying vulnerable populations, agencies, service providers, and local government authorities can better target their limited resources to those populations most at risk.

MATERIALS AND METHODS

Western Australia is Australia's largest state with an area of more than 2,500,000 km^2 and over 12,500 km of coastline. It has a population of approximately 2.6 million people (15). The southwest corner of the state has a mediterranean climate (i.e., hot dry summers and cooler wet winters) where about 85% of the WA population lives. The central four-fifths of the State are semiarid or desert and are lightly inhabited. An exception to this is the northern tropical region that has an extremely hot monsoonal climate.

Derive HW Intensity, Adjust for Delayed Effects of HW, and Identify Significant Health Service Usage Measures

Heat waves were measured using HW intensity at each geographical area represented by statistical local area (SLA) in WA. A HW day, defined by an EHF, was defined as the exceedance of the previous 3-day mean daily temperature (DT) above the 95th percentile threshold, multiplied by the difference between the 3-day mean DT and the mean of the prior 30 days. Nairn and Fawcett (16) provide the full equation. The EHF was then normalized and expressed as a heat wave severity index (HWSI), dividing the EHF by the long-term 85th percentile of positive EHF at every location. The HWSI data at SLA level were sourced from the Australian Bureau of Meteorology (BoM). The BoM identifies severe HWs when HWSI is greater than 1, which becomes extreme when HWSI is greater than 3. In our analysis, severe and extreme HW days were combined to severe/extreme HW days, as the counts for extreme HW days were very small and not suitable for a separate statistical analysis. Low-intensity HW days occur if the HWSI value was between 0 and 1; and non-heat wave days were defined as having a HWSI less than or equal to 0. The EHF was calculated over a 3-day period (16), and we applied the EHF value to the first day in an attempt to identify any possible delayed effects of HW.

Time series design was used for the study. The daily health service usage data from 1 November 2006 to 30 April 2015 for warm months (November to April in the following year) for the whole of WA was obtained and measured from following three datasets: (1) hospital admission data from WA hospital morbidity data system (HMDS), including overall (all admissions), cardiovascular diseases (defined as having a principal diagnosis of ICD-10-AM seventh Edition codes between I00-I99 plus G45), respiratory diseases (J00–J99), kidney diseases (N10–N19), and heat-related diseases (having a principal or any additional diagnosis of L55, L74.0, T67, X30, or X32); (2) overall emergency department (ED) attendance data from WA ED data collection; and (3) death data from WA registry of births, deaths and marriages. The chosen HMDS conditions were based on existing literature where conditions were identified as having a strong association with HWs (10, 17). The health service utilization rates in different HW intensities were compared with those during non-HW days for all aforementioned conditions.

Estimated resident populations (ERPs) by age group, gender, and SLA were sourced from Australian Bureau of Statistics. The monthly populations were computed using a linear interpolation method, based on mid-year ERPs. Such populations were then applied to all the days in the month of the study period. Daily health service usage rates were calculated by age group, gender, and SLA. The total population covered in the study period (i.e., warm months) from 1 November 2006 to 30 April 2015 was

11,698,702 person-years. To assess for the delayed effects of HW on health service usage, service usage rates were first derived by dividing daily service usage counts by daily populations on the same day as the HW day, or 2- to 30-day cumulative counts divided by corresponding cumulative populations.

A Pearson correlation analysis was then conducted between the EHF for a day (i.e., first day of the 3-day period) and its corresponding health service usage rate of that day. The rates or cumulative rates with the highest positive correlation with a significance value of 0.05 or less were then selected and used in the bivariate and multivariate statistical analyses to assess the potential risk factors of high service usage during HW exposure. Only health service usage measures with significant correlation with EHF were included in the further analyses below.

Sensitivity of datasets to HW was examined, and only results identified as having significant association with EHF will be reported in this paper.

Determine Risk Factors and Interactions between Risk Factors and HW Intensity

A literature review was conducted to identify potential risk factors of HW. Age, gender, HW intensity, SES [measured by the socioeconomic index for areas (SEIFA)], and service accessibility [measured by the accessibility/remoteness index of Australia (ARIA)] were identified as key risk factors in the WA context.

Health service usage measures with significant associations with EHF among different population groups during HW days were compared with those during non-heat wave days. *Via* bivariate analyses, the interactive effects of HW and risk factor were examined to identify vulnerable groups. Risk factors included age group (0–14, 15–59, and 60+ years), gender, SEIFA, ARIA for 2011, and geographical areas [local government areas (LGAs)] sourced from the ABS.

Poisson regression modeling was then used to evaluate the potential association between HW intensity and the number of presentations to EDs and inpatient admissions for heat-related causes. In the models, daily health service usage counts by age group, gender, and SLA were used as a dependent variable and regressed on all potential risk factors described above. The offset variable was daily populations by age group, gender, and SLA. Where an excess of 0 count was identified, zero-inflated Poisson regression was used. Where there was an over-dispersion of counts of health service usage, negative binomial regression was applied.

The interactions between each risk factor and HW intensity were assessed in the regression models. Variables such as public holidays and weekend days were also included in the model to adjust for their confounding effects when assessing the vulnerability of populations to HW.

Determine Geographical Variations Using Composite Rankings

To compare the health service utilization rates among different geographical regions, both crude rates and age standardized rates (ASRs) were calculated. The 2001 Australian standard population was used for standardization.

Where a health service usage indicator was identified as having a significant association with HW, it was further examined by LGAs. To summarize the overall impact (combined effect) of HW on three significant health service usage indicators (i.e., overall ED attendances, hospitalizations due to heat-related episode, and chronic kidney disease) in different LGAs, the following formula was used to derive a composite score for each LGA.

$$\text{Composite score} = \sum_{j=1}^{3} \text{DASR}_j \times \frac{\text{RR}_j}{\sum_{i=1}^{3} \text{RR}_i}$$

where DASR_j is the difference of ASRs for a particular health service usage indicator between HW days and non-HW days, and RR_j is the relative risk between HW and non-HW days for that health service usage indicator. Finally, the composite score was divided into five quantiles representing the least, small, median, high, and highest impact of HW for a particular LGA with the highest impact areas being defined as hotspots.

Significant difference was defined as having a p-Value <0.05. SAS Enterprise version 5.1 (SAS Institute Inc.) was used for statistical analysis.

Ethics approval for this project was obtained from the WA Department of Health Human Research Ethics Committee. Health service utilization and mortality data are routinely collected by the Department of Health WA. This study was given approval to access and analyze de-identified data to ensure that patient confidentiality was maintained.

RESULTS

Only results related to ED attendances and hospitalizations due to heat and kidney diseases are presented here, as measures in other datasets were not identified as having significant association with the EHF.

Association between Risk Factors and Health Usage Measures

Table 1 shows the association between each of the main risk factors and their associations with HW intensity for health service usage measures without adjusting for other risk factors. Only those measures that had a significant association with HW intensity were included. A dose–response relationship between measured health service usage rates and HW intensity was apparent regardless of age group, gender, SEIFA, and ARIA. The more intense the HW, the higher the health service usage rates. For hospitalization, there was also a strong dose–response relationship between age and rates under each HW intensity category. The older the population group, the higher the health service usage rates. However, young age (0–14 years) was more vulnerable to heat than the other two age groups in terms of ED attendance.

Males had higher heat-related hospitalization and ED attendance rates than females. However, females had higher rates of hospitalization due to kidney diseases.

There was an apparent dose–response relationship between health service usage rates and SEIFA categories. Overall, the more socially advantaged the population, the lower the rate.

TABLE 1 | Crude health service usage rates and 95% CIs by risk factors and HW intensity, November 2006–April 2015, Western Australia.

Risk factor	Level	HW intensity	Heat-related hospitalization (/10,000,000 per day)	Kidney disease hospitalization (/10,000,000 per day)	Emergency department attendance (/100,000 per day)
Age (years)	60+	No HW[a]	4.55 (4.31–4.79)	114.37 (113.83–114.91)	110.11 (109.96–110.27)
		Low intensity	**11.30 (10.04–12.55)**	**124.79 (122.92–126.66)**	108.83 (108.32–109.33)
		Severe/extreme	**26.26 (21.42–31.10)**	**126.62 (121.87–131.38)**	**115.61 (114.29–116.92)**
	15–59	No HW[a]	1.82 (1.74–1.90)	54.93 (54.74–55.13)	92.61 (92.54–92.68)
		Low intensity	**4.32 (3.91–4.72)**	**60.43 (59.75–61.11)**	92.81 (92.56–93.05)
		Severe/extreme	**7.56 (6.23–8.89)**	**61.23 (59.53–62.92)**	**99.60 (98.97–100.22)**
	0–14	No HW[a]	1.57 (1.43–1.70)	14.17 (13.99–14.35)	125.69 (125.53–125.84)
		Low intensity	2.22 (1.69–2.75)	**15.08 (14.47–15.70)**	**118.41 (117.91–118.91)**
		Severe/extreme	4.24 (2.43–6.06)	**16.50 (14.90–18.10)**	**129.27 (127.98–130.56)**
Gender	Male	No HW[a]	2.94 (2.83–3.05)	53.76 (53.55–53.98)	102.90 (102.82–102.99)
		Low intensity	**7.25 (6.66–7.84)**	**59.49 (58.74–60.25)**	**101.44 (101.16–101.73)**
		Severe/extreme	**12.50 (10.58–14.42)**	**58.84 (56.98–60.70)**	**108.01 (107.29–108.74)**
	Female	No HW[a]	1.53 (1.44–1.61)	60.94 (60.71–61.17)	101.14 (101.05–101.23)
		Low intensity	**2.95 (2.57–3.33)**	**66.21 (65.41–67.02)**	**99.55 (99.27–99.84)**
		Severe/extreme	**7.53 (6.02–9.04)**	**68.46 (66.42–70.50)**	**108.00 (107.26–108.74)**
Socioeconomic index for areas	Most disadvantaged area + Q2	No HW[a]	3.44 (3.22–3.67)	71.61 (71.14–72.07)	198.31 (198.09–198.53)
		Low intensity	**9.30 (8.04–10.55)**	**76.94 (75.33–78.56)**	**190.81 (190.08–191.55)**
		Severe/extreme	**13.08 (9.38–16.77)**	**76.68 (72.68–80.69)**	**213.52 (211.59–215.44)**
	Q3	No HW[a]	2.30 (2.14–2.45)	59.99 (59.63–60.34)	96.09 (95.96–96.22)
		Low intensity	**5.09 (4.32–5.86)**	**65.96 (64.72–67.20)**	**95.26 (94.83–95.69)**
		Severe/extreme	**11.21 (8.35–14.08)**	**66.13 (63.02–69.23)**	**100.72 (99.61–101.82)**
	Least disadvantaged area + Q4	No HW[a]	1.94 (1.86–2.02)	53.13 (52.94–53.32)	81.64 (81.58–81.71)
		Low intensity	**4.21 (3.82–4.61)**	**58.71 (58.05–59.37)**	**82.31 (82.08–82.53)**
		Severe/extreme	**9.03 (7.59–10.47)**	**59.89 (58.23–61.54)**	**87.14 (86.56–87.72)**
Accessibility/remoteness index of Australia	R and VR	No HW[a]	3.99 (3.64–4.34)	69.83 (69.17–70.48)	273.76 (273.38–274.13)
		Low intensity	**14.05 (11.80–16.30)**	69.64 (67.40–71.88)	**258.97 (257.73–260.22)**
		Severe/extreme	**16.81 (11.60–22.02)**	66.69 (62.05–71.32)	**258.88 (256.25–261.52)**
	MA	No HW[a]	3.40 (3.09–3.71)	56.82 (56.25–57.39)	186.01 (185.71–186.30)
		Low intensity	**8.65 (6.77–10.52)**	**61.65 (59.42–63.89)**	**192.51 (191.37–193.65)**
		Severe/extreme	**11.48 (6.57–16.39)**	61.29 (56.22–66.36)	**199.77 (197.13–202.41)**
	A	No HW[a]	2.12 (1.99–2.24)	57.79 (57.51–58.07)	97.58 (97.47–97.68)
		Low intensity	**4.41 (3.84–4.98)**	**63.26 (62.30–64.22)**	**100.37 (100.02–100.72)**
		Severe/extreme	**10.22 (7.98–12.46)**	**65.50 (62.96–68.03)**	**103.22 (102.00–104.14)**
	HA	No HW[a]	1.90 (1.82–1.99)	55.40 (55.18–55.61)	68.96 (68.89–69.03)
		Low intensity	**4.06 (3.64–4.49)**	**61.84 (61.10–62.58)**	**70.83 (70.60–71.06)**
		Severe/extreme	**8.60 (7.04–10.15)**	**62.22 (60.35–64.10)**	**72.06 (71.47–72.64)**

[a]*Reference category for HW intensity; HW, heat wave.*
Bold numbers denote a higher rate during for the low or severe/extreme HW intensity days compared to non-HW days.

The rates during low intensity or severe/extreme HW days were significantly higher than those during non-HW days.

There was also an apparent dose–response relationship between service accessibility and heat-related hospitalization rate. The less remote a population, the lower the health service usage rate.

Identify Vulnerable Populations through Adjusting for Risk Factors *via* Regression Analyses

Table 2 presents the final regression analysis results showing risk factors and their interaction with HW intensity when examining effects of HW on health service usage measures. Only risk factors with significant interaction with HW intensity were included in the final results.

First, we observed that there was an apparent dose–response relationship between the HW intensity and health service usage rates. The more intense the HW, the higher the health service usage rates. Those aged 15–59 and 60 years and over were more at risk of heat- or kidney disease-related hospital admissions than those aged 0–15 years. Meanwhile, those aged 0–14, and 60 years and over, had higher chance to attend ED than those aged 15–59 years.

Males had nearly two times higher heat-related hospitalization rates than females. However, females had higher kidney disease-related hospitalization rates and ED attendance rates than males with HW exposure.

TABLE 2 | Adjusted rate ratios and 95% CIs of risk and confounding factors for health service usage measures, November 2006 to April 2015, Western Australia.

Risk factor	Category	Interaction with	Heat-related hospitalization[a]	Kidney disease hospitalization[a]	Emergency department attendance[a]
HW intensity	Severe/extreme		2.120 (1.327–3.387)	1.157 (1.047–1.279)	1.046 (1.037–1.055)
	Low intensity		1.451 (1.223–1.824)	0.988 (0.945–1.032)	1.023 (1.019–1.026)
	No HW[a]				
Age group	60+ years		3.027 (2.737–3.348)	8.041 (7.934–8.151)	1.212 (1.210–1.214)
	15–59 years		1.172 (1.064–1.290)	3.887 (3.836–3.939)	
	0–14 years				1.315 (1.313–1.317)
Gender	Male		1.939 (1.814–2.072)	0.898 (0.893–0.903)	0.992 (0.991–0.993)
	Female				
SEIFA	Most disadvantaged + Q2		1.343 (1.242–1.452)	1.262 (1.252–1.272)	1.546 (1.544–1.548)
	Q3		1.166 (1.085–1.252)	1.119 (1.112–1.127)	1.200 (1.198–1.202)
	Least disadvantaged + Q4				
ARIA	Remote and very remote		2.132 (1.939–2.343)	1.255 (1.242–1.268)	3.269 (3.263–3.275)
	Moderately accessible		1.576 (1.426–1.742)	0.943 (0.933–0.954)	2.243 (2.238–2.247)
	Accessible		1.070 (0.999–1.147)	1.034 (1.027–1.040)	1.322 (1.320–1.324)
	Highly accessible				
Public holiday	Yes		1.102 (0.965–1.258)	1.009 (0.996–1.022)	1.121 (1.118–1.124)
	No				
Month	November		3.444 (2.984–3.975)	1.140 (1.129–1.151)	1.029 (1.027–1.031)
	December		3.636 (3.159–4.184)	1.072 (1.062–1.083)	1.042 (1.039–1.044)
	January		4.572 (3.990–5.238)	1.149 (1.138–1.159)	1.005 (1.003–1.008)
	February		3.135 (2.718–3.616)	1.174 (1.163–1.185)	1.013 (1.011–1.015)
	March		2.236 (1.930–2.589)	1.096 (1.086–1.106)	1.024 (1.022–1.026)
	April				
Year	2015		1.212 (1.070–1.374)	1.529 (1.508–1.549)	1.054 (1.051–1.057)
	2014		1.083 (0.967–1.213)	1.537 (1.519–1.556)	1.067 (1.064–1.070)
	2013		1.111 (0.992–1.244)	1.654 (1.634–1.674)	1.108 (1.105–1.111)
	2012		1.114 (0.997–1.246)	1.626 (1.606–1.646)	1.129 (1.126–1.131)
	2011		0.766 (0.676–0.868)	1.543 (1.523–1.562)	1.124 (1.121–1.127)
	2010		0.773 (0.682–0.876)	1.400 (1.382–1.418)	1.059 (1.056–1.061)
	2009		0.743 (0.652–0.847)	1.208 (1.192–1.224)	1.042 (1.039–1.045)
	2008		0.659 (0.576–0.755)	1.143 (1.127–1.158)	1.021 (1.018–1.024)
	2006		0.579 (0.469–0.715)	1.066 (1.046–1.088)	1.010 (1.006–1.013)
	2007				
Weekend	Weekend		1.042 (0.980–1.108)	0.994 (0.988–1.000)	1.068 (1.067–1.070)
	Weekday				
Age group[a] HW intensity	60+ years	Severe/extreme	2.142 (1.330–3.450)	0.950 (0.856–1.055)	1.013 (1.000–1.027)
	60+ years	Low intensity	1.757 (1.326–2.328)	1.023 (0.977–1.070)	0.990 (0.985–0.996)
	60+ years	No HW[a]			
	15–59 years	Severe/extreme	1.521 (0.948–2.440)	0.955 (0.863–1.057)	
	15–59 years	Low intensity	1.666 (1.268–2.189)	1.033 (0.989–1.080)	
	15–59 years	No HW[a]			
	0–14 years	Severe/extreme			0.969 (0.957–0.980)
	0–14 years	Low intensity			0.944 (0.939–0.949)
	0–14 years	No HW[a]			
Gender[a] HW intensity	Male	Severe/extreme	0.864 (0.665–1.122)	0.969 (0.927–1.012)	0.965 (0.955–0.974)
	Male	Low intensity	1.277 (1.081–1.508)	1.020 (1.001–1.039)	1.000 (0.996–1.004)
	Male	No HW[a]			
	Female	Severe/extreme			
	Female	Low intensity			
	Female	No HW[a]			

[a]*Under these headings, any cells without RRs and 95% confidence intervals (CIs) are reference categories, and in the brackets are 95% CIs; HW, heat wave.*

There was an apparent dose–response relationship between SEIFA and all three health service usage measures. The more disadvantaged the population, the higher the rate of health service usage.

There was also an apparent dose–response relationship between ARIA and heat-related hospitalization, ED attendance, and kidney disease-related hospitalization rates overall. The less accessible services were, the higher the health impact.

Emergency department attendance rates were higher during pubic holidays and weekend. However, there were no statistically significant differences in admission rates for heat- and kidney disease-related hospital admissions between these two periods. Other variables, such as year and month, were also used to adjust the possible impact of these confounding factors on the three health service utilization rates. Interactions of age and gender with HW effect were also examined. For details of their impact, refer to **Table 2**.

Identify Geographical Variation in Population Response to HW

Figure 1 shows the composite ranking of the effects of HW by LGA in WA. Only three significant health service usage measures were included in the calculation of the composite ranking. In the populous Perth metropolitan area (as shown in the insert in the map), the overall impacts of HW were between small to high. In the majority of the southern areas, there was a higher impact from HW than the northern areas. However, the highest impact areas were all located in regional and remote areas.

DISCUSSION

Sensitivity of Data Sources/Conditions

Outcomes from this study indicated that the heat-related hospitalizations and overall ED presentations were the two most sensitive measures for assessing the impact of HW on health services. Hospital admissions due to kidney diseases were also sensitive. However, overall hospital admissions, hospital admissions due to cardiovascular and respiratory diseases, and all-cause deaths were not sensitive to HW. Similar findings were observed in other studies between HW and ED attendances and hospital admissions due to kidney diseases (18, 19). We also found that the effect of HW on health service indicators examined were not usually immediate and different data sources and conditions had diverse delayed effects of HW. Overall ED attendances and heat-related hospitalizations showed an early effect of HW within 3 and 5 days of a HW event, respectively. This is consistent with some previous studies where lag effects of HW were apparent with a short lag effect for ED attendance data (14, 20, 21). However, kidney disease-related hospital admissions reached their peak rate 25 days after a HW event.

The different lag effect in different data sources is most likely due to varying patient case-mix and structure of the general population involved. In heat-related hospitalizations, only records with heat-related conditions were included. These data sources may potentially fail to identify patients affected by HW but who present to hospital due to exacerbation of pre-existing comorbidities. Although we have excluded elective patients from hospitalization data, in an attempt to identify hospitalizations potentially related to heat exposure, we could not identify an apparent association between all-cause hospitalizations and HW intensity. In ED attendance data, however, all patients were included and potentially heat-related conditions would be included.

Indicators such as heat-related hospitalizations and overall ED attendances can provide responding agencies with insight into the impact of HW on health services. ED datasets are rapidly accessible and could be used for syndromic surveillance. However, hospitalization and mortality data are usually not available for up to 6 months or even longer, which render them unsuited for timely identification of HW-related vulnerable populations and activation of emergency response strategies. Findings from this study reinforce the response strategy of using rapidly accessible ED data to monitor heat-related health impacts during HW events. Therefore, the design of HW service provision must take into account the sensitivity and timeliness of data sources.

Resilience and Vulnerability to HW

Our study confirmed that age was an important risk factor for HW: people aged 60 years and over were more vulnerable to HW than other age groups and attended health services more frequently, and young people aged 14 and less were more vulnerable to HW for ED services. Gabriel and Endlicher (10) and Tong et al. (11) indicated that the elderly may suffer more due to poor thermoregulation and hormonal changes. Older people with chronic diseases such as cardiovascular and respiratory diseases were particularly vulnerable (22, 23). Previous studies also found that children were at high risk of morbidity and mortality during HWs (8, 9, 14, 24) and children's inability to lose heat through sweating could cause convulsions and disorientation (17).

Anderson et al. (25) found that there was no significant difference between the vulnerability of males and females during HWs in relation to respiratory hospitalizations. However, our study did identify a significant difference between males and females in heat- and kidney disease-related hospitalizations. Our study observed a higher impact on males than females in heat-related hospitalizations while the study from Rainham and Smoyer-Tomic (26) observed that females had a higher relative risk of mortality than males. This may be due to more men working outside when there is a HW; however, the exact reason warrants further exploration.

Previous studies found that chronic diseases are also risk factors for increased health service utilization among people in extreme heat weather (12–14). People with chronic kidney and cardiovascular conditions are among the most susceptible to heat due to hyperthermia and dehydration. Although our study did not identify a strong association between the rate of hospitalization due to cardiovascular conditions and heat, we did find a strong association between the rate of hospitalization due to chronic kidney diseases and HW intensity, consistent with findings of Nitschke et al. (18) and Williams et al. (19).

Our findings on the main risk factors for HW morbidity were consistent with those identified by Reid et al. (27), which included SES (as indicated by education and poverty), social isolation, and

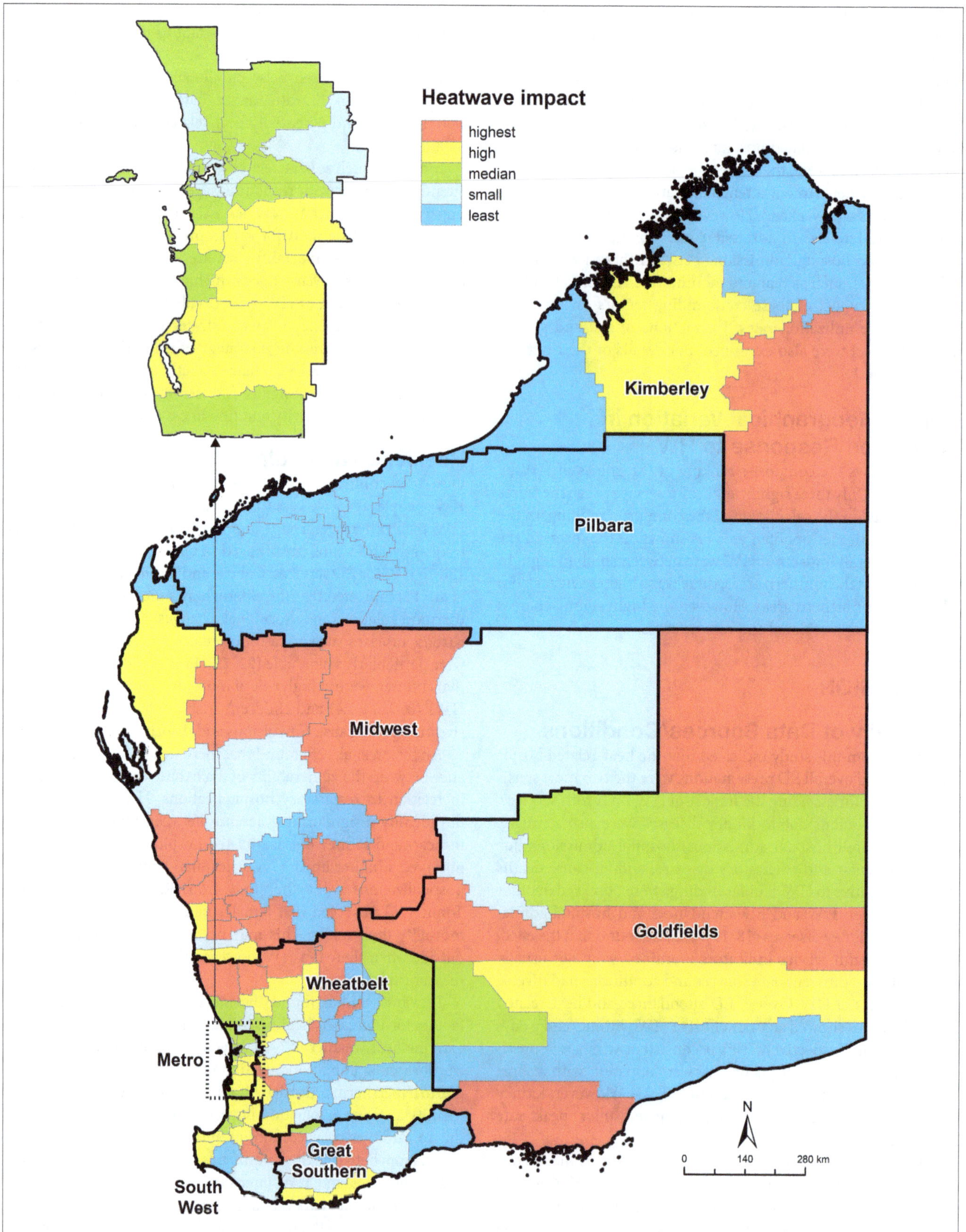

FIGURE 1 | Heat wave (HW) impact based on composite scores of difference in age standardized rates between HW and non-HW days by local government areas, November 2006 to April 2015, Western Australia.

proportion of elderly. The importance of SES in the evaluation of effects of HW was highlighted in several studies of vulnerability to HW (11, 28). Overall, populations with lower SES, poor accessibility to services, and older or younger age groups have higher vulnerability to HWs. The more risk factors in a population, the higher its vulnerability due to the additive feature of the regression models we applied. That means, the contribution of each risk factor would be added up to create a greater health utilization rate. Such vulnerable groups should be the main focus in the development and implementation of HW-related health promotion programs by relevant government and non-government agencies.

The possible joint effects of HW and age or gender were examined in this study and the regression modeling results showed in **Table 2**. The associations of risk factors and HW intensity were more complicated than expected. For example, the interaction between those aged over 60 years and the intensity of HW on heat-related hospitalization showed a clear dose–response relationship. However, the interaction between the two did not show an apparent dose–response relationship in age group 15–59 years. Instead, the heat-related hospitalization rate increased significantly in age group 15–59 years during low intensity HW exposure. Similarly, patterns were observed on interaction analysis between HW and males on heat-related hospitalization and kidney diseases-related hospitalization. Whether such a pattern was due to the impact from other unexamined risk factors warrants further exploration.

Regional Differences

This study was able to reinforce some assumptions on HW vulnerability and resilience in regional areas. Depending upon the data sources and conditions, regional responses to HW varied. For example, residents living in far north LGA regions (those with blue colors in **Figure 1**) with hot dry summer/cool or cold winter climate were least impacted by HWs. However, those living in LGAs with hot dry summer/mild winter climate were more vulnerable to HWs. Physiological acclimatization is likely to be an important factor limiting heat-related health service usage in hot humid or hot dry environment (4), and our study partially confirmed such an observation. However, the sensitivity of data should also be considered for obtaining most suitable health service indicators to explore the effect of HW on health service utilization.

All these regional differences in the study are most likely related to residents' acclimatization, the region's SES, accessibility to services, and age/gender and ethnicity distribution of the population as described in other studies (29–31). Which of these factors have played the most important role, and how they interact with each other, warrants further study.

The use of weighted ranking of difference in ASRs between HW and non-HW days by LGA allows us to combine the effects of HW on three data sources/conditions that showed a strong association with effects of HW. Local governments are the main government agencies who would implement the HW strategies. The hotspots identified *via* composite scores will be more reliable than a single health service usage measure in assisting local government agencies to allocate limited resources to those in most need.

Policy Implications for Emergency Management

As Michelozzi et al. (32) indicated in the consideration of global climate change that the impacts of heat on health will assume greater public health significance in future. The results from this study have significant policy implications for emergency management of HW. This study identified at risk population groups and provided a visual display mapping tool of HW vulnerability and resilience to assist local governments and emergency management regions.

By demonstrating the areas of greatest vulnerability, responding agencies are able to better target prevention and preparedness programs to those most in need. The findings from this study can also be used by local government authorities to better target, engage, and represent the needs of identified at risk groups within their boundaries. The geographical breakdown of HW risk factors will allow responding agencies to better understand and contextualize areas of vulnerability to HWs within their community and appropriately tailor community awareness programs, appropriate risk communication, and HW response plans to the needs of the community.

It is also worth noting that, in the design of the health promotion programs to tackle HWs, identified risk factors should be considered together, so that the programs can be implemented effectively and in an integrated fashion.

Limitations and Future Directions

The study did not include factors such as air quality measures and their potential interaction with HW intensity measures, as indicated in several studies (33, 34). This study did not include aboriginality as a risk factor, although this is a population group that experiences high rates of chronic kidney and cardiovascular disease (35), and social disadvantage (36). In addition, we did not adjust for the effect of green space on the health outcomes due to unavailability of such data in a vast state such as WA.

Limited diagnostic information in ED data prevented further examination of HW effects on populations with different causes of ill health. Improvements in ED data collection, particularly of diagnostic information, should be considered so that health education messages can effectively target higher risk groups.

Further studies are needed to explore the effects of HW on various disease conditions and on possible mechanisms that explain why populations living in different geographic locations have varied responses to HW. It is also important to conduct evaluation studies to assess the effectiveness of current preventative programs in relation to HW.

AUTHOR CONTRIBUTIONS

JX, TS, LJ, GY, and CS designed the study and contributed to draft and revision. JX, LJ, GY, and CS analyzed this work. JN and RF compiled the meteorological data used in the study. JN, RF, AR, and TW provided contribution to drafts and also revisions. All the authors confirmed the last version.

ACKNOWLEDGMENTS

The authors thank Peter Somerford and Shannon Carter of Epidemiology Branch, Department of Health WA for their support to the study; Dimpal Patel, master student of Curtin University of Technology for identifying relevant literature; and National Extreme Heat Warnings project members from University of Adelaide, Departments of Health New South Wales and South Australia for fruitful discussion on the methodology and issues in relation to the study.

REFERENCES

1. Australian Government. *State of Australian Cities 2013*. Canberra: Government of Australia (2013).
2. Coates L, Haynes K, O'Brien J, McAneney J, Dimer de Oliveira F. Exploring 167 years of vulnerability: an examination of extreme heat events in Australia 1844–2010. *Environ Sci Policy* (2014) 42:33–44. doi:10.1016/j.envsci.2014.05.003
3. Scalley B, Spicer T, Jian L, Xiao J, Nairn J, Robertson A, et al. Responding to heatwave intensity: excess heat factor is a superior predictor of health service utilisation and a trigger for heatwave plans. *Aust N Z J Public Health* (2015) 39:582–7. doi:10.1111/1753-6405.12421
4. Keatinge WR, Donaldson GC, Cordioli E, Marinelli M, Kunst AE, Mackenback JP, et al. Heat related mortality in warm and cold regions of Europe: observational study. *BMJ* (2000) 321:670–3. doi:10.1136/bmj.321.7262.670
5. Patz JA, Campbell-Lengrum D, Holloway T, Foley JA. Impact of regional climate change on human health. *Nature* (2005) 438:310–7. doi:10.1038/nature04188
6. Anderson BG, Bell ML. Weather-related mortality: how heat, cold, and heat waves affect mortality in the United States. *Epidemiology* (2009) 20:205–13. doi:10.1097/EDE.0b013e318190ee08
7. Fischer EM, Schar C. Consistent geographical patterns of changes in high-impact European heatwaves. *Nat Geosci* (2010) 3:398–403. doi:10.1038/ngeo866
8. Dalip J, Phillips GA, Jelinek GA, Weiland TJ. Can the elderly handle the heat? A retrospective case-control study of the impact of heat waves on older patients attending an inner city Australian emergency department. *Asia Pac J Public Health* (2015) 27:N1837–46. doi:10.1177/1010539512466428
9. Knowlton K, Rotkin-Ellman M, King G, Margolis HG, Smith D, Solomon G, et al. The 2006 California heat wave: impacts on hospitalizations and emergency department visits. *Environ Health Perspect* (2009) 117:61–7. doi:10.1289/ehp.11594
10. Gabriel KMA, Endlicher WR. Urban and rural mortality rates during heat waves in Berlin and Brandenburg, Germany. *Environ Pollut* (2011) 159:2044–50. doi:10.1016/j.envpol.2011.01.016
11. Tong S, Wang XY, Yu W, Chen D, Wang X. The impact of heatwaves on mortality in Australia: a multicity study. *BMJ Open* (2014) 4:2. doi:10.1136/bmjopen-2013-003579
12. Gronlund CJ, Zanobetti A, Schwartz JD, Wellenius GA, O'Neill MS. Heat, heat waves, and hospital admissions among the elderly in the United States, 1992-2006. *Environ Health Perspect* (2014) 122:1187. doi:10.1289/ehp.1206132
13. Turner LR, Connell D, Tong S. The effect of heat waves on ambulance attendances in Brisbane, Australia. *Prehosp Disaster Med* (2013) 28:482–7. doi:10.1017/S1049023X13008789
14. Wang X, Barnett AG, Yu W, Fitzgerald G, Tippett V, Aitken P, et al. The impact of heatwaves on mortality and emergency hospital admissions from non-external causes in Brisbane, Australia. *Occup Environ Med* (2012) 69:163–9. doi:10.1136/oem.2010.062141
15. Australian Bureau of Statistics. *Australian Demographic Statistics*. Canberra: Australian Bureau of Statistics (2016). Available from: http://www.abs.gov.au/ausstats/abs@.nsf/PrimaryMainFeatures/3101.0?OpenDocument
16. Nairn J, Fawcett RJB. The excess heat factor: a metric for heatwave intensity and its use in classifying heatwave severity. *Int J Environ Res Public Health* (2015) 12:227–53. doi:10.3390/ijerph120100227
17. Glasper A. Planning for a heat wave: the implications for health care. *Br J Nurs* (2011) 20:834–5. doi:10.12968/bjon.2011.20.13.834
18. Nitschke M, Tucker GR, Hansen AL, Williams S, Zhang Y, Bi P. Impact of two recent extreme heat episodes on morbidity and mortality in Adelaide, South Australia: a case-series analysis. *Environ Health* (2011) 10:42. doi:10.1186/1476-069X-10-42
19. Williams S, Nitschke M, Weinstein P, Pisaniello D, Parton K, Bi P. The impact of summer temperatures and heatwaves on mortality and morbidity in Perth, Australia 1994-2008. *Environ Int* (2012) 40:33–8. doi:10.1016/j.envint.2011.11.011
20. Khalaj B, Lloyd G, Sheppeard V, Dear K. The health impacts of heat waves in five regions of New South Wales, Australia: a case-only analysis. *Int Arch Occup Environ Health* (2010) 83:833–42. doi:10.1007/s00420-010-0534-2
21. Sun X, Sun Q, Yang M, Zhou X, Li X, Yu A, et al. Effects of temperature and heat waves on emergency department visits and emergency ambulance dispatches in Pudong New Area, China: a time series analysis. *Environ Health* (2014) 13:76–84. doi:10.1186/1476-069X-13-76
22. Schaffer A, Muscatello D, Broome R, Corbett S, Smith W. Emergency department visits, ambulance calls, and mortality associated with an exceptional heat wave in Sydney, Australia, 2011: a time-series analysis. *Environ Health* (2012) 11:3. doi:10.1186/1476-069X-11-3
23. Bustinza R, Lebel G, Gosselin P, Bélanger D, Chebana F. Health impacts of the July 2010 heat wave in Québec, Canada. *BMC Public Health* (2013) 13:1–7. doi:10.1186/1471-2458-13-56
24. Kovats RS, Hajat S, Wilkinson P. Contrasting patterns of mortality and hospital admissions during hot weather and heat waves in Greater London, UK. *Occup Environ Med* (2004) 61:893. doi:10.1136/oem.2003.012047
25. Anderson GB, Dominici F, Wang Y, McCormack MC, Bell ML, Peng RD. Heat-related emergency hospitalizations for respiratory diseases in the medicare population. *Am J Respir Crit Care Med* (2013) 187:1098. doi:10.1164/rccm.201211-1969OC
26. Rainham DGC, Smoyer-Tomic KE. The role of air pollution in the relationship between a heat stress index and human mortality in Toronto. *Environ Res* (2003) 93:9–19. doi:10.1016/S0013-9351(03)00060-4
27. Reid CE, O'Neill MS, Gronlund CJ, Brines SH, Brown DG, Diez-Roux AV, et al. Mapping community determinants of heat vulnerability. *Environ Health Perspect* (2009) 117:1730–6. doi:10.1289/ehp.0900683
28. Toloo GS, Yu W, Aitken P, FitzGerald G, Tong S. The impact of heatwaves on emergency department visits in Brisbane, Australia: a time series study. *Crit Care* (2014) 18:R69. doi:10.1186/cc13826
29. Betancourt JR, Green AR, Carrillo JE, Ananeh-Firempong HO II. Defining cultural competence: a practical framework for addressing racial/ethnic disparities in health and health care. *Public Health Rep* (2003) 118:293–302. doi:10.1016/S0033-3549(04)50253-4
30. Mechanic D, Tanner J. Vulnerable people, groups, and populations: societal view. *Health Aff (Millwood)* (2007) 26:1220–30. doi:10.1377/hlthaff.26.5.1220
31. Matthies F, Bickler G, Cardenosa Marin N, Hales S. *Heat Health Action Plans*. Copenhagen, Denmark: WHO Regional Office for Europe (2008).
32. Michelozzi P, De Sario M, Accetta G, de'Donato F, Kirchmayer U, D'Ovidio M, et al. Temperature and summer mortality: geographical and temporal variations in four Italian cities. *J Epidemiol Community Health* (2006) 60:417–23. doi:10.1136/jech.2005.040857
33. De Sario M, Katsouyanni K, Michelozzi P. Climate change, extreme weather events, air pollution and respiratory health in Europe. *Eur Respir J* (2013) 42:826. doi:10.1183/09031936.00074712
34. Jian L, Zhao Y, Zhu Y-P, Zhang M-B, Bertolatti D. An application of ARIMA model to predict submicron particle concentrations from meteorological factors at a busy roadside in Hangzhou, China. *Sci Total Environ* (2012) 426:336–45. doi:10.1016/j.scitotenv.2012.03.025
35. AIHW. *Cardiovascular Disease, Diabetes and Chronic Kidney Disease – Australian Facts: Aboriginal and Torres Strait Islander People*. Australian Government: Australian Institute of Health and Welfare (2015). Available from: http://www.aihw.gov.au/publication-detail/?id=60129553629
36. Mitrou F, Cooke M, Lawrence D, Povah D, Mobilia E, Guimond E, et al. Gaps in Indigenous disadvantage not closing: a census cohort of social

8

Expression of the Biologically Active Insulin Analog SCI-57 in *Nicotiana benthamiana*

*Adriana Muñoz-Talavera[1], Miguel Ángel Gómez-Lim[2], Luis A. Salazar-Olivo[3], Jörg Reinders[4], Katharina Lim[5], Abraham Escobedo-Moratilla[6], Alberto Cristian López-Calleja[2], María Cristina Islas-Carbajal[1] and Ana Rosa Rincón-Sánchez[7]**

[1] Department of Physiology, Institute of Experimental and Clinical Therapeutics, University Center for Health Sciences, University of Guadalajara, Guadalajara, Mexico, [2] Department of Genetic Engineering, Center for Research and Advanced Studies of the National Polytechnic Institute, Irapuato, Mexico, [3] Division of Molecular Biology, Institute for Scientific and Technological Research of San Luis Potosí, San Luis Potosí, Mexico, [4] Scientific Support Unit Analytical Chemistry, Leibniz Research Centre for Working Environment and Human Factors, Dortmund, Germany, [5] Institute of Functional Genomics, University of Regensburg, Regensburg, Germany, [6] CONACYT-Consortium for Research, Innovation, and Development of the Drylands (CIIDZA), IPICYT, San Luis Potosí, Mexico, [7] Institute of Molecular Biology and Gene Therapy, Department of Molecular Biology and Genomic, University Center for Health Sciences, University of Guadalajara, Guadalajara, Mexico

***Correspondence:**
Ana Rosa Rincón-Sánchez
anarosarincon@yahoo.com.mx

Diabetes mellitus is a growing problem worldwide; however, only 23% of low-income countries have access to insulin, and ironically it costs higher in such countries than high-income ones. Therefore, new strategies for insulin and insulin analogs production are urgently required to improve low-cost access to therapeutic products, so as to contain the diabetes epidemic. SCI-57 is an insulin analog with a greater affinity for the insulin receptor and lower thermal degradation than native insulin. It also shows native mitogenicity and insulin-like biological activity. In this work, SCI-57 was transiently expressed in the *Nicotiana benthamiana* (*Nb*) plant, and we also evaluated some of its relevant biological effects. An expression plasmid was engineered to translate an N-terminal ubiquitin and C-terminal endoplasmic reticulum-targeting signal KDEL, in order to increase protein expression and stability. Likewise, the effect of co-expression of influenza M2 ion channel (M2) on the expression of insulin analog SCI-57 (SCI-57/M2) was evaluated. Although using M2 increases yield, it tends to alter the SCI-57 amino acid sequence, possibly promoting the formation of oligomers. Purification of SCI-57 was achieved by FPLC cation exchange and ultrafiltration of *N. benthamiana* leaf extract (NLE). SCI-57 exerts its anti-diabetic properties by stimulating glucose uptake in adipocytes, without affecting the lipid accumulation process. Expression of the insulin analog in agroinfiltrated plants was confirmed by SDS-PAGE, RP-HPLC, and MS. Proteome changes related to the expression of heterologous proteins on *N. benthamiana* were not observed; up-regulated proteins were related to the agroinfiltration process. Our results demonstrate the potential for producing a biologically active insulin analog, SCI-57, by transient expression in *Nb.*

Keywords: diabetes, insulin analog SCI-57, proteomic profile, *Nicotiana benthamiana*, transient expression, 3T3-L1 adipocytes

INTRODUCTION

Diabetes is a public health problem, as it has been estimated that the number of patients with diabetes in 2040 will be 642 million, representing 10% of world population (Ogurtsova et al., 2017).

In order to manage the autoimmune destruction of insulin-producing pancreatic beta cells in type 1 diabetes (DM1), it is necessary to administer insulin *via* lifelong daily injection. Currently, worldwide, DM1 represents 5% to 10% of all diabetes cases (You and Henneberg, 2016), however, the use of insulin is not limited to only those people afflicted with DM1. A prospective study on diabetes in the UK (UKPDS) showed that to achieve better glycemic control, after five years, more than 50% of people with type 2 diabetes (DM2) required additional medication such as insulin (King et al., 1999). Similarly, general recommendations for patients with DM2, published by the American Diabetes Association (ADA) and the European Association for the Study of Diabetes (EASD), include insulin and insulin analogs as treatment options in dual and triple anti-hyperglycemic therapy (Inzucchi et al., 2015).

As a consequence of the increasing incidence of diabetes, the need for insulin and insulin analogs will augment exponentially. Therefore, new strategies for insulin and insulin analog production are urgently required, in order to increase the availability of therapeutic products for containing the diabetes epidemic. Likewise, globally, only 23% of low-income countries reported that insulin is generally available, although at higher costs than high-income countries (WHO, 2016). The average insulin cost increased three-fold from 2002 to 2013, with availability and rising costs having an impact on diabetes patients and health systems worldwide (Hua et al., 2016). For these reasons, the study of new platforms for the expression of insulin and insulin analogs costs is of utmost importance.

Recombinant human insulin is predominantly produced using *Escherichia coli* and yeast. *E. coli*, as expression system implicates several disadvantages; insulin is obtained *via* the production of insulin precursors (IP), therefore *in vitro* cleavage and oxidative refolding are necessary. In addition, some IP forms inclusion bodies requiring solubilization. With regard to yeast-based expression systems, although the insulin is correctly folded and directly secreted in the culture supernatant, the standard recovery and purification process may require numerous steps (Mollerup et al., 2002).

Plants are considered to be safe, effective, and affordable alternative systems for producing a wide variety of recombinant proteins such as enzymes, vaccines, and other biopharmaceuticals (Ma et al., 2005; Redwan, 2007; Castillo-Esparza, 2014). Their most important advantage over bacterial, yeast or mammal systems relates to the low cost of large-scale production (Twyman et al., 2003; Ma et al., 2005), partly because the necessary processes comprise existing agricultural systems, thus reducing operating and capital costs (Lico et al., 2008). Studies carried out by Tuse and collaborators have shown that costs can be as high as 1.00–2.00 dollars per kilogram of protein (Tuse et al., 2014). Plant-based expression systems hold tremendous potential for high-capacity production of insulin, in a very cost-effective manner, and may also contend with bacterial and yeast disadvantages such as extensive purification requirements (Baeshen et al., 2014). Recombinant human insulin has been successfully produced in transgenic *Arabidopsis thaliana* (Nykiforuk et al., 2006), and human proinsulin in transgenic tobacco and lettuce chloroplasts (Boyhan and Daniell, 2011), creating a natural cell store with long-term stability that provides storage until required.

Recombinant proteins can be produced in plants by genetic transformation or transient expression. Stable transformation involves the chromosomal integration of the gene of interest. This process can therefore take substantial time (often years) and require considerable resources. Likewise, the expressed protein yield is relatively low, and the release of a transgenic plant implies biosecurity problems (Edelbaum et al., 1992; Kusnadi et al., 1997). Recent studies have shown that proteins generated by transient expression (magnifection) have benefits, as human pathogens are not involved; thus, sterility is not required during production, meaning expression is rapid and high-level, with the potential to provide gram quantities of product in less than 4 weeks to use in clinical trials for FDA approval (Buyel, 2018). Phase I of the clinical study to produce immunoglobulins for the treatment of non-Hodgkin's lymphoma, by transient expression in *Nicotiana benthaminana*, has been completed (Klimyuk et al., 2014). Another recent development in this field is the production of ZMapp, a combination of three chimeric monoclonal antibodies destined to the treatment of Ebola virus disease. This combination is being developed as a product of molecular agriculture by the Leaf Biopharmaceutical Company and is produced by transient expression in *N. benthamiana* (Budzianowski, 2015; Hiatt et al., 2015). ZMapp was approved by the FDA and WHO during the Ebola outbreak in West Africa in 2014, because the transient expression system allowed rapid production, and previous studies had shown positive results among primates (Qiu et al., 2014). Subsequently, ZMapp began formal clinical development and recently completed phase II trials in Liberia, Sierra Leone, Guinea, and the United States (Na et al., 2015; Davey et al., 2016).

SCI-57 is an insulin analog that has a ten-fold affinity for the insulin receptor, higher resistance to thermal degradation than insulin, native mitogenicity and biological effect. The objective of this work was to transiently express the insulin analog SCI-57 in *N. benthamiana* leaves, purify, and characterize the protein by Reversed-Phase High-Performance Liquid Chromatography (RP-HPLC), mass spectrometry (MS), Diagonal two-dimensional electrophoresis (D-2DE) and enzyme-linked immunosorbent assay (ELISA). Here, we developed a new strategy for the production and purification of SCI-57 in plant leaves, evaluating some of its diabetes-relevant biological effects such as triglyceride accumulation and 2-NBDG uptake in 3T3-L1 adipocytes.

MATERIALS AND METHODS

Construction of Expression Vectors

The native version of the protein was obtained from the Protein Data Base (PDBID: 2JZQ). Three molecular strategies were used to increase the expression and accumulation of the insulin analog SCI-57: 1) The addition of a retention signal (KDEL peptide) at the carboxyl-terminus end to direct the recombinant protein to the endoplasmic reticulum, ensuring its correct folding and accumulation (Fischer and Emans, 2000; Cabrera et al., 2003; Conley et al., 2011; Giritch et al., 2015; Lacombe et al., 2018). 2) Ubiquitin fusion at amino-terminus to increase protein expression levels (Hondred et al., 1999; Streatfield, 2007; Benchabane et al., 2008); the ubiquitin at the plasmid construct was located on the 5' end, downstream of the translationally silent *BsaI* site, and 10 bp from the start codon (**Supplementary Figure S1**). 3) Co-expression of the ion channel of the influenza virus (M2) to increase the yield and quality of the recombinant protein (Sainsbury et al., 2013; Jutras et al., 2015); M2 was on the pMDC85 plasmid (PMDC85-M2). For optimal expression in plants, the gene encoding SCI-57 was codon optimized and synthesized (GenScript, USA). The 451 bp fragment corresponding to SCI-57 gene, KDEL peptide, and ubiquitin was digested with *BsaI* and subcloned in the *BsaI* site of pICH31070, in order to obtain the pICH31070-SCI-57 expression vector. pICH31070 containing green fluorescent protein (GFP) was used as positive control (pICH31070-GFP).

The vectors were introduced—the 5′ module (pICH15879), the 3′ module (pICH31070-SCI-57, pICH31070-GFP, PMDC85-M2), and the integrase module (pICH14011)—in *Agrobacterium tumefaciens* GV3101 strain by electroporation.

Agroinfiltration of *N. Benthamiana* Plants

The infiltration procedure was carried out, following our laboratory procedure (Coconi-Linares et al., 2013). In brief, GV3101 cells were incubated at 28°C with constant agitation (180 rpm) in YEB liquid medium with 50 mg/l kanamycin until the OD 600_{nm} = 1.0. Subsequently, cultures were diluted with infiltration buffer (10 mM MES (4-morpholineethanesulfonic acid) pH 5.5, 10 mM $MgSO_4$ and 100 μM acetosyringone) to achieve an OD 600_{nm} = 0.6.

The bacterial suspension containing pICH31070-GFP was mixed with equal volumes of the 5′ module and integrase module suspension. The bacterial suspension containing pICH31070-SCI-57 was mixed with equal volumes of the 5′ module and integrase module suspension, with or without pMDC85-M2 suspension to evaluate the M2 role in SCI-57 expression.

Bacterial suspension mixtures were infiltrated into plant leaves using syringes (**Figure 1A**). After infiltration, the plants were grown at 25°C during a 16-hour light/8-hour dark photoperiod, until GFP expression was observed over most of the leaf surface area (**Figure 1B**). After 4–5 days, the leaves were harvested and macerated using a mortar and pestle, in the presence of liquid nitrogen and stored at −80°C.

Extraction of Total Soluble Proteins (TSP) and SDS-PAGE

The macerated tissue was mixed and homogenized with the extraction buffer: 100 mM citrate buffer pH 4.3, 1 μl of protease inhibitor cocktail (Sigma-Aldrich, USA), and 10 μl of cellulases per ml (Roche, USA) at a ratio of 1 g leaf tissue to 1.5 ml buffer. Subsequently, this was incubated at 37°C for 1 h and afterwards centrifuged at 10,000 rpm for 15 min at 4°C. The resulting solution was filtered with cellulose acetate membranes of 0.8, 0.45, and 0.22 μm (Millipore Corporation, USA) in order to remove solids and pigments. The NLE was stored at 4°C for subsequent analysis.

We used a low pH extraction buffer to precipitate contaminants such as cell debris and photosynthetic pigments present in green tissues like the leaves of *N. benthamiana*. In addition, this method was also useful for precipitating the protein ribulose-1,5-bisphosphate carboxylase/oxygenase (RuBisCO) which represents approximately 50% of the TSP present in the leaves and usually complicates the generation of highly pure recombinant proteins (Bendandi et al., 2010; Lai et al., 2010; Tuse et al., 2015).

In order to measure the TSP in NLE, we conducted the Bradford analysis. A standard protein curve was constructed using bovine serum albumin (Sigma-Aldrich, USA) from 0 to 1.5 mg/ml, using the extraction buffer as diluent. The absorbance of the standards and samples was measured at 595 nm.

TSP were separated by 13% Tricine–SDS-PAGE under reducing conditions (5% β-mercaptoethanol) and samples were heated for 5 min at 95°C. Electrophoresis was performed for 90 min at 120V. Gels were visualized with Coomassie blue stain (Sigma-Aldrich, USA).

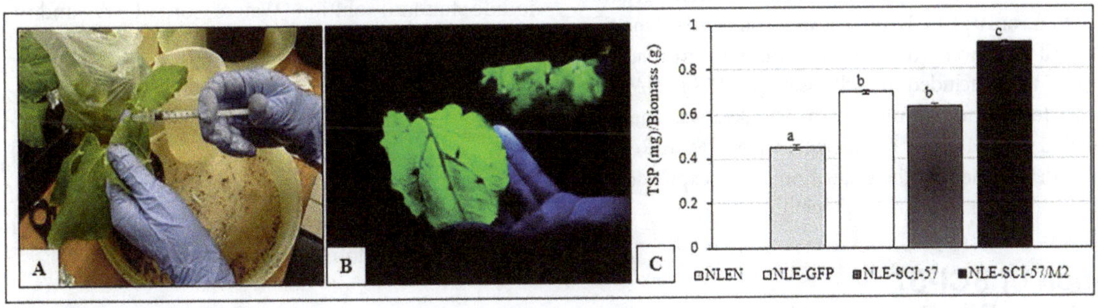

FIGURE 1 | (A) Syringe agroinfiltration of *Nicotiana benthamiana* leaves with *Agrobacterium tumefaciens*. **(B)** Transient expression of GFP in leaves of *N. benthamiana* 4 days after the agroinfiltration. **(C)** Bradford analysis of the total soluble proteins (TSP). Leaves were harvested four days post-agroinfiltration. Results are presented as the mean ± S.D. of three independent experiments in triplicate. Lowercase letters indicate significant differences according to the Mann-Whitney test ($p \leq 0.05$). NLEN, *N. benthamiana*-leaf extract from non-agroinfiltrated plants; NLE-GFP, *N. benthamiana*-leaf extract from GFP expressing plants; NLE-SCI-57, *N. benthamiana*-leaf extract from SCI-57 expressing plants; NLE-SCI-57/M2, *N. benthamiana*-leaf extract from SCI-57 expressing plants and co-expressing M2.

Extraction of Total RNA and cDNA Preparation

Total RNA was extracted from 100–200 mg of frozen agroinfiltrated leaves, following the manufacturer's procedure for TRIzol (Invitrogen, USA). The quality of these samples was evaluated by the presence of ribosomal bands on the ethidium bromide-stained agarose gel electrophoresis. Accordingly, total RNA was treated with DNase (Invitrogen, USA). RNA samples (5 µg) were reverse transcribed to generate single-stranded cDNA using an oligo (dT)18 Primer and 200 units of SuperScript III reverse transcriptase, as described by the manufacturer (Invitrogen, USA).

Gene Analysis by Endpoint PCR and Quantitative Real-Time PCR (qRT-PCR)

Primers were designed using the Primer select software (Graham and Holland, 2005) and validated with the help of the OligoAnalyzer program (Owczarzy et al., 2008) (data available in **Supplementary Table S1**). They were synthesized by the T4 Oligo company (T4 Oligo, México). Endpoint PCR was performed to amplify 18S rRNA, GFP and SCI-57, whereas qRT-PCR assays were performed to amplify 18S rRNA and SCI-57.

End-point PCR samples were amplified by applying the following program: initial denaturation at 98°C for 3 min, followed by 30 cycles of denaturation for 45 s at 94°C, annealing for 30 s at 60.4°C, and elongating for 30 s at 72°C. End-point PCR assays were performed on MultiGene™ OptiMax Thermal Cycler (Labnet International Inc., USA), and the enzyme Taq polymerase was used as described by the manufacturer (Invitrogen, USA) for a reaction volume of 25 µl with 250 ng of cDNA. No template controls (NTCs) were included with each instrument run for quality control, and 18S rRNA was chosen as the housekeeping gene. Samples were analyzed by 2% ethidium bromide-stained agarose gel electrophoresis.

qRT-PCR samples were diluted to a 100 ng/µl single-stranded cDNA concentration with sterile water. The CFX96 real-time PCR detection system (Bio-Rad, USA) was used for all qRT-PCRs. Samples were amplified using SYBR Green with the following program: initial denaturation at 95°C for 3 min, followed by 40 cycles of denaturation for 5 s at 98°C, annealing for 30 s at 60.4°C, and elongating for 30 s at 72°C. Amplification reactions were prepared using a total volume of 10 µl. PCR was followed by a standard melting curve analysis. All PCRs were run in triplicate, and control reactions without template were included in each assay. The 18S rRNA gene was used as a reference for normalization. The data was analyzed using the Bio-Rad CFX Manager 3.1 management software. Relative expression was determined by the evaluation of the expression by the $2^{-\Delta\Delta CT}$ (Livak and Schmittgen, 2001) method.

Purification of SCI-57

Cation Exchange Fast Protein Liquid Chromatography (FPLC)

Analysis was carried out with a column of SP-Sepharose Fast Flow (GE Healthcare, Sweden) connected to the FPLC equipment (ÄKTA avant 25, Amersham Biosciences, USA). Recombinant human insulin (PISA pharmaceutical, México) on citrate buffer was used as positive control (1.75 mg/ml). The column was equilibrated with 10 ml of binding buffer (100 mM citrate buffer pH 4.3). Then, 5 ml of NLE or insulin solution was passed through the column. The column was washed with 5 ml of washing buffer (100 mM citrate buffer pH 4.3). The mobile phases were buffer A (100 mM citrate buffer pH 4.3) and buffer B (100 mM citrate buffer pH 4.3 with 1M NaCl). The elution profile to achieve the separation constituted a gradient of 100% B for 60 min with a continuous flow rate of 0.4 ml/min; samples were collected in 1 ml fractions. Elution fractions were monitored by a single path ultraviolet monitor at 280 nm. SCI-57 presence on the fractions was evaluated by 13% Tricine SDS-PAGE.

The fractions containing SCI-57 were filtrated through centrifugal filter devices with a cutoff of 3 kDa (Millipore, USA).

Reversed-Phase High-Performance Liquid Chromatography (RP-HPLC) Analysis

Samples were analyzed using the HPLC System Agilent 12900 Infinity II (Agilent Technologies, USA). The diode array detector was set to collect signals within the spectral range of 200–400 nm. Chromatographic separation was performed on the chromatographic column (15 cm × 0.21 cm) Vydac 218MS C18 with a 5µ particle size and 300 A° pore size (Vydac, Hesperia, USA). The column was kept at 30°C in a column oven. During chromatographic separation, the mobile phase was in gradient elution from 100% A: H_2O 0.1% trifluoroacetic acid (TFA) to 100% B: acetonitrile (ACN) 0.1% TFA over 1 h at a flow rate of 0.5 ml/min. The sample injection volume was 20 µL. Agilent ChemStation software was used for collecting and processing the data.

Ionization Pattern and Exact Molecular Weight Determination

SCI-57

A 30 µM purified SCI-57 sample obtained from A2–A7 fraction concentration and solvent exchange into formic acid 0.1% by 3 kDa filter was analyzed using the SYNAPT-HDMS system (Waters Corp., USA) with ESI-Lockspray interphase. Prior to the experiments, the system was calibrated with a sodium iodide standard solution (Waters Corp., USA), and the European Pharmacopoeia Reference standard insulin (EP insulin) sample was analyzed as a positive control (30 µM).

In the experiment, data was acquired by injecting the protein solution directly into the interphase. We used a scan interval of 50–2,000 m/z with an ionizing spray voltage of 3.2 kV in positive ionization mode and a desolvation temperature of 110°C to acquire data. Molecular weight estimations were generated by the UniDec GUI versión 1.1.10 (Marty et al., 2015).

SCI-57 M2

The A2–A4 and A5–A7 fractions from SCI-57/M2 purification were concentrated by ultrafiltration with 3 kDa membranes and subsequently lyophilized. The resulting sample was dissolved in 0.1% TFA (16 µM), and the NaCl content was removed using

C18 Zip-Tips (Millipore Corp., USA). The EP insulin standard (18 µM) was used as a positive control. Hence, the samples were dissolved in alpha-cyano-4-hydroxycinnamic acid (3.5 mg/ml in 50% acetonitrile, 0.1% TFA) and left to dry at room temperature. Molecular weight analysis was performed in the MALDI TOF/TOF Analyzer 4800 plus mass spectrophotometer (Applied Biosystems/MDS SCIEX, USA) in linear mode and with a laser intensity of 3,800 Hz.

Identification of SCI-57 and Proteomic Profile by Gel-Assisted Sample Preparation (GASP), Using Liquid Chromatography-Tandem Mass Spectrometry (LC-MS/MS) and Applying Sequential Windowed Acquisition of All Theoretical Fragment Ion Mass Spectra (SWATH)

We used the FluoroProfile protein quantification kit to determine concentration of samples (Sigma-Aldrich Corporation), with BSA as standard. Equal amounts of protein (50 µg) were prepared in compliance with the GASP protocol, which was published by Fischer and Kessler (2015). The sample was dissolved on GASP buffer (8M urea, 2M thiourea, and 0.1 M DTT). Acrylamide/bis-acrylamide solution was added to reach a final concentration of 20%. The gel was formed by the TEMED and ammonium persulfate addition. Gel pieces were obtained by centrifugation through a plastic mesh and then fixed overnight by adding ethanol/acetic acid/water (40/10/50). In order to dehydrate the gel pieces, 1 ml of acetonitrile (ACN) was added, and then to rehydrate gel pieces, 0.5 ml 50 mM ammonium carbonate was added and shaken for 10 min. Gel pieces were dried in the speedvac for 2 h at 30°C. Trypsin solution 1:40 in 50 mM ammonium carbonate was added to the gel pieces at 37°C overnight for proteolysis. The addition of ACN and 5% formic acid were subsequently used to facilitate peptide extraction. The supernatant was dried using the speedvac and after the sample was resuspended in 5% formic acid.

From the sample containing the digested proteins, 8 µl were injected into the NanoLC 425 (AB Sciex) for peptide separation. Peptides were then separated on the YMC-Triart C18 1.9 µm, 3.0 × 150 mm column (YMC GmbH, Germany). The flow rate was set to 6 µL/min over 120-min multi-segment gradient: 0 min 98% A-2% B, 100 min 60% A-40% B, 102 min 20% A-80% B, 108 min 20% A-80% B, 110 min 98% A-2% B, 120 min 98% A-2% B (solvent A: 0.1% formic acid; solvent B: acetonitrile with 0.1% formic acid). The data set was generated when the fractionated peptides were transferred to the Q-TOF MS mass analyzer (TripleTOF 5600+, Sciex). The instrument was operated using positive ion with a mass resolution of ~30,000 for TOF MS scan (m/z 400–1,000) and ~15,000 for MS/MS; it was automatically calibrated after every two injections, using RePLiCal (Holman et al., 2016). A TOP20 method was used for the library runs, and variable SWATH-windows (60 windows from 400 to 1,000 m/z) were used for SWATH-MS-runs. The accumulation time for IDA was set to 250 ms for an MS1 scan and 50 ms per MS2 scan; the total cycle time was approximately 1.3 s. The accumulation time for SWATH was set to 50 ms for an MS1 scan and 35 ms per MS2 scan; the total cycle time was approximately 1.3 s (Reinders et al., 2016; Feist et al., 2018). The SWATH-library was built using the NCBI database, trypsin as protease, fragment ion mass tolerance of 0.055 Da, maximum one missed cleavage site, oxidation of methionine, pGlu for N-terminal Gln as variable modifications, only doubly and triply charged ions with the Protein Pilot 4.5 software (Sciex GmbH, Germany), and employing a 1% false discovery rate. In Skyline, a scoring model using the second best peaks for each peptide was employed using MProphet (Reiter et al., 2011). Furthermore, peak intensity, retention time difference, retention time difference squared, library intensity dot product, weighted peak shape, weighted co-elution, co-elution count, signal to noise ratio, and product mass error were factored in.

For the comparison in protein expression of the different *N. benthamiana* leaf extract, skyline MSstats was used. *N. benthamiana* leaf extract from non-agroinfiltrated plants (NLEN) were determined as a control group. *N. benthamiana* leaf extract from plants expressing GFP (NLE-GFP), *N. benthamiana* leaf extract from plants expressing SCI-57 (NLE-SCI-57), *N. benthamiana* leaf extract from plants expressing SCI-57, and co-expressing M2 (NLE-SCI-57/M2) were compared to the control group at a confidence level of 95%, resulting in the generation of a file for comparing protein expression levels. Data from Skyline software (3.7) were analyzed using Microsoft Excel 2016.

Diagonal Electrophoresis for the Detection of Disulfide Bridges

SDS-PAGE Tricine gel was run under non-reducing conditions (Schagger, 2006). The strip of gel containing the protein sample was cut from the gel slab of the first-dimensional electrophoresis. Following treatment with 10 mM DTT + 50% glycerol and 50 mM iodoacetamide, the band was embedded into another polyacrylamide gel slab for the second-dimensional electrophoresis, under reducing conditions. The gel was silver stained according to Blum et al. (1987). The EP insulin (1 µg) was used as positive control.

SCI-57 Detection by ELISA

SCI-57 concentration was assessed with the help of the Enzyme-Linked Immunosorbent Assay (ELISA) on the strength of the double binding test (Sandwich ELISA), using DRG Iso-Insulin ELISA Kit (No cat. EIA-2336) DRG Instruments GmbH (Germany). All technical procedures, described by the manufacturer, were adhered to.

3T3-L1 Adipogenesis

Confluent cultures of 3T3-L1 preadipocytes were induced to adipose differentiation with adipogenic medium (AM; L15 medium added with 10% (v/v) fetal bovine serum (FBS), 0.25 µM dexamethasone, 0.1 mM 3-isobutyl-1-methylxanthine, 1 µM d-biotin, 80 U/ml penicillin, 80 µg/ml streptomycin and 5 µg/ml insulin) (Herrera-Herrera et al., 2009). After three days, the cells were fed with maintenance medium (MM; L15 added with 10%

(v/v) FBS, 100 nM insulin, 1 μM d-biotin, 80 U/ml penicillin and 80 μg/ml streptomycin). 3T3-L1 preadipocytes were cultured with non-adipogenic medium to act as negative controls (NAM; L15 added to 10% (v/v) FBS).

Effect of SCI-57 on 3T3-L1 Adipogenesis

3T3-L1 preadipocytes were incubated with insulin-lacking adipogenic medium (AMI–) in the presence or the absence of 50 μl/ml NLE-SCI-57 or NLE-SCI-57/M2 or NLEN. Three days later, the cells were refed with insulin-lacking maintenance medium added to the respective NLE preparations. As a positive control, 3T3-L1 preadipocytes were incubated with insulin-containing AM and MM. Parallel experiments evaluated the synergic effects of insulin and NLE, by adding NLE preparations to insulin-containing medium.

After seven days in MM, the extent of lipid accumulation was estimated by staining intracellular triglycerides with oil red O (Ramirez-Zacarias et al., 1992).

Effect of SCI-57 on 2-NBDG Uptake by 3T3-L1 Adipocytes

Cell monolayers of terminally differentiated 3T3-L1 adipocytes cultured on 96-well fluorescence plates were incubated for 60 min with PBS containing BSA 1 mg/ml and 80 μM of the fluorescent glucose analog 2-NBDG (Zapata-Bustos et al., 2014b) in the presence of NLE-SCI-57, NLE-SCI-57/M2, NLEN (50 μl/ml each), or FPLC purified fractions (25 μl/ml). Positive controls received 100 nM insulin or 10 pM oral hypoglycemic rosiglitazone (RGZ). Afterward, cell monolayers were washed with PBS to remove free 2-NBDG, and the fluorescence retained in the cells was measured on a Tecan-GENios (Tecan, Austria) fluorescence reader at an excitation wavelength of 460 nm and emission at 540 nm, using the Magellan 4.0 program. The values of 2-NBDG incorporation in the absence of insulin were subtracted from those obtained with 100 nM insulin to establish 100% specific 2-NBDG incorporation.

Statistical Analysis

The data from most of the experiments was expressed as the mean ± the standard deviation for each group. The significant differences between groups were evaluated using non-parametric statistics. Kruskal–Wallis and Mann–Whitney U test were performed using SPSS Statistics version 20 (SPSS Inc., Chicago, IL, USA) where a p-value < 0.05 was considered statistically significant. Statistical analysis was applied to results from TSP, quantitative real-time PCR, intracellular triglycerides and 2-NBDG uptake.

RESULTS

Expression of Recombinant Proteins in *N. Benthamiana*.

The 451 bp coding sequence for SCI-57 was cloned into the pICH31070 plasmid. The *Bgl*II restriction analysis confirmed their presence with a resulting plasmid of 5,393 bp in size, as anticipated (**Supplementary Figure S1**).

It was necessary to recombine pro-vector modules within the cell of the plant in order to produce SCI-57. It was thus essential to ascertain that pro-vector assembly was carried out correctly, and that the transient expression of recombinant proteins in *N. benthamiana* was not affected by external factors. GFP was used as a visible tool to confirm the pro-vector assembly *in vivo* and therefore the SCI-57 expression. Four days after agroinfiltration (**Figure 1A**), GFP could be observed on the majority of leaf surfaces (**Figure 1B**). Leaves were thus harvested to obtain NLE. The quantity of TSP on NLE was determined by the Bradford assay. The Bradford assay revealed a TSP concentration which was at least 1.4 times higher in NLE from plants expressing heterologous proteins compared to NLEN. The greatest amount of TSP was observed on NLE-SCI-57/M2, followed by NLE-GFP and NLE-SCI-57. The results were presented as the mean ± S.D. of three independent experimental values for TPS (mg)/biomass (g) (**Figure 1C**).

To confirm the expression of SCI-57 in *Nb* plants, TSP extracts (TSPE) were separated by SDS-PAGE. A protein ~6.4 kDa in size, corresponding to SCI-57 molecular weight, was observed. The band was identified on NLE-SCI-57 and NLE-SCI-57/M2. However, band intensity was greater when M2 was co-expressed (**Figure 2**). The band was not detectable in NLEN or NLE-GFP (**Figure 2**).

Gene Analysis by Endpoint PCR and Quantitative Real-Time PCR (qRT-PCR)

First, total RNA was extracted from the different *Nb* plants and reverse transcribed with random primers. The cDNA was then subjected to PCR with specific primer pairs: 18S rRNA (149 bp), GFP (158 bp) and SCI-57 (196 bp). The 18S rRNA was chosen as a housekeeping gene. The presence of 18S rRNA was confirmed in agroinfiltrated and non-agroinfiltrated plants, as expected. The presence of GFP was observed on lane 3 when GFP primers were used. This lane corresponds to *Nb* agroinfiltrated with pICH31070-GFP. Whereas SCI-57 was observed on lane 4 when SCI-57 primers were used, a lane which corresponds to *Nb* agroinfiltrated with pICH31070-SCI-57 (**Figure 3A**).

In **Figure 3B**, a slight difference in band intensity between SCI-57 expression in the presence and absence of M2 co-expression is apparent. Our observations indicate that M2 co-expression increases SCI-57 yield.

Relative expression quantitative real-time PCR was employed in order to quantify SCI-57, using cDNA from agroinfiltrated plants, both with and without co-expressed M2. Final relative quantification was carried out using the comparative $2^{-\Delta\Delta CT}$ method. Expression levels were normalized using the 18S rRNA constitutive endogenous gene. The cDNA from agroinfiltrated plants with co-expressed M2 showed approximately two-fold change difference in SCI-57 level of expression compared with agroinfiltrated plants without co-expressed M2 (**Figure 3C**).

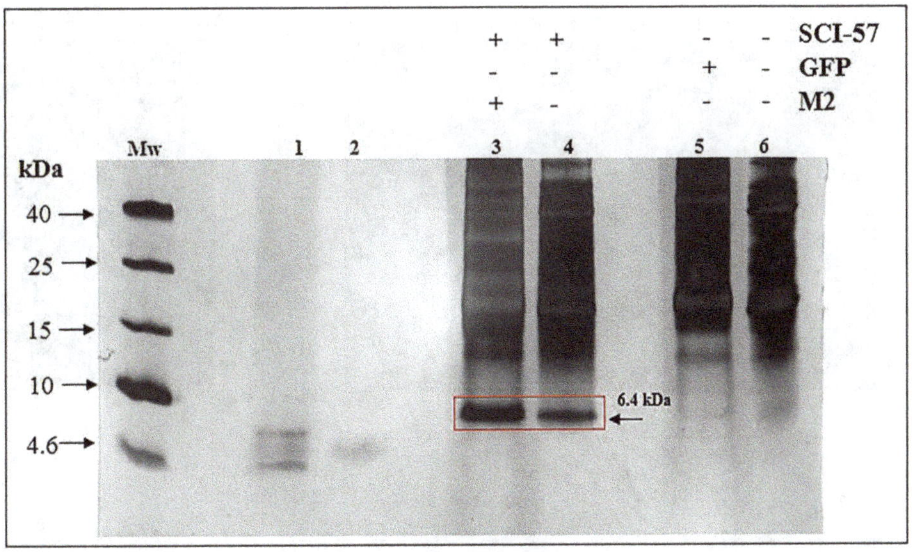

FIGURE 2 | TSP analysis from NLEN and NLE from agroinfiltrated plants by SDS-PAGE. Twenty micrograms of TSP were loaded per lane. Mw, Molecular weight marker; lane 1, Insulin 0.01 µg; lane 2, Insulin 0.001µg; lane 3, NLE-SCI-57/M2; lane 4, NLE-SCI-57; lane 5, NLE-GFP; lane 6, NLEN. Side numbers indicate molecular mass markers in kDa. Red Square and black arrow indicates the protein corresponding to SCI-57.

SCI-57 Purification

Purification of SCI-57 was carried out with a cation exchange column from the NLE-SCI-57 and NLE-SCI-57/M2 samples. The equipment allowed us to monitor the relative intensity at 280 nm of each fraction obtained (**Figures 4A** and **5A**).

High purity of SCI-57 is crucial when administered through direct injection into the blood of the diabetes patient. Correspondingly, SCI-57 purification was accomplished by cation exchange FPLC. The recombinant human insulin as a positive control was purified using ÄKTA avant 25 with prepacked SP-Sepharose Fast Flow. Insulin was eluted, displaying one peak on the chromatogram, from the fraction A4 to fraction A11 (**Supplementary Figure S2**). The aforementioned fractions corresponded to 0.17 M to 0.42 M NaCl. This is consistent with previous publications which establish that, under similar experimental conditions, insulin captured by the column was eluded from 0.10 to 0.45 M NaCl, recovering up to 70% (Jagschies et al., 2018). It was thus probable that SCI-57 would be eluted with a similar concentration of NaCl.

With respect to NLE-SCI-57 purification, two peaks were observed: one from A2–A6 and another from A7–A10, both eluting at the same NaCl concentration range as the insulin peak (**Figure 4A**). SDS-PAGE analysis from fraction A2–A5 (**Figure 4B**) displays one band corresponding to the insulin analog molecular weight ~ 6.4 kDa. SDS-PAGE analysis from the fractions conforming to the second peak (A6–A10) show a band corresponding to SCI-57 molecular weight, as well as several bands that may represent higher molecular weight proteins (**Figure 4C**). The SCI-57 recovery was greater than 60% of the protein captured by the column (**Table 2**). Regarding NLE-SCI-57/M2 purification, two peaks were observed in the chromatograms (**Figure 5A**). The first peak goes from fraction A1–A3 and the second peak from A4–A10. The A1–A10 fraction analysis (**Figures 5B, C**) detected a band corresponding to a protein with the size ~6.4 kDa and the presence of proteins with a molecular weight greater than 14 kDa, which was similar to the proteins observed on A7–A10 NLE-SCI-57 purification. The SCI-57/M2 recovery was 46% of the protein captured by the column (**Table 2**).

After identifying the fractions containing SCI-57, the elution fractions in which the protein is present were combined, and the resultant solution was concentrated twenty-fold in a 3-kDa cutoff filter (Millipore, Bedford, MA, USA). The resultant solution contains pure SCI-57, as revealed by the gel (**Figure 4D**, lane 8).

Reversed-Phase High-Performance Liquid Chromatography (RP-HPLC) Analysis

Once SCI-57 has been identified in the NLE-SCI-57, samples are evaluated by RP-HPLC. As a positive control, EP insulin, commercial insulin and bovine insulin were used. NLE-SCI-57 (**Figure 6D**) and NLE-SCI-57/M2 (**Figure 6E**) samples exhibit a peak with a retention time (RT) = 12.96 ± 1.30 and RT = 13.02 ± 1.30 min, which is similar to commercial insulin RT = 12.61 ± 1.26 (**Figure 6A**), EP insulin RT = 12.83± 1.28 (**Figure 6B**), and bovine insulin RT = 12.51± 1.25 (**Figure 6C**). The peak was not detectable in extracts of non-agroinfiltrated plants (**Figure 6F**).

After evaluating NLE-SCI-57, a purified SCI-57 sample from A2–A7 fractions was analyzed with the help of HPLC (**Figure 4D**, lane 8) to confirm that the peak observed on NLE-SCI-57 corresponds to the insulin analog SCI-57. The chromatogram (**Figure 6G**) displays a peak with a rt = 13.011, corresponding to the SCI-57 retention time previously observed on non-purified NLE-SCI-57.

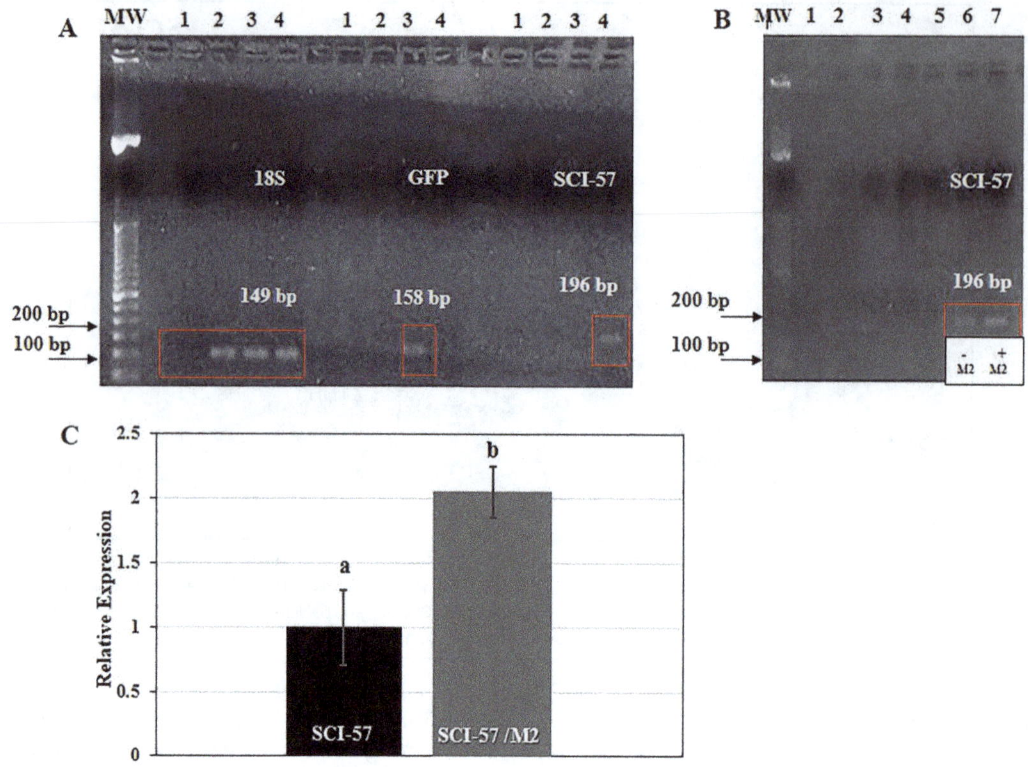

FIGURE 3 | (A) RT-PCR analysis of 18S, GFP and SCI-57 gene expression. Reactions were performed in the same conditions for all lanes, with specific primer pairs: 18S (149 bp), GFP (158 bp) and SCI-57 (196 bp). Mw: Molecular weight marker; lane 1: No template controls (NTCs); lane 2: No-agroinfiltrated N.b; lane 3: Plants agroinfiltrated with GFP; lane 4: Plants agroinfiltrated with SCI-57. The red square indicates the location of the amplification products. **(B)** RT-PCR analysis of SCI-57 gene expression with and without M2 co-expression. Reactions were performed in the same conditions for all lanes, with specific primer pairs: SCI-57 (196 bp). Mw, Molecular weight marker; lane 3, NTCs; lane 4, No-agroinfiltrated N.b; lane 5, Plants agroinfiltrated with GFP; lane 6, Plants agroinfiltrated with SCI-57; lane 7, Plants agroinfiltrated with SCI-57 co-expressing M2. The red square indicates the location of the amplification products. **(C)** Analysis of the relative expression of SCI-57 with and without the M2 co-expression by qRT-PCR. Relative expression was evaluated employing the RT-PCR primers (**Supplementary Table S1**). Expression was normalized against 18S rRNA gene expression. Results are presented as the mean ± S.D. of three independent experiments in triplicate. Lowercase letters indicate significant differences according to the Mann-Whitney U test ($p \leq 0.05$).

Ionization Pattern and Exact Molecular Weight Determination

An SCI-57 purified protein sample (A2–A7 fractions) was analyzed using a SYNAPT-HDMS system (Waters Corp.) with ESI-Lockspray interphase. Molecular weight estimations were generated by the UniDec GUI tool version 1.1.10 (Marty et al., 2015). Two SCI-57 proteins variants were identified from the sample (**Figure 7**). The protein variant with highest intensity had a molecular weight corresponding to SCI-57 (~6.4 kDa). The second protein variant had a molecular weight of ~ 7.1 kDa. The difference of mass units between the SCI-57 insulin analog and the protein mass identified is likely to refer to the addition of KDEL peptide to the protein sequence. The EP insulin experimental molecular weight was ~5.8 kDa (**Supplementary Figure S4**).

The samples from fractions A2–A4 and A5–A7 NLE-SCI-57/M2 and EP insulin were analyzed using a MALDI TOF/TOF Analyzer 4800 plus mass spectrophotometer (Applied Biosystems/MDS SCIEX, USA), using a linear mode with a laser intensity of 3,800 Hz. On the A2–A4 purified fractions, the presence of three proteins was identified; the most abundant on the sample had a molecular weight of ~7.1 kDa (**Figure 8A**). The protein was previously identified on the purified protein sample from NLE-SCI-57, probably representing the one corresponding to a molecular weight of SCI-57 + KDEL peptide. On the A5–A7 purified sample, the ~7.1 kDa protein was also identified (**Figure 8B**). The EP insulin molecular weight was ~5.8 kDa (**Supplementary Figure S5**).

Identification of SCI-57 and Proteomic Profile by Gel-Assisted Sample Preparation (GASP), Using Liquid Chromatography-Tandem Mass Spectrometry (LC-MS/MS) and Applying Sequential Windowed Acquisition of All Theoretical Fragment Ion Mass Spectra (SWATH)

We performed a differential proteomic NLE analysis on plants expressing heterologous proteins (GFP, SCI-57, and SCI-57/

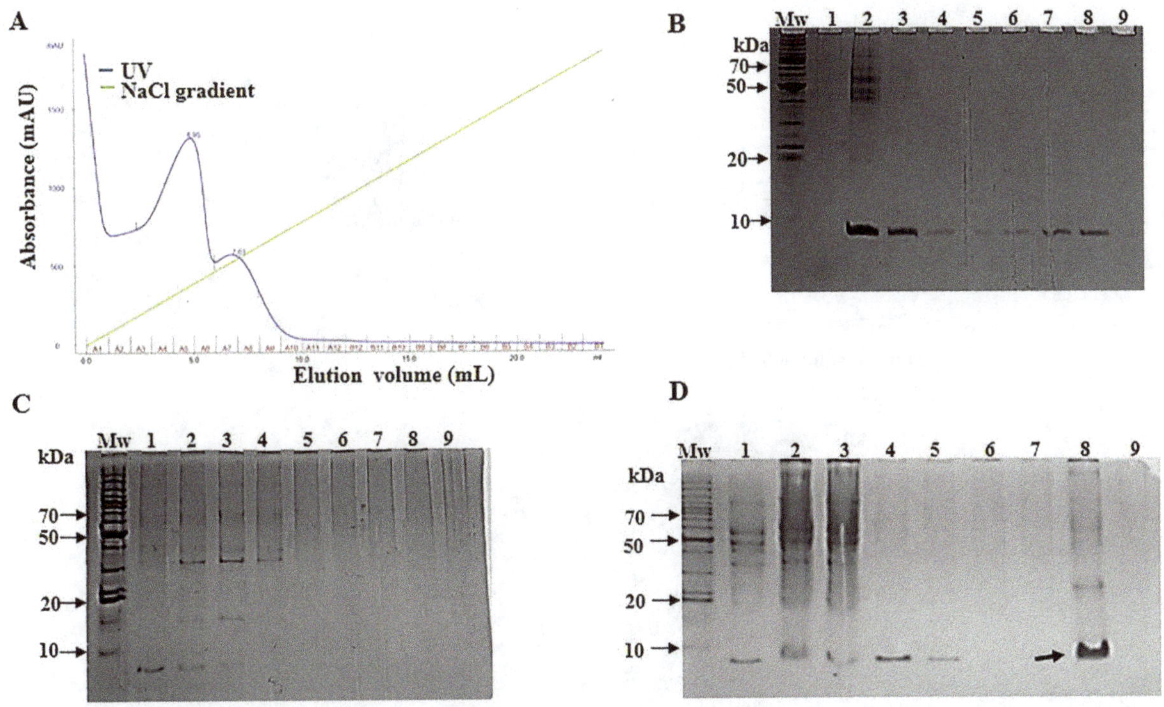

FIGURE 4 | NLE-SCI-57 purification and fraction analysis. **(A)** NLE SCI-57 cation exchange separation performed on SP-Sepharose Fast Flow. Five ml of the sample was loaded. Elution fractions were 1 ml, and the flow rate was set at 0.4 ml/min 100 mM citrate buffer pH 4.3 (elution with 0–1 M linear NaCl gradient). Absorbance was expressed in milli-absorbance units for the A280 (blue line). Fractions were labeled by the A–B letters from 1–12 numbers. **(B)** 13% Coomassie stained Glycine SDS-PAGE gel, on which NLE-SCI-57 elution fractions were resolved. Mw: Molecular weight marker; lane 1:3.5 µg recombinant human insulin (PISA pharmaceutical, México); lane 2,3: Flow through from the column; from lane 4 to 8: Fraction A1 to A5 respectively from SCI-57 purification by cation exchange. **(C)** 13% Coomassie stained Glycine SDS-PAGE gel, on which NLE-SCI-57 elution fractions were resolved. Mw: Molecular weight marker; from lane 1 to 9: Fraction A6 to B11 respectively from SCI-57 purification by cation exchange. **(D)** 13% Coomassie stained Glycine SDS-PAGE gel, displaying ultrafiltrated A2–A7 fractions obtained by the SCI-57 purification by FPLC. Mw, Molecular weight marker, lane 1; NLE SCI-57, lane 2, NLE SCI-57 concentrated with 3 kDa membrane, lane 3: Flow through from the column, lane 4 to 7: Fraction A1 to A4, lane 8: Sample containing A2–A7 fractions ultrafiltrated with 3 kDa membrane, and analyzed by HPLC. 5 µL molecular weight marker and 20 µL of each fraction were loaded on the gel. Arrow indicates the protein corresponding to SCI-57.

M2) and NLEN to identify the proteomic changes related to heterologous protein expression on the TSP extract. A total of 280 plant proteins were detected with at least two unique peptides. The 280 protein intensities on NLEN sample were used to normalize protein intensities on NLE of plants expressing heterologous proteins in order to determine relative protein expression.

On a TSP basis, 102 proteins were up-regulated, and 82 down-regulated in NLE-GFP, compared to non-agroinfiltrated leaves; similar to NLE-SCI-57, with 89 up-regulated proteins and 102 down-regulated. NLE-SCI-57/M2 manifested 103 up-regulated and 44 down-regulated proteins. The plants expressing heterologous proteins (GFP, SCI-57 and SCI-57/M2) share 48 up-regulated and 23 down-regulated proteins by at least twofold (**Supplementary Tables S2, S3**), work is also underway to address these proteins to the most affected biological processes in leaves. Interestingly, all the plants expressing heterologous proteins showed up to five-fold up regulated pathogenesis-related and stress-inducible proteins (**Table 1**) which are related to agroinfiltration as previously reported (Pruss et al., 2008; Goulet et al., 2010; Robert et al., 2015); for example: protease inhibitors (Kunitz 2 trypsin inhibitor), cell wall modifying enzymes (Expansin) and proteins related to the pathogenesis (PR) induced by *Agrobacterium* mainly PR-1 proteins (antimicrobial activity), PR-2 (β-glucanases) and PR-3 (chitinases).

Label-free analysis made it possible to identify the peptide FVNQHLCGSDLVEALYLVCERG on samples from plants expressing SCI-57 by measuring the intensity of the seven most intensive peptide fragment ions of the peptide. This peptide is also one of the identified peptides for the peptide map of insulin digestion with trypsin. The peptide was not detected on NLEN (**Supplementary Figure S6**).

Diagonal Electrophoresis for Detecting Disulfide Bridges

Figure 9 exhibited diagonal electrophoresis gels stained with silver, evaluating the presence of disulfide bridges in the NLE-SCI-57, NLE-SCI-57/M2, NLEN, and insulin samples. Spots or bands that ran off the diagonal and to the left of the slope indicated proteins containing disulfide bridges. Therefore, NLE-SCI-57 (**Figure 9A**) showed a protein corresponding to SCI-57 molecular weight, running off the diagonal to the left of the slope and indicating the presence of disulfide bridges. The NLE-SCI-57/M2 displayed

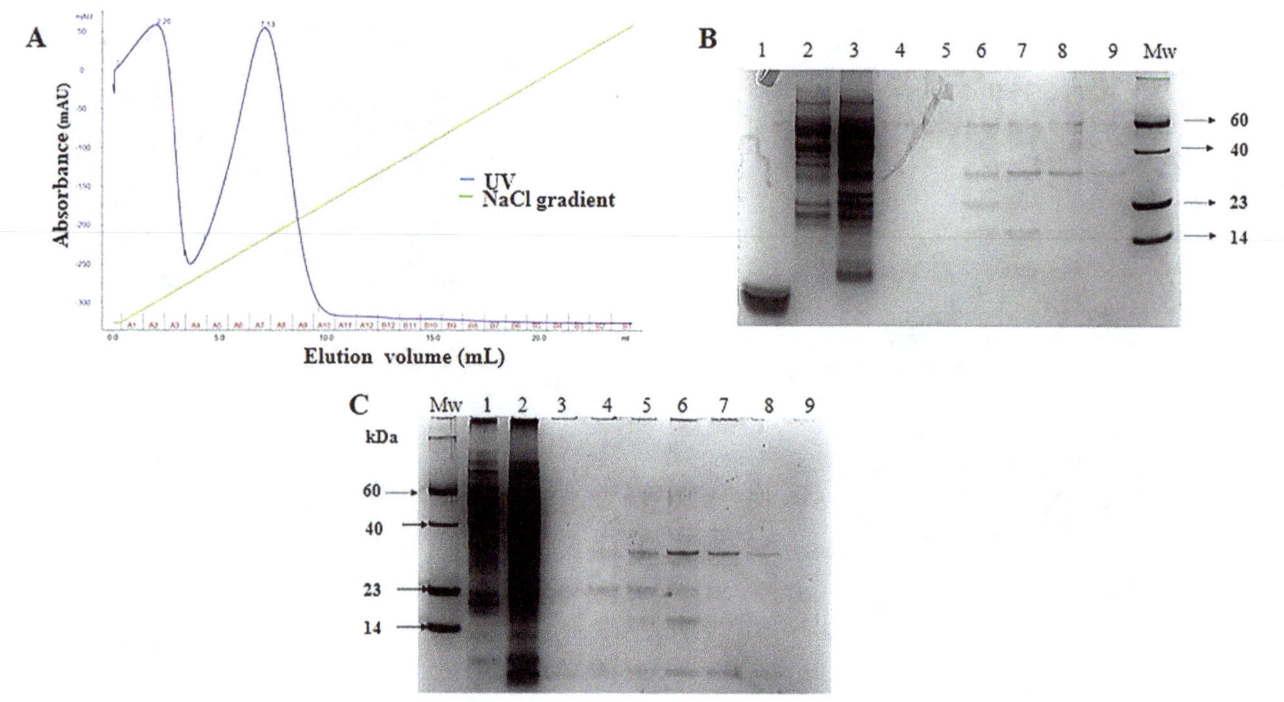

FIGURE 5 | NLE-SCI-57/M2 purification and fraction analysis. **(A)** NLE-SCI-57/M2 cation exchange separation performed on SP-Sepharose Fast Flow 5 ml of the sample was loaded. Elution fractions were 1 ml, and the flow rate was set at 0.4 ml/min 100 mM citrate buffer pH 4.3 (elution with 0–1 M linear NaCl gradient). Absorbance was expressed in milli-absorbance units for the A280 (blue line). Fractions were labeled by the A–B letters from 1–12 numbers. **(B)** 13% Coomassie stained Glycine SDS-PAGE gel, on which SCI-57/M2 elution fractions were resolved. Lane 1, Insulin 10 μg, lane 2, NLEN, lane 3, NLE SCI-57/M2, lane 4, A1 fraction, lane 5, A2 fraction, from lane 6 to 9, -Fraction A5 to A8 respectively obtained by the purification with cation exchange FPLC, Mw, Molecular weight marker. **(C)** 13% Coomassie stained Glycine SDS-PAGE gel, on which SCI-57/M2 elution fractions were resolved. Mw, Molecular weight marker, lane 1, NLEN, lane 2, NLE SCI-57/M2, from lane 3 to 9, A3 to A9 fractions. 5 μL molecular weight marker and 20 μL of each fraction were loaded on the gel.

a protein corresponding to SCI-57 molecular weight, however, it did not run off the diagonal (**Figure 9C**).

SCI-57 Detection by Anti-Insulin Antibodies

Quantitative determination of SCI-57 was accomplished by applying the enzyme-linked immunosorbent assay (ELISA) method. The response was measured using the commercially available insulin ELISA kit (DRG Insulin ELISA EIA-2935). The SCI-57 concentration was obtained by equation $y = 38.867x - 26.925$. The equation was obtained by plotting the absorbance values against insulin concentrations from the calibrator solutions provided in the kit, with a correlation coefficient of 0.9967. Purified SCI-57 obtained from NLE-SCI-57 A2–A7 fractions manifested a concentration of 1.16^{-6} mg/ml (26.65 mU/L). The sample was measured using the Bradford method with a concentration of 0.086 mg/ml. This concentration corresponds to 19.11% of total soluble protein (%TSP) or 0.1505 mg/g leaves fresh weight (LFW) (**Table 2**).

SCI-57 Affects 3T3-L1 Adipogenesis

In order to determine whether *Nb* preparations affect the development of adipose tissue, we evaluated their effects on 3T3 adipogenesis. When added to preadipocytes exposed to insulin-lacking adipogenic medium (AMI^-), NLE-SCI-57 stimulated the accumulation of lipids in these cells significantly compared to the insulin-lacking control (AMI^-), although to a lesser extent than the positive control adipogenic medium (AM). This proadipogenic effect was stronger in NLE-SCI-57/M2 treated cells and was not observed in cells treated with (NLEN) (**Figure 10**).

We then assayed the effects of NLE-SCI-57 and NLE-SCI-57/M2 in insulin-containing medium or adipogenic medium (AM) to determine whether the extracts have synergic effect on adipogenesis stimulation (**Figure 10**). Under these conditions, NLE-SCI-57 and NLE-SCI-57/M2 increased the pro-adipogenic effect of insulin. As in the previous assay, NLEN did not show proadipogenic effects.

SCI-57 Stimulates 2-NBDG Uptake

We evaluated the effect of SCI-57 on 2-NBDG incorporation in terminally differentiated 3T3-L1 cells to establish whether it stimulates glucose uptake by adipocytes (**Figure 11**). NLE-SCI-57 exerted a marked ~15.3-*fold* increase in the 2-*NBDG* uptake in comparison to insulin, whereas NLE-SCI-57/M2 exhibited a 5.3-fold increase. The NLEN stimulated 2-NBDG incorporation, causing a 6.5-fold increase.

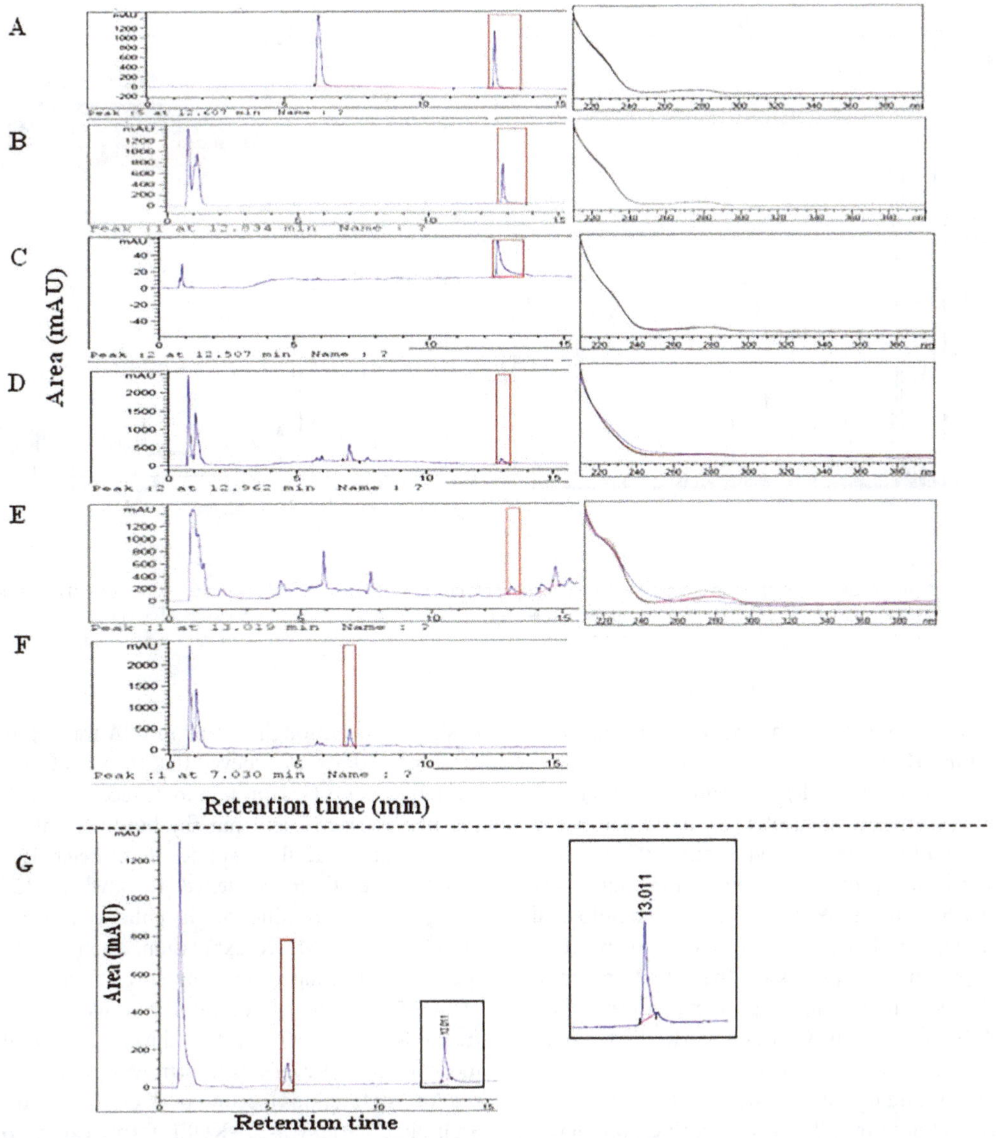

FIGURE 6 | Chromatograms and UV spectra respectively from: **(A)** Commercial insulin 0.12 mg/ml (PISA, pharmaceutics); **(B)** EP insulin 0.2 mg/ml; **(C)** Bovine insulin 0.125 mg/ml; **(D)** NLE SCI-57; **(E)** NLE SCI-57 M2; **(F)** NLEN; **(G)** Chromatogram from NLE-SCI-57 (A2–A7 fractions) purification and concentration by ultrafiltration with 3 kDa membranes. All samples were diluted on citrate buffer pH 4.3.

A purified NLE-SCI-57 sample (A2–A7 fractions) stimulated 2-NBDG incorporation by a 6.4-fold increase; the sample was previously analyzed by HPLC (**Figure 6G**). The purified fraction A1–A3 from NLE-SCI-57/M2 had a lower 2-NBDG uptake (3.7-fold increase) compared to the A4–A9 fraction (5.1-fold increase).

DISCUSSION

In this work, we have demonstrated that it is feasible to produce biologically active insulin analog SCI-57 by transient expression in *N. benthamiana* with a yield of 19.11% of TSP (**Table 2**). Furthermore, the number of plants for the production of one gram of the recombinant protein was calculated by considering leaf biomass yield per plant (Lai and Chen, 2012). Then, it will be necessary at least 2293 plants to get a gram of the insulin analog SCI-57, which is comparable to previous reports where the best-performing plant-based platforms (Merlin et al., 2014).

A ~6.4 kDa band, which was expected to be the size of the insulin analog SCI-57, was detectable in the *N. benthamiana* leaf extract (NLE) from agro-infiltrated plants with SCI-57 constructions (**Figure 2**). Unpurified SCI-57 was readily detectable by SDS-PAGE according to Virgen-Ortiz and colleagues, although only abundant proteins are detected when using this technique (Virgen-Ortiz et al., 2013). Therefore, SCI-57 was expressed at significant levels. Furthermore, M2 co-expression tends to increase SCI-57 levels on leaf extracts. This was corroborated by gene analysis,

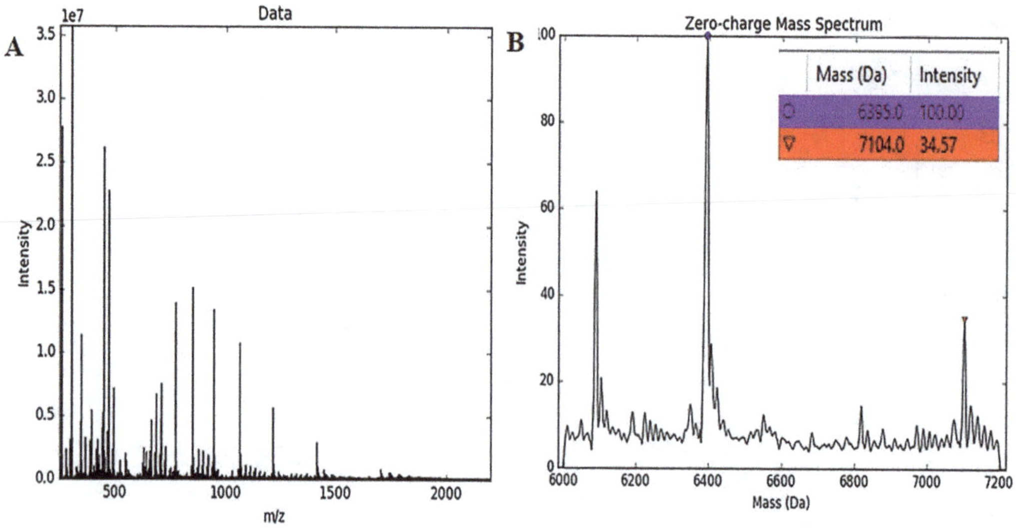

FIGURE 7 | MS spectra and molecular weight of native protein. **(A)** The spectrum obtained by MS of the SCI-57 purified fractions (A2–A7) containing SCI-57 in its native form. **(B)** Molecular weight of proteins contained in SCI-57 purified fractions, by applying the deconvolution to the spectrum obtained by MS.

as twice as much SCI-57 seemed to be expressed when M2 is co-expressed (**Figure 3C**).

The endoplasmic reticulum (ER) of plant cells is able to accumulate a high concentration of proteins with the addition of a retention signal (KDEL) at the carboxyl terminal (C-terminal) end of the recombinant protein; this retention signal was included in the SCI-57 gene sequence. However, Okomoto et al. (Okomoto et al., 1999) found that, on the second day of infection, the recombinant protein still possessed the KDEL retention sequence. From the third day onwards, a protein mixture without KDEL and with KDEL was present. On day 4, the KDEL sequence was removed from the recombinant protein.

Based on Okomoto's findings and the MS analysis of the sample containing A2–A7 fractions from NLE-SCI-57 purification (**Figure 7**), we presume that the addition of a retention signal (KDEL) generates a mixture of two proteins: SCI-57 and SCI-57+KDEL. This concurs with the findings on the FPLC, where two peaks were observed (**Figure 4A**). Therefore, the band observed on the SDS-PAGE analysis (**Figure 4B**) from the fractions conforming to the first peak (A2-A6) corresponds to SCI-57 ~6.4 kDa, whereas the bands with higher molecular weight observed on A7-A10 may be SCI-57+KDEL ~7.1 kDa, which tends to form molecular aggregates (**Figure 4C**). Thus, SDS-PAGE was not capable of separating proteins with similar weights: SCI-57 and SCI-57+KDEL. Diagonal electrophoresis results (**Figure 9**) indicate that SCI-57 structure had disulfide bonds; hence, transient expression did not affect proper SCI-57 folding or disulfide bond formation.

M2 co-expression was used to enhance the yield and quality of SCI-57. However, the results from molecular weight determination (**Figure 8**) and diagonal electrophoresis suggested the presence of a 7.1 kDa protein with no disulfide bridges (**Figure 9**). Previous publications reported that M2 co-expression increases the pH in the Golgi apparatus (Jutras et al., 2015). Although SCI-57 mRNA was higher when M2 was co-expressed, it was believed that the use of M2 interferes in the binding of the KDEL protein to its receptor, neutralizing the acid pH necessary to carry out the binding. Basic pH inhibits the cleavage of the KDEL peptide (Reithmeier, 1996; Lodish et al., 2008) in the SCI-57 sequence. Thus, when M2 is co-expressed, SCI-57+KDEL production is enhanced, when compared to SCI-57 with no M2 co-expression. Therefore, the two peaks on the FPLC chromatogram may correspond to different degrees of SCI-57+KDEL aggregation. It is likely that on the A1–A4 fractions (first peak on the chromatogram, **Figure 5A**), the monomeric SCI-57+KDEL form was predominant; whereas on the A4–A9 fractions (second peak on the chromatogram, **Figure 5A**), oligomeric SCI-57+KDEL forms can be observed on the SDS-PAGE. Insulin self-assembly and aggregation were induced by our working conditions for purification (**Supplementary Figure S3**); previous publications reported that buffer citrate, chloride ions from NaCl, and the presence of zinc promote insulin aggregation (Carpenter, 1966; Nettleton et al., 2000). High NaCl concentration and zinc presence on the NLE-SCI-57/M2 could stimulate greater oligomeric formation on SCI-57+KDEL; thereby, interfering with the insulin analog SCI-57 recovery on the purification method.

From RP-HPLC, it was established that the band detected on SDS-PAGE gel from NLE-SCI-57 corresponded to a protein with similar retention time and UV spectra as the insulins that we evaluated (**Figure 6**). These findings were corroborated by the analysis of purified A2–A7 fractions (**Figure 6G**). In the case of the NLE-SCI-57/M2 sample, the presence of a peak with a similar retention time is also observed (**Figure 6E**). However, the UV spectrum differs slightly from the NLE-SCI-57 sample. Therefore, M2 protein interferes with the appropriate processing of the SCI-57 insulin analog.

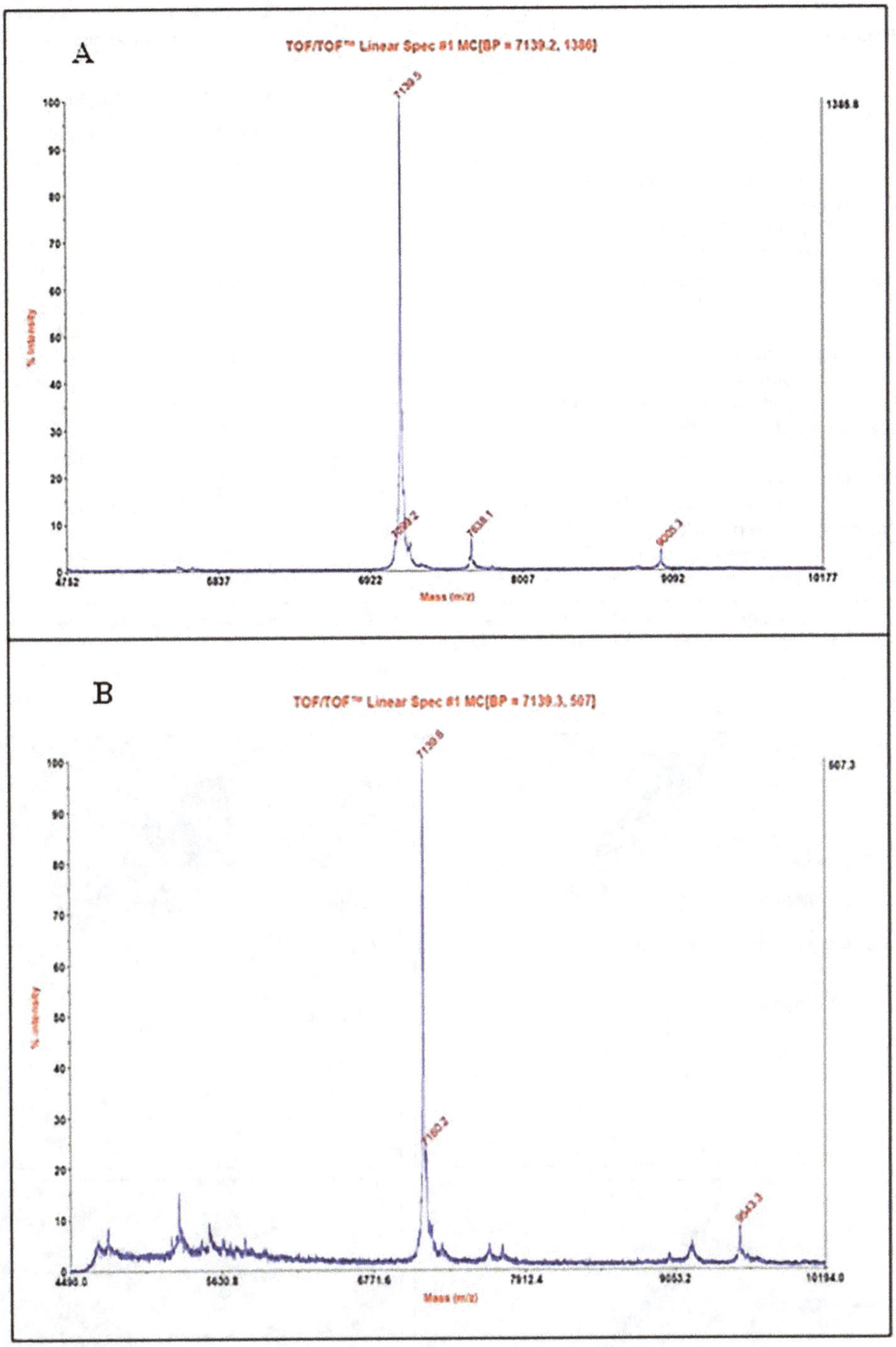

FIGURE 8 | MALDI-TOF mass spectrum from **(A)** A2–A4 fractions obtained by FPLC of NLE SCI-57/M2. **(B)** A5–A7 fractions obtained by FPLC of NLE SCI-57/M2. Molecular masses were determined by MS using vendor-provided software (Applied Biosystems/MDS SCIEX, USA).

The peptide FVNQHLCGSDLVEALYLVCGER was identified on NLE-SCI-57 (**Supplementary Figure S6**). This reinforces the evidence that SCI-57 is functionally expressed in *N. benthamiana*.

Recombinant proteins expressed in plants usually maintain their native structural properties, facilitating recognition by antibodies. Specific recognition of SCI-57 was observed by two monoclonal antibodies, which were directed against separate antigenic determinants on the insulin molecule by ELISA. Although the ELISA test did not show a concentration similar to the Bradford method, results confirm that when SCI-57 is expressed without M2 and purified by FPLC, it is functionally active. Furthermore, most commercial insulin assays fail to detect

TABLE 1 | Relative abundance of up-regulated proteins[1] by at least 5-fold in NLE GFP, NLE SCI-57 and NLE SCI-57/M2 compared with NLEN.

NCBI accession	Protein name	Relative abundance (n-fold)		
		NLE GFP / NLEN	*NLE SCI-57 / NLEN*	*NLE SCI-57 / M2 / NLEN*
XP_009760305.1	Glucan endo-1,3-beta-glucosidase, basic vacuolar isoform isoform X2	56.6	15.4	19.7
XP_009617302.1	Endochitinase A	69.5	37.6	36.2
XP_019225618.1	Pathogenesis-related R major form	6.8	6.3	7.1
XP_009781670.1	Pathogenesis-related protein R minor form	15.6	18.8	15.5
XP_016495116.1	Suberization-associated anionic peroxidase-like	58.7	8.8	64.5
XP_019244706.1	Kunitz trypsin inhibitor 2-like	72.4	50.5	53.1
XP_009593782.1	Peroxidase P7-like	31.1	8.7	24.0
AAA34078.1	Beta(1,3)-glucanase regulator	32.5	34.5	37.3
CBK52316.1	Nb cell deth marker	9.3	13.3	15.2
XP_019238089.1	Basic form of pathogenesis-related protein 1	27.7	5.8	43.6
XP_019261786.1	Wound-induced protein WIN1	31.7	7.4	49.1
XP_009768114.1	Expansin-like A2	7.7	13.8	9.1
OIT28720.1	Basic endochitinase	23.2	10.6	6.7
XP_019265536.1	Non-specific lipid transfer protein GPI-anchored 1	15.1	15.5	9.7
XP_019241188.1	Aquaporin PIP-type pTOM75	13.3	20.3	6.6
XP_009787159.1	Basic form of pathogenesis-related protein 1-like	313.3	81.0	128.3
prf||1202235A	protein 1a,pathogenesis related	22.1	35.2	10.9

[1]Proteins were listed base on the n-fold expression normalized with NLEN. Ratios were inferred from MS/MS peptide abundance values determined for each protein. Red numbers indicate the group with the highest value and blue values indicate the group with the lowest value.

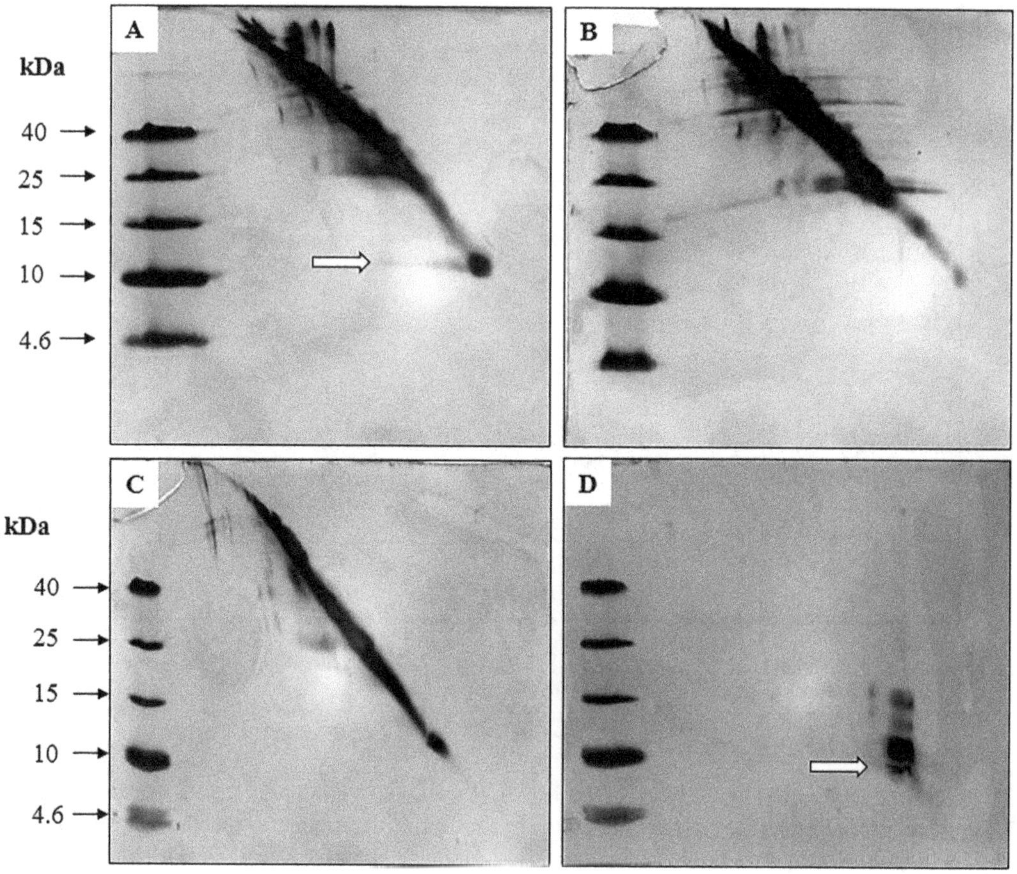

FIGURE 9 | Silver-stained diagonal gel, identifying intermolecular protein disulfides in **(A)** NLE SCI-57, **(B)** NLEN, **(C)** NLE SCI-57/M2 and **(D)** EP insulin. Eight microgram of the samples and 1 µg of insulin were loaded on the gel. White arrows indicate proteins with disulfide bridges.

TABLE 2 | Yield of the SCI-57 expression and purification.

Protein	Recovery from the purification method (%)	Highest expression level	Plants/g recombinant protein
SCI-57	62.52	19.11% TSP or 0.1505 mg/g LFW	2,293[1]
SCI-57/M2	46.39	ND	ND

The expression levels are reported as mass of the insulin analog SCI-57 per unit of biomass (LFW, leaves fresh weight.). The recombinant protein productivity values were calculated by considering leaf biomass yield per plant [[1] (Lai and Chen, 2012)]. ND, not determined.

recombinant insulin analogs (Heald et al., 2006); therefore, SCI-57 may tend to be underestimated.

As insulin and insulin analogs stimulate the development of adipose tissue (Hartman, 2008), we evaluated the effect of *Nb* preparations on the adipose differentiation of 3T3-L1 cells induced with an insulin-lacking adipogenic medium. Our results indicate that NLE-SCI-57 partially, and NLE-SCI-57/M2 advantageously, replace insulin's role on 3T3 adipogenesis, whereas NLEN did not stimulate lipid accumulation in these cells. When the effect of *Nb* preparations on lipid accumulation was evaluated in the presence of insulin, both NLE-SCI-57 and NLE-SCI-57/M2 samples showed a synergic effect with the hormone stimulating more than twice the lipid accumulation in 3T3-L1 cells. As in the insulin-lacking condition, NLEN sample did not stimulate 3T3 lipid accumulation in the presence of the hormone (**Figure 10**). These results prove that our agroinfiltrated *Nb* preparations possess insulin-mimetic properties.

Hypoglycemic drugs exert their effects by any of the following three mechanisms: by diminishing intestinal glucose, increasing insulin secretion, or stimulating glucose uptake by insulin-targeted tissues such as adipose or skeletal muscle tissues. This last hypoglycemic mechanism is the most promising therapeutic target for both Type 1 and Type 2 diabetes.

In order to determine whether SCI-57 has an insulin-mimetic effect by stimulating the incorporation of glucose in adipocytes, we evaluated its effects on the uptake of 2-NBDG in 3T3-L1 adipocytes (**Figure 11**). NLE-SCI-57 promoted 2-NBDG incorporation by adipocytes almost at the same level as RGZ. In contrast, NLE-SCI-57/M2 exhibit a lower 2-NBDG incorporation than RGZ. We also evaluated the effect of purified fractions from agroinfiltrated *Nb* preparations on the incorporation of glucose. The purified NLE-SCI-57 fractions (**HPLC, Figure 11**) stimulates the incorporation of 2-NBDG to a greater extent than insulin; whereas purified NLE-SCI-57/M2 fractions (**A1–A3 and A4–A9, Figure 11**) are incorporated to a lesser extent than purified NLE-SCI-57 fractions. The high capacity of NLE-SCI-57 to stimulate the uptake of glucose in terminal adipocytes, and its low adipogenic capacity (pro-obesity), make it an optimal candidate for replacing native insulin. Whereas the NLE-SCI-57/M2 sample, has low (relative) incorporation of 2-NBDG and a marked pro-adipogenic effect (**Figure 10**).

Surprisingly, NLEN stimulated glucose uptake to the same extent as NLE-SCI-57/M2 (**Figure 11**), suggesting the *Nb* extract itself can incorporate glucose in 3T3-L1 adipocytes. Currently, we have no explanation for this effect. Although we and others

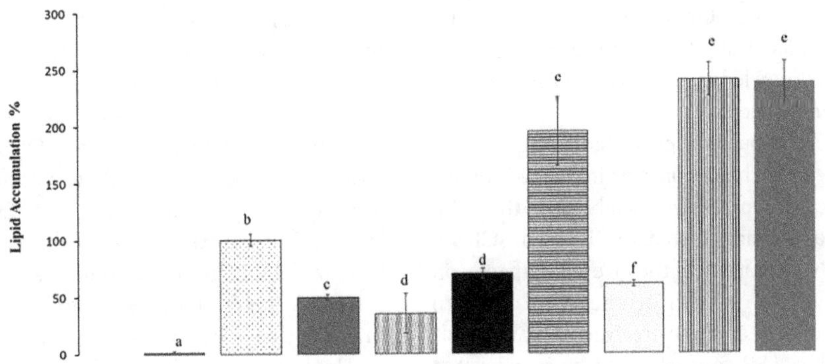

NAM	+	-	-	-	-	-	-	-	-
AM	-	+	-	-	-	-	+	+	+
AMI-	-	-	+	+	+	+	-	-	-
NLEN (50 µl/ml)	-	-	-	+	-	-	+	-	-
NLE SCI-57 (50 µl/ml)	-	-	-	-	+	-	-	+	-
NLE SCI-57/M2 (50 µl/ml)	-	-	-	-	-	+	-	-	+

FIGURE 10 | Effect of SCI-57 on 3T3 adipogenesis. Adipose differentiation of 3T3-L1 preadipocytes was induced in the presence (AM) or the absence (AMI-) of 5 µg/ml insulin. Control cultures received a non-adipogenic medium (NAM). Effects of NLE preparations on 3T3-L1 adipogenesis were evaluated under both induction conditions by quantitation of intracytoplasmic lipid accumulation with oil red O. Results are presented as the mean ± S.D. of experiments in triplicate. Lowercase letters indicate significant differences according to the Mann-Whitney U test ($p \leq 0.05$).

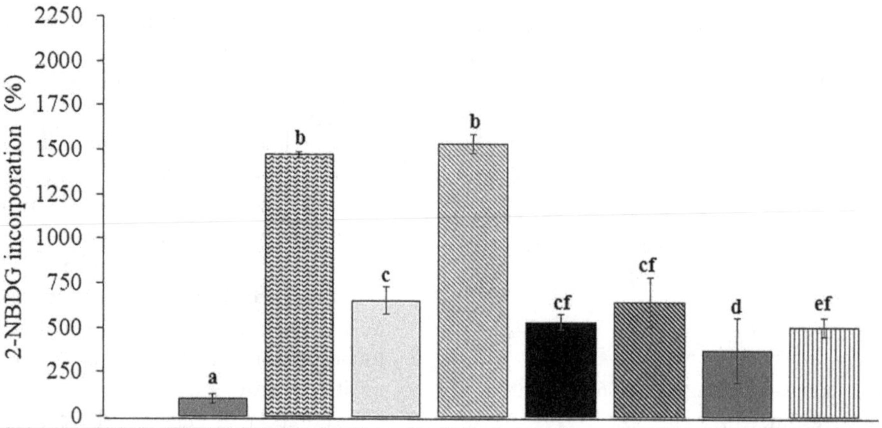

INS (nM)	100	-	-	-	-	-	-	-
RGZ (μM)	-	10	-	-	-	-	-	-
NLEN (μl/ml)	-	-	50	-	-	-	-	-
NLE SCI-57 (μl/ml)	-	-	-	50	-	-	-	-
NLE SCI-57/M2 (μl/ml)	-	-	-	-	50	-	-	-
HPLC (μl/ml)	-	-	-	-	-	25	-	-
A1-A3 (μl/ml)	-	-	-	-	-	-	25	-
A4-A9 (μl/ml)	-	-	-	-	-	-	-	25

FIGURE 11 | Effect of NLEN, NLE SCI-57, NLE SCI-57/M2 and purified samples on 2-NBDG uptake in 3T3-L1 adipocytes. Mature 3T3-L1 adipocytes were incubated as described (Zapata-Bustos et al., 2014b). Control treatments were incubated with insulin 100 nM (INS) or rosiglitazone 10μM (RGZ). Results are presented as the mean ± S.D. of experiments in quadruplicate. Lowercase letters indicate significant differences according to the Mann-Whitney U test ($p \leq 0.05$). HPLC: Purified NLE-SCI-57 sample (A2–A7 fractions) analyzed by HPLC (**Figure 6G**). A1–A3 and A4–A9: NLE-SCI-57/M2 fractions.

have documented insulino-mimetic effects in diverse plant extracts (Naowaboot et al., 2012; Ortiz-Andrade et al., 2012; Khattak et al., 2013; Eddouks et al., 2014; Zapata-Bustos et al., 2014a), to the best of our knowledge, this property has not yet been evaluated for *Nicotiana* species.

Plants expressing heterologous proteins manifested at least 1.4 greater quantity of TSP than non-agroinfiltrated plants (**Figure 1C**). We conducted a proteomic analysis of the NLE of the different protein expression systems (GFP and SCI-57) using as control a NLEN to estimate the overall impacts on the biochemical pathways and protein synthesis in order to characterize the specific effects of these treatments at the cell-wide scale. However higher TSP content could be only related with pathogenesis and stress-related proteins produced as response of agroinfiltration (**Table 1**).

Targeted depletion pathogenesis-related and stress-inducible proteins may improve *N. benthamiana* as a protein expression platform and help identify the proteome changes in *N. benthamiana* when expressing different heterologous proteins with the aim to improve protein yield.

CONCLUSIONS

For the first time, the results presented here show that *N. benthamiana* plants are capable of producing a biologically active insulin analog; SCI-57. The purification process enables us to extract pure SCI-57, in its active form, from a complex matrix of plant proteins, applying a time effective procedure. From the protein characterization experiments, we conclude that strategies to increase SCI-57 expression and accumulation may interfere with proper folding and the KDEL cleavage, generating the absence on disulfide bond formation and the KDEL peptide presence on the protein sequence. Even though SCI-57 in the lack of M2 co-expression produces a mixture of SCI-57 and SCI-57+KDEL, glycemic control was demonstrated through the 2-NBDG uptake by 3T3-L1 adipocytes, without any apparent pro-adipogenic or anti-adipogenic effects.

However, when SCI-57 is co-expressed with M2, it appears that M2 inhibits the cleavage of KDEL from SCI-57, and tends to encourage the formation of oligomeric forms, although further experiments are required to fully validate these findings.

When M2 is not co-expressed, the insulin analog SCI-57 displayed a lower pro-adipogenic effect and had a higher 2-NBDG uptake compared to when M2 is co-expressed. Overall our observations suggest that SCI-57 exerts its anti-diabetic properties, stimulating glucose uptake, without affecting the development of adipose tissue.

Proteome changes related to the expression of heterologous proteins on *N. benthamiana* were not observed; up-regulated proteins were related to the agroinfiltration process. However, further experiments are required, employing leaves agroinfiltrated with an empty vector.

AUTHOR CONTRIBUTIONS

AM-T: Conceived of this idea, carried out the experiments, processed the experimental data, performed the analysis, drafted the manuscript, and designed the figures. JR and KL: Label-free proteomic analysis experimental design, assessment of the structural analyses by diagonal electrophoresis. MI-C: Contributed to the interpretation of the results and English revision, final approval of the version for submission. LS-O: Conceived, planned, financed the adipocyte experiments, and provided a critical review of the final manuscript. AE-M: Design and technical execution of MS analysis, interpretation of analytical assays, A critical review of the final manuscript. AL-C: Technical support for molecular cloning, transient expression in *N. benthamiana* and qRT-PCR for gene expression analysis, data acquisition and revision of the manuscript. MG-L: Key role in the study design, editing the manuscript and critical revision for important intellectual content, a critical review of the final manuscript. AR-S: Study design and concept, financial support for part of the study, drafting and editing the manuscript and critical revision for important intellectual content, final approval of the version for submission. All authors discussed the results and commented on the manuscript.

FUNDING

This work was supported in part by PROINPEP 2015, 2016 (AR-S), awarded to support Ph.D. students of the pharmacology program PROSNI 2016, 2017 to AR-S, and by own resources of the Doctors MG-L, LS-O, JR, and AR-S.

ACKNOWLEDGMENTS

AM-T thanks CONACYT for national and international scholarship No. 398200. AM-T gratefully acknowledges the multidisciplinary Department of Genetic Engineering laboratory team for their support of this project. The authors would like to Francisco Pérez (Centro de Biociencias, UASLP, México) for his technical assistance in MS experiments.

REFERENCES

Baeshen, N. A., Baeshen, M. N., Sheikh, A., Bora, R. S., Ahmed, M. M., Ramadan, H. A., et al. (2014). Cell factories for insulin production. *Microb. Cell Fact* 13, 141. doi: 10.1186/s12934-014-0141-0

Benchabane, M., Goulet, C., Rivard, D., Faye, L., Gomord, V., and Michaud, D. (2008). Preventing unintended proteolysis in plant protein biofactories. *Plant Biotechnol. J.* 6 (7), 633–648. doi: 10.1111/j.1467-7652.2008.00344.x

Bendandi, M., Marillonnet, S., Kandzia, R., Thieme, F., Nickstadt, A., Herz, S., et al. (2010). Rapid, high-yield production in plants of individualized idiotype vaccines for non-Hodgkin's lymphoma. *Ann. Oncol.* 21 (12), 2420–2427. doi: 10.1093/annonc/mdq256

Blum, H., Beier, H., and Gross, H. J. (1987). Improved silver staining of plant proteins, RNA and DNA in polyacrylamide gels. *Electrophoresis* 8 (2), 93–99. doi: doi:10.1002/elps.1150080203

Boyhan, D., and Daniell, H. (2011). Low-cost production of proinsulin in tobacco and lettuce chloroplasts for injectable or oral delivery of functional insulin and C-peptide. *Plant Biotechnol. J.* 9 (5), 585–598. doi: 10.1111/j.1467-7652.2010.00582.x

Budzianowski, J. (2015). Tobacco against Ebola virus disease. *Przegl Lek* 72 (10), 567–571.

Buyel, J. F. (2018). Plant molecular farming - integration and exploitation of side streams to achieve sustainable biomanufacturing. *Front. Plant Sci.* 9, 1893. doi: 10.3389/fpls.2018.01893

Cabrera, M., Muñiz, M., Hidalgo, J., Vega, L., Martín, M. E., and Velasco, A. (2003). The retrieval function of the kdel receptor requires pka phosphorylation of its C-Terminus. *Mol. Biol. Cell* 14 (10), 4114–4125. doi: 10.1091/mbc.E03-04-0194

Carpenter, F. H. (1966). Relationship of structure to biological activity of insulin as revealed by degradative studies. *Am. J. Med.* 40 (5), 750–758. doi: 10.1016/0002-9343(66)90156-2

Castillo-Esparza J. F., Monroy García A., and Gómez-Lim M. A. (2014). "Chapter 6. Expression of the Capsid protein on human papillomavirus in plants as alternative for the production of vaccines," in *plant-derived pharmaceuticals: principles and applications for developing countries*. Ed. K. L. Hefferon (CAB International). 91–104.

Coconi-Linares, N., Ortega-Davila, E., Lopez-Gonzalez, M., Garcia-Machorro, J., Garcia-Cordero, J., Steinman, R. M., et al. (2013). Targeting of envelope domain III protein of DENV type 2 to DEC-205 receptor elicits neutralizing antibodies in mice. *Vaccine* 31 (19), 2366–2371. doi: 10.1016/j.vaccine.2013.03.009

Conley, A. J., Joensuu, J. J., Richman, A., and Menassa, R. (2011). Protein body-inducing fusions for high-level production and purification of recombinant proteins in plants. *Plant Biotechnol. J.* 9 (4), 419–433. doi: 10.1111/j.1467-7652.2011.00596.x

Davey, R. T. Jr., Dodd, L., Proschan, M. A., Neaton, J., Neuhaus Nordwall, J., Koopmeiners, J. S., et al. (2016). A randomized, controlled trial of zmapp for ebola virus infection. *N Engl. J. Med.* 375 (15), 1448–1456. doi: 10.1056/NEJMoa1604330

Eddouks, M., Bidi, A., El Bouhali, B., Hajji, L., and Zeggwagh, N. A. (2014). Antidiabetic plants improving insulin sensitivity. *J. Pharm. Pharmacol.* 66 (9), 1197–1214. doi: 10.1111/jphp.12243

Edelbaum, O., Stein, D., Holland, N., Gafni, Y., Livneh, O., Novick, D., et al. (1992). Expression of active human interferon-beta in transgenic plants. *J. Interferon. Res.* 12 (6), 449–453. doi: 10.1089/jir.1992.12.449

Feist, M., Schwarzfischer, P., Heinrich, P., Sun, X., Kemper, J., von Bonin, F., et al. (2018). Cooperative STAT/NF-κB signaling regulates lymphoma metabolic reprogramming and aberrant GOT2 expression. *Nat. Commun.* 9 (1), 1514. doi: 10.1038/s41467-018-03803-x

Fischer, R., and Emans, N. (2000). Molecular farming of pharmaceutical proteins. *Transgenic Res.* 9 (4–5), 279–299. doi: 10.1023/A:1008975123362

Fischer, R., and Kessler, B. M. (2015). Gel-aided sample preparation (GASP)—A simplified method for gel-assisted proteomic sample generation from protein extracts and intact cells. *Proteomics* 15 (7), 1224–1229. doi: 10.1002/pmic.201400436

Giritch, A., Marillonnet, S., Klimyuk, V., and Gleba, Y. (2015). "Production of hetero-oligomeric proteins in plants," in *Google Patents*.

Goulet, C., Goulet, C., Goulet, M. C., and Michaud, D. (2010). 2-DE proteome maps for the leaf apoplast of Nicotiana benthamiana. *Proteomics* 10 (13), 2536–2544. doi: 10.1002/pmic.200900382

Graham, K. J., and Holland, M. J. (2005). "PrimerSelect: a transcriptome-wide oligonucleotide primer pair design program for kinetic RT-PCR–based transcript profiling," in *Methods in enzymology.* (Elsevier BV: Academic Press), 544–553.

Hartman, I. (2008). Insulin analogs: impact on treatment success, satisfaction, quality of life, and adherence. *Clin. Med. Res.* 6 (2), 54–67. doi: 10.3121/cmr.2008.793

Heald, A. H., Bhattacharya, B., Cooper, H., Ullah, A., McCulloch, A., Smellie, S., et al. (2006). Most commercial insulin assays fail to detect recombinant insulin analogues. *Ann. Clin. Biochem.* 43 (Pt 4), 306–308. doi: 10.1258/000456306777695690

Herrera-Herrera, M. L., Zapata-Bustos, R., and Salazar-Olivo, L. A. (2009). Simplified culture techniques for growth and differentiation of murine and human pre-adipocytes for translational applications. *Cytotherapy* 11 (1), 52–60. doi: 10.1080/14653240802495963

Hiatt, A., Pauly, M., Whaley, K., Qiu, X., Kobinger, G., and Zeitlin, L. (2015). The emergence of antibody therapies for Ebola. *Hum. Antibodies* 23 (3-4), 49–56. doi: 10.3233/hab-150284

Holman, S. W., McLean, L., and Eyers, C. E. (2016). RePLiCal: a QconCAT protein for retention time standardization in proteomics studies. *J. Proteome Res.* 15 (3), 1090–1102. doi: 10.1021/acs.jproteome.5b00988

Hondred, D., Walker, J. M., Mathews, D. E., and Vierstra, R. D. (1999). Use of ubiquitin fusions to augment protein expression in transgenic plants. *Plant Physiol.* 119 (2), 713–724. doi: 10.1104/pp.119.2.713

Hua, X., Carvalho, N., Tew, M., Huang, E. S., Herman, W. H., and Clarke, P. (2016). Expenditures and prices of antihyperglycemic medications in the United States: 2002–2013. *JAMA* 315 (13), 1400–1402. doi: 10.1001/jama.2016.0126

Inzucchi, S. E., Bergenstal, R. M., Buse, J. B., Diamant, M., Ferrannini, E., Nauck, M., et al. (2015). Management of hyperglycemia in type 2 diabetes, 2015: a patient-centered approach: update to a position statement of the american diabetes association and the european association for the study of diabetes. *Diabetes Care* 38 (1), 140–149. doi: 10.2337/dc14-2441

Jagschies, G., Lindskog, E., Lacki, K., and Galliher, P. M. (2018). "Chapter 4. Process Capability Requirements," in *Biopharmaceutical processing: development, design, and implementation of manufacturing processes.* (Eds. G. Jagschies, E. Lindskog, K. Lacki, and P. M. Galliher. Elsevier Science), 73–94

Jutras, P. V., D'Aoust, M. A., Couture, M. M., Vezina, L. P., Goulet, M. C., Michaud, D., et al. (2015). Modulating secretory pathway pH by proton channel co-expression can increase recombinant protein stability in plants. *Biotechnol. J.* 10 (9), 1478–1486. doi: 10.1002/biot.201500056

Khattak, M. M. A. K., Taher, M., Ichwan, S., and Azahari, N. (2013) *Selected Herbal Extracts Improve Diabetes Associated Factors in 3T3-L1 Adipocytes.* Elsevier.

King, P., Peacock, I., and Donnelly, R. (1999). The UK Prospective Diabetes Study (UKPDS): clinical and therapeutic implications for type 2 diabetes. *Br. J. Clin. Pharmacol.* 48 (5), 643–648. doi: 10.1046/j.1365-2125.1999.00092.x

Klimyuk, V., Pogue, G., Herz, S., Butler, J., and Haydon, H. (2014). Production of recombinant antigens and antibodies in Nicotiana benthamiana using 'magnifection' technology: GMP-compliant facilities for small- and large-scale manufacturing. *Curr. Top. Microbiol. Immunol.* 375, 127–154. doi: 10.1007/82_2012_212

Kusnadi, A. R., Nikolov, Z. L., and Howard, J. A. (1997). Production of recombinant proteins in transgenic plants: practical considerations. *Biotechnol. Bioeng.* 56 (5), 473–484. doi: 10.1002/(sici)1097-0290(19971205)56:5<473::aid-bit1>3.0.co;2-f

Lacombe, S., Bangratz, M., Brizard, J.-P., Petitdidier, E., Pagniez, J., Sérémé, D., et al. (2018). Optimized transitory ectopic expression of promastigote surface antigen protein in Nicotiana benthamiana, a potential anti-leishmaniasis vaccine candidate. *J. Biosci. Bioeng.* 125 (1), 116–123. doi: 10.1016/j.jbiosc.2017.07.008

Lai, H., and Chen, Q. (2012). Bioprocessing of plant-derived virus-like particles of Norwalk virus capsid protein under current Good Manufacture Practice regulations. *Plant Cell Rep.* 31 (3), 573–584. doi: 10.1007/s00299-011-1196-6

Lai, H., Engle, M., Fuchs, A., Keller, T., Johnson, S., Gorlatov, S., et al. (2010). Monoclonal antibody produced in plants efficiently treats West Nile virus infection in mice. *Proc. Natl. Acad. Sci. U.S.A.* 107 (6), 2419–2424. doi: 10.1073/pnas.0914503107

Lico, C., Chen, Q., and Santi, L. (2008). Viral vectors for production of recombinant proteins in plants. *J. Cell. Physiol.* 216 (2), 366–377. doi: 10.1002/jcp.21423

Livak, K. J., and Schmittgen, T. D. (2001). Analysis of relative gene expression data using real-time quantitative PCR and the 2(-Delta Delta C(T)) Method. *Methods* 25 (4), 402–408. doi: 10.1006/meth.2001.1262

Lodish H. (2008). "Chapter 14. Vesicular traffic, secretion and endocytosis," in *Molecular cell.* Eds. H. Lodish, A. Berk, C. A. Kaiser, M. Krieger, M. P. Scott, A. Bretscher, et al., 8th Edn. (New York: Macmillan Learning), 631–672.

Ma, J. K. C., Barros, E., Bock, R., Christou, P., Dale, P. J., Dix, P. J., et al. (2005). Molecular farming for new drugs and vaccines: Current perspectives on the production of pharmaceuticals in transgenic plants. *EMBO Rep.* 6 (7), 593–599. doi: 10.1038/sj.embor.7400470

Marty, M. T., Baldwin, A. J., Marklund, E. G., Hochberg, G. K. A., Benesch, J. L. P., and Robinson, C. V. (2015). Bayesian deconvolution of mass and ion mobility spectra: from binary interactions to polydisperse ensembles. *Anal Chem.* 87 (8), 4370–4376. doi: 10.1021/acs.analchem.5b00140

Merlin, M., Gecchele, E., Capaldi, S., Pezzotti, M., and Avesani, L. (2014). Comparative evaluation of recombinant protein production in different biofactories: the green perspective. *BioMed. Res. Int.* 2014, 14. doi: 10.1155/2014/136419

Mollerup, I., Weber Jensen, S., Larsen, P., Schou, O., and Snel, L. (2002). "Insulin, purification," in *Encyclopedia of bioprocess technology.* (Wiley Online Library) doi: 10.1002/0471250589.ebt121

Na, W., Park, N., Yeom, M., and Song, D. (2015). Ebola outbreak in Western Africa 2014: what is going on with Ebola virus? *Clin. Exp. Vaccine Res.* 4 (1), 17–22. doi: 10.7774/cevr.2015.4.1.17

Naowaboot, J., Chung, C. H., Pannangpetch, P., Choi, R., Kim, B. H., Lee, M. Y., et al. (2012). Mulberry leaf extract increases adiponectin in murine 3T3-L1 adipocytes. *Nutr. Res.* 32 (1), 39–44. doi: 10.1016/j.nutres.2011.12.003

Nettleton, E. J., Tito, P., Sunde, M., Bouchard, M., Dobson, C. M., and Robinson, C. V. (2000). Characterization of the oligomeric states of insulin in self-assembly and amyloid fibril formation by mass spectrometry. *Biophys. J.* 79 (2), 1053–1065. doi: 10.1016/S0006-3495(00)76359-4

Nykiforuk, C. L., Boothe, J. G., Murray, E. W., Keon, R. G., Goren, H. J., Markley, N. A., et al. (2006). Transgenic expression and recovery of biologically active recombinant human insulin from Arabidopsis thaliana seeds. *Plant Biotechnol. J.* 4 (1), 77–85. doi: 10.1111/j.1467-7652.2005.00159.x

Ogurtsova, K., da Rocha Fernandes, J. D., Huang, Y., Linnenkamp, U., Guariguata, L., Cho, N. H., et al. (2017). IDF diabetes atlas: global estimates for the prevalence of diabetes for 2015 and 2040. *Diabetes Res. Clin. Pract.* 128, 40–50. doi: 10.1016/j.diabres.2017.03.024

Okomoto, T., Minamikawa, T., Edward, G., Vakharia, V., and Herman, E. (1999). Posttranslational removal of the carboxyl-terminal KDEL of the cysteine protease SH-EP occurs prior to maturation of the enzyme. *J. Biol. Chem.* 274 (16), 11390–11398. doi: 10.1074/jbc.274.16.11390

Ortiz-Andrade, R., Cabanas-Wuan, A., Arana-Argaez, V. E., Alonso-Castro, A. J., Zapata-Bustos, R., Salazar-Olivo, L. A., et al. (2012). Antidiabetic effects of Justicia spicigera Schltdl (Acanthaceae). *J. Ethnopharmacol* 143 (2), 455–462. doi: 10.1016/j.jep.2012.06.043

Owczarzy, R., Tataurov, A. V., Wu, Y., Manthey, J. A., McQuisten, K. A., Almabrazi, H. G., et al. (2008). IDT SciTools: a suite for analysis and design of nucleic acid oligomers. *Nucleic Acids Res.* 36 (suppl_2), W163–W169. doi: 10.1093/nar/gkn198

Pruss, G. J., Nester, E. W., and Vance, V. (2008). Infiltration with Agrobacterium tumefaciens induces host defense and development-dependent responses in the infiltrated zone. *Mol. Plant Microbe Interact.* 21 (12), 1528–1538. doi: 10.1094/mpmi-21-12-1528

Qiu, X., Wong, G., Audet, J., Bello, A., Fernando, L., Alimonti, J. B., et al. (2014). Reversion of advanced Ebola virus disease in nonhuman primates with ZMapp. *Nature* 514 (7520), 47–53. doi: 10.1038/nature13777

Ramirez-Zacarias, J. L., Castro-Munozledo, F., and Kuri-Harcuch, W. (1992). Quantitation of adipose conversion and triglycerides by staining intracytoplasmic lipids with Oil red O. *Histochemistry* 97 (6), 493–497. doi: 10.1007/bf00316069

Redwan, E.-R. M. (2007). Cumulative updating of approved biopharmaceuticals. *Hum. Antibodies* 16 (3–4), 137. doi: 10.3233/HAB-2007-163-408

Reinders, Y., Voller, D., Bosserhoff, A. K., Oefner, P. J., and Reinders, J. (2016). Testing suitability of cell cultures for silac-experiments using SWATH-mass spectrometry. *Methods Mol. Biol.* 1394, 101–108. doi: 10.1007/978-1-4939-3341-9_8

Reiter, L., Rinner, O., Picotti, P., Hüttenhain, R., Beck, M., Brusniak, M.-Y., et al. (2011). mProphet: automated data processing and statistical validation for large-scale SRM experiments. *Nat. Methods* 8, 430. doi; 10.1038/nmeth.1584

Reithmeier, R. A. F. (1996). "Chapter 16 - Assembly of proteins into membranes," in Biochemistry of Lipids. Lipoproteins and Membranes. *New Comprehensive Biochemistry*. Eds. Vance, D. E., and Vance, J. E. (Elsevier B.V.), 425–471.

Robert, S., Goulet, M. C., D'Aoust, M. A., Sainsbury, F., and Michaud, D. (2015). Leaf proteome rebalancing in Nicotiana benthamiana for upstream enrichment of a transiently expressed recombinant protein. *Plant Biotechnol. J.* 13 (8), 1169–1179. doi: 10.1111/pbi.12452

Sainsbury, F., Varennes-Jutras, P., Goulet, M. C., D'Aoust, M. A., and Michaud, D. (2013). Tomato cystatin SlCYS8 as a stabilizing fusion partner for human serpin expression in plants. *Plant Biotechnol. J.* 11 (9), 1058–1068. doi: 10.1111/pbi.12098

Schagger, H. (2006). Tricine-SDS-PAGE. *Nat. Protoc.* 1 (1), 16–22. doi: 10.1038/nprot.2006.4

Streatfield, S. J. (2007). Approaches to achieve high-level heterologous protein production in plants. *Plant Biotechnol. J.* 5 (1), 2–15. doi: 10.1111/j.1467-7652.2006.00216.x

Tuse, D., Ku, N., Bendandi, M., Becerra, C., Collins, R. Jr., Langford, N., et al. (2015). Clinical safety and immunogenicity of tumor-targeted, plant-made id-klh conjugate vaccines for follicular lymphoma. *BioMed. Res. Int.* 2015, 15. doi: 10.1155/2015/648143

Tuse, D., Tu, T., and McDonald, K. A. (2014). Manufacturing economics of plant-made biologics: case studies in therapeutic and industrial enzymes. *BioMed. Res. Int.* 2014, 256135. doi: 10.1155/2014/256135

Twyman, R. M., Stoger, E., Schillberg, S., Christou, P., and Fischer, R. (2003). Molecular farming in plants: host systems and expression technology. *Trends Biotechnol.* 21 (12), 570–578. doi: 10.1016/j.tibtech.2003.10.002

Virgen-Ortiz, J. J., Ibarra-Junquera, V., Escalante-Minakata, P., Osuna-Castro, J. A., Ornelas-Paz Jde, J., Mancilla-Margalli, N. A., et al. (2013). Improving sodium dodecyl sulfate polyacrylamide gel electrophoresis detection of low-abundance protein samples by rapid freeze centrifugation. *Anal. Biochem.* 443 (2), 249–251. doi: 10.1016/j.ab.2013.09.015

WHO (2016). *Global Report on Diabetes*. World Health Organization.

You, W.-P., and Henneberg, M. (2016). Type 1 diabetes prevalence increasing globally and regionally: the role of natural selection and life expectancy at birth. *BMJ Open Diabetes Res. Care* 4 (1), e000161. doi: 10.1136/bmjdrc-2015-000161

Zapata-Bustos, R., Alonso-Castro, A. J., Gomez-Sanchez, M., and Salazar-Olivo, L. A. (2014a). Ibervillea sonorae (Cucurbitaceae) induces the glucose uptake in human adipocytes by activating a PI3K-independent pathway. *J. Ethnopharmacol* 152 (3), 546–552. doi: 10.1016/j.jep.2014.01.041

Zapata-Bustos, R., Alonso-Castro, Á. J., Gómez-Sánchez, M., and Salazar-Olivo, L. A. (2014b). Ibervillea sonorae (Cucurbitaceae) induces the glucose uptake in human adipocytes by activating a PI3K-independent pathway. *J. Ethnopharmacolsss* 152 (3), 546–552. doi: 10.1016/j.jep.2014.01.041

9

The Problem with Big Data: Operating on Smaller Datasets to Bridge the Implementation Gap

Richard P. Mann[1], Faisal Mushtaq[2]*, Alan D. White[2,3], Gabriel Mata-Cervantes[2], Tom Pike[2], Dalton Coker[3], Stuart Murdoch[4], Tim Hiles[4], Clare Smith[4], David Berridge[4], Suzanne Hinchliffe[4], Geoff Hall[2,4], Stephen Smye[2,4], Richard M. Wilkie[2], J. Peter A. Lodge[2,4] and Mark Mon-Williams[2]

[1] School of Mathematics, University of Leeds, Leeds, UK, [2] Faculty of Medicine and Health, University of Leeds, Leeds, UK, [3] Big Data and Analytics Unit, Institute of Global Health Innovation, Imperial College London, London, UK, [4] Leeds Teaching Hospitals NHS Trust, Leeds, UK

***Correspondence:**
Faisal Mushtaq
f.mushtaq@leeds.ac.uk

Big datasets have the potential to revolutionize public health. However, there is a mismatch between the political and scientific optimism surrounding big data and the public's perception of its benefit. We suggest a systematic and concerted emphasis on developing models derived from smaller datasets to illustrate to the public how big data can produce tangible benefits in the long term. In order to highlight the immediate value of a small data approach, we produced a proof-of-concept model predicting hospital length of stay. The results demonstrate that existing small datasets can be used to create models that generate a reasonable prediction, facilitating health-care delivery. We propose that greater attention (and funding) needs to be directed toward the utilization of existing information resources in parallel with current efforts to create and exploit "big data."

Keywords: big data, small data, surgery, health economics, length of stay

The "big data" revolution is central to the long-term vision of health services across the globe (1). For example, big data are central to the UK's Department of Health plans to save £5bn by 2020 through improved operational productivity (2). However, there is a mismatch between the political and scientific optimism surrounding big data and the public's perception of its benefit (3). In this regard, Big Data constitute a deceptively difficult health-care policy. The research community needs to persuade a skeptical public whose personal health data should be made available for analysis if the big data recommendations are to be realized (4, 5) – see for example, the controversial NHS England "care.data" program. Our concern is that the lack of demonstrable *benefits* from data analytics in the short-term may reinforce skepticism and erode government enthusiasm (and support) for big data projects. The UK, where national policy on Big Data is currently under review (6), might serve as a useful test-bed for other countries. We propose that one of the solutions to the many problems facing Big Data could be bridged by demonstrating the benefits of data analytics using smaller, readily available data.

There are already many examples of local and regional routinely collected data sets being used to improve health-care services (4). In fact, the idea of health service research providing useful information to hospital management is, of course, far from new. These cases suggest that analyzing existing, routinely available health data ("small data") might be a good starting point for altering public perception, given the difficult strategy of exploiting larger datasets. However, progress in these domains often proceeds in an *ad hoc* manner and success is self-contained. We suggest a systematic and concerted emphasis on developing *models* from these data could illustrate how data science can produce tangible benefits. In order to demonstrate the value of a small data model-based approach, we produced a proof-of-concept model predicting hospital length of stay (LOS).

We chose LOS because the average cost of an excess bed is approximately £273 per day, and the average cost of an elective inpatient stay is £3,366 (7). A model that could predict LOS with some accuracy would mean that fewer operations would be canceled at short notice because of a lack of bed space, thus saving staff and equipment costs, and crucially, provide an improved service for patients.

The current system of bed planning stands as a testament to the remarkable abilities of staff within a hospital – individuals who use extensive insight and knowledge to juggle beds in an environment where both acute and emergency operations can change the requirements on a moment-to-moment basis. The complex, dynamical nature of the hospital is analogous to a weather system and shows similar characteristics (for example, "chaotic" features such as a sensitive dependence on initial conditions). The difference between the weather forecaster and the hospital bed planner lies in the quality of the models they can run to simulate the system of interest. Cognitive science has shown that humans are poor at making decisions under conditions of high uncertainty (8) and tend to prioritize immediate problems over longer-term planning (9, 10), whereas mathematical models can assist in optimizing decision making (11). We therefore studied whether we could utilize existing NHS data to build a simple predictive model as a precursor to one who could help forecast the need for beds following elective surgery (as the scheduling of elective operations in a very large acute NHS Trust, Leeds Teaching Hospitals, has an element of flexibility that offers a degree of control to those running hospitals). We used available data that had been routinely collected by clinicians, health service practitioners, and administrators on an internal system on a daily basis.

For illustrative purposes, we created a model (see Datasheet S2 in Supplementary Material) that could use predictors known *a priori*, and *post hoc* knowledge (e.g., operation time) to provide estimations of LOS for patients undergoing laparoscopic cholecystectomy (LC). We focused on this procedure because it is estimated that 10 and 15% of the adult western population have gallstones (12) – the most common and costly digestive disease (13) – and LC is the preferred treatment option for symptomatic gallstones (14). Due to its prevalence, we reasoned that a predictive model might complement individual intuition and help hospitals plan elective procedures and associated beds in a more efficient manner. This could be beneficial as the costs associated with discharging patients too early can be greater than the initial investment of bed stay and a day-case surgery policy is not suitable across all specialties and procedures – despite demonstrable success in some areas (15). Previous research indicates that modeling LOS is technically feasible (16, 17), yet these approaches are rarely used in practice. This is particularly surprising given the costs associated with sub-optimal bed allocation and the nature of current approaches to scheduling – even the most rudimentary model should provide information of value – that could ultimately translate to economic benefits in the long run.

Our analysis revealed that month, weekday, year, patient age, and operation time were all predictive of LOS using data from 2004 to 2012. **Figure 1** shows how each predictor influences LOS, if all other predictors are held constant.

Since patient age and operation time were the strongest predictors of stay duration (**Figures 1C,D**), we extracted a two-dimensional plot of their partial effect in combination (see **Figure 2**). Note that operation time is a variable only known post-surgery [though surgeon expertise and difficulty are correlates (18)]. The pseudo-R^2 for this model was 0.29. Based on 1,000 permutations where stay durations were permuted and the model refitted, this model reached statistical significance at a threshold of $p < 0.001$. For younger patients (<55 years), we found a relatively weak relationship between operation length and LOS up to the 3-h mark, but for older patients (>55 years), stay duration increased strongly with surgery length.

There is, of course, substantial between-patient variation unaccounted for by our model (given data limitations), and there is considerable room for further predictive improvement. Intrinsic (but unrecorded) differences between patients are always likely to make prediction difficult. In reality, decision makers face scheduling problems on different time horizons; here, we included operation length as a predictor, but this is clearly not known until the operation is complete. Without this predictor, the best-fit model selects month, year, and patient age as factors, with a pseudo-R^2 value of 0.17. It is remarkable that a simple five-factor model can account for this amount of variance in the data given the complexity of the system.

The results of this exercise demonstrate that existing small data sets could be used to create models that allow a reasonable prediction of hospital LOS after surgery. It is notable that the data we used had considerable limitations. For instance, we focused on one procedure with data from one (albeit, large) NHS Trust, and we did not identify the incidence of complications. These issues could be addressed and may have a substantial impact. If this process is replicated across multiple procedures and hospitals, we could be in a better position to plan for 23 h, 5.5-day facilities instead of full in-patient facilities. This information could ultimately influence how hospitals plan and flex their bed-base.

In summary, we have demonstrated a "proof of concept" that a proportion of the variance associated with patient LOS can be predicted from a limited number of factors. Many applications of medical statistics, such as tests for the efficacy of drugs, require careful experimental design to determine causal effects of putative interventions. In contrast, scheduling problems only require accurate prediction given the observable traits of the patient, since no intervention is proposed. This is where predictive modeling from existing small data sets has the lowest barrier

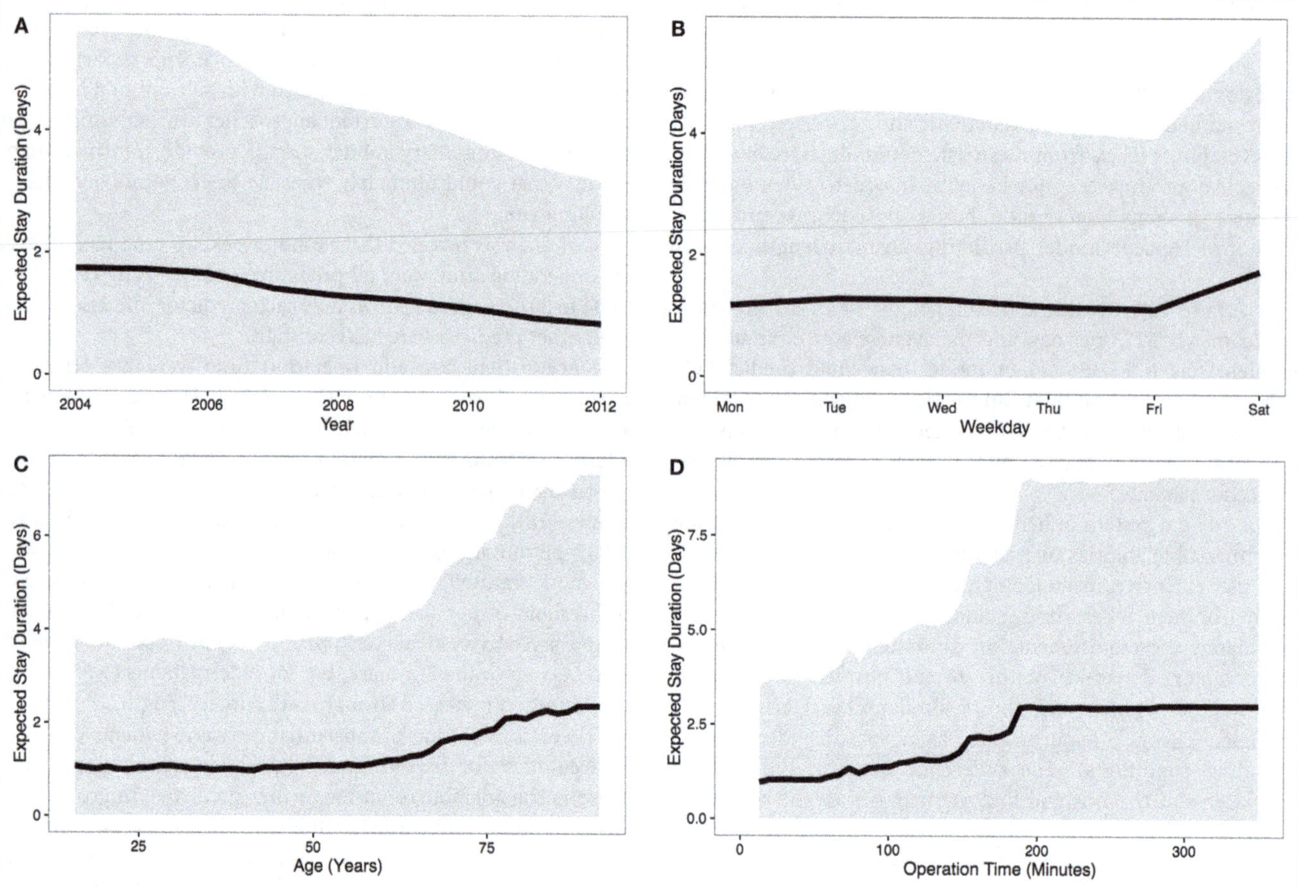

FIGURE 1 | Predicting patient stay duration. The results from the model are presented using line plots (the median prediction is represented by a solid black line and the gray region represents the 95% quantile). **(A)** These data show a steady downwards trend in stay duration over the nine relevant years; **(B)** the duration of stay is longer for operations on Saturdays – most likely due to weekday discharge; **(C)** for patients above 55 years of age, stay duration rapidly increases with age; and finally, **(D)** stay duration also increases with operation time – presumably an indicator of complications in surgery or intrinsically more difficult cases. Interestingly, stay duration reaches a plateau for operations over ~3 h, though there are relatively few data points for surgeries of this length – and as such, this relationship should be treated with caution.

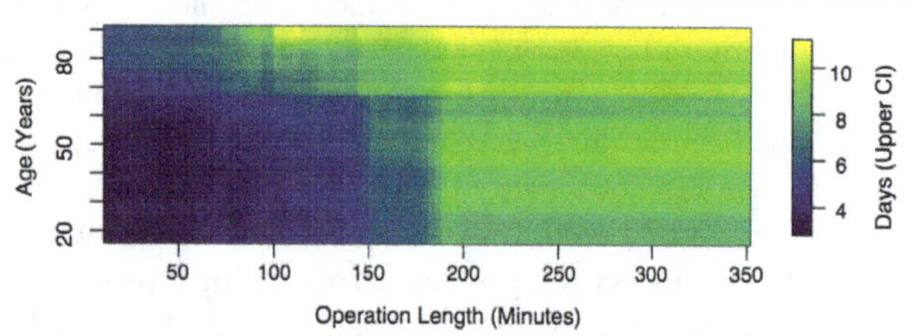

FIGURE 2 | Upper 95% confidence interval of predicted stay duration. This figure shows that while, for younger patients, the effect of surgery length on length of stay is relatively weak up to the 3-h mark, for older patients (>55 years), stay duration increases strongly with duration length across all time scales.

to entry. Systematically recording and utilizing more of these data would allow these data to inform the best computational model and allow schedulers to use the model ahead of time when it can be most efficacious. Crucially, these models could be rapidly developed and deployed from existing datasets. Providing, for example, fewer cancelations of elective operations as a result of the effective implementation of a small data LOS model would provide a tangible example of the benefits of data analytics to the public. We suggest that this could provide *one* solution to the reticence of a public who are skeptical about the benefits of their data being collected, particularly if existing datasets can be utilized in novel and clinically beneficial ways.

Finally, while our example is from the UK NHS – an organization that is the largest health-care provider and one of the largest global producers of health data – the resulting predictive model could be used across other health-care systems. Moreover, a demonstration of the usefulness of data analytics in any country can help change the public's (and clinicians) perception of the value of big data. The UK NHS Hospital Trusts data systems provide an opportune vehicle by which the big data implementation gap can be addressed and, if successful, could serve as a model for others to follow. We therefore propose that greater attention (and funding) needs to be directed toward the utilization of existing data resources, in parallel with current efforts to create and exploit "big data" sets. It is probable that smaller analytical projects yielding efficiency in the short-term ("small data") will persuade society of the longer-term merits of exploiting data, as well as identify the challenges and opportunities in analytics in a more tractable fashion than is afforded by still-to-be-created big data repositories.

AUTHOR CONTRIBUTIONS

ADW collected the data. RPM analyzed the data. FM, RPM, GM-C, TP, DC, SM, TH, CS, DB, GH, SH, SS, RMW, JPAL, and MM-W wrote the paper.

FUNDING

This work was supported by funding from the Leeds Teaching Hospitals Charitable Foundation to ADW, RMW, JPAL and MM-W and an MRC Grant (R17427) to MM-W.

REFERENCES

1. NHS England. *High Quality Datasets: Our Vision*. (2014). Available from: http://www.nhs.uk/NHSEngland/thenhs/records/healthrecords/Pages/care-data.aspx
2. Carter P. *Operational Productivity and Performance in English NHS Acute Hospitals: Unwarranted Variations: An Independent Report for the Department of Health by Lord Carter*. London: Department of Health (2016). Available from: https://www.gov.uk/government/uploads/system/uploads/attachment_data/file/499229/Operational_productivity_A.pdf (accessed 1 April 2016).
3. Raghupathi W, Raghupathi V. Big data analytics in healthcare: promise and potential. *Health Inf Sci Syst* (2014) 2:1–10. doi:10.1186/2047-2501-2-3
4. Ipsos MORI Social Research Institute. *The One-Way Mirror: Public Attitudes to Commercial Access to Health Data*. (2016). Available from: https://www.ipsos-mori.com/Assets/Docs/Publications/sri-wellcome-trust-commercial-access-to-health-data.pdf (accessed 1 April 2016).
5. Parliamentary Office of Science & Technology. Big data and public health. *POSTnote*. London: The Parliamentary Office of Science and Technology (2014). p. 1–4.
6. National Data Guardian. *Caldicott Review: Information Governance in the Health and Care System*. London: Department of Health (2013).
7. Department of Health. *Reference Costs 2012–13*. London: Department of Health (2013).
8. Tversky A, Kahneman D. Judgment under uncertainty: heuristics and biases. *Science* (1974) 185:1124–31. doi:10.1126/science.185.4157.1124
9. Anderson LR, Stafford SL. Individual decision-making experiments with risk and intertemporal choice. *J Risk Uncertain* (2009) 38:51–72. doi:10.1007/s11166-008-9059-4
10. Mischel W, Grusec J. Waiting for rewards and punishments: effects of time and probability on choice. *J Pers Soc Psychol* (1967) 5:24–31. doi:10.1037/h0025699
11. Cresswell KM, Bates DW, Sheikh A, Morrison Z, Robertson A, Cresswell K, et al. Ten key considerations for the successful implementation and adoption of large-scale health information technology. *J Am Med Inform Assoc* (2013) 20:e9–13. doi:10.1136/amiajnl-2013-001684
12. Vaughan J, Gurusamy KS, Davidson BR. Day-surgery versus overnight stay surgery for laparoscopic cholecystectomy. *Cochrane Database Syst Rev* (2013) 7:CD006798. doi:10.1002/14651858.CD006798.pub4
13. Gollan J, Bulkley G, Diehl A, Elashoff J, Federle M, Hogan W. Gallstones and laparoscopic cholecystectomy. *JAMA* (1993) 269:1018–24. doi:10.1001/jama.1993.03500080066034
14. Ballal M, David G, Willmott S, Corless DJ, Deakin M, Slavin JP. Conversion after laparoscopic cholecystectomy in England. *Surg Endosc* (2009) 23:2338–44. doi:10.1007/s00464-009-0338-1
15. Appleby J. Day case surgery: a good news story for the NHS. *BMJ* (2015) 351:h4060. doi:10.1136/bmj.h4060
16. Chuang M-T, Hu Y-H, Lo C-L. Predicting the prolonged length of stay of general surgery patients: a supervised learning approach. *Int Trans Oper Res* (2016):1–16. doi:10.1111/itor.12298
17. Hachesu PR, Ahmadi M, Alizadeh S, Sadoughi F. Use of data mining techniques to determine and predict length of stay of cardiac patients. *Healthc Inform Res* (2013) 19:121–9. doi:10.4258/hir.2013.19.2.121
18. Yasunaga H, Tsuchiya K, Matsuyama Y, Ohe K. Analysis of factors affecting operating time, postoperative complications, and length of stay for total knee arthroplasty: nationwide web-based survey. *J Orthop Sci* (2009) 14:10–6. doi:10.1007/s00776-008-1294-7

10

Situation, Impacts and Future Challenges of Tobacco Control Policies for Youth: An Explorative Systematic Policy Review

Chhabi Lal Ranabhat[1,2,3,4]*, Chun-Bae Kim[2,5]*, Myung Bae Park[4] and Mihajlo (Michael) Jakovljevic[6,7]

[1] Policy Research Institute, Kathmandu, Nepal, [2] Institute for Poverty Alleviation and International Development, Yonsei University, Wonju, South Korea, [3] Manmohan Memorial Institute of Health Science, Kathmandu, Nepal, [4] Department of Gerontology, Pai Chai University, Daejeon, South Korea, [5] Department of Preventive Medicine, Yonsei University Wonju College of Medicine, Wonju, South Korea, [6] Department of Global Health Economics and Policy, University of Kragujevac, Kragujevac, Serbia, [7] Division of Health Economics, Lund University, Lund, Sweden

***Correspondence:**
Chhabi Lal Ranabhat
chhabir@gmail.com
Chun-Bae Kim
kimcb@yonsei.ac.kr

Background: Tobacco use in youths is a major public health challenge globally, and approaches to the challenge have not been sufficiently addressed. The existing policies for tobacco control are not well specified by age.

Objective: Our study aims to systematically investigate existing tobacco control policies, potential impacts, and national and international challenges to control tobacco use targeting the youth.

Data sources: We used the statistics of the Global Youth Tobacco Survey (GYTS), studies, and approaches of tobacco control policies targeting youth. Considering country, continent, age, and significance, PubMed, Health Inter-Network Access to Research Initiative (HINARI), Scopus, the Cochrane Library, Google, and Google Scholar were searched. The related keywords were tobacco control, youth, smoking, smoking reduction policies, prevalence of tobacco use in youth, classification of tobacco control policies, incentives to prevent young people from using tobacco, WHO Framework Convention on Tobacco Control (FTCT), etc. The search strategy was by timeline, specific and popular policies, reliability, significance, and applicability.

Results: We found 122 studies related to this topic. There were 25 studies focusing on situation, significance, and theoretical aspects of tobacco control policies associated with youth; 41 studies on national population polices and challenges; and 7 studies for global challenges to overcome the youth tobacco epidemic. All national policies have been guided by WHO-MPOWER strategies. Increases in tobacco tax, warning signs on packaging, restriction of tobacco product advertisements, national law to discourage young people, and peer-based approaches to quit tobacco are popular policies. Smuggling of tobacco products by youth and ignorance of smokeless tobacco control approach are major challenges.

Limitation: Our study was flexible for the standard age of youth and we were not able to include all countries in the world and most of the studies focused on smoking control rather than all smokeless tobaccos.

Conclusion: The policies of tobacco control adopted by many countries are based on the WHO Framework Convention on Tobacco Control but not necessarily focused on youth. Due to the physical and economic burden of tobacco consumption by youth, this is a high priority that needs to be addressed. Youth-focused creative policies are necessary, and more priority must be given to tobacco prevention in youth. Tobacco control should be a social, public health, and quality-of-life concern rather than a business and trade issue.

Implication of key findings: There is limited research on how and in what ways tobacco control policies reach young people and their engagement with these policies from physical, physiological, and psychological aspects. Analysis of these aspects, popular polices practiced in different countries, and creative strategies support the need to review current practices and future ways to discourage youth from tobacco use.

Keywords: tobacco control, smoking, policies, youth, preventive measure, tobacco products

INTRODUCTION

Tobacco consumption is a major challenge for the 21st century because tobacco-related deaths are increasing, destroying the young generation and promoting an environmental threat. Globally, tobacco has killed 100 million people in the 20th century, much more than all deaths in World Wars I and II combined, and tobacco-related deaths will number around 1 billion in the 21st century if current tobacco use patterns continue (Eriksen et al., 2015). Of the 100 million projected tobacco-related deaths over the next 20 years, about half will be of people in the productive ages of 35–69 (Centers for Disease Control and Prevention, 2000). Regardless of many national bans on tobacco sales to minors, approximately 25% of people under 18 years old are using tobacco and 12.6% are using more than two types of tobacco products (Arrazola et al., 2014). There are multiple impacts (economic, health, social, family, and peer groups) of tobacco use in youth because they are losing high amount of money, as the tax on tobacco increases year by year, risk factors for many disease, vulnerability to alcohol use and drugs, and copying his/her tobacco use by juniors in schools and sibling in family put them at risk for tobacco use.

There are a variety of programs and policies for tobacco control, but policy analyses on age-specific tobacco control are very rare. It is important because the resources, efforts, and approaches to quitting tobacco for people 60 years of age and those 16 years age do not have a similar impact. A study pointed out that there is a need for a comprehensive multifaceted approach to tobacco control policies for youth (Grimsaw and Stanton, 2017; Cancer Council., 2017a). There is a need to observe that as a foundation and productive age group, youth should be a high priority because interventions would be cost-effective and more productive to family and the nation. Moreover, approaches to controlling tobacco in youth are easy in comparison with late adults and the elderly because nicotine addiction in the late stage is difficult to overcome. From the point of its effectiveness, preventive and nominal remedial approaches are sufficient for youth. In contrast, more resources and complex medical approaches are necessary in late-stage addiction. Likewise, different kinds of medical risk can be prevented in the early stage (youth) but are hardly possible in the late stage. Previous studies, research, policies, and programs are not clearly distinctly age-specific tobacco control approaches, and in our study, we explore the different dynamics of tobacco control policies focusing on youth.

Prevalence of Tobacco Use Among Youth

Tobacco use among youth remains a major public health concern worldwide. Globally, there are about 1.2 billion smokers, of whom more than 50% are young people; the prevalence varies by region, country, and gender (Khuder et al., 2008; Lim et al., 2010; Al-Sadat et al., 2010). By gender, smoking among boys (16%) is almost three times than that among girls (6%) globally. In the West Pacific, the prevalence of smoking among boys (18%) is four times than that among girls (4%), whereas in the United States and Europe, the gap between boys and girls is less than double. Smokeless tobacco is also gaining popularity and is currently used globally by 8% (6% in boys and 2% in girls). The highest proportion of girls using smokeless tobacco (17%) is found in the West Pacific and the lowest (2%) is found in Europe (World Health Organization., 2012). India, with 327 million adolescents, has one of the youngest populations in the world; the number of adolescents using tobacco is approximately 21% of the country's population (Vidhubala

---

Abbreviations: CDC, Centers for Disease Control and Prevention; FCTC, Framework Convention on Tobacco Control; GYTS, Global Youth Tobacco Survey; NRF, National Research Foundation; STM, Sales to minor; WHO, World Health Organization; IARC, International Agency for Research on Cancer; BAT, British American Tobacco.

et al., 2014). Since 1980, large reductions in the estimated prevalence of daily smoking have been observed at the global level for both boys and girls (e.g., in the United States, about 10% from 1980 to 1990 of 12th-grade students), (Nelson et al., 2008) but because of population growth, the gross number of smokers has increased significantly (Ng et al., 2014). According to the Global Youth Tobacco Survey (GYTS) 2011, the top three countries for tobacco consumption rates were Papua New Guinea (43.8%), Chile (31.5%), and Lithuania (30.8%), while Cambodia consumption rate was the lowest (0.2%) (World Health Organization, 2011). Prevalence of youth tobacco use reduces life expectancy (Ranabhat et al., 2018; Ranabhat et al., 2019). Socially, youth from disadvantaged groups are more vulnerable to smoking because of their social context (Hefler and Chapman, 2014). Despite the variation in statistics between different classifications of youth, youth smoking is a major threat in every aspect.

Understanding Youth

Youth is a critical and foundation period of human life; however, there is no consistent definition. Youth is the time of life when one is young, but often means the time between childhood and adulthood (maturity) (Walker et al., 2013). Around the world, the English terms youth, adolescent, teenager, kid, and young person are interchanged, often meaning the same thing (Konopka, 1973). The United Nations has defined the contextual definition of youth: age between 15 and 24 by UN secretaries, UNESCO, and ILO; age of 15–32 by UN habitat; age of 10–24 by UNFPA and WHO; child until 18 by UNICEF; and age between 15 and 35 by the African youth charter (United Nation., 2016). Beyond this, different countries have defined the youth in their context, and we have used the term youth as a wide concept as used by different scholars and organization. The focus of this study is on tobacco control policies applicable for youth despite the age variation.

Youth Period and Risk for Tobacco Use/Smoking

There are theoretical and empirical studies about the risk of youth tobacco use/smoking. Youth may initiate smoking by i) social learning theory; youth are eager to try something new, i.e., attention, retention, motor reproduction, and reproduction and motivation process; (Bandura and McClelland, 1977) ii) psychological development theory; they decide whether they should use or not, i.e., age, self-control, academic achievement, growth trend, and distal structure (parents or peer); (Jessor and Jessor, 1977) iii) behavior theory; the attitude of acceptance and to continue or not, i.e., person's behavior is a function of behavioral intention, which is determined by attitude toward the act; (Ajzen and Fishbein, 1970), and iv) self-conceiving theory; every activity of human is determined by self-conception (Rosenberg, 1986). Blum has explored different aspects of human emotions, motivation, and perceptions, particularly during the period of youth (Blum, 2009). Due to their age, physiological changes, and family and social environments, youth often perpetuate smoking practices, and they ultimately become addicted. Indeed, youth tobacco use is a primary source of substance use and other social deviations. High school male students who have smokers in family and school, smoker friends, media and advertisement influence, and easy access to the purchase of cigarettes are factors to youth smoking; smokers often lack self-control even though they know smoking is harmful (Simons-Morton et al., 1999; Alexander et al., 2001; Ertas, 2007).

Key Questions

KQ1—What is the current situation of youth tobacco use in terms of prevalence and control policy pattern?
KQ2—What are the major and popular policies to control tobacco in the national and global context targeting youth?
KQ3—What could be the best creative policies for tobacco control for youth?

Objective of the Study

The aim of this study is to systematically investigate the situation regarding youth tobacco use, existing policies, effectiveness, and challenges in the national and global context.

METHODS

Eligibility Criteria

We focused precisely on tobacco control policies, targeting youth, policies adopted by countries, challenges to implementing those policies, publications in English, and availability of latest prevalence data.

Studies were included based on the following PICOS strategies.

1) Population: Youth population and age limit vary between countries.
2) Intervention: Popular and successful intervention policies to control tobacco use targeting for youth.
    a. Disconnect youth from tobacco
    b. Smoking/tobacco use cessation
3) Comparison: Comparison of tobacco control policies by country and intervention time duration.
4) Outcomes: Prevalence of tobacco use before intervention and after intervention.
5) Study types: Interventional studies, surveys (cross-sectional and follow up), cohort and randomized control trials, core contents related to study from official web pages and some gray materials.

Exclusion:

1) Did not meet the inclusion criteria.
2) General tobacco control not applicable for youth; data available are not in English; mixed studies with tobacco use; coffee, alcohol, and other substance use/abuse; and data with mixed/overlap of age (youth and adult/youth and elder).

The details of excluded data with reason are available in the PRISMA flowchart (**Figure 1**).

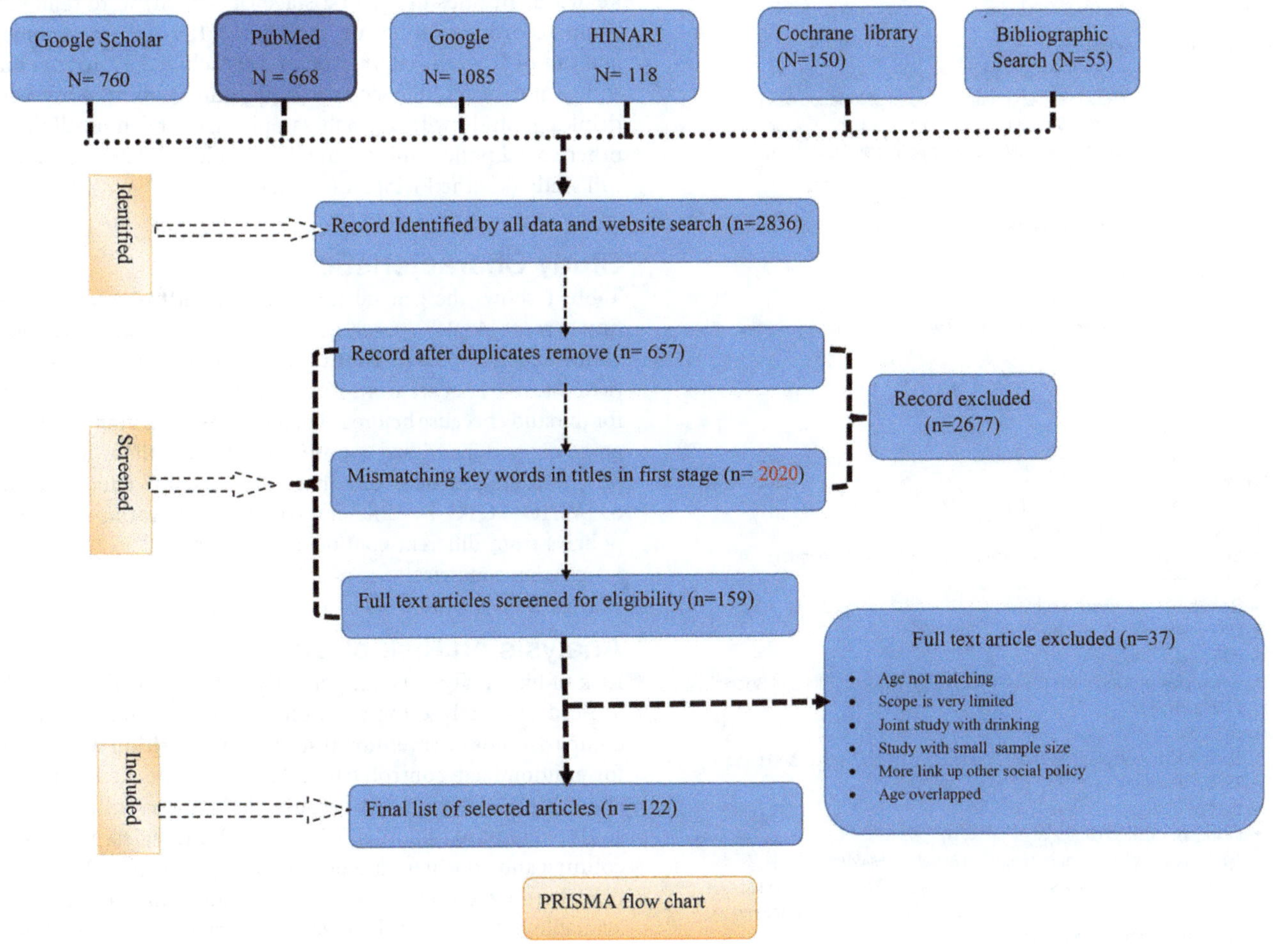

FIGURE 1 | PRISMA flow chart of research strategy.

Data Searching Strategy

Literature search strategies were developed using Medical Subjects Headings (MeSH) terms and keywords. Different health and social science search engines and databases were used (PubMed, Scopus, the Cochrane Library, HINARI, Google, and Google Scholar) to find sources regarding global and national policies mostly focusing on youth tobacco use. We used single, double, or multiple MeSH terms, free text, and specific terms under a subheading to identify relevant studies from the online data sources. Search strategy also included content, synonyms, year, and country names (**Box 1**). We downloaded and analyzed relevant journal articles, books, survey results, analytical views related to the WHO FCTC, and unpublished reports.

Data Source Management

We, all authors, established the inclusion and exclusion criteria and data search strategies. CR and MBP searched all data and CBK and MJ verified those data. There were some data that were ambiguous and less relevant to our study but we decided to include some in our study.

Ways of Screening and Selection of Data Sources

The title of the study was screened by search engines using major keywords and titles. Many times, search engines were used to find the appropriate titles. After that, the titles were selected. In a second step, abstract and full-length studies were selected by database search engines. In the third stage, full-length articles were screened based on inclusion criteria. Studies were assessed using criteria developed, for example, effective for public health implications, representativeness of study samples, comparability, credibility of data collection tools, and attributability to the intervention. An additional criterion of "generalizability" assessed whether findings were likely to be transferable at a global, regional, or national level. Particular attention was paid to internal and external validity; important quality and validity issues are discussed alongside study results.

Quality Assessment

For quality assessment of resources, we used the Effective Public Health Practice Project (EPHPP) Quality Assessment Tool for

BOX 1 | Electronic data search strategy.

Terminology used for search
Tobacco control policies, Smoking reduction policy, Youth and smoking, Tobacco use by adolescents, Comparative studies of tobacco use by boys and girls, Systemic review of tobacco control policies, Classification of tobacco control policies, Incentives on preventing and cessation of smoking, Legal provision for tobacco control, Effectiveness of WHO FCTC, Interventions for tobacco control on youth, MPOWER strategies, tobacco control policies by country continent, age gender, Effectiveness of MPOWER etc.

PubMed Search Options
- Search by: Terminology mentioned above
- Search Details: Single, double or multiple MeSH terms as mentioned in terminology
- Article type: All
- Text availability: Abstract and all text
- Publication date: Any time
- Complementary search: Similar articles

Scopus search options
- Search by: Subject area and title
- Display options: All available
- Source type: Journal, Book Series and Conference preceding

Cochrane library
- Search by: Key words and titles
- Date: before 2005 and between 2005 – 2019
- Language: English
- Search folder: Cochrane review, Cochrane protocol, Trial and Special collection

Google Scholar
- Search terminologies: As mentioned above by key words and titles
- Time: Any times
- Sort by: Relevance
- Included: Related citations

Health Inter Network Access to Research Initiative (HINARI)
- Search terminologies: As mentioned above by key words and titles
- Content type: Journal article, Publication, Book Chapter, Conference preceding, Data, Government documents
- Publication date: Before 2005 and between 2005 – 2019
- Discipline: Medicine, Public health, Policy
- Language: English

Google
- Key words: As mentioned above by key words and titles
- Display: all
- Purpose: Screening key titles

Intervention (Higgins and Green, 2011) as reference. All research studies applied in this paper were searched and screened by two authors (Chhabi Ranabhat and Myung-Bae Park), with any disagreement resolved by consensus or arbitration of authors during meetings. For the risk of bias, we considered only selection bias and data collection method.

RESULTS

Search Outcome

The cumulative total records found in our search screen were 2,836 from PubMed (n = 668) Google Scholar (n = 760), Google (n = 1,085), Health Inter-Network Access to Research Initiative (HINARI n = 118), Cochrane library (n = 150), and Bibliographic Search (n = 55). The total excluded 2677 records in the first stage: duplicates (n = 657) and mismatching keywords in titles in the first stage (n = 2020) were removed. From record screening, we found n = 159 full text sources, and out of 159 full-length articles, we excluded 37 articles due to age not matching, scope is very limited, joint study with drinking, study with a small sample size, and more links to other social policy, and we finally included 122 articles in our full study (see the PRISMA flowchart).

Study Characteristics

Table 1 shows the general characteristics of the study. Almost fifty percent (44.94%, n = 89) of our retrieved studies were about youth-targeted tobacco control in youth and most of the data (87.60%, n = 121) are from 2005 to 2019. We set the time frame for the study because before 2005, there was a situation of tobacco epidemic and individual countries were doing their own efforts on controlling tobacco use after 2005 (actually after signature on WHO FCTC by different countries). Regarding national policies from different continents, more than 1/3 (41.46%) are from Asian countries.

Analysis on Risk of Bias

Risk of bias analysis is not perfectly attractive with our study. We did not analyze the attrition bias because our study is a comparison of interventional studies and attrition bias occurs for randomized control trials. Moreover, we had very low influence of selection bias because all the interventions in this study were based on WHO MPOWER strategies. Studies by country and continent are not in equal proportion. We found that there were few studies in Africa, and more studies were available for Asia, but the creative policies we presented have no geographical boundaries. The number of studies for Asian countries is more than that from other continents because Asia has more than 2/3 of the world population and there are

TABLE 1 | General characteristics of included studies based on key questions, time interval, and region.

Characteristics	N	%
Characteristics of studies by key questions (*n* = 88)		
Situation of youth tobacco use	15	17.04
Nature of tobacco control policies focusing youth	21	23.86
Popular policies by different countries and major challenges	41	46.59
Way forward and creative policies	12	13.63
Characteristics of studies by year (time) (*n* = 122)		
Before 2005	15	12.29
2006 to 2019	107	87.70
Characteristics of study by continent (*n* = 43)		
Australia	6	13.95
Asia	17	39.53
Africa	4	9.30
Europe	4	9.30
North America	7	16.27
South America	5	11.62

a higher number of countries compared to other continents. Most importantly, we focused on the policies related to youth and policies applicable to all age groups; gender and location were not prioritized. We applied almost all national representative survey results and global studies. There were no significant issues on data collection from the aspect on risk of bias.

Synthesis of Result

We synthesized the results *via* a descriptive approach in three perspectives. The first one is youth-targeted current pattern of tobacco control policies and their impact. We have divided the policy pattern into two categories: i) protect the youth form tobacco use and ii) help the youth quit tobacco use. Likewise, we compared the effectiveness and challenges of tobacco control in different countries. Other important aspects are global challenges and ways on controlling tobacco use among youth.

Patterns of Youth Tobacco Control Policies

Over the past two decades, a number of tobacco control policies have been implemented to prevent smoking initiation and encourage cessation among adolescents. To expand the fight against the tobacco epidemic, WHO introduced MPOWER, an initiative that includes six strategies: monitor tobacco use and prevention policies; protect people from tobacco smoke; offer help to people who want to quit using tobacco; warn about the dangers of tobacco; enforce bans on tobacco advertising, promotion, and sponsorship; and raise taxes on tobacco (World Health Organization, 2008). The effectiveness of MPOWER on youth is distinct. The International Agency for Research on Cancer (IARC) found that after increasing the tax and price of tobacco, there was significant reduction in tobacco use because youth are price sensitive and have a limited amount of resources (World Health Organization, 2011). Similarly, the smoke-free air law has a protective effect on young people and reduced smoking prevalence among boys of high socioeconomic status (Tauras et al., 2013). Most youth are influenced by tobacco advertisements, and according to the WHO, 24 countries have implemented a complete ban on direct and indirect tobacco advertising, promotion and sponsorship (TAPS) (World Health Organization, 2013). A study in 19 developing countries showed that there was a positive correlation between smoking and exposure to advertising (Kostova and Blecher, 2013). There were no appropriate research examining the effectiveness of offering to quit tobacco/smoking and warning of the harmful effects of tobacco applicable for youth. Therefore, in high-, (Dupont and Ward, 2002) low-, and middle-income countries, (Joseph, 2010) raising the price of tobacco and the tax on tobacco is more effective in reducing youth tobacco use than other strategies. The US Centers for Disease Control and Prevention (CDC) identified seven basic principles for tobacco control; three of these policies are relevant to youth: reducing tobacco use among adolescents; reducing the initiation of tobacco use among children, adolescents, and young adults; and increasing smoking cessation attempts among adolescent smokers (Centers for Disease Control Prevention (CDC)., 2007). A tobacco control plan in the United Kingdom has implemented three strategies to protect youth from tobacco use: reducing tobacco consumption, supporting parents and youths, and reinforcing the benefits of clean air spaces (National Health Service., 2015). Policy researchers have classified tobacco control initiatives into two groups: those intending to prevent first-time tobacco users (adolescents) and those aiming for cessation of tobacco use among current users, including both occasional and frequent users. These initiatives are based on multipronged approach, described below.

Disconnect Youth From Tobacco and Use Advertising Campaigns and Laws to Demotivate Youth From Tobacco Consumption

Popular policies within this guideline include cigarette tax increases, smoke-free air laws, and youth access laws (laws on sales to minors and laws against youth possession, use, and purchase) (Warner et al., 2003). Ross and Chaloupka highlighted that in the United States, higher cigarette prices reduced the probability of youth smoking, and the teen-specific perceived price of cigarettes had a negative effect on demand (Ross and Chaloupka, 2003). Similar findings have been reported by other researchers, and some have found that increased price decreased current smoking prevalence and the number of cigarettes smoked per day among youth and young adult smokers (Wasserman et al., 1991; Tauras, 2004; Levy et al., 2004). Other approaches to discourage adolescent smoking are restrictions on smoking at home, more extensive bans on smoking in public places, and enforced bans on smoking at school (Wakefield et al., 2000; Farkas et al., 2000). Sales to minors (STM) laws, which penalize merchants and retailers for selling tobacco to youth, and possession, use, and purchase laws, which punish youth themselves for possessing, using, or purchasing tobacco products, have also been applied (Rabin and Sugarman, 2001). Some studies have revealed an association between youth access and STM laws, but a sustained relationship between those laws and decreased youth smoking prevalence has been questioned. A study from Bangladesh shows that youth are more vulnerable due to a tobacco-friendly environment in school (Kabir et al., 2013). When the price increase policy was endorsed in the United States, it had a mixed impact, but a systematic review revealed no significant change in youth smoking. This law was also controversial, and cases were brought to court (Jason et al., 2005). Raising taxes on tobacco and STM laws have thus shown mixed effects, along with legal restrictions on adolescent smoking in the United States.

Increasing Smoking Cessation

Tobacco cessation, especially smoking cessation, depends on patterns of smoking such as age, peer pressure, influences of electronic media, and effective counseling to users. Among youth, quitting smoking has had no special program, and only 2–8% of youth smokers have attempted to quit in the Grimshaw et al., 2003 study. Hodder et al. suggested that universal school-based interventions could be an effective way to get youth to quit using tobacco and alcohol (Hodder et al., 2014).

In family and school, both approaches can be equally useful because some family members, teachers, and seniors need to quit smoking and pupils at risk must be disconnected from the first puff of smoking. Preventing youth from starting tobacco use is more effective and costs less than helping users quit, but no proper comparative studies have examined the different patterns and effects of youth tobacco control policies.

Major National Tobacco Control Policies Intervention, Outcomes, and Challenges

Table 2 shows the national tobacco control policies targeting youth. In 26 studies, researchers explored the overview and impact of youth-related tobacco control policies from China, India, Nepal, Thailand, Japan, South Korea, Namibia, Chad, Seychelles, Mauritius, Niger, Eritrea, Madagascar, South Africa, North Africa, France, United Kingdom, Australia, Uruguay, Panama, Colombia, Guatemala, Brazil, United States, and Canada. Likewise, in 15 studies, the challenges to control tobacco use in those countries were investigated. Seven studies were used as representative of global situations and challenges.

The direction of current policies has shifted significantly after WHO FCTC in tobacco control movement. The average strength of policies adopted varies significantly by country efforts. Cultural diversity leads to different pros and cons of tobacco control initiatives to any age, gender, geography, etc., and these subtleties must be taken into account when forming policies, and the FCTC was implemented on a national and local level.

A report of the US Surgeon General in 2012 showed that the global youth tobacco use rate was decreasing satisfactorily; the rate was 28% in 2000 and had declined to 8% by 2013 (Health UDo, Services H., 2012), but that survey did not match the GYTS of 2011. WHO FCTC has a comprehensive and global impact, specific to reducing the burden of youth tobacco use, but countries are reluctant to take proactive roles and prepare specific strategies due to lack of strong monitoring by WHO (Warner and Tam, 2012). Nevertheless, taxation, clean indoor air policies, and warning labels are ranked as the highest priorities but are general approaches, and there is still a need for more specific guidelines, integrated approaches, and age-specific tobacco control initiatives.

Tobacco companies around the world are focusing on strategic plans to block the implementation of Article 11 of the WHO FCTC, which sets guidelines on packaging and labeling of tobacco products (Sebrié et al., 2010) because youth are their target group as after they have become addicted, youth become regular customers. Tobacco companies have the power and money to influence legislators (Patel et al., 2007) and challenge the government's legislative powers through litigation (Holden and Lee, 2009). The British American Tobacco (BAT) company's former quality controller appealed against the ban on public smoking in Uganda; however, it was not successful. The tobacco industry in Kenya went to court to challenge the Tobacco Control Act of 2007, which created challenges for public smoking ban in public places (Tumwine, 2011). Similar cases have also been seen in the US high courts without decisions, representing a challenge to implement the WHO FCTC. Tobacco companies have litigated against new cigarette labeling policies in Uruguay, Brazil, and Paraguay to stop or delay the implementation of pictorial warnings (Sebrié et al., 2010) Thus, tobacco control stakeholders and tobacco production, manufacturing, and distribution companies need to continue to fight. It shows that tobacco companies may be a negative influence on youth-friendly tobacco control policies in the future.

DISCUSSION

The WHO FCTC sought to substantially reduce and sustain reductions in indoor smoking and had high levels of public support and a strong public commitment with close monitoring in France, (Fong et al., 2013) China, (Levy et al., 2014) the United States and Canada, (House of Representative, USA., 2009; Levy et al., 2011; Hitchman et al., 2013) South Africa, (Reddy et al., 2013) South Korea, (Levy et al., 2010) and Brazil (Levy et al., 2012) (**Table 1**). The popular policies were tax increase, restriction on advertisement, and smoking ban in public places, but the most effective policy is raising the tax on tobacco products (Health NCfCDPaHPUOoSa., 2012) Abuse of youth to promote smoking by companies and smuggling are major challenges, particularly in Africa and South America. The above policies showed that hard policies (legal provision) could be more effective and long lasting. Some creative soft policies (program and interventions) were also equally effective but policies related to tobacco cessation are not enough. Primarily, strong monitoring and creative preventive policies led to satisfactory reduction on prevalence on youth tobacco use.

In our study, we explored the need to formulate tobacco control policies by age groups, and the vulnerable age group is the youth; there is a need for a preventive way that is cost-effective and a lesser burden to the disease both clinically and economically. There are some similar conclusions in our studies. Saleheen et al. suggested that there is need for targeted policies for youth and burden of diseases produced by tobacco (Saleheen et al., 2014). Another systematic review by Jawad with 36 studies from 15 countries yielding 125 elasticity estimates found that a 10% price increase would reduce demand by 8.3% for cigars, 6.4% for roll your owns, 5.7% for bidis, and 2.1% for smokeless tobacco (Jawad et al., 2018), mostly to youth (Levy et al., 2018). Another systematic review from 16 studies by Duncan found that a tobacco control approach in health care settings is more effective than in school and at home (Duncan et al., 2018). A policy review by Glantz concluded that e-cigarettes are replacing conventional cigarettes, but it is not a good approach to reducing nicotine dependency (Glantz and Bareham, 2018). Now, the JUUL lab's mission is to eliminate cigarettes, but it does not relieve nicotine dependency as it only replaces traditional tobaccos; the challenge for JUUL is to eliminate nicotine dependency in the future. The tobacco control project period is also a significant factor because comprehensive tobacco control programs lead to an 8% short-term relative reduction, increasing to a 12% long-term relative reduction in smoking prevalence through the greater impact on youth smoking (Levy et al., 2018).

TABLE 2 | National tobacco policies and challenges to control.

Policy intervention and outcomes by countries	Current challenges
China applied a tax increase, smoke-free policies, health warnings, media campaigns, and cessation incentives targeting youth with strong monitoring mechanisms. Youth tobacco use dropped from 10% to 3% from 2001 to 2011(World Health Organization, 2011).	The tobacco companies are not honest in implementing the warning message and pictures on packets because the letter size are small and in English (Hu et al., 2013). Only 1/4 of youth know about the harmful effect of tobacco use, and annual average cigarette sales per capita is increasing (Katanoda et al., 2013).
India and Thailand have implemented graphic health warnings on various tobacco products, and other countries in the region are in the process of implementing warnings targeting youth because it is the most cost-effective approach (World Health Organization, 2011). According to the Global Youth Tobacco Survey (GYTS), the situation of youth smoking before and after implementation was 10.8–4.4% in India and smokeless tobacco is very high.	Easy use of pocket money to purchase of tobacco and use of smokeless tobacco without tax in India (Kaur and Jain, 2011; Oswal, 2015).
Nepal government endorsed the National Tobacco Control Strategic Plan (2013–2016) special provision of youth(Ministry of Health and Population., 2013). Those provisions are raising tax on tobacco products, complete ban on advertising for tobacco products, and incentive to youth who want to quit tobacco use. The prevalence of youth tobacco use in Nepal decreased slightly from 18% to 12% in a 6-year period of time.	There is a great challenge that smokeless tobacco prevalence is increasing due to the comparative low price of cigarettes (Hawkins et al., 2018), poor implementation of health- and tobacco-related laws, (Ranabhat et al., 2019) and indigenous youth from hill areas are more likely to use tobacco (Pradhan et al., 2013).
Japan has endorsed a smoking control policy by law with four components including a smoking ban in public places, governmental offices, taxis, and schools. They have also implemented a reward strategy for youth who quit smoking, which has focused on girls and has demonstrated positive impact (Kim et al., 2013). According to WHO report 2016, youth tobacco use in 2002 was 17%, and in 2016, it reduced in 3.1% (World Health Organization, 2017).	Higher prevalence of smoking in part-time high school children, parent smoking, and alcohol use together are major challenges in Japan (Watanabe et al., 2013).
In South Korea, tobacco tax increases, mass media campaign, Health Promotion Act, and Juvenile Protection Act helped to protect youth from smoking (Do and Farooqui, 2012; Durkin et al., 2012) Youth tobacco prevalence decreased from 17.5% to 8% between 2000 and 2008 after an adjustment for gender (Korean Association on Smoking or Health., 2010).	Only 30% of cigarette packets are covered by mild and light warning signs and 30% youth suffer from secondhand smoke (Cho, 2014).
Namibia and Chad banned smoking in public places with no exceptions (i.e., no designated smoking areas), thereby creating 100% smoke-free environments and fully meeting the standards of the FCTC and its guidelines (Tumwine, 2011).	In most African countries, youth have been using cigarettes in spite of warning activities, like girls have been using in night clubs (Doku, 2010). Warning message from mass media have been highly ignored (Islami et al., 2015).
Chad further restricts smoking in vehicles carrying minors or pregnant women (Tumwine, 2011).	
Seychelles banned smoking in public places, workplaces, and public transport without designated smoking rooms. Its law does not apply to hotel rooms, although the owner may prohibit or restrict smoking (Tumwine, 2011).	
Mauritius has legislation on packaging and labeling of tobacco products, but in other countries, such legislation has only been partially adopted (Tumwine, 2011).	
Niger, Chad, Eritrea, and Madagascar have legislation against all forms of direct and indirect advertisement of tobacco (Tumwine, 2011).	
South Africa has the most comprehensive ban on tobacco advertising, promotion, and sponsorship, but the ban does not extend to advertising in books, magazines, newspapers, films, or video transmissions made outside South Africa (Tumwine, 2011) Youth tobacco decreased from 24% to 12% according to GYTS in 2011.	
The most successful approaches in North Africa include raising taxes and banning advertising (Madkour et al., 2013).	
Tobacco excise taxes and increased prices reduced tobacco consumption and prevented young people from beginning to smoke in France and some other countries. As a consequence, public health has improved (Chaloupka et al., 2011).	High prevalence of girls smoking, high socioeconomic health inequality, and parent's smoking are becoming major challenges in the European region (Lorant et al., 2015).
Less attractive cigarette packaging, warning signs about smoking, and restrictions on advertisement have been successful in reducing youth smoking in the UK (Asamura et al., 2015).	
Stead et al. recommended nicotine replacement therapy to help youth in the UK quit smoking, citing success rates of 50–70% (Stead et al., 2008).	
First-world country using plain packaging, long anti-smoking advertisements (White et al., 2013), smoking bans in hospitals and prisons (Sullivan and Rees, 2014), and utilization of social media (Maddox et al., 2013) have all been implemented in Australia. Likewise, multi-component community education interventions and peer-based approach (Cancer Council., 2017b) are effective in influencing smoking behavior and preventing the uptake of smoking in young people. The prevalence of tobacco use by youth in 2005 was 12%, and in 2017, it declined to 6.5% (Greenhalgh EaW MH., 2019)	Australia has mostly focused on smoking cessation. Dennis Thomas has explored 21 challenges to quit smoke; youths start smoking from friends and family also but there is sufficient support to quit (Thomas et al., 2016).

(Continued)

TABLE 2 | Continued.

Policy intervention and outcomes by countries	Current challenges
Comprehensive smoke-free laws have been implemented in four countries (Uruguay, Panama, Colombia, and Guatemala), and in many cities, states, and provinces (Griffith et al., 2010). Colombia has forwarded the tobacco control law from the senate (Ruiz et al., 2009), imposed higher tobacco taxation, taken control of illegal tobacco smuggling, and reimburses medical smoking cessation interventions (Müller and Wehbe, 2008). Brazil applied tax increases, smoke-free airway laws, a mass media campaign, and a cessation program (Horta et al., 2001). The situation of youth tobacco users dropped from 11.1% to 10% between 1997 and 2011 according to the GYTS.	Tobacco smuggling is a serious problem in Latin America, and youth are at high risk and the price of cigarettes is low in Latin America and the result is youths easily start smoking using their pocket money(Muller and Wehbe, 2008).
The US applied higher tobacco taxes and well-funded tobacco prevention and cessation programs that include mass media campaigns, strong smoke-free laws, and effective regulation of tobacco products and marketing, warning pictures on tobacco packaging, a family smoking prevention law, and removed of different flavors (like chocolate) (Winickoff et al., 2011; Campaign for Tobacco-Free kids, 2013). Tobacco price and prevalence of youth smoking are inversely proportional (Carpenter and Cook, 2008) and if prices were 10% higher, 12–17 incidence (youth smoking) would be 11.9% lower (Boonn, 2016). A study showed the reduction in prevalence of youth smoking from 35% to 16% from 1999 to 2013 (Rondeau et al., 2008). Similar policies were applied by Canada and reduced the youth smoking from 25%–12% from 2002–2011 (Canadian tobacco use monitoring survey 2011; current smoking from 1985 to 2011; youth aged 15-19, 2011).	Water pipe smoking has become epidemic in North American youth; particularly in US (Soule et al., 2015). There is still insufficient strategy to overcome menthol flavor, and pictures of warning in packets and secondhand smoking, and there is increasing smoking pattern in colleges and universities.

Way Forward

We discussed the situation of youth tobacco use, its effectiveness, and major challenges. Now, there is the question of the way forward. UN sustainable development goal 3a indicates strengthening the implementation of the WHO Framework Convention on Tobacco Control in all countries, as appropriate. Multiple impacts of tobacco control focusing on youth directly reduce adult and premature mortality rate (Ranabhat et al., 2017). Thus, there is a need for specific policies by age because growth and development, psychology, social environment, responsibilities, and pathophysiology are not similar for all ages. In this line, there should be different policies, programs, interventions, and remedies. Similarly, the priority of tobacco control should be different because intervention for youth and the elderly does not provide similar outcomes. Other public health projects like maternal health, child reproductive health, disease control, etc., are a matter of resource allocation, and we expect measurable outcomes in each micro activity. There is no debate that tobacco prevention for youth ensures low cost and higher output. The funding organizations for tobacco control have not encouraged or disappointed because such organizations have not provided significant outcomes. If we distinguish by age, specific tobacco control, and prevention program, funding projects may revisit their policies and invest more on youth due to their economic productive life. It is possible because youth have short exposure to tobacco addiction, can make strong commitments to quit tobacco, are easy to motivate to quit tobacco, and have family and social pressure in comparison with adults and the elderly. A similar analysis can be found in *The State of Youth Tobacco Prevention and Control Spending in Alabama: Struggles, Consequences, and Solutions* report 2014 (Dunlap and McCallum, 2014).

The average strength of policies varied significantly by country. The success of tobacco control initiatives was significantly associated with the number and types of policy adopted (Wipfli and Huang, 2011). In European countries, limiting youth exposure to smoking in movies might be an effective way to prevent adolescent smoking onset (Morgenstern et al., 2013). In addition, a family smoking prevention law in the United States has reduced the prevalence of youth smoking (Ribisl, 2012). Recently, Nepal drafted a clear provision that people who use tobacco (including smokeless tobacco) will not be eligible as government employees; this policy is appealing because it directly affects unemployed youth (Sinha et al., 2012). Peer-based approach projects are best models in youth tobacco control in Australia. Youth are active users of social media such as Facebook, Twitter, YouTube, Messenger, and other apps. Creative mobilization of information technology could be useful for implementation and monitoring of youth tobacco use (Freeman, 2012). Social drama, documentary, family movies, cartoons about tobacco use impact on youth from elementary school could also discourage youth from using tobacco (Merchant, 2013). Hence, appropriate use of mass media and social network is more effective. The e-cigarette is another option for tobacco control, but regulatory issues surrounding audit of electronic cigarettes is unknown (Jovanovic and Jakovljevic, 2015). A systematic review by Park et al. concluded that the use of multimedia, tailored approaches, personalized feedback, and interactive feature programs could positively affect tobacco prevention and cessation (Park and Drake, 2015). Likewise, receptivity to tobacco advertising was significantly associated with progression toward use in adolescents (Pierce et al., 2018).

Strengths and Limitations

This article describes tobacco control policies with a focus on the younger generation. This is an issue that is significant but often neglected. This article is intended for a wide range of readers (basic readers to policy makers, policy researchers, and other stakeholders related to tobacco control). However, this paper also has some limitations. We used the term youth as used by different authors in their articles and context than any fixed age. Here, we have used terms such as boys, girls, adolescents, elder children, and teenagers synonymously with youth. Tobacco use is focused mostly on smoking, though smokeless tobacco is also a major problem that the world also needs to face. Being a comprehensive review, all components of systematic review and meta-analysis are not applicable to use.

CONCLUSION

About 1/5 of youth used tobacco globally and it has multiple impacts on health economy and family integrity. The prevalence of tobacco use is decreasing but not at a satisfactory rate. The policies of tobacco control adopted by many countries are based on the WHO Framework Convention on Tobacco Control but have not necessarily focused on youth. Due to the physical and economic burden of tobacco consumption by youth, this is a high priority that needs to be addressed. In this digital age, creative tobacco control policies focusing on youth must be applied. Successful policies of tobacco control for youth that need to be replicated by context, country, region, and gender can be recommended. Tobacco control should be a social, public health, and quality-of-life concern rather than a business and trade issue.

AUTHOR CONTRIBUTIONS

CR prepared the research concept and framework, collected the articles, prepared the manuscript, and overall pursued the article. C-BK verified the concept, verified the reference, and reviewed the manuscript. MBP verified all references and prepared the composition of contents. MJ reviewed the manuscript and rearranged some parts.

FUNDING

This study was supported by a National Research Foundation Grant of Korea, Korean Government (NRF-2016S1A5B892520) and the Korean Medical Association (RIHP-2015-02).

ACKNOWLEDGMENTS

We sincerely acknowledge Prof. Indeok Kong, Dr. Shambu Prasad Acharaya (WHO), Dr. Nabin Baral and Arthur Atkinson for their quick review and Margaret Storey for English language improvement.

REFERENCES

Agaku, I., King, B., and Dube, S. R., Office on Smoking and Health, National Center for Chronic Disease Prevention and Health Promotion, CDC. (2013). Current cigarette smoking among adults—United States, 2011. *JAMA*. 309(6):539–541. doi 10.1001/jama.201.114523

Ajzen, I., and Fishbein, M. (1970). The prediction of behavior from attitudinal and normative variables. *J. Exp. Soc. Psychol.* 6 (4), 466–487. doi: 10.1016/0022-1031(70)90057-0

Alexander, C., Piazza, M., Mekos, D., and Valente, T. (2001). Peers, schools, and adolescent cigarette smoking. *J. Adolesc. Health* 29 (1), 22–30. doi: 10.1016/S1054-139X(01)00210-5

Al-Sadat, N., Misau, A., Zarihah, Z., Maznah, D., and Su, T. T. (2010). Adolescent tobacco use and health in South East Asia. *Asia-Pac. J. Public Health* 22 (3 suppl), 175S–180S. doi: 10.1177/1010539510372835

Arrazola, R. A., Neff, L. J., Kennedy, S. M., Holder-Hayes, E., and Jones, C. D.; Centers for Disease and Control Prevention (CDC). (2014). Tobacco use among middle and high school students—United States, 2013. *MMWR Morb. Mortal. Wkly. Rep.* 63 (45), 1021–1026.

Asamura, H., Chansky, K., Crowley, J., Goldstraw, P., Rusch, V. W., Vansteenkiste, J. F., et al. (2015). The International Association for the Study of Lung Cancer Staging Project: proposals for the revision of the N descriptors in the forthcoming 8th edition of the TNM classification for lung cancer. *J. Thorac. Oncol.* 10 (12), 1675–1684. doi: 10.1097/JTO.0000000000000678

Bandura, A. (1976). *Social learning theory*. Stanford University. New York, USA: General Learning Press.

Blum, L. A. (2009). *Friendship, altruism and morality (Routledge Revivals)*. New York, USA: Routledge (Taylor & Francis Group). doi: 10.4324/9780203857304

Boonn, A. (2016). Raising cigarette taxes reduces smoking, especially among kids (and the cigarette companies know it). *Campaign Tob. Free Kids*. https://www.tobaccofreekids.org/assets/factsheets/0146.pdf

Campaign for Tobacco-Free Kids. New survey shows U.S. youth smoking rates fell to record lows in 2013. (2013) http://www.tobaccofreekids.org/press_releases/post/2013_12_18_youth_rates. Accessed May 05, 2015.

Canada. (2011). Canadian Tobacco Use Monitoring Survey (CTUMS) 2011: https://www.canada.ca/en/health-canada/services/publications/healthy-living/canadian-tobacco-use-monitoring-survey-ctums-2011.html?wbdisable=true. Accessed August 14 2018.

Cancer Council. (2017a). Approaches to youth smoking prevention.

Cancer Council. (2017b). Peer Based Approach. http://www.tobaccoinaustralia.org.au/chapter-5-uptake/5-28-peer-based-approaches.

Carpenter, C., and Cook, P. J. (2008). Cigarette taxes and youth smoking: new evidence from national, state, and local youth risk behavior surveys. *J. Health Econ.* 27 (2), 287–299. doi: 10.1016/j.jhealeco.2007.05.008

Centers for Disease Control and Prevention., *Cigarette smoking among adults and trends in smoking cessation—United States 2012*. (2000).

Centers for Disease Control Prevention (CDC) (2007). *Best practices for comprehensive tobacco control programs* 2007. Atlanta: U.S. Department of Health and Human Services, National Center for Chronic Disease Prevention and Health Promotion, Office on Smoking and Health.

Chaloupka, F. J., Straif, K., and Leon, M. E. (2011). Effectiveness of tax and price policies in tobacco control. *Trop. Biomed.* 20 (3), 235–238. doi: 10.1136/tc.2010.039982

Cho, H. J. (2014). The status and future challenges of tobacco control policy in Korea. *J. Prev. Med. Public Health* 47 (3), 129. doi: 10.3961/jpmph.2014.47.3.129

Do, Y. K., and Farooqui, M. A. (2012). Differential subjective responsiveness to a future cigarette price increase among South Korean youth smokers. *Nicotine Tob. Res.* 14 (2), 209–216. doi: 10.1093/ntr/ntr187

Doku, D. (2010). The tobacco industry tactics—a challenge for tobacco control in low and middle income countries. *Afr. Health Sci.* 10 (2), 201–203.

Duncan, L. R., Pearson, E. S., and Maddison, R. (2018). Smoking prevention in children and adolescents: a systematic review of individualized interventions. *Patient Educ. Couns.* 101 (3), 375–388. doi: 10.1016/j.pec.2017.09.011

Dunlap, S. T., and McCallum, D. M. (2014). *The state of youth tobacco prevention and control spending in Alabama: struggles, consequences, and solutions*. Alabama: The Institute for Social Science Research, University of Alabama.

Dupont, D., and Ward, A. J. (2002). *The economic impacts of cigarette tax reductions on youth smoking in Canada*. Ste-Catherines: Brock University.

Durkin, S., Brennan, E., and Wakefield, M. (2012). Mass media campaigns to promote smoking cessation among adults: an integrative review. *Trop. Biomed.* 21 (2), 127–138. doi: 10.1136/tobaccocontrol-2011-050345

Eriksen, M., Mackay, J., and Schluger, N. (2015). *The tobacco atlas*. Fifth Atlanta: The American Cancer Society.

Ertas, N. (2007). Factors associated with stages of cigarette smoking among Turkish youth. *Eur. J. Public Health* 17 (2), 155–161. doi: 10.1093/eurpub/ckl095

Farkas, A. J., Gilpin, E. A., White, M. M., and Pierce, J. P. (2000). Association between household and workplace smoking restrictions and adolescent smoking. *J. Am. Med. Assoc.* 284 (6), 717–722. doi: 10.1001/jama.284.6.717

Fong, G. T., Craig, L. V., Guignard, R., Nagelhout, G. E., Tait, M. K., Driezen, P., et al. (2013). Evaluating the effectiveness of France's indoor smoke-free law 1 year and 5 years after implementation: findings from the ITC France survey. *PloS One* 8 (6), e66692. doi: 10.1371/journal.pone.0066692

Freeman, B. (2012). New media and tobacco control. *Trop. Biomed.* 21 (2), 139–144. doi: 10.1136/tobaccocontrol-2011-050193

Glantz, S. A., and Bareham, D. W. (2018). E-cigarettes: Use, effects on smoking, risks, and policy implications. *Annu. Rev. Public Health* 39, 215–235. doi: 10.1146/annurev-publhealth-040617-013757

Greenhalgh EaW, MH. (2019). Tobacco in Australia: comprehensive online sources. https://www.tobaccoinaustralia.org.au/chapter-1-prevalence/1-6-prevalence-of-smoking-teenagers.

Griffith, G., Cardone, A., Jo, C., Valdemoro, A., and Sebrié, E. (2010). Implementation of smokefree workplaces: challenges in Latin America. *SciElo Public Health* 52, S347–S354. doi: 10.1590/S0036-36342010000800033

Grimsaw, G., and Stanton, A. (2017). Tobacco cessation interventions for young people.

Grimshaw, G., Stanton, A., Blackburn, C., Andrews, K., Grimshaw, C., Vinogradova, Y., et al. (2003). Patterns of smoking, quit attempts and services for a cohort of 15-to 19-year-olds. *Child Care Health Dev.* 29 (6), 457–464. doi: 10.1046/j.1365-2214.2003.00365.x

Hawkins, S. S., Bach, N., and Baum, C. F. (2018). Impact of tobacco control policies on adolescent smokeless tobacco and cigar use: a difference-in-differences approach. *BMC Public Health* 18 (1), 154. doi: 10.1186/s12889-018-5063-z

Health NCfCDPaHPUOoSa . (2012). *Preventing tobacco use among youth and young adults.* Atalanta, USA.

Health UDo, Services H. (2012). *Preventing tobacco use among young people: a report of the Surgeon General.* Atlanta, GA: US Department of Health and Human Services, Public Health Service, Centers for Disease Control and Prevention, National Center for Chronic Disease Prevention and Health Promotion, Office on Smoking and Health.

Hefler, M., and Chapman, S. (2014). Disadvantaged youth and smoking in mature tobacco control contexts: a systematic review and synthesis of qualitative research. *Trop. Biomed.* 5 (17), 56. doi: 10.1136/tobaccocontrol-2014-051756

Higgins, J., and Green, S. (2011). *Cochrane handbook for systematic reviews of interventions version 5.1. 0.* London, UK: the cochrane collaboration.

Hitchman, S. C., Driezen, P., Logel, C., Hammond, D., and Fong, G. T. (2013). Changes in effectiveness of cigarette health warnings over time in Canada and the United States, 2002–2011. *Nicotine Tob. Res.* 16 (5), 536–543. doi: 10.1093/ntr/ntt196

Hodder, R. K., Freund, M., Wolfenden, L., Bowman, J., Gillham, K., Dray, J., et al. (2014). Systematic review of universal school-based resilience interventions targeting adolescent tobacco, alcohol or illicit drug use: review protocol. *BMJ Open* 4 (5), e004718. doi: 10.1136/bmjopen-2013-004718

Holden, C., and Lee, K. (2009). Corporate power and social policy the political economy of the transnational tobacco companies. *Glob. Soc. Policy* 9 (3), 328–354. doi: 10.1177/1468018109343638

Horta, B. L., Calheiros, P., Pinheiro, R. T., Tomasi, E., and Amaral, K. D. (2001). Tobacco smoking among teenagers in an urban area in Southern Brazil. *Rev. Saúde. Pública.* 35 (2), 159–164. doi: 10.1590/S0034-89102001000200009

House of Representative, USA. (2009). A family smoking prevention and tobacco control act. *In: Public Law.*

Hu, T. W., Lee, A. H., and Mao, Z. (2013). WHO Framework Convention on Tobacco Control in China: barriers, challenges and recommendations. *Glob. Health Promot.* 20 (4), 13–22. doi: 10.1177/1757975913501910

Islami, F., Stoklosa, M., Drope, J., and Jemal, A. (2015). Global and regional patterns of tobacco smoking and tobacco control policies. *Eur. Urol. Focus* 1 (1), 3–16. doi: 10.1016/j.euf.2014.10.001

Jason, L. A., Pokorny, S. B., Muldowney, K., and Velez, M. (2005). Youth tobacco sales-to-minors and possession-use-purchase laws: a public health controversy. *J. Drug Educ.* 35 (4), 275–290. doi: 10.2190/1F1R-KGTL-PVDE-V9EJ

Jawad, M., Lee, J. T., Glantz, S., and Millett, C. (2018). Price elasticity of demand of non-cigarette tobacco products: a systematic review and meta-analysis. *Tob. Control* 27 (6), 689–695. doi: 10.1136/tobaccocontrol-2017-054056

Jessor, R., and Jessor, S. L. (1977). *Problem behavior and psychosocial development: a longitudinal study of youth.* New York, USA: Academic Press.

Joseph, R. A. (2010). *The economics of youth tobacco use in India.* Chicago: University of Illinois.

Jovanovic, M., and Jakovljevic, M. (2015). Regulatory issues surrounding audit of electronic cigarette charge composition. *Front. Psychiatry* 6, 133. doi: 10.3389/fpsyt.2015.00133

Kabir, M., Goh, K.-L., and Khan, M. (2013). Adolescent tobacco use and its determinants evidence from Global Youth Tobacco Survey. *Asia-Pac. J. Public Health* 27 (2), 1579–1589. doi: 10.1177/1010539512472357

Katanoda, K., Jiang, Y., Park, S., Lim, M. K., Qiao, Y. L., and Inoue, M. (2014). Tobacco control challenges in East Asia: proposals for change in the world's largest epidemic region. *Tob. Control* 23 (4), 359–368. doi: 10.1136/tobaccocontrol-2012-050852

Kaur, J., and Jain, D. (2011). Tobacco control policies in India: implementation and challenges. *Indian J. Public Health* 55 (3), 220. doi: 10.4103/0019-557X.89941

Khuder, S. A., Price, J. H., Jordan, T., Khuder, S. S., and Silvestri, K. (2008). Cigarette smoking among adolescents in Northwest Ohio: correlates of prevalence and age at onset. *Int. J. Environ. Res. Public Health* 5 (4), 278–289. doi: 10.3390/ijerph5040278

Kim, J. A., Lee, C. Y., Lim, E. S., and Kim., G. S. (2013). Smoking cessation and characteristics of success and failure among female high-school smokers. *Jpn. J. Nurs. Sci.* 10 (1), 68–78. doi: 10.1111/j.1742-7924.2012.00212.x

Konopka, G. (1973). Requirements for healthy development of adolescent youth. *Adolescence* 8 (31), 291-316. https://psycnet.apa.org/record/1974-22647-001

Korean Association on Smoking or Health. (2010). Smoking Prevalence of Youth http://www.kash.or.kr/user_new/pds_view.asp.

Kostova, D., and Blecher, E. (2013). Does advertising matter? Estimating the impact of cigarette advertising on smoking among youth in developing countries. *Contemp. Econ. Policy* 31 (3), 537–548. doi: 10.1111/j.1465-7287.2012.00323.x

Levy, D. T., Chaloupka, F., and Gitchell, J. (2004). The effects of tobacco control policies on smoking rates: a tobacco control scorecard. *J. Public Health Manage. Pract.* 10 (4), 338–353. doi: 10.1097/00124784-200407000-00011

Levy, D. T., Cho, S. I., Kim, Y. M., Park, S., Suh, M. K., and Kam, S. (2010). SimSmoke model evaluation of the effect of tobacco control policies in Korea: the unknown success story. *Am. J. Public Health* 100 (7), 1267–1273. doi: 10.2105/AJPH.2009.166900

Levy, D. T., Pearson, J. L., Villanti, A. C., Blackman, K., Vallone, D.M., Niaura, R. S., et al. (2011). Modeling the future effects of a menthol ban on smoking prevalence and smoking-attributable deaths in the United States. *Am. J. Public Health* 101 (7), 1236–1240. doi: 10.2105/AJPH.2011.300179

Levy, D., de Almeida, L. M., and Szklo, A. (2012). The Brazil SimSmoke policy simulation model: the effect of strong tobacco control policies on smoking prevalence and smoking-attributable deaths in a middle income nation. *PLoS Med.* 9 (11), e1001336. doi: 10.1371/journal.pmed.1001336

Levy, D., Rodríguez-Buño, R. L., Hu, T. W., and Moran, A. E. (2014). The potential effects of tobacco control in China: projections from the China SimSmoke simulation model. *Br. Med. J.* 348 (10), g1134. doi: 10.1136/bmj.g1134

Levy, D. T., Tam, J., Kuo, C., Fong, G. T., and Chaloupka, F. (2018). Research full report: the impact of implementing tobacco control policies: the 2017 tobacco control policy scorecard. *J. Public Health Manage. Pract.* 24 (5), 448. doi: 10.1097/PHH.0000000000000780

Lim, K. H., Sumarni, M., Kee, C. C., Christopher,, V. M., Noruiza Hana, M., Lim, K. K., et al. (2010). Prevalence and factors associated with smoking among form four students in Petaling District, Selangor, Malaysia. *Trop. Biomed.* 27 (3), 394–403.

Lindblom, E. (2005). Raising cigarette taxes reduces smoking, especially among kids (and the cigarette companies know it). *Campaign for Tobacco-Free Kids, January 31. (Smoke Free South Carolina).* https://www.tobaccofreekids.org/microsites/passthebuck_sc/resources/sccigtaxandkids.pdf. Accessed May 05, 2015.

Lorant, V., Soto, V. E., Alves, J., Federico, B., Kinnunen, J., Kuipers, M., et al. (2015). Smoking in school-aged adolescents: design of a social network survey in six European countries. *BMC Res. Notes* 8 (1), 91. doi: 10.1186/s13104-015-1041-z

Maddox, R., Davey, R., Cochrane, T., Lovett, R., and van der Sterren, A. (2013). Study protocol—Indigenous Australian social networks and the impact on smoking policy and programs in Australia: protocol for a mixed-method prospective study. *BMC Public Health* 13 (1), 879. doi: 10.1186/1471-2458-13-879

Madkour, A. S., Ledford, E. C., Andersen, L., and Johnson, C. C. (2013). Tobacco advertising/promotions and adolescents' smoking risk in Northern Africa. *Trop. Biomed.* 23, 244–252. doi: 10.1136/tobaccocontrol-2012-050593

Merchant, Z. F. (2013). *A study on the depiction of drug usage, alcohol consumption and cigarette smoking in movies and its perceived effect on a young audience. A comparative study of American and Indian cinema and their respective Audiences.* South Florida: Department of Mass Communications University of South Florida.

Ministry of Health and Population. (2013). *National Tobacco Control Strategic Plan (2013–2016).* Teku, Kathmandu, Nepal: National Health Education Information and Communication Center.

Morgenstern, M., Sargent, J. D., Engels, R. C. M. E., Scholte, R. H. J., Florek, E., Hunt, K., et al. (2013). Smoking in movies and adolescent smoking initiation: Longitudinal study in six European countries. *Am. J. Prev. Med.* 44 (4), 339–344. doi: 10.1016/j.amepre.2012.11.037

Muller, F., and Wehbe, L. (2008). Smoking and smoking cessation in Latin America: a review of the current situation and available treatments. *Int. J. Chron. Obstruct. Pulmon. Dis.* 3 (2), 285. doi: 10.2147/COPD.S2654

Müller, F., and Wehbe, L. (2008). Smoking and smoking cessation in Latin America: a review of the current situation and available treatments. *Int. J.COPD* 3 (2), 285–293. doi: 10.2147/COPD.S2654

National Health Service. (2015). Smokefree. 2015/03/15; https://www.nhs.uk/smokefree. Accessed 2015/03/15.

Nelson, D. E., Mowery, P., Asman, K., Pederson, L. L., O'Malley, P. M., Malarcher, A., et al. (2008). Long-term trends in adolescent and young adult smoking in the United States: metapatterns and implications. *Am. J. Public Health* 98 (5), 905–915. doi: 10.2105/AJPH.2007.115931

Ng, M., Freeman, M. K., Fleming, T. D., Robinson, M., Dwyer-Lindgren, L., Thomson, B., et al. (2014). Smoking prevalence and cigarette consumption in 187 countries, 1980–2012. *J. Am. Med. Assoc.* 311 (2), 183–192. doi: 10.1001/jama.2013.284692

Organization WH. (2011). *WHO Report on The Global Tobacco Epidemic: Global youth tobacco survey data 2011.* Geneva: World Health Organization.

Organization WH. (2011). *Effectiveness of tax and price policies for tobacco control.*

Organization WH. (2013). *WHO report on the global tobacco epidemic, 2013: Enforcing bans on tobacco advertising, promotion and sponsorship.* World Health Organization.

Organization WH. (2017). *WHO report on the global tobacco epidemic, 2017: Monitoring tobacco use and prevention policies.* World Health Organization.

Oswal, K. C. (2015). Factors associated with tobacco use among adolescents in India results from the Global Youth Tobacco Survey, India. *Asia-Pac. J. Public Health* 27 (2), NP203–NP211. doi: 10.1177/1010539511436322

Park, E., and Drake, E. (2015). Systematic review: internet-based program for youth smoking prevention and cessation. *J. Nurs. Scholarsh.* 47 (1), 43–50. doi: 10.1111/jnu.12104

Patel, P., Collin, J., and Gilmore, A. B. (2007). The law was actually drafted by us but the Government is to be congratulated on its wise actions: British American Tobacco and public policy in Kenya. *Trop. Biomed.* 16 (1), e1–e1. doi: 10.1136/tc.2006.016071

Pierce, J. P., Sargent, J. D., Portnoy, D. B., White, M., Noble, M., Kealey, S., et al. (2018). Association between receptivity to tobacco advertising and progression to tobacco use in youth and young adults in the PATH Study. *JAMA Pediat.* 172 (5), 444–451. doi: 10.1001/jamapediatrics.2017.5756

Pradhan, P. M. S., Niraula, S. R., Ghimire, A., Singh, S. B., and Pokharel, P. K. (2013). Tobacco use and associated factors among adolescent students in Dharan, Eastern Nepal: a cross-sectional questionnaire survey. *BMJ Open* 3 (2), e002123. doi: 10.1136/bmjopen-2012-002123

Rabin, R. L., and Sugarman, S. D. (2001). *Regulating tobacco.* New York: Oxford University Press.

Ranabhat, C. L., Kim, C. B., Park, M. B., and Acharaya, S. (2017). Multiple disparities in adult mortality in relation to social and health care perspective: results from different data sources. *Glob. Health* 13 (1), 57. doi: 10.1186/s12992-017-0283-z

Ranabhat, C. L., Atkinson, J., Park, M. B., Kim, C. B., and Jakovljevic, M. (2018). The influence of universal health coverage on life expectancy at birth (LEAB) and healthy life expectancy (HALE): a multi-country cross-sectional study. *Front. Pharmacol.* 9, 960. doi: 10.3389/fphar.2018.00960

Ranabhat, C. L., Park. M. B., Kim. C. B., Kim, C. S., Jeong, H. S., Koh, S. B., et al. (2018). Influence of key health related indicators on adult mortality: result from UN member countries. *Iran. J. Public Health* 47 (6), 794–802.

Ranabhat, C. L., Kim, C. B., Singh, A., Acharya, D., Pathak, K., Sharma, B., et al. (2019). Challenges and opportunities towards the road of universal health coverage (UHC) in Nepal: a systematic review. *Arch. Public Health* 77 (1), 5. doi: 10.1186/s13690-019-0331-7

Reddy, P., James, S., Sewpaul, R., Yach, D., Resnicow, K., Sifunda, S., et al. (2013). A decade of tobacco control: the South African case of politics, health policy, health promotion and behaviour change. *S. Afr. Med. J.* 103 (11), 835–840. doi: 10.7196/samj.6910

Ribisl, K. M. (2012). Research gaps related to tobacco product marketing and sales in the family smoking prevention and tobacco control act. *Nicotine Tob. Res.* 14 (1), 43–53. doi: 10.1093/ntr/ntr098

Rondeau, V., Allain, H., Bakchine, S., Bonet, P., Brudon, F., Chauplannaz, G., et al. (2008). General practice-based intervention for suspecting and detecting dementia in France: a cluster randomized controlled trial. *Dementia* 7 (4), 433–450. doi: 10.1177/1471301208096628

Rosenberg, M. (1979). *Conceiving The Self.* 1st ed, New York, USA: Basic Books.

Ross, H., and Chaloupka, F. J. (2003). The effect of cigarette prices on youth smoking. *Health Econ.* 12 (3), 217–230. doi: 10.1002/hec.709

Ruiz, M. A., Rivera-Rodríguez, D. E., Marín, Y., González, J. C., and Moreno, R. H. (2009). Tobacco control initiatives in Colombia's congress, 1992-2007. *Rev. Panam. Salud Publica/Pan. Am. J. Public Health* 25 (6), 471–480.

Saleheen, D., Zhao, W., and Rasheed, A. (2014). Epidemiology and public health policy of tobacco use and cardiovascular disorders in low- and middle-income countries. *Arterioscler. Thromb. Vasc. Biol.* 34 (9), 1811–1819. doi: 10.1161/ATVBAHA.114.303826

Sebrié, E. M., Blanco, A., and Glantz, S. A. (2010). Cigarette labeling policies in Latin America and the Caribbean: progress and obstacles. *Salud Pública Méx.* 52, S233–S243. doi: 10.1590/S0036-36342010000800019

Simons-Morton, B., Crump, A. D., Haynie, D. L., Saylor, K. E., Eitel, P., and Yu, K. (1999). Psychosocial, school, and parent factors associated with recent smoking among early-adolescent boys and girls. *Prev. Med.* 28 (2), 138–148. doi: 10.1006/pmed.1998.0404

Sinha, D., Bajracharya, B., Khadka, B., Rinchen, S., Bhattad, V., and Singh, P. (2012). Smokeless tobacco use in Nepal. *Indian J. Cancer* 49 (4), 352. doi: 10.4103/0019-509X.107728

Soule, E. K., Lipato, T., and Eissenberg, T. (2015). Waterpipe tobacco-smoking: a new smoking epidemic among the young? *Curr. Pulmonol. Rep.* 4 (4), 163–172. doi: 10.1007/s13665-015-0124-6

Stanton, A,, and Grimshaw, G. (2013). Tobacco cessation interventions for young people. *Cochrane Database Syst. Rev.* (8), CD003289. doi: 10.1002/14651858 CD003289.pub5

Stead, L. F., Perera, R., Bullen, C., Mant, D., and Lancaster, T. (2008). Nicotine replacement therapy for smoking cessation. *Cochrane Database Syst. Rev.* 1 (1). CD000146. doi: 10.1002/14651858.CD000146.pub3

Sullivan, D. H., and Rees, M. A. (2014). Smoking bans in secure psychiatric hospitals and prisons. *J. Law Med.* 22 (1), 22–30.

Tauras, J. A. (2004). Public policy and smoking cessation among young adults in the United States. *Health Policy* 68 (3), 321–332. doi: 10.1016/j.healthpol.2003.10.007

Tauras, J. A., Huang, J., and Chaloupka, F. J. (2013). Differential impact of tobacco control policies on youth sub-populations. *Int. J. Environ. Res. Public Health* 10 (9), 4306–4322. doi: 10.3390/ijerph10094306

Thomas, D., Mackinnon, A. J., Bonevski, B., Abramson, M. J., Taylor, S., Poole, S. G., et al. (2016). Development and validation of a 21-item challenges to stopping smoking (CSS-21) scale. *BMJ Open* 6 (3), e011265. doi: 10.1136/bmjopen-2016-011265

Tumwine, J. (2011). Implementation of the framework convention on tobacco control in Africa: current status of legislation. *Int. J. Environ. Res. Public Health* 8 (11), 4312–4331. doi: 10.3390/ijerph8114312

United Nation. (2016) Definition of Youth 2009; http://www.un.org/esa/socdev/documents/youth/fact-sheets/youth-definition.pd. Accessed 05/22.

United States Congress House of Represen. (2010). Family Smoking Prevention and Tobacco Control ACT. BiblioGov. Washington DC, USA.

Vidhubala, E., Sahaya, G., Vijayalakshmi, S., Bharathi, P., and Quarishy, Z. B. (2014). Prevalence of tobacco use among school children, exposure to passive smoking and their knowledge level about tobacco control in Chennai city,

Tamil Nadu-A School Based Survey. *J. Indian Assoc. Child Adolesc. Ment. Health* 10 (2), 110–131.

Wakefield, M. A., Chaloupka, F. J., Kaufman, N. J., Orleans, C. T., Barker, D. C., and Ruel, E. E. (2000). Effect of restrictions on smoking at home, at school, and in public places on teenage smoking: cross sectional study. *Br. Med. J.* 321 (7257), 333–337. doi: 10.1136/bmj.321.7257.333

Walker, S., Sanci, L., and Temple-Smith, M. (2013). Sexting: young women's and men's views on its nature and origins. *J. Adolesc. Health* 52 (6), 697-701. doi: 10.1016/j.jadohealth.2013.01.026

Warner, K. E., and Tam, J. (2012). The impact of tobacco control research on policy: 20 years of progress. *Trop. Biomed.* 21 (2), 103–109. doi: 10.1136/tobaccocontrol-2011-050396

Warner, K., Jacobson, P., and Kaufman, N. (2003). Innovative approaches to youth tobacco control: introduction and overview. *Trop. Biomed.* 12 (suppl 1), i1–i5. doi: 10.1136/tc.12.suppl_1.i1

Wasserman, J., Manning, W. G., Newhouse, J. P., and Winkler, J. D. (1991). The effects of excise taxes and regulations on cigarette smoking. *J. Health Econ.* 10 (1), 43–64. doi: 10.1016/0167-6296(91)90016-G

Watanabe, I., Shigeta, M., Inoue, K., Matsui, D., Ozaki, E., Kuriyama, N., et al. (2013). Personal factors associated with smoking among marginalized and disadvantaged youth in Japan. A strong relationship between smoking and convenience store use. *Int. J. Behav. Med.* 20 (4), 504–513. doi: 10.1007/s12529-012-9268-8

White, V. M., Durkin, S. J., Coomber, K., and Wakefield, M. A. (2013). What is the role of tobacco control advertising intensity and duration in reducing adolescent smoking prevalence? Findings from 16 years of tobacco control mass media advertising in Australia. *Trop. Biomed.* 05 (09), 45. doi: 10.1136/tobaccocontrol-2012-050945

Winickoff, J. P., McMillen, R. C., Vallone, D. M., Pearson, J. L., Tanski, S.E., Dempsey, J. H., et al. (2011). US attitudes about banning menthol in cigarettes: results from a nationally representative survey. *Am. J. Public Health* 101 (7), 1234–1236. doi: 10.2105/AJPH.2011.300146

Wipfli, H., and Huang, G. (2011). Power of the process: Evaluating the impact of the Framework Convention on Tobacco Control negotiations. *Health Policy* 100 (2), 107–115. doi: 10.1016/j.healthpol.2010.08.014

World Health Organization. (2008) *WHO Report on the global tobacco epidemic, 2008: The MPOWER package.* Geneva: World Health Organization.

World Health Organization. (2011) *WHO report on the global tobacco epidemic, 2011: warning about the dangers of tobacco.* Geneva: World Health Organization.

World Health Organization. (2011). *WHO report on the global tobacco epidemic: Global youth tobacco survey data 2011.* Geneva: World Health Organization.

World Health Organization. (2011). *Effectiveness of tax and price policies for tobacco control.* Geneva: World Health Organization.

World Health Organization. (2012). *Global progress report on implementation of the WHO Framework Convention on Tobacco Control.* Geneva: World Health Organization.

World Health Organization. (2013). *WHO report on the global tobacco epidemic, 2013: Enforcing bans on tobacco advertising, promotion and sponsorship.* Geneva: World Health Organization.

World Health Organization. (2017). *WHO report on the global tobacco epidemic, 2017: Monitoring tobacco use and prevention policies.* Geneva: World Health Organization.

11

Physical Activity and Survival among Long-Term Cancer Survivor and Non-Cancer Cohorts

*Anthony S. Gunnell[1,2], Sarah Joyce[3], Stephania Tomlin[3], Dennis R. Taaffe[1,4,5], Prue Cormie[6], Robert U. Newton[1,4,7], David Joseph[1,8,9], Nigel Spry[1,9,10], Kristjana Einarsdóttir[11] and Daniel A. Galvão[1,4]**

[1] *Exercise Medicine Research Institute, Edith Cowan University, Joondalup, WA, Australia,* [2] *School of Population Health, University of Western Australia, Nedlands, WA, Australia,* [3] *Public Health and Clinical Services Division, Western Australian Department of Health, East Perth, WA, Australia,* [4] *School of Medical and Health Sciences, Edith Cowan University, Joondalup, WA, Australia,* [5] *School of Human Movement and Nutrition Sciences, The University of Queensland, St. Lucia, QLD, Australia,* [6] *Institute for Health and Ageing, Australian Catholic University, Melbourne, VIC, Australia,* [7] *University of Queensland Centre for Clinical Research, The University of Queensland, Brisbane, QLD, Australia,* [8] *Department of Radiation Oncology, Sir Charles Gairdner Hospital, Nedlands, WA, Australia,* [9] *Faculty of Medicine, University of Western Australia, Nedlands, WA, Australia,* [10] *Genesis Cancer Care, Joondalup, WA, Australia,* [11] *Centre of Public Health Sciences and Unit for Nutrition Research, School of Health Sciences, University of Iceland, Reykjavik, Iceland*

***Correspondence:**
Daniel A. Galvão
d.galvao@ecu.edu.au

Evidence suggests physical activity improves prognosis following cancer diagnosis; however, evidence regarding prognosis in long-term survivors of cancer is scarce. We assessed physical activity in 1,589 cancer survivors at an average 8.8 years following their initial diagnosis and calculated their future mortality risk following physical activity assessment. We also selected a cancer-free cohort of 3,145 age, sex, and survey year group-matched cancer-free individuals from the same source population for comparison purposes. Risks for cancer-specific mortality and all-cause mortality in relation to physical activity levels were estimated using Cox regression proportional hazard regression analyses within the cancer and non-cancer cohorts. Physical activity levels of 360+ min per week were inversely associated with cancer-specific mortality in long-term cancer survivors [hazard ratios (HR) = 0.30 (95% confidence intervals (CI) 0.13–0.70)] and participants without prior cancer [HR = 0.16 (95% CI 0.05–0.56)] compared with no reported physical activity. Physical activity levels of 150–359 and 360+ min were inversely associated with all-cause mortality in long-term cancer survivors [150–359 min; HR = 0.55 (95% CI 0.31–0.97), 360+ min; HR = 0.41 (95% CI 0.21–0.79)] and those without prior cancer [150–359 min; HR = 0.52 (95% CI 0.32–0.86), 360+ min; HR = 0.50 (95% CI 0.29–0.88)]. These results suggest that meeting exercise guidelines of 150 min of physical activity per week were associated with reduced all-cause mortality in both long-term cancer surviving and cancer-free cohorts. Exceeding exercise oncology guidelines (360+ min per week) may provide additional protection in terms of cancer-specific death.

Keywords: physical activity, cancer, survival, longitudinal, cohort study

INTRODUCTION

Identification and management of lifestyle risk factors affecting prognosis in cancer survivors is becoming increasingly important as cancer screening and treatments continue to improve. In Australia, the number of cancers diagnosed almost doubled between 1991 and 2009, with a corresponding increase in age-standardized incidence of 12% (1). During a similar period of time, 5-year relative survival following any cancer diagnosis increased from 47% in 1982–1987 to 66% in 2006–2010 (1).

Assessment of physical activity levels and their effects in those who survived cancer has been undertaken by a number of researchers (2, 3); however, the usual period of assessment has been within a relatively short period following cancer diagnosis (almost exclusively less than 2 years). These studies have generally shown positive associations between increasing levels of physical activity and improved quality of life, cancer-specific mortality, and all-cause mortality for survivors of certain cancer types, particularly breast (4), colorectal (5–7), and prostate (8) cancer. Additionally, it has been suggested that cancer recurrence might be positively impacted by physical activity levels post-diagnosis, although evidence appears contradictory (9–12). To date, however, assessment of physical activity levels in terms of their effects on mortality in long-term survivors has been almost non-existent, although a recent study by Inoue-Choi et al. (13) suggested improved survival benefits for cancer survivors may be associated with adherence to the recommended physical activity guidelines. With improved long-term survival in those diagnosed with cancer, it is important to understand whether the survival benefits associated with physical activity extend beyond the immediate rehabilitation stage associated with cancer (and treatment) recovery. Moreover, it is important to assess whether physical activity behaviors contribute similar benefits in these long-term cancer survivors, compared to cancer-naive individuals. By linking the Western Australian Cancer Registry dataset with the Western Australian Health and Wellbeing Surveillance System (HWSS) dataset, we were able to obtain self-reported leisure-time physical activity (LTPA) levels at time points between 2 and 28 years following first recorded cancer diagnosis. This allowed us to investigate whether long-term survivors of "any cancer" benefited from increased physical activity, in terms of future cancer-specific and all-cause mortality risk.

MATERIALS AND METHODS

Ethics Statement

The study was approved by the Human Research Ethics Committees of Edith Cowan University and the Western Australian Department of Health and has therefore been performed in accordance with the ethical standards laid down in the 1964 Declaration of Helsinki and its later amendments.

Study Design

This population-based cohort study utilized self-reported lifestyle survey information (from the HWSS) individually linked with cancer registry data (both held by the Western Australian Department of Health). The HWSS is a comprehensive monthly survey commissioned by the Western Australian Department of Health to provide information on a wide range of issues pertaining to the Western Australian population's physical and mental well-being. It utilizes computer-assisted telephone interviewing to assess approximately 6,000 Western Australians each year who are selected from the WA White Pages® telephone directory using a stratified random process with over-sampling representative to the population in rural and remote areas. Each year since its inception, more than 75% of those contacted completed the survey (14) and a majority (77% in 2010) of participants provided their name, address, and date of birth for the purpose of linkage with administrative health data. Only those HWSS participants who provided consent for their information to be used in this manner were linked to other registries for this study. The probabilistic matching procedures used to link individuals are based on full name and address, phonetic compression algorithms, and other identifiers, and they have been estimated to be 99.89% accurate (15). This linkage allowed identification of incident cancer diagnoses prior to an initial survey date and provided information on behavioral factors and demographics at the time of survey. Mortality data were obtained through linking to the Western Australian Mortality Registry for the entire study period (2004–2011).

Study Population

Between May 1, 2004 and January 1, 2011, some 44,317 surveys for which consent was provided for data linkage were completed as part of the HWSS. Where participants had been surveyed more than once (1,616 people) during the study period, their last survey was included for analysis. Upon further restriction to those aged 40+ years, to target adult cancers only, 25,433 participants remained. Those with a diagnosed cancer (other than non-melanoma skin cancer) after 1982 and more than 2 years prior to their survey date were identified (1,813). Their first cancer within this period was considered their incident cancer. After further exclusion of cancer survivors with multiple cancers diagnosed prior to the survey, a cohort of 1,667 cancer survivors was selected. Exclusion of a further 78 individuals with missing information for body mass index (BMI), alcohol consumption, and/or SF-8 questions (**Table 1**) left a cancer survivor cohort of 1,589. These participants were surveyed on average 8.8 years (quartile 1 = 4 years, quartile 3 = 12 years) following their first recorded cancer diagnosis.

A non-cancer cohort (NCC) was selected from the same source population of 44,317 individuals. Stratified random sampling without replacement at a ratio of 2:1 was performed using the age (10-year age blocks from 40 years onward), sex, and survey year frequency distributions of the 1,667 cancer survivors identified previously. This was performed using the "proc surveyselect" function within SAS Inc. software (version 9.3). The resulting 3,334 individuals had no cancer diagnosis prior to their survey (**Table 2**). After exclusion of 189 individuals with missing data for BMI and SF-8 questions, a final 3,145 cancer-free individuals were included in the final analyses.

TABLE 1 | Cancer survivor cohort: baseline characteristics by level of leisure-time physical activity (LTPA), in participants surveyed an average of 8.8 years following initial reported cancer diagnosis.

	No LTPA (*n* = 439)	<150 min LTPA (*n* = 460)	150–359 min LTPA (*n* = 384)	360+ min LTPA (*n* = 384)
	n (%)	*n* (%)	*n* (%)	*n* (%)
Male	205 (46.7)	187 (40.6)	173 (45.0)	184 (47.9)
Age at survey (years)*				
40–49	18 (4.1)	28 (6.1)	26 (6.8)	35 (9.1)
50–59	58 (13.2)	86 (18.7)	75 (19.5)	76 (25.8)
60–69	111 (25.3)	133 (28.9)	122 (31.8)	137 (27.2)
70–79	146 (33.3)	138 (30.0)	114 (29.7)	102 (26.6)
80+	106 (24.2)	75 (16.3)	47 (12.2)	34 (8.8)
Body mass index (kg/m²)*				
<25	131 (29.8)	168 (36.5)	137 (35.7)	134 (34.9)
25–29	157 (35.8)	155 (33.7)	159 (41.4)	162 (42.2)
30+	119 (27.1)	120 (26.1)	74 (19.3)	76 (19.8)
Missing	32 (7.3)	17 (3.7)	14 (3.6)	12 (3.1)
Daily fruit and/or vegetable intake*				
<4 servings	129 (29.4)	106 (23.0)	87 (22.7)	63 (16.4)
4–5 servings	172 (39.2)	191 (41.5)	126 (32.8)	142 (37.0)
6 servings	64 (14.6)	84 (18.3)	69 (18.0)	63 (16.4)
7+ servings	74 (16.9)	79 (17.2)	102 (26.6)	116 (30.2)
Smoking status				
Never	187 (42.6)	220 (47.8)	188 (49.0)	176 (45.8)
Ex-smoker	202 (46.0)	194 (42.2)	161 (41.9)	181 (47.1)
Current	50 (11.4)	46 (10.0)	35 (9.1)	27 (7.0)
Alcohol consumption (# drinks on any given day)*				
None	165 (37.6)	169 (36.7)	104 (27.1)	95 (24.7)
≤2 standard drinks	199 (45.3)	223 (48.5)	197 (51.3)	197 (51.3)
>2 standard drinks	75 (17.1)	67 (14.6)	83 (21.6)	92 (24.0)
Missing	0	1 (0.2)	0	0
SF-8 physical health component score*				
PCS < 50	300 (68.3)	267 (58.0)	180 (46.9)	127 (33.1)
PCS ≥ 50	137 (31.2)	193 (42.0)	204 (53.1)	256 (66.7)
Missing	2 (0.5)	0	0	1 (0.3)
SF-8 mental health component score*				
MCS < 54	231 (52.6)	247 (53.7)	181 (47.1)	154 (40.1)
MCS ≥ 54	206 (46.9)	213 (46.3)	203 (52.9)	229 (59.6)
Missing	2 (0.5)	0	0	1 (0.3)
Diabetes mellitus (% yes)*	77 (17.5)	62 (13.5)	34 (8.8)	24 (6.2)
Previous cancer type				
Breast	98 (22.3)	107 (23.3)	88 (22.9)	79 (20.6)
Prostate	75 (17.1)	78 (17.0)	57 (14.8)	70 (18.2)
Colorectal	50 (11.4)	56 (12.2)	55 (14.3)	43 (11.2)
Melanoma	76 (17.3)	84 (18.3)	70 (18.2)	91 (23.7)
Other	140 (33.9)	135 (29.4)	114 (29.7)	101 (26.3)
Years from diagnosis to survey [mean (Q1–Q3)] (mean = 8.82; 4–12)	9.2 (5–13)	8.7 (4–12)	8.6 (4–12)	8.7 (4–13)

Significantly associated with LTPA ($p < 0.05$).

TABLE 2 | Non-Cancer cohort: baseline characteristics by level of leisure-time physical activity (LTPA) in survey participants without a prior recorded cancer diagnosis.

	No LTPA (*n* = 886)	<150 min LTPA (*n* = 882)	150–359 min LTPA (*n* = 801)	360+ min LTPA (*n* = 765)
	n (%)	*n* (%)	*n* (%)	*n* (%)
Male*	407 (45.9)	353 (40.0)	339 (42.3)	399 (52.2)
Age at survey (years)*				
40–49	42 (4.7)	49 (5.6)	55 (6.9)	68 (8.9)
50–59	108 (12.2)	149 (16.9)	165 (20.6)	168 (22.0)
60–69	239 (27.0)	232 (26.3)	267 (33.3)	268 (35.0)
70–79	286 (32.3)	284 (32.2)	225 (28.1)	205 (26.8)
80+	211 (23.8)	168 (19.0)	89 (11.1)	56 (7.3)
Body mass index (kg/m²)*				
<25	290 (32.7)	315 (35.7)	359 (44.8)	336 (43.9)
25–29	315 (35.6)	303 (34.4)	284 (35.5)	306 (40.0)
30+	197 (22.2)	208 (23.6)	132 (16.5)	102 (13.3)
Missing	84 (9.5)	56 (6.4)	26 (3.2)	21 (2.8)
Daily fruit and/or vegetable intake*				
<4 servings	276 (31.2)	234 (26.5)	167 (20.8)	146 (19.1)
4–5 servings	323 (36.5)	336 (38.1)	283 (35.3)	276 (36.1)
6 servings	125 (14.1)	157 (17.8)	152 (19.0)	129 (16.9)
7+ servings	162 (18.3)	155 (17.6)	199 (24.8)	214 (28.0)
Smoking status*				
Never	393 (44.4)	479 (54.3)	411 (51.3)	370 (48.4)
Ex-smoker	349 (39.4)	307 (34.8)	330 (41.2)	338 (44.2)
Current	144 (16.2)	96 (10.9)	60 (7.5)	57 (7.4)
Alcohol consumption (# drinks on any given day)*				
None	335 (37.8)	316 (35.8)	220 (27.5)	170 (22.2)
≤2 standard drinks	417 (47.1)	441 (50.0)	441 (55.1)	415 (54.2)
>2 standard drinks	134 (15.1)	125 (14.2)	140 (17.5)	180 (23.5)
Missing	0	0	0	0
SF-8 physical health component score*				
PCS < 50	563 (63.5)	446 (50.6)	305 (38.1)	224 (29.3)
PCS ≥ 50	322 (36.3)	436 (49.4)	495 (61.8)	541 (70.7)
Missing	1 (0.1)	0	1 (0.1)	0
SF-8 mental health component score*				
MCS < 54	443 (50.0)	421 (47.7)	338 (42.2)	293 (38.3)
MCS ≥ 54	442 (49.9)	461 (52.3)	462 (57.7)	472 (61.7)
Missing	1 (0.1)	0	1 (0.1)	0
Diabetes mellitus (% yes)*	129 (14.6)	120 (13.6)	80 (10.0)	62 (8.1)

Significantly associated with LTPA ($p < 0.05$).

Study Variables

Participants were asked to estimate the number of sessions and minutes per session of LTPA during the past week, in terms of walking 10 or more minutes consecutively, performing moderate physical activity (e.g., golf, gentle swimming, and lawn bowls), or vigorous physical activity (e.g., tennis, jogging, and cycling). Using recommendations of the Australian Institute of Health and Welfare (16), total LTPA was calculated using the formula [total LTPA = walk-time + moderate-time + (2 × vigorous-time)]. Sufficient LTPA was defined as follows: no LTPA, <150 min LTPA, 150–359 min LTPA, or 360+ min LTPA per week. While Australian physical activity guidelines (16) collapse the upper two categories (150–359 min and 360+ min), given the approximately equal number of participants in the two upper categories, stratification was preferable in this instance. For those aged 65+ years, no weighting was applied for vigorous physical activity in order to improve comparability between years due to the question not being asked for that age group prior to 2008. Few respondents aged 65+ years reported being vigorously active from 2008 onward. For those whose total LTPA per week exceeded 1,680 min, their summed value was re-coded to 1,680 min for analysis as recommended in the Australian Health and Welfare guidelines (16).

Confounding variables included in the adjusted Cox regression analyses were sex, age at survey, previous cancer type (none, breast, prostate, colorectal, melanoma, other), smoking status (never more than 100 cigarettes, ex-smoker, current-smoker), fruit and/or vegetable intake (<4, 4–5, 6, 7+ servings daily; based on quintile distribution), BMI (<25, 25–29, 30+ kg/m^2; adapted from World Health Organization classifications), long-term risky alcohol intake (none, ≤2 standard drinks, 3+ standard drinks on a drinking day; based on National Health and Medical Research Council guidelines), SF-8 physical health component score (<50, 50+; based on median values), SF-8 mental health component score (<54, 54+; based on median values), year of survey, and self-reported diabetes status. The SF-8 Health Survey component of the HWSS is an eight item version of the SF-36®. Higher SF-8 scores correspond to better functioning.

Two outcomes were investigated following the participants' surveys, namely cancer-specific mortality and all-cause mortality. Cancer death was identified using the International Classification of Diseases version 10 codes C00-D48, present as either principal or other cause of death.

Statistical Analyses

Differences in baseline characteristics in relation to level of LTPA were assessed using the Kruskall–Wallis (for ordinal variables) and chi square (for nominal variables) tests.

Person-time was calculated from the date of survey until death, or end of follow-up (January 1, 2011), whichever occurred first. Cox proportional hazards regression models were used to estimate hazard ratios (HR) with 95% confidence intervals (CI) for future mortality. Separate analyses were performed for the two outcome types (cancer-specific and all-cause mortality), with non-cancer mortality being censored in cancer-related analyses.

The final adjusted Cox models, which incorporated a stratum of "time from cancer diagnosis until survey" for the cancer survivor cohort, included LTPA, previous cancer type, age, sex, smoking status, BMI, daily fruit and vegetable intake, survey year, long-term risky alcohol use, SF-8 physical and mental health component scores, and self-reported diabetes. Socioeconomic index for areas and region (metro or regional residence) were not included in the adjusted model as they were not significantly associated with the outcome in crude Cox models.

Differences in survival as a function of prior cancer status (yes/no) were assessed by combining the CCs and NCCs, and introducing a variable denoting prior cancer status to the adjusted Cox regression model. All aforementioned covariates were also included in this model.

Trends for the effects of LTPA on the two outcomes were estimated by excluding the categorical LTPA variable from the class statement in the adjusted Cox regression model. To test for interaction between LTPA and prior cancer status, the two cohorts were combined, and interaction terms [LTPA × prior cancer status (yes/no)] were added to the models.

The proportional hazards assumption that the ratio of mortality rates according to the exposure variable remained constant for the adjusted models was tested by inclusion of an interaction term between the LTPA variable and log(survival time). No violation of the proportional hazards was observed.

For all analyses, a two sided $p < 0.05$ was considered statistically significant. The statistical software SAS 9.3 was used to perform all analyses.

RESULTS

Baseline Characteristics

At time of survey, the median age for both the CC (n = 1,589) and the NCC (n = 3,145) was 68 years [interquartile range (IQR): 60–76 years]. Median BMI was similar between cohorts (CC = 26.6 kg/m^2, IQR = 23.8–29.9; NCC = 26.0 kg/m^2, IQR = 23.4–29.2), as was median fruit/vegetable servings per day (CC = 5.0 servings, IQR = 4.0–6.0; NCC = 5.0 servings, IQR = 4.0–6.0), median SF-8 physical health component score (CC = 49.6, IQR = 39.9–54.4; NCC = 51.1, IQR = 42.3–55.6), median SF-8 mental health component score (CC = 54.1, IQR = 48.1–57.7; NCC = 54.8, IQR = 49.3–57.7), and percentage with self-reported diabetes (CC = 11.8%; NCC = 11.5%). Percentage of current smokers (CC = 9.5%; NCC = 10.5%) and long-term risky drinking (>2 standard drinks on any given day) (CC = 19.8%; NCC = 18.0%) varied slightly between cohorts.

LTPA-Stratified Baseline Characteristics in the CC

Compared with those who reported no LTPA per week, those reporting increased levels of LTPA tended to be younger, have lower BMI, greater fruit/vegetable and alcohol intake, and were less likely to be current smokers (**Table 1**). Mental health component scores from SF-8 questions were appreciably higher in the 360+ min of LTPA group and an apparent dose-response between increasing levels of LTPA and percentage of those with SF-8 physical health component scores above the median was observed (**Table 1**). All of the aforementioned factors were significantly associated with LTPA aside from gender and smoking status. In terms of time from first cancer diagnosis until survey, a slightly higher mean number of years were observed in the "no LTPA" group compared to the other LTPA levels. However, no significant association between LTPA and "years from cancer diagnosis until survey" was observed.

LTPA-Stratified Baseline Characteristics in the NCC

The relationships between LTPA-stratified baseline characteristics for the NCC (**Table 2**) appeared to mirror those observed in the CC; however, significant associations between LTPA and gender, and LTPA and smoking status were observed in the NCC that were not present within the CC. This may relate in part to the greater number of individuals present in the NCC.

Cohort Follow-up

The median duration of follow-up after survey was 2.6 years (out to 7.6 years) for the cancer survivor cohort, during which time 83 cancer-specific deaths and 135 all-cause deaths occurred. In comparison, a median duration of 2.8 years (out to 7.6 years) for the NCC was observed, during which time 52 cancer-specific deaths and 152 all-cause deaths occurred.

Survival in Relation to Prior Cancer Status

Prior cancer was associated with a threefold increased risk [HR = 3.05 (95% CI 2.15–4.33)] for cancer-specific mortality, compared to those without prior cancer after adjustment for LTPA, age, sex, smoking status, BMI, daily fruit and vegetable intake, survey year, long-term risky alcohol use, SF-8 physical and mental health component scores, and self-reported diabetes. Adjusted estimates of risk for all-cause mortality were 72% higher [HR = 1.72 (95% CI 1.36–2.17)] in those with a prior reported cancer, compared to those with no prior cancer reported.

LTPA and Cancer-Specific Mortality

Risks for cancer-specific mortality in participants with prior cancer [HR = 0.30 (95% CI 0.13–0.70)] and without prior cancer [HR = 0.16 (95% CI 0.05–0.56)] were significantly reduced in those reporting 360 min or more of LTPA per week, compared to those reporting none (**Table 3**). For both prior-CCs and NCCs there appeared to be an inverse dose–response relationship between level of LTPA and risk of cancer-specific mortality (CC p_{trend} = 0.0024; NCC p_{trend} = 0.0016). However, no significant interaction was observed between prior cancer status and LTPA in relation to cancer-specific mortality ($p_{interaction}$ = 0.8341) risk.

LTPA and All-Cause Mortality

All-cause mortality during the follow-up period was significantly reduced by 45–59% (**Table 3**) for those reporting 150–359 or 360+ min per week of LTPA, regardless of prior cancer status. While not significant, results also suggested some reduction in risk for those performing less than 150 min LTPA per week. Significant trends were observed in terms of effects from increasing levels of LTPA on reduction in all-cause mortality, for the cancer (p = 0.0178) and non-cancer (p = 0.0215) cohorts. No significant interaction was observed between prior cancer status and LTPA in relation to all-cause mortality ($p_{interaction}$ = 0.9932) risk.

DISCUSSION

This observational study aimed to investigate the relationship between LTPA and cancer-specific mortality, and between LTPA and all-cause mortality, in two cohorts; a long-term cancer survivor cohort and a cohort without prior recorded cancer who were frequency matched on age, gender, and survey year to those in the CC. Results confirmed an association between 150 min or more LTPA and reduced all-cause mortality in both cohorts. In relation to cancer-specific mortality, physical activity exceeding 360 min per week was associated with survival benefits regardless of a person's prior cancer status. Lower levels of physical activity (<150, 150–359 min per week) were not significantly associated with reductions in cancer-specific mortality in those with or without a prior cancer.

Physical activity has previously been shown to provide immediate beneficial effects for cancer survivors, including improvements in physiological markers, body composition, physical function, fatigue, and psychological outcomes (2, 17–20). Although evidence related to long-term cancer survivors is sparse, a recent study by Inoue-Choi et al. (13) suggested adherence to recommended levels of physical activity in long-term

TABLE 3 | Risk for cancer-specific death and all-cause death by weekly leisure-time physical activity (LTPA) levels, in cohorts with and without previously reported cancer diagnosis.

		Outcomes following physical activity assessment					
		Cancer-specific death			All-cause death		
	At risk (n)	No. of events	Hazards ratio (HR)[a]	95% confidence intervals (CI)	No. of events	HR[a]	95% CI
LTPA (minutes per week)							
Cancer cohort (CC)							
None	405	40	Ref.	Ref.	67	Ref.	Ref.
<150	443	24	0.62	0.36–1.06	38	0.70	0.46–1.08
150–359	370	12	0.55	0.28–1.08	18	0.55	0.31–0.97
360+	371	7	0.30	0.13–0.70	12	0.41	0.21–0.79
Total participants	1,589	83			135		
Non-cancer cohort							
None	801	26	Ref.	Ref.	73	Ref.	Ref.
<150	826	13	0.66	0.33–1.31	41	0.78	0.52–1.15
150–359	774	10	0.54	0.25–1.15	21	0.52	0.32–0.86
360+	693	3	0.16	0.05–0.56	17	0.50	0.29–0.88
Total participants	3,145	52			152		

[a]*Cox model includes age at survey, sex, smoking category, long-term risky drinking category, body mass index category, daily fruit and vegetable intake, survey year, self-reported diabetes, SF-8 mental health component score, SF-8 physical health component score, and previous cancer type (for CC).*

cancer survivors may improve all-cause, CVD-specific, and cancer-specific mortality. While the study variables and design used by Inoue-Choi et al. differed to those in our study in that we included men and women, a comparative non-cancer group, and different doses of physical activity (e.g., 150, 150–359, and 360+ min per week), it was of interest to note the clear protective (adjusted) effects of physical activity that existed for both cancer-specific and all-cause mortality outcomes in their study. Similarly, a recent prospective cohort study (21) of 830 long-term prostate cancer survivors assessed physical activity at 2.5, 4.7, and 6.8 years post-diagnosis (comparable to the 8.8-year assessment time point in our study) showed a protective effect of increased physical activity and prostate cancer mortality. In our study, the likelihood of cancer-related death for cancer survivors appeared to decrease for increasing levels of physical activity culminating in a significant 70% reduced risk for those performing 360+ min of LTPA per week. In the same exposure group (360+ min), all-cause mortality in cancer survivors was reduced by almost 60%.

In our cohort containing individuals with and without prior cancer, we observed a 72% increased all-cause mortality risk over the follow-up period in cancer survivors compared to those without a prior cancer. We also observed a threefold increased risk for cancer-specific mortality in those with prior cancer compared to cancer-naive participants. Higher risk of non-cancer-related mortality may in part be explained by an overrepresentation of CVD risk factors being observed in cancer survivors (22). Although it would have been interesting to test for CVD-specific mortality, we did not investigate this due to the relatively low numbers of cancer survivors having a CVD-specific death recorded and the likelihood of competing risks between the CVD and cancer mortality outcomes.

For long-term cancer survivors, previous evidence suggests an increased risk for both cancer and non-cancer-related mortality compared to that of the general population (23, 24). A number of studies have highlighted the above average incidence of second primary or recurrent cancers in those surviving an initial cancer (25). This increased risk for subsequent cancer appears to depend upon cancer type and/or cancer treatment, and other individual-specific risk profiles (e.g., lifestyle, genetics, and other exposures) (25). In addition, increases in all-cause and non-cancer-related mortality in cancer survivors have been reported (13). There are a number of mechanisms by which physical activity may further improve cancer-specific survival in long-term cancer survivors as well as those without prior cancer. Since both cohorts (those with and those without prior cancer) observed apparent cancer-specific survival benefits from physical activity, one explanation might be that physical activity reduces the likelihood of cancer incidence, resulting in fewer cancer deaths. However, in some unpublished analyses from this study we observed no significant relationship between physical activity and cancer incidence (or second primary cancer incidence in the prior-CC). An alternative explanation is that physical activity may play a role in improving prognosis of those who develop an incident or second primary cancer. Evidence supporting this has been reported by a number of researchers (26). Although the biological mechanisms through which this is achieved are still unclear, there are a number of promising avenues. The influence of exercise on host factors such as metabolic hormones, inflammation/cytokines, and immune surveillance have been suggested, as have exercise's effects on certain tumor-related factors such as p27, CTNNB1, CACNA2D3, and L3MBTL1 (26).

By selecting an NCC from the same source cohort who possessed similar age and gender distributions as the cancer survivors, we investigated whether differential physical activity-related effects on our two outcomes (cancer mortality and all-cause mortality) might exist. Certainly, physical activity has been associated with reduced all-cause mortality rates (27) and cardiovascular-related disease (28–30) or cardiovascular-death (31) in population-based cohorts. Results from our study of a positive association between physical activity and decreasing cancer-specific and all-cause mortality in our NCC reflected previous findings. Moreover, our results suggested the benefits of moderate to high levels of physical activity in decreasing cancer-specific and all-cause mortality were comparable between those with or without a prior cancer. From a health promotion and management perspective, this provides a degree of confirmation that physical activity recommendations for the general public are applicable and beneficial for cancer survivors. Moreover, these benefits were observed in an aggregate cancer survivor group and, while cancer type was accounted for in the analyses, it is likely these benefits of physical activity would apply broadly to survivors of most cancer types.

There are a number of strengths attributable to this study. Foremost was our ability to gain all recorded retrospective and post-survey cancer and mortality records for those who participated in the survey. This allowed an assessment of physical activity levels an average 8.8 years following cancer survivors' initial cancer diagnoses. Second, the in-depth survey of participants allowed adjustment of numerous confounding variables associated with lifestyle, physical, and mental health, which provides a greater reliability in estimating the association between physical activity and the outcomes of interest. In addition, access to non-cancer survey participants (at time of survey) enabled comparison of physical activity influences on the outcomes in participants with and without a prior cancer. It is unlikely there would be many instances of misclassification of cancer outcomes as these were mostly derived from pathology laboratories or radiation oncologists (32). For similar reasons, mortality records are unlikely to be a basis for misclassification bias.

Some limitations exist with this study. Given the self-reported nature of the physical activity measurements, some misclassification of the exposure might exist. Any associated bias is likely reduced by the use of quite broad categories for physical activity (0, <150, 150–59, 360+ min per week) and is unlikely to relate to the outcomes due to the prospective nature of the study. While it made sense to classify physical activity based on recommendations and health promotion messages, our aggregation of low, moderate, and vigorous physical activity in calculating amount of LTPA per week excluded our ability to measure differences in effectiveness between low, moderate, and vigorous levels of physical activity. Moreover, although we adjusted for a number of potential confounders in our analyses, possible confounding may still exist and contribute to the identified associations. In addition, loss to follow-up (between survey and outcome) would likely have been minimal since the individuals were followed up through the Western Australian Health registries—in terms of cancer and/or death. This means that virtually all deaths and cancers reported throughout the follow-up period would be included; however, those occurring outside of Western Australia would presumably be lost to follow-up. Finally, the observational nature of the study does not permit us to infer cause and effect.

In summary, this study suggests physical activity is associated with improved cancer-specific and all-cause survival in long-term survivors of cancer. These associations were comparable in magnitude to those seen in a NCC of similar age and gender, selected from the same source population. Evidence also suggested further benefits in survival may be achieved by those exceeding 360 min of LTPA per week, regardless of an individual's prior cancer status.

AUTHOR CONTRIBUTIONS

AG, SJ, ST, DT, PC, RN, DJ, NS, KE, and DG: substantial contributions to the conception or design of the work or the acquisition, analysis, or interpretation of data for the work; drafting the work or revising it critically for important intellectual content; final approval of the version to be published; agreement to be accountable for all aspects of the work in ensuring that questions related to the accuracy or integrity of any part of the work are appropriately investigated and resolved.

ACKNOWLEDGMENTS

We wish to thank the Western Australian Department of Health for providing the data used for this investigation. We are furthermore grateful to the Data Linkage Branch of the WA Department of Health for linking the data and facilitating the extractions. DG is funded by a Movember New Directions Development Award obtained through Prostate Cancer Foundation of Australia's Research Program and by the Cancer Council Western Australia Research Fellowship.

FUNDING

This study was supported by Edith Cowan University internal research.

REFERENCES

1. Australian Institute of Health and Welfare. *Australian Institute of Health and Welfare and Australasian Association of Cancer Registries 2012. Cancer in Australia: An Overview, 2012. Cancer Series No. 74. Cat. No. CAN 70.* Canberra: AIHW (2012).
2. Fong DY, Ho JW, Hui BP, Lee AM, Macfarlane DJ, Leung SS, et al. Physical activity for cancer survivors: meta-analysis of randomised controlled trials. *BMJ* (2012) 344:e70. doi:10.1136/bmj.e70
3. Ballard-Barbash R, Friedenreich CM, Courneya KS, Siddiqi SM, McTiernan A, Alfano CM. Physical activity, biomarkers, and disease outcomes in cancer survivors: a systematic review. *J Natl Cancer Inst* (2012) 104(11):815–40. doi:10.1093/jnci/djs207
4. Holmes MD, Chen WY, Feskanich D, Kroenke CH, Colditz GA. Physical activity and survival after breast cancer diagnosis. *JAMA* (2005) 293(20):2479–86. doi:10.1001/jama.293.20.2479
5. Meyerhardt JA, Giovannucci EL, Holmes MD, Chan AT, Chan JA, Colditz GA, et al. Physical activity and survival after colorectal cancer diagnosis. *J Clin Oncol* (2006) 24(22):3527–34. doi:10.1200/JCO.2006.06.0855
6. Je Y, Jeon JY, Giovannucci EL, Meyerhardt JA. Association between physical activity and mortality in colorectal cancer: a meta-analysis of prospective cohort studies. *Int J Cancer* (2013) 133(8):1905–13. doi:10.1002/ijc.28208
7. Meyerhardt JA, Giovannucci EL, Ogino S, Kirkner GJ, Chan AT, Willett W, et al. Physical activity and male colorectal cancer survival. *Arch Intern Med* (2009) 169(22):2102–8. doi:10.1001/archinternmed.2009.412
8. Kenfield SA, Stampfer MJ, Giovannucci E, Chan JM. Physical activity and survival after prostate cancer diagnosis in the health professionals follow-up study. *J Clin Oncol* (2011) 29(6):726–32. doi:10.1200/JCO.2010.31.5226
9. Patterson RE, Cadmus LA, Emond JA, Pierce JP. Physical activity, diet, adiposity and female breast cancer prognosis: a review of the epidemiologic literature. *Maturitas* (2010) 66(1):5–15. doi:10.1016/j.maturitas.2010.01.004
10. Ibrahim EM, Al-Homaidh A. Physical activity and survival after breast cancer diagnosis: meta-analysis of published studies. *Med Oncol* (2011) 28(3):753–65. doi:10.1007/s12032-010-9536-x
11. Beasley JM, Kwan ML, Chen WY, Weltzien EK, Kroenke CH, Lu W, et al. Meeting the physical activity guidelines and survival after breast cancer: findings from the after breast cancer pooling project. *Breast Cancer Res Treat* (2012) 131(2):637–43. doi:10.1007/s10549-011-1770-1
12. Meyerhardt JA, Heseltine D, Niedzwiecki D, Hollis D, Saltz LB, Mayer RJ, et al. Impact of physical activity on cancer recurrence and survival in patients with stage III colon cancer: findings from CALGB 89803. *J Clin Oncol* (2006) 24(22):3535–41. doi:10.1200/JCO.2006.06.0863
13. Inoue-Choi M, Robien K, Lazovich D. Adherence to the WCRF/AICR guidelines for cancer prevention is associated with lower mortality among older female cancer survivors. *Cancer Epidemiol Biomarkers Prev* (2013) 22(5):792–802. doi:10.1158/1055-9965.EPI-13-0054
14. Davis P, Joyce S. *Health and Wellbeing of Adults in Western Australia 2010, Overview and Trends.* Western Australia: Department of health (2011).
15. Holman CD, Bass AJ, Rouse IL, Hobbs MS. Population-based linkage of health records in Western Australia: development of a health services research linked database. *Aust N Z J Public Health* (1999) 23(5):453–9. doi:10.1111/j.1467-842X.1999.tb01297.x
16. Australian Institute of Health and Welfare. *Australia Survey: A Guide and Manual for Implementing Analysis and Reporting.* AIHW cat. no CVD 22 (2003).
17. Knols R, Aaronson NK, Uebelhart D, Fransen J, Aufdemkampe G. Physical exercise in cancer patients during and after medical treatment: a systematic review of randomized and controlled clinical trials. *J Clin Oncol* (2005) 23(16):3830–42. doi:10.1200/JCO.2005.02.148
18. Conn VS, Hafdahl AR, Porock DC, McDaniel R, Nielsen PJ. A meta-analysis of exercise interventions among people treated for cancer. *Support Care Cancer* (2006) 14(7):699–712. doi:10.1007/s00520-005-0905-5
19. Schmitz KH, Courneya KS, Matthews C, Demark-Wahnefried W, Galvão DA, Pinto BM, et al. American College of Sports Medicine roundtable on exercise guidelines for cancer survivors. *Med Sci Sports Exerc* (2010) 42(7):1409–26. doi:10.1249/MSS.0b013e3181e0c112
20. Galvao DA, Newton RU. Review of exercise intervention studies in cancer patients. *J Clin Oncol* (2005) 23(4):899–909. doi:10.1200/JCO.2005.06.085
21. Friedenreich CM, Wang Q, Neilson HK, Kopciuk KA, McGregor SE, Courneya KS. Physical activity and survival after prostate cancer. *Eur Urol* (2016) 70(4):576–85. doi:10.1016/j.eururo.2015.12.032
22. Weaver KE, Foraker RE, Alfano CM, Rowland JH, Arora NK, Bellizzi KM, et al. Cardiovascular risk factors among long-term survivors of breast, prostate, colorectal, and gynecologic cancers: a gap in survivorship care? *J Cancer Surviv* (2013) 7(2):253–61. doi:10.1007/s11764-013-0267-9
23. Baade PD, Fritschi L, Eakin EG. Non-cancer mortality among people diagnosed with cancer (Australia). *Cancer Causes Control* (2006) 17(3):287–97. doi:10.1007/s10552-005-0530-0
24. Fosså SD, Gilbert E, Dores GM, Chen J, McGlynn KA, Schonfeld S, et al. Noncancer causes of death in survivors of testicular cancer. *J Natl Cancer Inst* (2007) 99(7):533–44. doi:10.1093/jnci/djk111

25. Ng AK, Travis LB. Subsequent malignant neoplasms in cancer survivors. *Cancer J* (2008) 14(6):429–34. doi:10.1097/PPO.0b013e31818d8779
26. Betof AS, Dewhirst MW, Jones LW. Effects and potential mechanisms of exercise training on cancer progression: a translational perspective. *Brain Behav Immun* (2013) 30(Suppl):S75–87. doi:10.1016/j.bbi.2012.05.001
27. Zhao G, Li C, Ford ES, Fulton JE, Carlson SA, Okoro CA, et al. Leisure-time aerobic physical activity, muscle-strengthening activity and mortality risks among US adults: the NHANES linked mortality study. *Br J Sports Med* (2014) 48(3):244–9. doi:10.1136/bjsports-2013-092731
28. Anand SS, Islam S, Rosengren A, Franzosi MG, Steyn K, Yusufali AH, et al. Risk factors for myocardial infarction in women and men: insights from the INTERHEART study. *Eur Heart J* (2008) 29(7):932–40. doi:10.1093/eurheartj/ehn018
29. Gunnell AS, Einarsdóttir K, Galvão DA, Joyce S, Tomlin S, Graham V, et al. Lifestyle factors, medication use and risk for ischaemic heart disease hospitalisation: a longitudinal population-based study. *PLoS One* (2013) 8(10):e77833. doi:10.1371/journal.pone.0077833
30. Li J, Siegrist J. Physical activity and risk of cardiovascular disease – a meta-analysis of prospective cohort studies. *Int J Environ Res Public Health* (2012) 9(2):391–407. doi:10.3390/ijerph9020391
31. Yang Q, Cogswell ME, Flanders WD, Hong Y, Zhang Z, Loustalot F, et al. Trends in cardiovascular health metrics and associations with all-cause and CVD mortality among US adults. *JAMA* (2012) 307(12):1273–83. doi:10.1001/jama.2012.339
32. Threlfall TJ, Thompson JR. *Cancer Incidence and Mortality in Western Australia, 2011*. Perth, WA: Department of Health (2013).

12

Adverse Events in Patients with Rheumatoid Arthritis and Psoriatic Arthritis Receiving Long-Term Biological Agents in a Real-Life Setting

Mayara Costa de Camargo[1]*, Bruna Cipriano Almeida Barros*[2]*, Izabela Fulone*[1]*, Marcus Tolentino Silva*[1]*, Miriam Sanches do Nascimento Silveira*[1]*, Iara Alves de Camargo*[1]*, Silvio Barberato-Filho*[1]*, Fernando de Sá Del Fiol*[1] *and Luciane Cruz Lopes*[1]*

[1] *Pharmaceutical Sciences Graduate Program, University of Sorocaba (UNISO), Sorocaba, Brazil,*

[2] *Hematology Graduate Program, Federal University of São Paulo (UNIFESP), São Paulo, Brazil*

***Correspondence:**
Luciane Cruz Lopes
luslopesbr@gmail.com;
luciane.lopes@prof.uniso.br

Background: Biological agents used for the treatment of psoriatic arthritis (PsA) and rheumatoid arthritis (RA) are associated with serious adverse effects (SAEs). Although several biologics have demonstrated good efficacy and tolerability in short-term trials, treatment guidelines recommend them as third line therapies due to a relative lack of long-term safety data.

Objective: To determine the frequency and severity of adverse effects associated with the long-term use of biologics in the treatment of PsA and RA, and possible risk factors for such events in a real-life setting.

Methods: We conducted a longitudinal study in PsA and RA patients only taking long-term biological agents from 2003 to 2011. Sources of information included dispensing pharmacy data and interviews with patients. Research staff conducted telephone interviews with patients inquiring about any apparent medication-related adverse drug reactions (ADRs) or SAEs. ADR/SAE's data was based on pharmacy reports. We conducted a multivariate analysis to identify the factors associated with the risk of ADRs.

Results: Of the 305 patients identified, we interviewed 268 patients. Most of these were taking adalimumab 127 (47.4%), 52 (19.4%) etanercept, 42 (15.7%) infliximab, 25 (9.3%) rituximab, 10 (3.7%) abatacept, 9 (3.4%) efalizumab, and 3 (1.1%) tocilizumab. Of the 268 patients, 116 (43.3%) experienced one or more adverse events related to biological agents with 1.6 events per patient, and of these 29 (25%) experienced one or more SAEs, with majority subjected to hospitalizations. The most frequently reported ADRs were administration site reactions as observed in 73 patients (27.2%), infections in 30 patients (11.2%), effects on nervous system in 22 patients (8.2%), and 15 (5.6%) patients withdrew due to ADRs. The use of rituximab was related with less risk of ADR [PR 0.42, 95% CI 0.18–0.96; $p = 0.04$] than other agents. No other predisposing factors were associated with risk of ADR. The monitoring of patients (medical consultation and laboratory test) was only completed by 48 patients (30.4%).

Conclusion: These data showed the early biological experience in Brazil that were associated with ADRs, withdrawals due to ADRs and SAEs. The quantification of adverse effects (serious or nonserious) considering close monitoring and patients' perceptions are increasingly important for future decision-making.

Keywords: adverse reaction, biologic agents, psoriatic arthritis, rheumatoid arthritis, safety

INTRODUCTION

Biologic agents, introduced in the late 1990s, have improved the treatment outcomes of autoimmune disease, inflammatory disease, and tumour therapy (Chen et al., 2006; NICE, 2012; Coates et al., 2013). Additionally, the application of biological processes involving recombinant DNA technology, which allowed the production of proteins like cytokines and humanized antibodies, must be credited (Mazurek and Jahnz-Rozyk, 2012).

These drugs include tumour necrosis factor (TNF) inhibitors (e.g. adalimumab, certolizumab, etanercept, golimumab and infliximab), anti-CD28 agent (abatacept), anti-cytokine agents (anakinra and tocilizumab), anti-B-cell agent (rituximab), T-cell modulating agent (alefacept), and inhibitors of interleukin (IL)-12 and IL-23 (ustekinumab) (Rosman et al., 2013). Indications for use vary between the countries in which they have been approved for marketing.

The wide use of biological agents in modern medicine is a challenge for physicians and requires constant learning, with distinct knowledge and familiarity of the disease to be treated. Additionally, these biological agents are expensive and compel the physicians to consider the economic burden on patients. Biologic agents have been associated with high rates of total adverse events and withdrawals due to adverse events (Singh et al., 2011).

Tumor Necrosis Factor-alpha (TNFα) is essential for increasing phagocytic activity of macrophages and other killer cells; therefore, anti-TNFα medication can lead to common and opportunistic infections (Curtis et al., 2011). These include tuberculosis, atypical mycobacteriosis, listeriosis, histoplasmosis, aspergillosis, pneumocystis, and legionellosis (Murdaca et al., 2015).

There is increasing evidence of the paradoxical induction of autoimmune processes associated with biological agents (Lee and Kavanaugh, 2005; Katz and Zandman-Goddard, 2010; Karmacharya et al., 2015). Autoimmune diseases secondary to biological therapies comprise a variety of both, systemic illnesses including lupus, vasculitis, sarcoidosis, and antiphospholipid syndrome (Pichler, 2006). Biological agents have also been associated with organ-specific autoimmune processes including interstitial lung disease, uveitis, optic neuritis, peripheral neuropathies, multiple sclerosis, and autoimmune hepatitis (Hausmann et al., 2010).

The majority of adverse effects manifest between one month to one year after initiating the therapy with a biological agent; however, they may also manifest years after treatment suspension (Mazurek and Jahnz-Rozyk, 2012). Biological agents may also manifest adverse effects that are yet unknown, suggesting that monitoring of ongoing patients is essential (NICE, 2012; Silveira et al., 2014; Gonzalez-Alvaro et al., 2015; Deighton et al., 2009).

Patient reports are an important source of information on patient safety (Fowler et al., 2008; Kuzel et al., 2004) and are useful in evaluating the adverse events (Hibbard et al., 2005; Zhu et al., 2011). In Brazil, patients reported one or more adverse reactions associated with biological agents in 67% of the cases. These patients had no close clinical monitoring (Lopes et al., 2014; Camargo et al., 2016).

To further elucidate the adverse effects and predisposing factors associated with the use of biologics in clinical practice, we performed an observational study in patients with psoriatic arthritis (PsA) and/or rheumatoid arthritis (RA) who had been using the same biological agent for at least six months. The main objective was to evaluated the medium- and long-term safety of biologics in patients from a middle-income country.

METHODS

Design and Setting

We utilized a retrospective longitudinal design to investigate the adverse drug reactions (ADRs) (Gonzalez-Alvaro et al., 2015) occurring in patients using long-term biologics (abatacept, adalimumab, efalizumab, etanercept, infliximab, rituximab, and tocilizumab) for treatment of PsA and RA in Brazil. The protocol was authorized by the Health State Department and approved by the Ethics Committee for Clinical Research of University of Sorocaba (August 17, 2009; protocol number 011/2009). Each patient provided an informed consent.

Definitions

We defined ADR as "a response to a medicine or medicinal product that is noxious and unintended, and which occurs in doses normally used in humans for the prophylaxis, diagnosis, or therapy of disease or for the modification of physiological function" (WHO, 2002). Therefore, we excluded events that resulted from drug errors, therapeutic failures, intentional or accidental poisoning, and drug abuse.

A serious adverse event (SAEs) was defined under the same code as 'any untoward medical occurrence that at any dose results in death; is life threatening; requires inpatient hospitalization or prolongation of existing hospitalization; creates persistent or significant disability/incapacity, or a congenital anomaly/birth defect' (International Council on Harmonisation, 1994).

Eligibility Criteria

Eligible patients were those who underwent treatment with biologics for PsA/RA for at least 6 months, during 2003–2011.

Identification of Patients and Collection of Patient Data

To identify eligible patients, two researchers abstracted data from all the dispensing orders from the database of the government (CODES-SP). The patients with PsA were identified by ICD code M07, and those with RA were identified by ICD code M05. Patient details such as name, address, telephone number, gender, age, healthcare provider, type of biologic dispensed, and duration of treatment and diagnoses were collected.

We contacted these patients by telephone, and if they proved eligible and agreed to participate in the study, we conducted interviews by telephone using a questionnaire. The questionnaire included the following: name of the drug that patient was using for the treatment of PsA and RA; time of diagnosis of the disease; comorbidities; adverse drug reaction and whether it led to discontinuing medications; and whether patients was informed about the risk of taking such drugs.

Interviews were conducted by telephone using computer-assisted telephonic interview technology with a microcomputer handset with headphones. This system allows recording and monitoring of the conversation. Research staff working in pairs independently recorded data from the interviews, with discrepancies (if any) resolved by the principal investigator (LCL). This interview approach was developed by local dermatologists and rheumatologists in accordance with the recommendations of Brazilian and others important guidelines. Each interviewer (pharmacists) received training on use of language, related to each question in the interview schedule.

In order to dispense the biologics drugs in the pharmacy of the government, all pharmacists monitoring the patients with a formal structured checklist for ADR validated by rheumatologist and dermatologists.

We crosschecked patients' reports with data obtained from pharmacy records and from the database of the government. If discrepancies were found between sources of information, we considered the information from the pharmacy records as definitive. Definitive information about the name of the biologic and the duration of its use was obtained from the pharmacy, and definitive information regarding the time of diagnosis, use of previous medicines, and laboratory results were obtained from the patient.

This study is a part of a protocol published elsewhere (Camargo et al., 2016; Silveira et al., 2014).

ADR Reporting

We collected information regarding the reported ADRs to understand their onset, nature of the reaction (system or organ affected), causality (Naranjo et al., 1981), and severity (ICH, 1994). The Naranjo algorithm (Naranjo et al., 1981) provided guidance for establishing causality and ADRs were ranked in three categories (definite, probable, and possible). The ADRs ranked as "definite" and "probable" were classified as likely caused by the biological agent. Pairs of reviewers (SBF, BCAB, FSDF, MCC) independently classified potential ADRs as "present" or "absent," and if present, classified them according to the causality classification. In case of disagreement a third reviewer (LL) provided adjudication.

Predisposing Factors

We considered the following variables as possible predisposing factors for ADRs. For each factor, we priori postulated the direction of the possible effects: i) **age** (older [≥60 years] versus younger [19–59 years], with a higher risk in older) (Girolomoni et al., 2012), ii) **presence of comorbidities** (none versus one or more, with a higher risk in one or more illnesses) (Mazurek and Jahnz-Rozyk, 2012), iii) **diagnosis of more than one immunosuppressive disease** (only one versus more than one, with a higher risk for diagnostic with one or more) (Coates et al., 2013), iv) **concomitant use of other medications** (none versus one versus two or more, with a higher risk with more than one medication) (Girolomoni et al., 2012), v) **concomitant use of disease modifying anti rheumatic drugs—DMARD** (none versus one or more, with a higher risk with more than one DMARD) (Mazurek and Jahnz-Rozyk, 2012), vi) **physician provided warnings regarding risk of medication** (higher risk when warnings were provided) (Girolomoni et al., 2012), vii) **health insurance** (private versus public health insurance, with a higher risk for private insurance) (Mariette et al., 2011), viii) **biological agent**, iv) **duration of use of biologics** (6 to 12 months versus 13 months or more).

Follow-Up and Clinical Monitoring

Clinical monitoring was done only in patients who were taking biologics during the interviews. We referred the guidelines of a few countries, such as Brazil (BRAZIL, 2014; BRAZIL, 2006), England (Smith et al., 2009), Canada (Bykerk et al., 2012), Germany (Wollenhaupt et al., 2013), European League against Rheumatism - EULAR (Gossec et al., 2016), Group for Research and Assessment of Psoriasis and Psoriatic Arthritis - GRAPPA (Coates et al., 2016) and took into account the common recommendations such as medical consults, laboratory blood examination, and radiograph.

As there is lack of consensus regarding the best interval for patient monitoring, we adopted the recommendations present in the Brazilian clinical protocols of the time, which considers as follows: **i) number of consults** (at least two annual medical consults); **ii) laboratory blood examination** (complete Blood Count, liver function tests and C-Reactive Protein test performed once a year) and **iii) radiography** (at least once a year). The IGRA sign test (interferon gamma release assay) was only introduced in public health service in 2014.

Owing to their high cost, biologics are only provided by government pharmacies, and therefore the follow-up was in accordance with the Brazilian official protocol. At the time of the study, annual radiography was considered as a test for monitoring tuberculosis progression, a condition common in Brazil, given the high number of patients acquired immunodeficiency syndrome (AIDS) in the general population.

Statistical Analysis

Initially, we obtained the descriptive statistics of the variables studied through frequencies. Later, the variables were stratified by patients, with and without ADRs and SAEs. We calculated the prevalence ratio (PR) to detect factors associated with the risk of ADRs using a Poisson regression.

We used with bivariate analysis (unadjusted) as a first step, and then, the analysis was adjusted for age, presence of comorbidities and use of other concomitant drugs. A significance level of $p < 0.05$ and a confidence interval of 95% were adopted. All analyses were performed using STATA software.

RESULTS

Of the 305 patients identified for using biologics for PsA or RA, 10 patients refused to participate, 13 were deceased and 14 used biological agent for less than 6 months. The resulting group of interviewees included, 268 plaintiffs of whom 158 (58.9%) were still using a biological agent at the time of the interview (**Figure 1**).

Table 1 presents characteristics of the patients with PsA and RA. Most of the patients were female (73.1%), less than 60 years old (mean age 55.8 ± 13), with rheumatoid arthritis only (73.1%), with one or more comorbidity (51.5%), using the biologic for 13 to 36 months (mean duration 35.7 ± 20).

Patients with RA showed different comorbidities as compared to those with PsA. Approximately, 102 (52%) patients with RA showed comorbidities and 46 (45.1%) had cardiovascular diseases. Twenty-two (21.5%) patients had metabolic diseases (mainly diabetes and obesity), while 17 (16.6%) had muscle pain that rendered work disabilities. On the other hand, 16 (25%) patients with PsA showed comorbidities and 8 (50%) had cardiovascular disease, 6 (37.5%) had dermatological problems, 4 (25%) had inflammatory bowel disease, 3 (18.8%) had metabolic disease, 3 (18.8%) had musculoskeletal problems including osteoporosis and ophthalmic disorders was observed in 2 patients (12.5%).

Table 2 depicts the characteristics of the adverse events in patients taking biological agents. Of the 268 patients, 116 (43.3%) experienced one or more adverse events related to the use of biological agents, at the rate of 1.6 events per patient. The most frequently [n = 73 (27.2%)] reported ADRs were administration site reactions (hypersensitivity reactions and cytokine-release syndrome), followed by incidences of respiratory and other types of infections [n = 30 (11.2%)] (opportunistic infections, urinary tract infections, skin infections, other systemic fungal infections and meninges infection)and effects on nervous system [n = 22 (8.2%)] (headaches and neuropathies). Of 116 patients with at least one ADR, 29 (25%) experienced SAE. The main causes for SAE included serious infections, malignancies and major cardiovascular events. There was no case of tuberculosis.

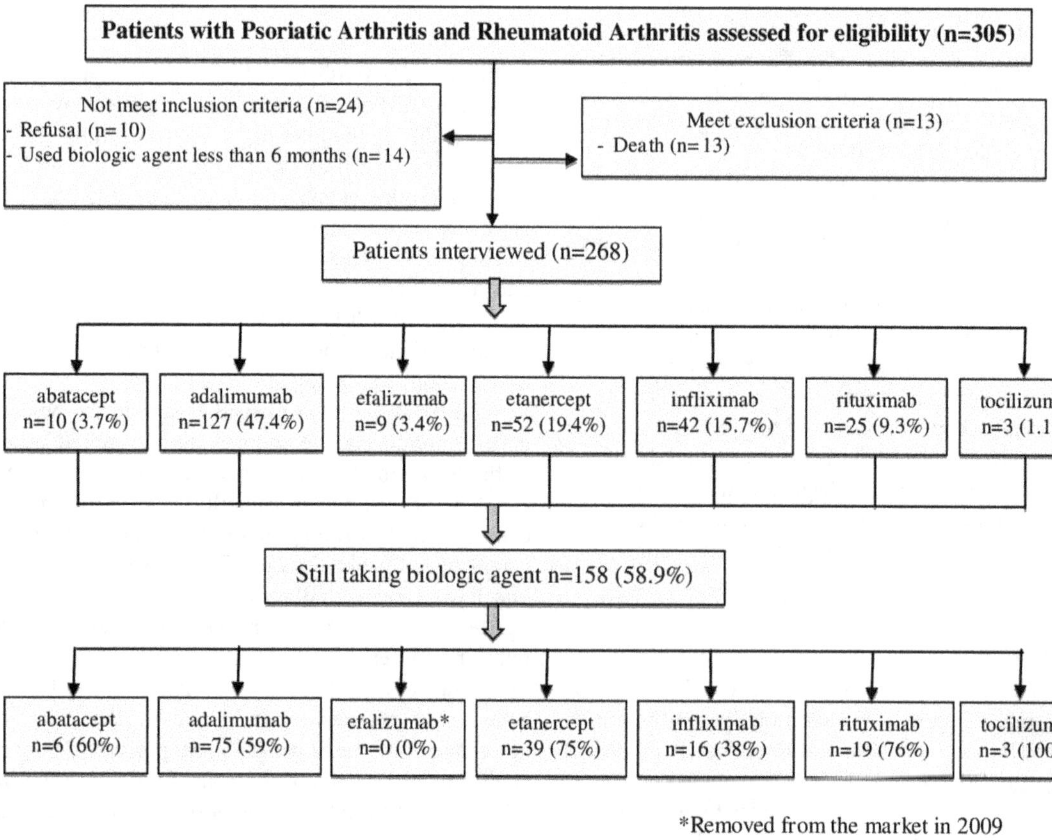

FIGURE 1 | Flow diagram of the steps of the sample composition.

TABLE 1 | Characteristics of the patients with psoriatic arthritis and rheumatoid arthritis.

Patients	n (%) 268 (100%)
Sex	
Female	196 (73.1)
Male	72 (26.9)
Age	
19–59	156 (58.2)
60 or more	112 (41.8)
mean ± sd	55.8 ± 13
Diagnostic	
Psoriatic arthritis only	63 (23.6)
Rheumatoid arthritis only	196 (73.1)
RA+PsA	9 (3.3)
Comorbidity*	
None	130 (48.5)
1 or more	138 (51.5)
Psoriasis	52 (37.7)
Cardiovascular	61(44.2)
Metabolic	34 (24.6)
Skeletal muscle	35 (25.4)
Others	28 (20.3)
Duration use of biologic agents (months)	
6 – 12	40 (14.9)
13 – 36	133 (49.6)
37 or more	95 (35.4)
mean ± sd	35.7 ± 20
Health care	
Private	56 (20.9)
Public	212 (79.1)
Concomitant use of drugs with biologic agent	
None	81 (30.2)
1	73 (27.2)
2 or more	114 (42.6)
DMARD used with biologic agent	
metrotexate	57 (21.3)
corticosteroids	24 (8.9)
Others	64 (23.9)
Time since diagnostic of disease RA/PSAR	
<1 years	5 (1.9)
1–3 years	9 (3.3)
3–5 years	31 (11.6)
>6 years	223 (83.2)

**Patients may have more than one comorbidity.*
PsA, Psoriatic arthritis; RA, rheumatoid arthritis.

We could not access the medical records to gain further details about these events. Eight patients required hospitalization, 6 had prolongation in existing hospitalization and 8 experienced life-threatening events.

Table 3 shows the characteristics of population of the study with respect to predisposing factors of ADR and the association with ADRs. Overall, rituximab showed less risk to ADR [PR 0.42, 95% CI (0.18–0.96); $p = 0.04$] than other agents. The factors such as age, private healthcare assistance, provision of information about risk of ADRs, showed no association with ADRs.

Table 4 presents the clinical follow-up and outcome in patients with on-going biologic treatments. One hundred fifty-one (95.6%) patients visited a doctor at least once a year, however, 48 patient (30.4%) did not undergo the laboratory tests (complete blood count, liver function test, reactive protein test), while 75 (47.5%) did get radiography done, whereas 58 (36.7%) patients had at least two medical consultations, underwent a laboratory blood test at least once, and had a radiography examination once a year.

DISCUSSION

Main Findings

The typical long-term users of biological drugs in this study were women aged 19–59 years, with one or more comorbidities, using biological drugs for 13–36 months and having access to public healthcare. Around 40% of the patients using biologics drugs for a long-term, had one or more ADR related to these agents, with 1.6 events per patient. The most common ADRs were administration site reactions, infections and symptoms related to nervous system (headache and neuropathic pain). The occurrence of SAEs was less than 10% of all patients. Nevertheless, the majority of SAEs did not lead to drug discontinuation. Notably, no case of tuberculosis or mortality were detected. None of other risk factors studied were associated with ADRs. Adalimumab was the biological agent most used for the majority of patients and ADRs related with this drug included serious infections disease and injections site reactions. The use of rituximab was related with lower risk of ADR than other agents. Complete clinical follow-up was done by 36.7% of patients, implying that remain the patients, despite receiving government medicines failed to follow-up, according to the official Brazilian guidelines.

Relation to Prior Literature

Biologicals have become potent and effective therapeutic alternative for many inflammatory and autoimmune diseases like RA and PsA, focus of this cohort population. Their direct and focused effect makes them superior to classic immunosuppressive, whose use is frequently limited by undesirable and often severe generalized adverse effect. Biologic agents targeting specific immune mediators have emerged as other treatment option for patients with RA, PsA and others immune disease who are unresponsive to, or intolerant of, non-biologic systemic agents. (Yazici, 2018; Michet, 2018).

Furthermore, conventional treatments for PsA have limited efficacy for nail disease, enthesitis or axial involvement, and some are unable to control moderate and severe peripheral joint and skin disease (Yazici, 2018). The introduction of biologic treatments offered the possibility of controlling multiple aspects of these diseases using a single drug, minimizing the need for additional therapies (Elyoussfi et al., 2016).

Although several biologics have demonstrated good efficacy and tolerability in short-term trials, treatment guidelines recommend them as third line therapies due to a relative lack of long-term safety data. Here, we have reviewed the long-term (>6 months) safety data. In our study, 35% of patients used biological agents for more than 37 months, reflecting the real scenario of its long-term use in Brazil.

Evidently, the harms of biologics must be balanced against their use benefits, when making a risk–benefit assessment of its use for a patient with systemic autoimmune conditions such as RA or PsA. Patients and physicians worry about risks including

TABLE 2 | Characteristics of adverse events in patients taking biological agents to treat psoriatic arthritis and rheumatoid arthritis.

Variables	abatacept (n = 10)		adalimumab (n = 127)		efalizumab (n = 9)		etanercept (n = 52)		infliximab (n = 42)		rituximab (n = 25)		tocilizumab (n = 3)		TOTAL (n = 268)	
	Number of Patients with ADR	**Number of Events**	**Number of Patients with ADR**	**Number of Events**	**Number of Patients with ADR**	**Number of Events**	**Number of Patients with ADR**	**Number of Events**	**Number of Patients with ADR**	**Number of Events**	**Number of Patients with ADR**	**Number of Events**	**Number of Patients with ADR**	**Number of Events**	**Number of Patients with ADR n (%)**	**Number of Events**
Adverse events* n (%)	6	9	91	188	5	9	37	73	24	55	16	27	2	6	181 (67.5)	367
Adverse event related with biologic agent**	3	3	65	115	2	3	23	27	15	37	7	9	1	2	116 (43.3)	186
Administration site reactions''	1	1	46	49	1	1	18	20	5	12	2	3	0	0	73 (27.2)	76
Respiratory infections and other types of infection[+]	1	1	22	30	1	1	1	1	5	5	0	0	0	0	30 (11.2)	38
Nervous System[§]	0	0	9	9	0	0	1	1	8	8	3	3	1	1	22(8.2)	22
Cardiovascular	0	0	3	11	0	0	2	4	1	5	1	1	1	1	8 (3.0)	22
Metabolic	0	0	3	5	0	0	1	1	1	1	0	0	0	0	5 (1.9)	7
Gastrointestinal tract	0	0	5	6	1	1	0	0	1	3	1	1	0	0	8 (3.0)	11
Immune	1	1	5	5	0	0	0	0	3	3	1	1	0	0	10 (3.7)	10
SAE (n = 29)																
Inpatient Hospitalization	0		10		1		3		1		0		0		15 (5.6)	
Prolongation of existing hospitalization	0		5		0		1		0		0		0		6 (2.2)	
Life-threatening[§§]	0		5		0		1		1		1		0		8 (3.0)	
Withdraw due ADRs	0		7		0		1		7		0		0		15 (5.6)	

A patient could have more than one event for system.
ADR, adverse drug reactions; SAE, serious adverse event.
**Adverse events ranked as possible, probable and definite.*
***Adverse event ranked as only definite or probable.*
''Hypersensitivity reactions and cytokine-release syndrome.
+Opportunistic infections, infections of the urinary tract, infections of the skin, other systemic fungal infections and infection of the meninges.
§Headache and neuropathies.
§§Life-threatening: requires inpatient hospitalization or prolongation of existing hospitalization; creates persistent or significant disability/incapacity, or a congenital anomaly/birth defect' (ICH, 1994).

TABLE 3 | Association between predisposing factors and ADRs.

Characteristics	N-ADR	ADR*	PR 95% IC Unadjusted	P value	PR 95% IC Adjusted	P value
Patients n (%)	153	115				
Age						
19–59	81	70	1.00	–	1.00	–
60 or more	72	45	0.81 (0.56–1.19)	0.277	0.82 (0.55–1.21)	0.323
Diagnostic (%)						
Rheumatoid arthritis only	105	91	1.00	–	1.00	–
Psoriatic arthritis only	41	22	0.52 (0.23–1.19)	0.123	0.66 (0.28–1.55)	0.342
RA+PsA	7	2	0.89 (0.55–1.41)	0.609	1.07 (0.64–1.78)	0.790
Comorbidity						
None	72	58	1.00	–	1.00	–
1 or more	81	57	0.99 (0.69–1.42)	0.946	0.94 (0.64–1.38)	0.735
Patient was guided about risk of medication						
No	135	95	1.00	–	1.00	–
Yes	18	20	0.79 (0.49–1.27)	0.325	0.81 (0.49–1.32)	0.393
Health insurance						
Private	31	25	1.00	–	1.00	–
Public	122	90	0.95 (0.61–1.48)	0.824	0.91 (0.58–1.43)	0.694
Biologic agent						
adalimumab	63	64	1.00	–	1.00	–
abatacept	7	3	0.60 (0.19–1.90)	0.380	0.52 (0.16–1.68)	0.277
efalizumab	7	2	0.44 (0.11–1.80)	0.254	0.57 (0.13–2.46)	0.454
etanercept	29	23	0.88 (0.55–1.41)	0.592	0.86 (0.53–1.40)	0.531
infliximab	27	15	0.71 (0.40–1.24)	0.230	0.73 (0.40–1.31)	0.286
rituximab	18	7	0.56 (0.26–1.21)	0.140	0.42 (0.18–0.96)	0.044
tocilizumab	2	1	0.66 (0.09–4.77)	0.682	0.56 (0.08–4.05)	0.565
Concomitant use of drugs with biologic agents**						
No	50	31	1.00	–	1.00	–
Yes	103	84	1.17 (0.78–1.77)	0.446	1.15 (0.75–1.76)	0.534
Concomitant use of DMARDs						
No	74	50	1.00	–	1.00	–
Yes	79	65	1.02 (0.61–1.70)	0.935	0.98 (0.58–1.67)	0.944
Duration use of biologic agents (months)						
6 to 12 months	24	16	1.00	–	1.00	–
13 months or more	129	99	1.08 (0.64–1.83)	0.777	0.95 (0.55–1.62)	0.839

*ADR ranked as definite or probable.
Adjusted to: age, comorbidity and concomitant use of others drugs.
***DMARDs not included.*

TABLE 4 | Clinical follow up and outcome judgment in patients with psoriatic arthritis and rheumatoid arthritis still taking biologics.

Outcomes	abatacept (n = 6) n (%)	adalimumab (n = 75) n (%)	etanercept (n = 39) n (%)	infliximab (n = 16) n (%)	rituximab (n = 19) n (%)	tocilizumab (n = 3) n (%)	Total** (n = 158) n (%)
Annual Review							
A) Consults[1]	6 (100.0)	69 (92.0)	38 (97.4)	16 (100.0)	19 (100.0)	3 (100.0)	151 (95.6)
B) Lab exams[2]	3 (50.0)	54 (72.0)	25 (64.1)	11 (68.7)	14 (73.7)	3 (100.0)	110 (69.6)
CBC	4 (66.7)	71 (94.7)	36 (92.3)	14 (87.5)	16 (84.2)	3 (100.0)	114 (72.1)
Liver function test	4 (66.7)	59 (78.7)	30 (76.9)	12 (75.0)	16 (84.2)	3 (100.0)	124 (78.5)
CRP test	3 (50.0)	58 (77.3)	26 (66.7)	11 (68.7)	14 (73.7)	3 (100.0)	115 (72.8)
C) Radiograph[3]	3 (50.0)	43 (57.3)	19 (48.7)	7 (43.7)	10 (52.6)	1 (33.3)	83 (52.5)
Adequate clinical monitoring							
D) A + B + C	3 (50.0)	33 (44.0)	9 (23.1)	5 (31.2)	7 (36.8)	1 (33.3)	58 (36.7)

efalizumab was removed from the market in 2009.
[1]At least two annual medical consults.
[2]Laboratory blood tests performed at least once a year (CBC – Complete Blood Count; Liver function tests; CRP test – C-Reactive Protoin test).
[3]Adiography performed at least once a year.
***Clinical follow up was checked in pts still taking the medication during the interview (n = 158).*

not only common ADRs such injection site reactions but also infections that may be less common.

The clinical representation of ADR to biologicals can be ambiguous with regard to pathogenesis of the reaction, because different pathomechanisms may lead to similar symptoms. This is especially important for infusion reactions, whereby no clear clinical distinction between allergic, IgE-mediated, and the more frequent no allergic, most probably complement-mediated reactions are possible. In our study, despite the long-term use of biological agents, mainly the anti-TNFα drugs (infliximab, etanercept and adalimumab) they still have reactions related with administrations. Infusions/Injections site reactions are a major complication of all anti-TNFα drugs with studies showing an incidence rate 3–40% (Henderson Berg and Carrasco, 2017).

The most common cutaneous side effects are injection site reactions, which are often defined as a constellation of symptoms, including swelling, erythema, pruritus, and pain around the site of injection (Zeltser et al., 2001; Clarke, 2010; Scherer et al., 2010). Administration site reactions can be divided into two types according to their mechanism of action: i. Type α - irritative reactions (immediate) commonly at the injection sites of subcutaneously administered biologics caused by proinflammatory actions of the substances (Corominas et al., 2014); ii. the Type hypersensitivity reactions categorized into Types I–IV, which are induced by IgE, IgG/IgM, complement or T-cells. Injection site reaction after etanercept injection produce a T-cell-mediated delayed-type hypersensitivity reaction, as approximately 8% of patients developed "recall injection site reaction," reactions at sites were medication was previously injected (Scherer et al., 2010).

The injections site reactions with etanercept, can occur in up to 37% of patients and characteristically these reactions consist of mild to moderate erythema, pain, pruritus and edema immediately evident or appear within 24–48 h and the mean duration of the reaction is 3–5 d and there is a gradual decrease in frequency and severity with continuation of injections (Kim et al., 2015; Murdaca et al., 2012). This didn't happen in the population of this cohort. Patients using adalimumab, etanercept and infliximab more than 6 months in our cohort had 36, 34 and 11% of infusion/injections site reactions. Data from the Hong Kong Biologics Registry that followed up 1,345 patients from 2005–2013 that reported the most frequent SAE (per 100-paties-year) was infusion/injection site reaction (0.75) (Mok et al., 2014).

We found that inappropriate injection techniques, injection close to blood vessels, the chemical and physical properties of the injected drug and a reaction to the vehicle component are several causes described in the literature resulting in irritative reactions (Corominas et al., 2014).

Severe infusion reactions, such as angioedema and shock, have been reported in patients under infliximab therapy. As infliximab is a chimeric human/mouse anti- TNF-α antibody, it may induce the synthesis of neutralizing antibodies which could reduce the efficacy of the drug. Therefore, methotrexate is usually co-administered to control both the rheumatic disease and the development of neutralizing antibodies (Murdaca et al., 2013). In spite of its fully human sequence, the production of antibodies to adalimumab has been also reported, which may reduce the efficacy of the drug and induce the development of adverse drug reactions and exanthema (Murdaca et al., 2012).

However, in the majority of cases the injections site reaction with adalimumab in our study were mild-to-moderate severity, and do not necessitated drug discontinuation.

Studies comparing the intravenous and subcutaneous route of administration of these two agents did not show any difference in clinical efficacy and safety, except that injection site reactions were more common with the subcutaneous access which is the case of adalimumab and etanercept use differently of infliximab that is indicate to infusion use (Gabay et al., 2013).

Few biologics are associated with a higher rate of some of the ADRs than others, and potential SAEs with short-term and long-term use (Singh et al., 2011). The safety of rituximab was consistent with earlier findings, which indicated that there was no increase in ADRs or SAE with its prolonged use (>5 years) (Van Vollenhoven et al., 2013; Winthrop et al., 2018).

This cohort is related to the use of long-term biologicals, which shows that the adverse effects may be different from those studies that indicate short-term adverse effects. The biologic use can increase the risk of serious infections in the first months of treatment with respect to disease-modifying antirheumatic drugs (DMARDs). Data from the British Society for Rheumatology Biologics Register (BSRBR) comparing the risk of serious infections between TNFi-treated patients and traditional DMARD-treated patients showed that the risk of serious infections with TNFi was increased in the first 6 months of initiating therapy for RA and that this risk was higher compared to traditional DMARDs (Galloway et al., 2011).

Another largest observational studies of infection in patients with autoimmune diseases found that compared to traditional DMARDs, the initiation of TNF-alpha antagonists was not associated with an increased risk of hospitalizations for serious infections (Grijalva et al., 2011).

Serious infections (such as infections requiring hospitalization or intravenous administration of antibiotics, opportunistic infections, including tuberculosis, systemic fungal infections and herpes zoster) were uncommon in population currently using the biological agents for more than six months.

Moreover, long-term use of biological could be related with non-serious infections, mainly of the upper respiratory tract. This ADR were common among the users of biologics in our study, endorsing the findings from earlier studies (Salliot et al., 2007; Winthrop et al., 2018).

Emerging data also suggest that the incidence of serious infections is dependent on, past history of serious infections, corticosteroids anti-inflammatory doses, and older age as important predictors of risk of serious infections in patients treated with biologics. The duration of treatment is also an important risk factor with the highest rate being observed during the first months of therapy and the risk of infection decreases over time (Singh, 2016). Our study included patients who used biologics for a prolonged period, which could explain the reduced number of opportunistic infections. No case of tuberculosis was reported.

A study in Latin America showed that the risk of serious infections may vary depending on the region and the characteristics of the patient (Ranza et al., 2019). This study compared a database not available publicly (BIOBADABRASIL) from Brazil versus a database of Argentina (BIOBADASAR) and showed that the risk of infections in Brazil was decreasing over time, corroborating our findings.

Nowadays, safety profile has changed mainly because we know more about the disease and about biologic agent. Furthermore, not only the function of these composites has to be understood, but also the subjacent immunology (which is very complex). Therefore, current patients do have less prolonged and severe chronic inflammation, key element for decrease of cardiovascular events or malignancy risk.

The delayed reactions related to dysfunction of the cellular response such as autoimmunity or cancer, may appear after many months or years of the cessation of the biologic therapy (Mazurek and Jahnz-Rozyk, 2012). However, recent cohort study showed no evidence of change in risk of solid cancer with increasing exposure to biologics in the first five years (Mercer et al., 2015).

The characteristics of the population of this study are similar to those found in studies carried out in Europe and USA (Sfriso et al., 2009; Schneeweiss et al., 2017). The most of patients were women, age around 50–55 years old, with at least one comorbidity.

Comorbidities in our study also were similar to those observed in other studies (Ruiz et al., 2014; Deus et al., 2015; Camargo et al., 2016; Ryan et al., 2011). Patients with RA had more cardiovascular diseases, metabolic diseases like type 2 diabetes mellitus and obesity, and muscle pain rendering in work disabilities. Patients with PsA also had more cardiovascular disease, metabolic disease, inflammatory bowel disease and autoimmune ophthalmic disease. Comorbidities in this study were not related to increase in risk of ADR, as found in patients with only psoriasis in other study (Lopes et al., 2014).

Considering the high costs of biologic therapies and their adverse events profile in long-term use, the follow up of the patients and individual monitoring is essential (Mazurek and Jahnz-Rozyk, 2012). The big problem here with the use of biologics is that the prescription is made by a private doctor and accessibility to the medicine is dependent on public service, disallowing appropriate monitoring.

Furthermore, the wide use of biological agents in modern medicine is a challenge in clinical practices, as it is a case of how fast new therapeutic principles based on novel knowledge and modern techniques can enter clinical practice, and that constant learning is required. Their use often requires a special knowledge and familiarity with the disease to be treated. Scientific data shows that ADRs to these drugs are clinically very heterogeneous. It makes clear, the monitoring of them seems essential (Pichler, 2006; Zemkova et al., 2007). Patients on biologic therapy should be monitored closely with routine blood tests, regular doctor's visit and outcome measures about effectiveness (considering the response to therapy), safety (presence of ADRs and SAEs) and quality of health for prolonged period (Emer et al., 2010; RCN, 2017).

There is a lack of data regarding the best interval for monitoring the patients. We would like to emphasize that we have adopted the recommendations of the Brazilian Clinical Protocols of the time. These are official government protocols, since these medications are only provided in government pharmacies. Most of the patients had medical consultations, and laboratory tests for liver function and blood cell counts, at least annually, according to the recommendations of several guidelines from England, Brazil, Canada, etc. (BRAZIL, 2006; Smith et al., 2009; Bykerk et al., 2012; BRAZIL, 2014; Michet, 2018, Coates et al., 2016; Gossec et al., 2016). The recommendations for radiography vary according to the adopted guideline. Usually, radiographic assessments are encouraged according to clinical manifestations and discretion of physician (Ritchlin et al., 2008). In this study, we decided to follow the Brazilian guideline, and the radiography was assumed as a test for monitoring the progression of tuberculosis.

The most appropriate way to monitor disease activity in PsA is under defined (Gossec et al., 2016). The recommended core set for PsA comprises of peripheral joints, pain, physical and global function assessment, quality of life and fatigue (Kimball et al., 2008). It is also recommended that radiographic monitoring for erosions and osteolysis of the hands and feet be done annually (Michet, 2018).

The effectiveness of the biologics in RA and PsA is unquestionable, but their association with potentially adverse effects can doubt the benefit risk ratio. Therefore, closer monitoring and education of patient and their caregivers about the nature of their condition, benefits and risks of treatment are essential for improving treatment outcome and overall patient satisfaction (Emer et al., 2010). The patients need to be advised to report any worsening of symptoms (neurological, cardiac, pulmonary, skin, uveitis and/or malignancies), avoid exposure to potential risk factors for infection, and to promptly communicate to their physician possible signs and symptoms of infection (RCN, 2017).

Strengths and Limitations

The strengths of this study included an extensive questionnaire, with questions about previous treatments, diagnosis, comorbidities, and if any adverse effects and its interference with the current treatment. Besides that, our sample size was relatively large, we contacted 305 patients and interviewed 268. Our data was checked twice, as we obtained data about use of medication from the pharmacy records and then confirmed the information from patient interview to ensure its accuracy.

This registry study has mounting importance in medical research and decision-making processes. In fact, despite the inherent limitations of such studies, including the lack of randomization, the relatively high frequency of missing data, and the presence of patients with different diseases, registries usually include larger populations than clinical trials, and therefore have a higher power to detect rare adverse events. In addition, registry studies may better reflect clinical practice with respect to randomized clinical trials, whose results may not immediately be extended to "real-life". Today, several registries in Europe are collecting data on the use of biological Drugs: ARTIS (Antirheumatic Therapies In Sweden), BIOBADASER (Base de Datos de Productos Biológicos de la Sociedad

Española de Reumatología, Spain), BSRBR (British Society for Rheumatology Biologics Register, United Kingdon), DANBIO (Danish Database for Biological Therapies in Rheumatology, Denmark), RATIO (Research Axed on Tolerance of Biotherapies, France) etc. Though most patients included in these registries are taking biologic agents for the treatment of RA/PsA, the safety information gained from these sources can be applied in clinical practices (Nikiphorou et al., 2017).

Brazil have had limited initiatives to build up an important national database linking with important clinical outcomes in RA/PsA/Psoriasis. There are databases restricted to a private insurance sustained by societies of rheumatologist and funding by pharmaceutical industry. An example of this is a multicentre prospective observational cohort in Brazil is the REAL (Rheumatoid arthritis in real life) that is following up 1,300 patients from 11 canters in 4 regions from Brazil, since 2015, funding by Bristol-Myers Squibb, Eli Lily and others pharmaceutical industries (Da Rocha Castelar-Pinheiro et al., 2018). Our study is one of the few studies in Brazil that had access to patients in public health sector, without any conflict of interest with long term follow-up.

Recall bias may have led to obtaining inaccurate information about previous treatments, side effects, and clinical monitoring. We try to reduce this limitation by only asking about the clinical monitoring to those who were still using the biological agents. Another limitation is the fact that ADR were not validated by a treating physician. However, some studies point that data reported by patients are potentially important to support and improve the care (Dawson et al., 2010; Nelson et al., 2015). Furthermore, in many countries, pharmacists are recognized as one of the most important healthcare providers in ADR reporting like in the Netherlands, Spain, Portugal, and Korea (Van Grootheest et al., 2004; Kim et al., 2010; Yu et al., 2016).

Implications

This study showed the association of biological agents with ADRs, withdrawals due to adverse events and SAEs in long-term use. Patients using biological agents must be aware of these risks and should be subjected to careful monitoring throughout the treatment to prevent or at least treat a possible ADR. Our data suggests that, patients need comorbidity warning of possible adverse events and recommended enhanced surveillance.

In the long-term, the possible risk of SAE requires caution and further monitoring and investigation. Therefore, review and further investigations of their safety are warranted.

AUTHOR CONTRIBUTIONS

LCL had the original idea and reviewed all of steps of the manuscript conception. MCC, IAC and MSNS collected the data. SBF, BCAB and FSDF performed the adverse reactions analysis and cross-checked the data. MTS performed data statistical analysis. BCAB and IF drafted the manuscript.

FUNDING

The authors have received support from FAPESP (Foundation for Research Support of the State of São Paulo, process number 2009/530841).

ACKNOWLEDGMENTS

Part of this work was shown as poster presentation in the European Drug Utilisation Research Group Conference 2017[1]. The correspondent author holds the copyright and has the permission for reuse of the published conference paper.

[1]Barros B, Camargo M, Silva MT, Castilho B, Mariano A, Lopes LC. Adverse events in patients with rheumatoid arthritis and psoriatic arthritis receiving long-term biological agents in a real-life setting. In: European Drug Utilisation Research Group Conference; 2017 Nov. 15–17; Glasgow, UK. p. 79.

REFERENCES

BRAZIL (2006). Portaria n°. 66, de 6 de novembro de 2006. Health Tecnology and Strategy Drugs Secretariat. Clinical Protocol and Guidelines- Rheumatoid Arthrist Diário Oficial da União. Available at: http://bvsms.saude.gov.br/bvs/saudelegis/sctie/2006/prt0066_ 01_11_2006_comp.html (Acessed January 06 2019).

BRAZIL (2014). Artrite Psoriática. Protocolo Clínico e Diretrizes Terapêuticas. Portaria SAS/MS n° 1.204, de 4 de novembro de 2014. Available at: http://conitec.gov.br/images/Protocolos/Artrite-Psoriaca.pdf (Accessed January 19, 2019).

Bykerk, V. P., Akhavan, P., Hazlewood, G. S., Schieir, O., Dooley, A., Haraoui, B., et al. (2012). Canadian Rheumatology Association recommendations for pharmacological management of rheumatoid arthritis with traditional and biologic disease-modifying antirheumatic drugs. *J. Rheumatol.* 39 (8), 1559–1582. doi: 10.3899/jrheum.110207

Camargo, I. A., Barros, B. C. A., do Nascimento Silveira, M. S., Osorio-de-Castro, C. G. S., Guyatt, G., and Lopes, L. C. (2016). Gap between official guidelines and clinical practice for the treatment of rheumatoid arthritis in São Paulo, Brazil. *Clin. Ther.* 38, 1122–1133. doi: 10.1016/j.clinthera.2016.02.020

Chen, Y. F., Jobanputra, P., Barton, P., Jowett, S., Bryan, S., Clark, W., et al. (2006). A systematic review of the effectiveness of adalimumab, etanercept and infliximab for the treatment of rheumatoid arthritis in adults and an economic evaluation of their cost-effectiveness. *Health Technol. Assess.* 10 (42), iii–iv, xi–xiii, 1–229. doi: 10.3310/hta10420

Clarke, J. B. (2010). Mechanisms of adverse drug reactions to biologics. *Handb. Exp. Pharmacol.* 196, 453–474. doi: 10.1007/978-3-642-00663 0_16

Coates, L. C., Tillett, W., Chandler, D., Helliwell, P. S., Korendowych, E., Kyle, S., et al. (2013). The 2012 BSR and BHPR guideline for the treatment of psoriatic arthritis with biologics. *Rheumatol. (Oxf. Engl.)* 52 (10), 1754–1757. doi: 10.1093/rheumatology/ket187

Coates, L. C., Kavanaugh, A., Mease, P. J., Soriano, E. R., Laura, Acosta-Felquer, M., Armstrong, A. W., et al. (2016). Group for Research and Assessment of Psoriasis and Psoriatic Arthritis 2015 Treatment Recommendations for Psoriatic Arthritis. *Arthritis Rheumatol.* 68 (5), 1060–1071. doi: 10.1002/art.39573

Corominas, M., Gastaminza, G., and Lobera, T. (2014). Hypersensitivity reactions to biological drugs. *J. Invest. Allergol. Clin. Immunol.* 24 (4), 212–225.

Curtis, J. R., Xie, F., Chen, L., Baddley, J. W., Beukelman, T., Saag, K. G., et al. (2011). The comparative risk of serious infections among rheumatoid arthritis patients starting or switching biological agents. *Ann. Rheum. Dis.* 70 (8), 1401–1406. doi: 10.1136/ard.2010.146365

Da Rocha Castelar-Pinheiro, G., Vargas-Santos, A. B., de Albuquerque, C. P., Bertolo, M. B., Junior, P. L., Giorgi, R. D. N., et al. (2018). The REAL study: a nationwide prospective study of rheumatoid arthritis in Brazil. *Adv. Rheumatol. (Lond. Engl.)* 58 (1), 9. doi: 10.1186/s42358-018-0017-9

Dawson, J., Doll, H., Fitzpatrick, R., Jenkinson, C., and Carr, A. J. (2010). The routine use of patient reported outcome measures in healthcare settings. *BMJ* 340, c186. doi: 10.1136/bmj.c186

Deighton, C., O'Mahony, R., Tosh, J., Turner, C., and Rudolf, M. (2009). Management of rheumatoid arthritis: summary of NICE guidance. *BMJ Br. Med. J.* 338, b702. doi: 10.1136/bmj.b702

Deus, R. S., Ferraz, A. L., Oesterreich, S. A., Schmitz, W. O., and Shinzato, M. M. (2015). Caracterização de pacientes com artrite reumatoide quanto a fatores de risco para doenças vasculares cardíacas no Mato Grosso do Sul. *Rev. Bras. Reumatol.* 55 (6), 493–500. doi: 10.1016/j.rbr.2015.02.001

Elyoussfi, S., Thomas, B. J., and Ciurtin, C. (2016). Tailored treatment options for patients with psoriatic arthritis and psoriasis: review of established and new biologic and small molecule therapies. *Rheumatol. Int.* 36 (5), 603–612. doi: 10.1007/s00296-016-3436-0

Emer, J. J., Frankel, A., and Zeichner, J. A. (2010). A practical approach to monitoring patients on biological agents for the treatment of psoriasis. *J. Clin. Aesthet. Dermatol.* 3 (8), 20–26.

Fowler, F. J., Jr., Epstein, A., Weingart, S. N., Annas, C. L., Bolcic-Jankovic, D., Clarridge, B., et al. (2008). Adverse events during hospitalization: results of a patient survey. *Jt. Comm. J. Qual. Patient Saf. Jt. Comm. Resour.* 34 (10), 583–590. doi: 10.1016/S1553-7250(08)34073-2

Gabay, C., Emery, P., van Vollenhoven, R., Dikranian, A., Alten, R., Pavelka, K., et al. (2013). Tocilizumab monotherapy versus adalimumab monotherapy for treatment of rheumatoid arthritis (ADACTA): a randomised, double-blind, controlled phase 4 trial. *Lancet (Lond. Engl.)* 381 (9877), 1541–1550. doi: 10.1016/S0140-6736(13)60250-0

Galloway, J. B., Hyrich, K. L., Mercer, L. K., Dixon, W. G., Fu, B., Ustianowski, A. P., et al. (2011). Anti-TNF therapy is associated with an increased risk of serious infections in patients with rheumatoid arthritis especially in the first 6 months of treatment: updated results from the British Society for Rheumatology Biologics Register with special emphasis on risks in the elderly. *Rheumatol. (Oxf. Engl.)* 50 (1), 124–131. doi: 10.1093/rheumatology/keq242

Girolomoni, G., Altomare, G., Ayala, F., Berardesca, E., Calzavara-Pinton, P., Chimenti, S., et al. (2012). Safety of anti-TNFα agents in the treatment of psoriasis and psoriatic arthritis. *Immunopharmacol. Immunotoxicol.* 34 (4), 548–560. doi: 10.3109/08923973.2011.653646

Gonzalez-Alvaro, I., Martinez-Fernandez, C., Dorantes-Calderon, B., Garcia-Vicuna, R., Hernandez-Cruz, B., Herrero-Ambrosio, A., et al. (2015). Spanish Rheumatology Society and Hospital Pharmacy Society Consensus on recommendations for biologics optimization in patients with rheumatoid arthritis, ankylosing spondylitis and psoriatic arthritis. *Rheumatol. (Oxf.)* 54 (7), 1200–1209. doi: 10.1093/rheumatology/keu461

Gossec, L., Smolen, J. S., Ramiro, S., de Wit, M., Cutolo, M., Dougados, M., et al. (2016). European League Against Rheumatism (EULAR) recommendations for the management of psoriatic arthritis with pharmacological therapies: 2015 update. *Ann. Rheum. Dis.* 75 (3), 499–510. doi: 10.1136/annrheumdis-2015-208337

Grijalva, C. G., Chen, L., Delzell, E., Baddley, J. W., Beukelman, T., Winthrop, K. L., et al. (2011). Initiation of tumor necrosis factor-alpha antagonists and the risk of hospitalization for infection in patients with autoimmune diseases. *Jama* 306 (21), 2331–2339. doi: 10.1001/jama.2011.1692

Hausmann, O. V., Seitz, M., Villiger, P. M., and Pichler, W. J. (2010). The complex clinical picture of side effects to biologicals. *Med. Clin. North America* 94 (4), 791–804, xi–ii. doi: 10.1016/j.mcna.2010.03.001

Henderson Berg, M. H., and Carrasco, D. (2017). Injection Site Reactions to Biologic Agents Used in Psoriasis and Psoriatic Arthritis. *J. Drugs Dermatol. JDD* 16 (7), 695–698.

Hibbard, J. H., Peters, E., Slovic, P., and Tusler, M. (2005). Can patients be part of the solution? Views on their role in preventing medical errors. *Med. Care Res. Rev. MCRR* 62 (5), 601–616. doi: 10.1177/1077558705279313

International Council on Harmonisation (1994). E2A Clinical safety data management: definition and standards for expedited reporting. 12 p. Available at: https://www.ich.org/fileadmin/Public_Web_Site/ICH_Products/Guidelines/Efficacy/E2A/Step4/E2A_Guideline.pdf (Accessed June 14 2019).

Karmacharya, P., Poudel, D. R., Pathak, R., Donato, A. A., Ghimire, S., Giri, S., et al. (2015). Rituximab-induced serum sickness: a systematic review. *Semin. Arthritis Rheum.* 45 (3), 334–340. doi: 10.1016/j.semarthrit.2015.06.014

Katz, U., and Zandman-Goddard, G. (2010). Drug-induced lupus: an update. *Autoimmun. Rev.* 10 (1), 46–50. doi: 10.1016/j.autrev.2010.07.005

Kim, W. B., Marinas, J. E., Qiang, J., Shahbaz, A., Greaves, S., and Yeung, J. (2015). Adverse events resulting in withdrawal of biologic therapy for psoriasis in real-world clinical practice: a Canadian multicenter retrospective study. *J. Am. Acad. Dermatol.* 73 (2), 237–241. doi: 10.1016/j.jaad.2015.04.023

Kim, J. Y., Ha, J.-H., Kim, B.-R., Jang, J., Hwang, M., Park, H.-J., et al. (2010). Analysis of Characteristics about Spontaneous Reporting—Reported in 2008. *JPERM* 3, 23–31.

Kimball, A. B., Gladman, D., Gelfand, J. M., Gordon, K., Horn, E. J., Korman, N. J., et al. (2008). National Psoriasis Foundation clinical consensus on psoriasis comorbidities and recommendations for screening. *J. Am. Acad. Dermatol.* 58 (6), 1031–1042. doi: 10.1016/j.jaad.2008.01.006

Kuzel, A. J., Woolf, S. H., Gilchrist, V. J., Engel, J. D., LaVeist, T. A., Vincent, C., et al. (2004). Patient reports of preventable problems and harms in primary health care. *Ann. Family Med.* 2 (4), 333–340. doi: 10.1370/afm.220

Lee, S. J., and Kavanaugh, A. (2005). Adverse reactions to biologic agents: focus on autoimmune disease therapies. *J. Allergy Clin. Immunol.* 116 (4), 900–905. doi: 10.1016/j.jaci.2005.03.028

Lopes, L. C., Silveira, M. S., de Camargo, M. C., de Camargo, I. A., Luz, T. C., Osorio-de-Castro, C. G., et al. (2014). Patient reports of the frequency and severity of adverse reactions associated with biological agents prescribed for psoriasis in Brazil. *Exp. Opin. Drug Safety* 13 (9), 1155–1163. doi: 10.1517/14740338.2014.942219

Mariette, X., Matucci-Cerinic, M., Pavelka, K., Taylor, P., van Vollenhoven, R., Heatley, R., et al. (2011). Malignancies associated with tumour necrosis factor inhibitors in registries and prospective observational studies: a systematic review and meta-analysis. *Ann. Rheum. Dis.* 70 (11), 1895–1904. doi: 10.1136/ard.2010.149419

Mazurek, J., and Jahnz-Rozyk, K. (2012). The variety of types of adverse side-effects during treatment with biological drugs. *Int. Rev. Allergol. Clin. Immunol. Family Med.* 18, 34–40.

Mercer, L. K., Lunt, M., Low, A. L., Dixon, W. G., Watson, K. D., Symmons, D. P., et al. (2015). Risk of solid cancer in patients exposed to anti-tumour necrosis factor therapy: results from the British Society for Rheumatology Biologics Register for Rheumatoid Arthritis. *Ann. Rheum. Dis.* 74 (6), 1087–1093. doi: 10.1136/annrheumdis-2013-204851

Michet, C.J. (last update Mar 2018). Psoriatic arthritis. BMJ Best Practice. Available at: bestpractice.bmj.com (Accessed 04/10/2019).

Mok, C. C., Chan, K. Y., Lee, K. L., Tam, L. S., and Lee, K. W. (2014). Factors associated with withdrawal of the anti-TNFalpha biologics in the treatment of rheumatic diseases: data from the Hong Kong Biologics Registry. *Int. J. Rheum. Dis.* 17 Suppl: 3, 1–8. doi: 10.1111/1756-185X.12264

Murdaca, G., Colombo, B. M., Cagnati, P., Gulli, R., Spano, F., and Puppo, F. (2012). Update upon efficacy and safety of TNF-alpha inhibitors. *Exp. Opin. Drug Safety* 11 (1), 1–5. doi: 10.1517/14740338.2012.630388

Murdaca, G., Spano, F., and Puppo, F. (2013). Selective TNF-alpha inhibitor-induced injection site reactions. *Exp. Opin. Drug Safety* 12 (2), 187–193. doi: 10.1517/14740338.2013.755957

Murdaca, G., Spano, F., Contatore, M., Guastalla, A., Penza, E., Magnani, O., et al. (2015). Infection risk associated with anti-TNF-alpha agents: a review. *Exp. Opin. Drug Safety* 14 (4), 571–582. doi: 10.1517/14740338.2015.1009036

Naranjo, C. A., Busto, U., Sellers, E. M., Sandor, P., Ruiz, I., Roberts, E. A., et al. (1981). A method for estimating the probability of adverse drug reactions. *Clin. Pharmacol. Ther.* 30 (2), 239–245. doi: 10.1038/clpt.1981.154

Nelson, E. C., Eftimovska, E., Lind, C., Hager, A., Wasson, J. H., and Lindblad, S. (2015). Patient reported outcome measures in practice. *BMJ* 350, g7818. doi: 10.1136/bmj.g7818

NICE (2012). National Clinical Guideline Centre (UK). National Institute for Health and Clinical Excellence: Guidance. Psoriasis: Assessment and Management of Psoriasis. London: Royal College of Physicians (UK) 2012. Available at: https://www.ncbi.nlm.nih.gov/books/NBK247829/ (Accessed 01/06/2019).

Nikiphorou, E., Buch, M. H., and Hyrich, K. L. (2017). Biologics registers in RA: methodological aspects, current role and future applications. *Nat. Rev. Rheumatol.* 13 (8), 503–510. doi: 10.1038/nrrheum.2017.81

Pichler, W. J. (2006). Adverse side-effects to biological agents. *Allergy* 61 (8), 912–920. doi: 10.1111/j.1398-9995.2006.01058.x

Ranza, R., de la Vega, M. C., Laurindo, I. M. M., Gómez, M. G., Titton, D. C., Kakehasi, A. M., et al. (2019). Changing rate of serious infections in biologic-exposed rheumatoid arthritis patients. *Clin. Rheumatol.* 38 (8), 2129–2139. doi: 10.1007/s10067-019-04516-2

RCN (2017). Royal College of Nursing. Assessing, Managing and Monitoring Biologic Therapies for Inflammatory Arthritis. RCN Guidance for Rheumatology Practitioners. Fourth edition. 96 p. Available at: https://www.rcn.org.uk/-/media/royal-college-of nursing/documents/publications/2017/september/pdf-005579.pdf (Accessed 01/19/2019).

Ritchlin, C. T., Kavanaugh, A., Gladman, D. D., Mease, P. J., Helliwell, P., Boehncke, W. H., et al. (2008). Treatment recommendations for psoriatic arthritis. *Ann. Rheum. Dis.* 68 (9), 1387–1394. doi: 10.1136/ard.2008.094946

Rosman, Z., Shoenfeld, Y., and Zandman-Goddard, G. (2013). Biologic therapy for autoimmune diseases: an update. *BMC Med.* 11, 88. doi: 10.1186/1741-7015-11-88

Ruiz, D. G., Azevedo, M. N. L., and Santos, O. L. R. (2014). Caracterização clínica de pacientes com artrite psoriásica. *Rev. Soc. Bras. Clin. Med.* 12 (2), 1–3.

Ryan, C., Leonardi, C. L., Krueger, J. G., Kimball, A. B., Strober, B. E., Gordon, K. B., et al. (2011). Association between biologic therapies for chronic plaque psoriasis and cardiovascular events: a meta-analysis of randomized controlled trials. *Jama* 306 (8), 864–871. doi: 10.1001/jama.2011.1211

Salliot, C., Gossec, L., Ruyssen-Witrand, A., Luc, M., Duclos, M., Guignard, S., et al. (2007). Infections during tumour necrosis factor — αblocker therapy for rheumatic diseases in daily practice: a systematic retrospective study of 709 patients. *Rheumatol. (Oxf.)* 46 (2), 327–334. doi: 10.1093/rheumatology/kel236

Scherer, K., Spoerl, D., and Bircher, A. J. (2010). Adverse drug reactions to biologics. *J. Dtsch. Dermatol. Ges. J. Ger. Soc. Dermatol. JDDG* 8 (6), 411–426. doi: 10.1111/j.1610-0387.2010.07339.x

Schneeweiss, M., Merola, J. F., Karlson, E. W., and Solomon, D. H. (2017). Rationale and desig of the Brigham cohort for psoriasis and psoriatic arthritis registy (COPPAR). *BMC Dermatology* 17 (1), 11, 1–9. doi: 10.1186/s12895-017-0063-8

Sfriso, P., Salaffi, F., Montecucco, C. M., Bombardieri, S., and Todesco, S. (2009). MonitorNet: the Italian multi-centre observational study aimed at estimating the risk/benefit profile of biologic agents in real-world rheumatology practice. *Reumatismo* 61 (2), 132–139. doi: 10.4081/reumatismo.2009.132

Silveira, M. S., de Camargo, I. A., Osorio-de-Castro, C. G., Barberato-Filho, S., Del Fiol F de, S., Guyatt, G., et al. (2014). Adherence to guidelines in the use of biological agents to treat psoriasis in Brazil. *BMJ Open* 4 (3), e004179. doi: 10.1136/bmjopen-2013-004179

Smith, C. H., Anstey, A. V., Barker, J. N., Burden, A. D., Chalmers, R. J., Chandler, D. A., et al. (2009). British Association of Dermatologists' guidelines for biologic interventions for psoriasis 2009. *Br. J. Dermatol.* 161 (5), 987–1019. doi: 10.1111/j.1365-2133.2009.09505.x

Singh, J. A., Wells, G. A., Christensen, R., Tanjong Ghogomu, E., Maxwell, L., Macdonald, J. K., et al. (2011). Adverse effects of biologics: a network meta-analysis and Cochrane overview. *Cochrane database Syst. Rev.* 2, CD008794. doi: 10.1002/14651858.CD008794.pub2

Singh, J. A. (2016). Infections With Biologics in Rheumatoid Arthritis and Related Conditions: a Scoping Review of Serious or Hospitalized Infections in Observational Studies. *Curr. Rheumatol. Rep.* 18 (10), 61. doi: 10.1007/s11926-016-0609-5

Van Grootheest, K., Olsson, S., Couper, M., and de Jong-van den Berg, L. (2004). Pharmacists' role in reporting adverse drug reactions in an international perspective. *Pharmacoepidemiol. Drug Saf.* 13 (7), 457–464. doi: 10.1002/pds.897

Van Vollenhoven, R. F., Emery, P., Bingham, C. O., Keystone, E. C., Fleischmann, R. M., Furst, D. E., et al. (2013). Long-term safety of rituximab in rheumatoid arthritis: 9.5-year follow-up of the global clinical trial programme with a focus on adverse events of interest in RA patients. *Ann. Rheum. Dis.* 72 (9), 1496–1502. doi: 10.1136/annrheumdis-2012-201956

WHO. (2002) World Health Organization. Department of Essential Drugs and Medicines Policy. Safety of medicines. A guide to detecting and reporting adverse drug reactions. Geneva: World Health Organization, 20 p. Available at: http://apps.who.int/iris/bitstream/handle/10665/67378/WHO_EDM_QSM_2002.2.pdf;jsessionid=F7D0B632670A3407829D860782550B58?sequence=1 (Accessed 01/06/2019).

Winthrop, K. L., Saag, K., Cascino, M. D., Pei, J., John, A., Jahreis, A., et al. (2018). Long-Term Safety of Rituximab in Rheumatoid Arthritis: analysis from the SUNSTONE Registry. *Arthritis Care Res.* 71 (8), 993–1003. doi: 10.1002/acr.23781

Wollenhaupt, J., Albrecht, K., Krüger, K., and Müller-Ladner, U. (2013). The new 2012 German recommendations for treating rheumatoid arthritis: differences compared to the European standpoint. *Z. Rheumatol.* 72 (1), 6–9. doi: 10.1007/s00393-012-1093-6

Yazici Y. (last update Jun 2018). Rheumatoid arthritis. BMJ Best Practice. Available at: bestpractice.bmj.com (Accessed 04/10/2019).

Yu, Y. M., Lee, E., Koo, B. S., Jeong, K. H., Choi, K. H., Kang, L. K., et al. (2016). Predictive factors of spontaneous reporting of adverse drug reactions among community pharmacists. *PloS One* 11 (5), e0155517. doi: 10.1371/journal.pone.0155517

Zemkova, M., Jebavy, L., Kotlarova, J., Vlcek, J., and Meyboom, R. H. (2007). The spectrum and types of adverse side effects to biological immune modulators: a proposal for new classification. *Folia Boil.* 53 (4), 146–155.

Zeltser, R., Valle, L., Tanck, C., Holyst, M. M., Ritchlin, C., and Gaspari, A. A. (2001). Clinical, histological, and immunophenotypic characteristics of injection site reactions associated with etanercept: a recombinant tumor necrosis factor alpha receptor: Fc fusion protein. *Arch. Dermatol.* 137 (7), 893–899. doi: 10-1001/pubs.ArchDermatol

Zhu, J., Stuver, S. O., Epstein, A. M., Schneider, E. C., Weissman, J. S., and Weingart, S. N. (2011). Can we rely on patients' reports of adverse events? *Med. Care* 49 (10), 948–955. doi: 10.1097/MLR.0b013e31822047a8.

13

Medicine Shortages: Gaps Between Countries and Global Perspectives

Angela Acosta[1,2], Egdda Patricia Vanegas[1,3], Joan Rovira[1,4], Brian Godman[1,5,6,7] and Tomasz Bochenek[1,8]*

[1] ISAGS, South American Institute of Government in Health, UNASUR, Rio de Janeiro, Brazil, [2] RAM Group, National University of Colombia, Bogotá, Colombia, [3] SEPRO Research Group, National University of Colombia, Bogotá, Colombia, [4] Andalusian School of Public Health, Granada, Spain, [5] Strathclyde Institute of Pharmacy and Biomedical Sciences, University of Strathclyde, Glasgow, United Kingdom, [6] Division of Clinical Pharmacology, Karolinska Institute, Karolinska University Hospital Huddinge, Stockholm, Sweden, [7] School of Pharmacy, Sefako Makgatho Health Sciences University, Garankuwa, South Africa, [8] Department of Drug Management, Faculty of Health Sciences, Jagiellonian University Medical College, Krakow, Poland

***Correspondence:**
Angela Acosta
angelaacosta@isags-unasur.org

Introduction: Over the last decade, global health policies and different research areas have focused on the relevance and impact of medicine shortages. Published studies suggest there have been difficulties with access to medicines since the beginning of the 20th century, and there have been advances in our understanding and management of the problem since then. However, in view of global and regional health care concerns with shortages, we believe this phenomenon needs to be characterized and described more fully regarding the types of medicines affected, possible causes, and potential strategies to address these. The aim of this scoping review was to identify, compare if possible, and characterize the recent literature regarding the situation of medicines shortages between countries, and provide different perspectives, including a global context and national approaches.

Methodology: A scoping study presented as a narrative review of the situation and findings principally based on published articles.

Results: Based on the reported cases in the literature, a typology of medicines shortage and supply interruption episodes and their causes were proposed; national approaches to notify and manage the medicines shortages cases were described and classified by update frequency; principal differences between market and supply chain management perspectives of the situation were identified and global and countries' perspectives were described.

Conclusion: Policy makers require solutions that prevent those cases in which the population's health is affected by episodes of medicine shortages and/or interruption in the supply chain. There is also a need to generate a glossary related to logistics management and the availability of medicines which will be useful to understand and overcome shortages. In addition, recognize that potential solutions are not only related with actions linked to research, development and innovation, but much wider. Overall, we believe this article can act as a basis for future discussions in this important area.

Keywords: medicine shortages, medicine access, pharmaceutical policy, medicine supply, South America, Europe, North America, Western Asia

INTRODUCTION

The World Health Organization (WHO) defined "access to medicines" as a multidimensional problem in view of the rising prices of new medicines and persisting problems of medicine shortages among others (World Health Organization, 2018). Other concerns include out-of-pocket payments, which are especially important in lower- and middle-income countries (LMICs) where expenditure of medicines can be up to 70% of total health care expenditure and potentially catastrophic for patients and their families if they become ill (Cameron et al., 2009; Ofori-Asenso and Agyeman, 2016; World Health Organization, 2018). However, this is outside the scope of this article, which principally deals with issues of shortages of medicines.

The last WHO Director-General's report included a variety of terms on global medicine shortages such as "shortage," "scarcity" (only in the Spanish version), and "stock outs" (only in the English version) that demand a comprehensive approach across countries (World Health Organization, 2018). Consequently, there is an urgent need to develop a set of terminologies related to the problems identified by countries regarding the continual availability of essential medicines.

There are different situations leading to out of stock of medicines. Some of them can be solved without causing obstacles to health care provision or in the availability of the best therapeutic option, whereas others may require additional efforts and ways to overcome affected health conditions. There have been several important efforts to document countries' experiences and potential ways forward to address concerns with medicine shortages. The study of ISAGS UNASUR published in 2017 characterized and analyzed the situation among eight South American countries: Bolivia, Chile, Colombia, Ecuador, Paraguay, Peru, Venezuela, and Uruguay (ISAGS, 2017). In 2018, Bochenek et al. (2018) systematically characterized, compared, and evaluated current measures, as well as legislative and organizational frameworks, to address medicines shortages among a wide range of European and Western Asian countries. These included 20 countries of the European Union (EU) and the European Free Trade Association (EFTA)—Austria, Belgium, Croatia, the Czech Republic, Estonia, France, Greece, Hungary, Ireland, Italy, Latvia, Lithuania, Malta, Norway, Poland, Portugal, Slovakia, Slovenia, Spain, and Switzerland. In addition, eight non-EU/EFTA countries: Albania, Azerbaijan, Israel, Kosovo, Montenegro, Republic of Srpska (Bosnia and Herzegovina), Serbia, and Turkey.

Both publications involving descriptions from different regions of the world with similar findings about formal definitions as well as strategies that had been developed to prevent or mitigate against medicine shortages. Both publications emphasized the urgent need to explore further the phenomena to identify mechanisms which introduce possible solutions for situations affected by medicine shortages, as well as facilitate the monitoring and assessing of signals and subsequent actions. However, there is a need to consolidate current findings to provide additional direction given current concerns, building on the experiences of other countries including Australia, Canada and the United States, as well as more recent research findings (Gupta and Huang, 2013; The Society of Hospital Pharmacists of Australian, SHPA, 2017; Videau et al., 2019).

Learning from other countries' experiences should not be underestimated or underutilized in shaping local or national pharmaceutical policies (Godman et al., 2010; Gupta and Huang, 2013; Godman et al., 2014; Moon et al., 2014; Godman et al., 2015; Moorkens et al., 2017; The Society of Hospital Pharmacists of Australian, SHPA, 2017; Godman et al., 2018; Kwon et al., 2018; Videau et al., 2019). Lessons can be drawn from cross-country comparisons, even if a given country's characteristics do not perfectly correspond in terms of geographical location, size, demography, economy, or type of health care system. Consequently, the objectives of this article are to consolidate current findings as well as characterize and describe more fully the situation across continents to provide further evidence about the types of affected medicines, identified causes, and potential strategies to address shortages. Subsequently, use the findings to provide suggestions to address this important topic.

MATERIALS AND METHODS

The design of this study is a scoping review. Scoping reviews have been useful to describe broad topic and provide an overview of diverse literature, including different study designs and methodologies, both widely available and gray scientific articles and reports (Pham et al., 2015).

Previous efforts have helped identify the main characteristics to describe the medicine shortage situation including potential definitions, general characteristics of the problem, description of information systems, potential and perceived causes of shortages, and implemented solutions (UNASUR, 2014; De Weerdt et al., 2015a; De Weerdt et al., 2015b; Pauwels et al., 2015; de Weerdt et al., 2017; Nurse-Findlay et al., 2017; Bochenek et al., 2018). We have built on this including the studies of Bochenek et al. (2018) and ISAGS (2017).

Full information on the content of the ISAGS survey form, including all the detailed questions which were posed in study on South American countries, can be found in the **Supplementary Material** to this paper. Likewise, detailed information on the content of the survey performed in European and Western Asian countries can be found in the **Supplementary Material** to the published study of Bochenek et al. Both surveys asked about existence of definitions of shortages of medicines, general characteristics of the problem, description of information systems, groups of medicines in shortage and particular molecules, potential and perceived causes of shortages, existence of processes, protocols and indicators to address shortages when they appear and to monitor their dynamics, and implemented solutions among others.

Search Process

First Step

Figure 1 shows the search process. In 2017, eligible studies were first identified from a search of PubMed with the following general MeSH terms strategy "DRUG OR MEDICINE AND SHORTAGE." The results were subsequently filtered by period (5 years from May 2012 to 2017), with references filtered by tittle and abstract taking into account representative descriptions of countries.

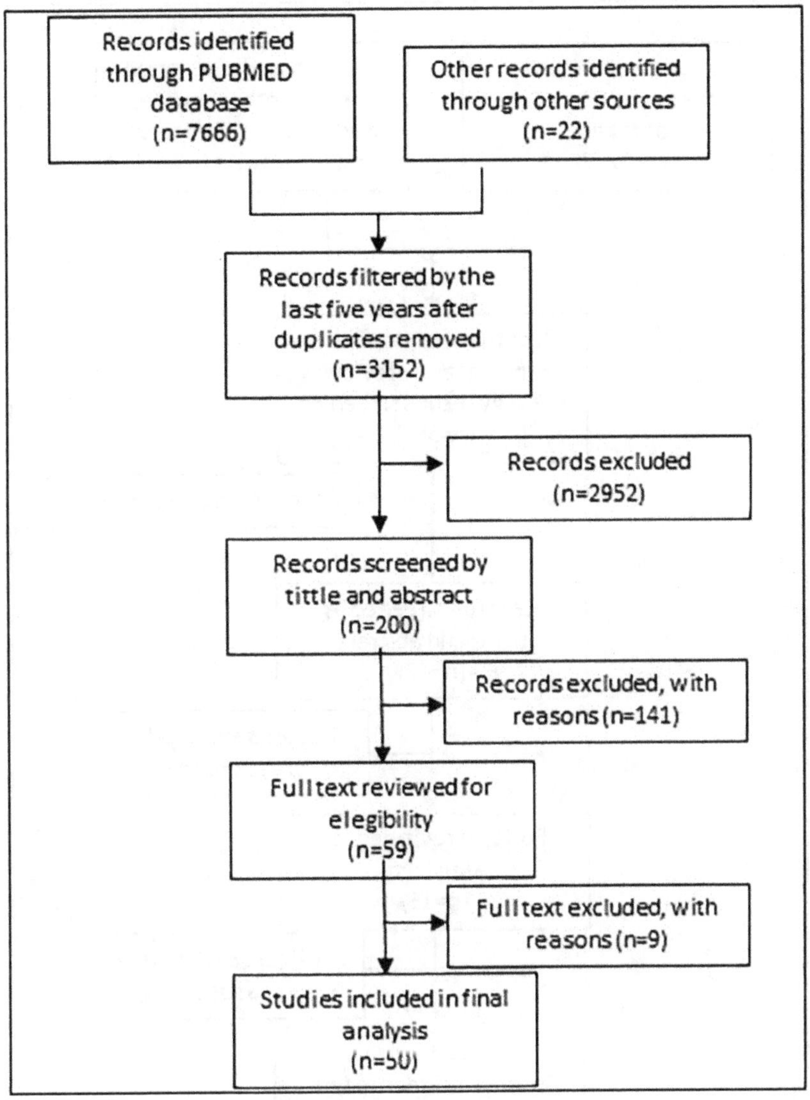

FIGURE 1 | Flow chart of first literature review process.

Other gray literature was retrieved from websites of the WHO, ministries of health and national health authorities. In addition, legal acts, as well as information gathered and disclosed within the public domain by organizations involved in pharmaceutical markets.

Second Step

Figure 2 shows the search process for the update implemented in 2019. The same search strategy was used filtered by period (January 2016 until April 2019) to help recover additional eligible studies. The strategy was also translated into Portuguese and Spanish to run a search in Lilacs, a specific database for Latin America countries.

To retrieve other potential studies, free text search terms and a snowball literature review was undertaken. We ran the term "SHORTAGE" with specific countries and continents including Africa, Australia, Canada, China, Costa Rica, Japan, Mexico, Panama and the United Kingdom.

Inclusion Criteria

This review includes studies that describe the medicines shortage situation within a large jurisdiction or system of care, and settings could be regional, national, or international.

Selection Process

Two reviewers (EV, AA) performed the screening of abstracts based on the tittle/abstract review. The full text of potential eligible studies was retrieved if one or both authors thought they were relevant. Disagreements were resolved by discussion and, when necessary, including a third author (TB) in the discussion.

Data Extraction

Data extracted from each study included the authors and year of publication, jurisdictional level, existence of definitions, general characteristics of shortages, medicines involved, description of information systems including four categories of frequencies of

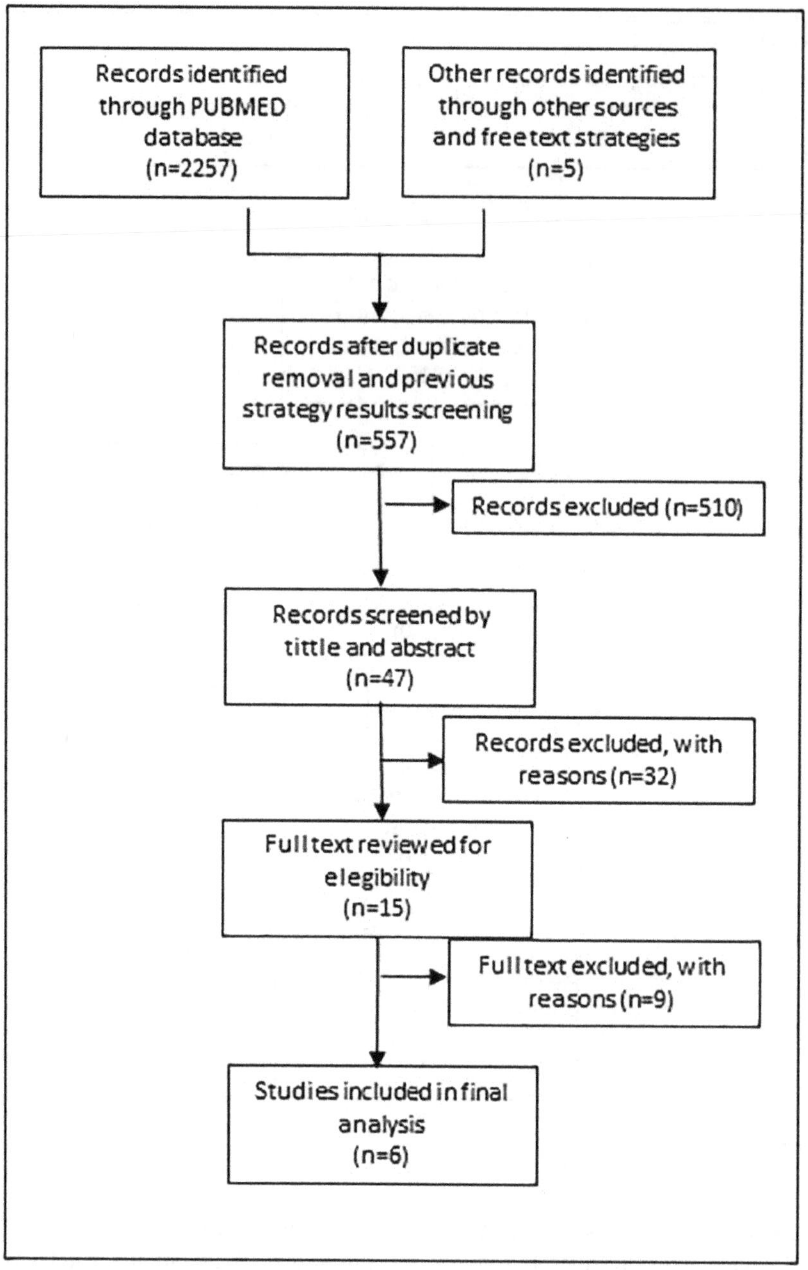

FIGURE 2 | Flow chart of second literature review process.

shortages reports (high, medium, low, unspecified), potential and perceived causes of shortages, and possible implemented solutions at jurisdictional levels.

RESULTS

Description of Studies

By 2017, the literature review had identified 50 references to include in this scoping review, and by 2019 another 6 new references where identified. Of these 56 references, 9 studies had a regional broad focus for Europe and Latin America. We found studies with country description of medicines shortage for one East Asia country (China), 7 European countries (Belgium, Finland, France, Ireland, Slovenia, Spain and the United Kingdom), two Latin America countries (Brazil and Venezuela); two North American countries (Canada and the United States); two Oceania countries (Australia and Fiji); and 4 Western Asia countries (Iran, Iraq, Jordan and Israel) (**Table 1**).

Three of the identified articles had developed surveys addressed to the ministries of health, state medicines agencies and local health authorities of various countries from three regions to discuss potential ways to address medicine shortages (Bogaert

TABLE 1 | Distribution of included references by geography.

Region/country	Number	Ref	Total by region
East Asia			**1**
China	1	• Yang, C., Wu, L., Cai, W., Zhu, W., Shen, Q., Li, Z., et al. (2016). Current situation,determinants, and solutions to drug shortages in Shaanxi Province, China: a qualitative study. PLoS ONE 11: e0165183. doi: 10.1371/journal.pone.0165183 (Yang et al., 2016)	
Europe			**16**
Europe (broad focus)	8	• Bochenek T, Abilova V, Alkan A, Asanin B, Beriain I de M, Besovic Z, et al. Systemic measures and legislative and organizational frameworks aimed at preventing or mitigating drug shortages in 28 European and Western Asian Countries. Front Pharmacol. 2018;8(JAN). (Bochenek et al., 2018) • Pauwels, K., Huys, I., Casteels, M., and Simoens, S. (2014). Drug shortages in European countries: a trade-off between market attractiveness and cost containment? BMC Health Serv Res. 14:438. doi: 10.1186/1472-6963-14-438 (Pauwels et al., 2014) • Pauwels, K., Simoens, S., Casteels, M., and Huys, I. (2015). Insights into European drug shortages: a survey of hospital pharmacists. PLoS ONE 10:e0119322.doi: 10.1371/journal.pone.0119322 (Pauwels et al., 2015) • Birgli, A. G. (2013). An Evaluation of Medicines Shortages in Europe with More In-Depth Review of These in France, Greece, Poland, Spain and the United Kingdom. Available online at: https://www.eaepc.org/images/pdf/evaluation.pdf (Birgli® ag, 2013) • Bogaert, P., Bochenek, T., Prokop, A., and Pilc, A. (2015). A qualitative approach to a better understanding of the problems underlying drug shortages, as viewed from Belgian, French and the European Union's perspectives. PLoS ONE 10:e0125691. doi: 10.1371/journal.pone.0125691 (Bogaert et al., 2015) • De Weerdt, E., Simoens, S., Casteels, M., and Huys, I. (2017b). Clinical, economic and policy implications of drug shortages in the European union. Appl. Health Econ. Health Policy 15, 441–445. doi: 10.1007/s40258-016-0264-z. (de Weerdt et al., 2017) • De Weerdt, E., Simoens, S., Hombroeckx, L., Casteels, M., and Huys, I. (2015b).Causes of drug shortages in the legal pharmaceutical framework. Regul. Toxicol.Pharmacol. 71, 251–258. doi: 10.1016/j.yrtph.2015.01.005 (De Weerdt et al., 2015b) • De Weerdt E, Simoens S, Casteels M, Huys I. Toward a European definition for a drug shortage: A qualitative study. Front Pharmacol. 2015;6(OCT):1–9. (De Weerdt et al., 2015a)	
Belgium	1	• Bauters T, Claus BO, Norga K, Huys I, Simoens S, Laureys G. Chemotherapy drug shortages in paediatric oncology: A 14-year single-center experience in Belgium. J Oncol Pharm Pract [Internet]. 2016;22(6):766–70. Available from: http://opp.sagepub.com/cgi/doi/10.1177/1078155215610915 (Bauters et al., 2016)	
Finland	1	• Heiskanen, K., Ahonen, R., Kanerva, R., Karttunen, P., and Timonen, J. (2017). The reasons behind medicine shortages from the perspective of pharmaceutical companies and pharmaceutical wholesalers in Finland. PLoS ONE 12:e0179479.doi: 10.1371/journal.pone.0179479. (Heiskanen et al., 2017)	
France	1	• Bocquet, F., Degrassat-Théas, A., Peigné, J., and Paubel, P. (2017). The new regulatory tools of the 2016 Health Law to fight drug shortages in France. Health Policy 121, 471–476. doi: 10.1016/j.healthpol.2017.03.007 (Bocquet et al., 2017)	
Ireland	1	• Kavanagh J. (2017). How Pharmaceutical Supply Chains Can Be Managed to Minimise the Number of Medicines Shortages, Unpublished Master's thesis, University College Dublin, Ireland. (Kavanagh, 2017) • Vella Bonanno, P., and Gavril, F. (2011). Seven years of EU Pharmaceutical regulation in Malta. WHO Drug Inf. 25, 341–412. (Bonnanno and Gavril, 2011)	
Slovenia	1	• Pfeffer, K., and Mozolová, B. (2017). Re-export of drugs in the Slovak Republic vol. 2 – the Act [Internet]. Available: https://www.twobirds.com/en/news/articles/2017/uk/ils/re-export-of-drugs-in-the-slovak-republic-vol-2-the-act (Pfeffer and Mozoľová, 2017)	
Spain	1	• Servicio Vasco de Salud -Osakidetza. Desabastecimiento De Medicamentos: Un Problema Sin Resolver [Internet]. Vol. 23, INFORMACIÓN FARMACOTERAPÉUTICA DE LA COMARCA. Vitoria - Gasteiz; 2016. Available from: http://www.osakidetza.euskadi.eus/contenidos/informacion/cevime_infac_2015/es_def/adjuntos/INFAC_Vol_23_N_7_Desabastecimientos.pdf (Servicio Vasco de Salud –Osakidetza, 2016)	
United Kingdom	2	• Costelloe, E. M., Guinane, M., Nugent, F., Halley, O., and Parsons, C. (2014). An audit of drug shortages in a community pharmacy practice. Ir. J. Med. Sci.435–440. doi: 10.1007/s11845-014-1139-7 (Costelloe et al., 2015) • Group AP. Why drug shortages occur. Drug Ther Bull [Internet]. 2015;53(3):33–6. Available from: https://dtb.bmj.com/content/53/3/33.full (All-party Pharmacy, 2015)	
Latin America			**3**
Latin America (broad focus)	1	• ISAGS. Situation of Essential Medicines at Risk of Supply Shortage with Emphasis on South American Countries [Internet]. Rio de Janeiro; 2017. Available from: http://isags-unasur.org/en/publicacao/situation-of-essential-medicines-at-risk-of-supply-shortage-with-emphasis-on-south-american-countries-2/ (ISAGS, 2017)	
Brazil	1	• Perini E, Rosa MB, Reis AMM, Perini E. Drug shortage: a public health problem. Cad Saude Publica [Internet]. 2016 Oct [cited 2017 Jul 10];32(10). Available from: http://www.scielo.br/scielo.php?script=sci_arttext&pid=S0102-311X2016001000301&lng=en&tlng=en (Rosa et al., 2016)	
Venezuela	1	• Aular de González Y. Escasez de medicamentos y su repercusión en la salud. Salus. 2014;18(2):5–6. (Aular de González, 2014)	

(Continued)

TABLE 1 | Continued

Region/country	Number	Ref	Total by region
North America			**29**
Canada	3	• Morrison, A. (2011). Drug Supply Disruptions [Environmental Scan Issue 17]Ottawa: Canadian Agency for Drugs and Technologies in Health. Available online at: https://www.cadth.ca/drug-supply-disruptions (Morrison, 2011) • Kaposy C. Drugs, money, and power: the Canadian drug shortage. J Bioeth Inq [Internet]. 2014 Mar [cited 2014 May 29];11(1):85–9. Available from: http://www.ncbi.nlm.nih.gov/pubmed/24357073 • Videau M, Lebel D, Bussières JF. Drug shortages in Canada: Data for 2016–2017 and perspectives on the problem. Ann Pharm Fr [Internet]. 2019; Available from: https://doi.org/10.1016/j.pharma.2018.11.007 (Videau et al., 2019)	
United States	26	• Schweitzer, S. O. (2013). How the US Food and Drug Administration can solve the prescription drug shortage problem. Am. J. Public Health. 10310–14. doi: 10.2105/AJPH.2013.301239 (Schweitzer, 2013) • Ventola, C. L. (2011). The drug shortage crisis in the United States: causes, impact, and management strategies. P T. 36, 740–757. (Ventola, 2011) • Goldsack, J. C., Reilly, C., Bush, C., McElligott, S., Bristol, M. N., Motanya, U. N., et al. (2014). Impact of shortages of injectable oncology drugs on patient care. Am. J. Heal. Pharm. 71, 571–578. doi: 10.2146/ajhp130569 (Goldsack et al., 2014) • Butterfield, L., Cash, J., and Pham, K. (2015). Position statement drug shortages and implications for pediatric patients. J. Pediatr. Pharmacol. Ther. 20, 149–152. doi: 10.5863/1551-6776-20.2.149 (Butterfield et al., 2015) • Mazer-Amirshahi, M., Goyal, M., Umar, S. A., Fox, E. R., Zocchi, M., Hawley, K.L., et al. (2017). U.S. drug shortages for medications used in adult critical care(2001-2016). J. Crit. Care. 41, 283–288. doi: 10.1016/j.jcrc.2017.06.005 (Mazer-Amirshahi et al., 2017) • McLaughlin,M.M., and Skoglund, E.W. (2015). Drug shortages and patient safety. J. Infus. Nurs. 38, 205–208. doi: 10.1097/NAN.0000000000000101 • McLaughlin, M., Kotis, D., Thomson, K., Harrison, M., Fennessy, G., Postelnick, M., et al. (2013). Effects on patient care caused by drug shortages: a survey. J. Manag. Care Pharm. 19, 783–788. doi: 10.18553/jmcp.2013.19.9.783 • McKeever AE, Bloch JR, Bratic A. Drug shortages and the burden of access to care: A critical issue affecting patients with cancer. Clin J Oncol Nurs. 2013; (McKeever et al., 2013) • Alevizakos M, Detsis M, Grigoras CA, Machan JT, Mylonakis E. The Impact of Shortages on Medication Prices: Implications for Shortage Prevention. Drugs. 2016;76(16):1551–8 (Alevizakos et al., 2016) • Griffith MM, Gross AE, Sutton SH, Bolon MK, Esterly JS, Patel JA, et al. The impact of anti-infective drug shortages on hospitals in the United States: Trends and causes. Clin Infect Dis. 2012;54(5):684–91. (Griffith et al., 2012) • Steers WD. Falling short: Causes and Implications of Drug Shortages in the United States. J Urol [Internet]. 2014;192(5):1315–7. Available from: http://www.ncbi.nlm.nih.gov/pubmed/25218647 (Steers, 2014) • Gabrielli A, Layon NT, Bones HL, Layon AJ. The Tragedy of the Commons - Drug Shortages and Our Patients' Health. Am J Med [Internet]. 2016;129(12):1237–8. Available from: http://linkinghub.elsevier.com/retrieve/pii/S0002934316310130%0A http://www.ncbi.nlm.nih.gov/pubmed/28029357 (Gabrielli et al., 2016) • Rinaldi F, de Denus S, Nguyen A, Nattel S, Bussières J-F. Drug Shortages: Patients and Health Care Providers Are All Drawing the Short Straw. Can J Cardiol [Internet]. 2016; Available from: http://linkinghub.elsevier.com/retrieve/pii/S0828282X1630842X%0A http://www.ncbi.nlm.nih.gov/pubmed/27923583 (Rinaldi et al., 2017) • Parsons HM, Schmidt S, Karnad AB, Liang Y, Pugh MJ, Fox ER, et al. Association Between the Number of Suppliers for Critical Antineoplastics and Drug Shortages: Implications for Future Drug Shortages and Treatment. J Oncol Pract [Internet]. 2016;12(3):249–50. Available from: http://jop.ascopubs.org/cgi/doi/10.1200/JOP.2015.007237 • Chen SI, Fox ER, Kennedy Hall M, Ross JS, Bucholz EM, Krumholz HM, et al. Despite federal legislation, shortages of drugs used in acute care settings remain persistent and prolonged. Health Aff. 2016;35(5):798–804. (Chen et al., 2016) • Fox ER, Tyler LS. Potential Association between Drug Shortages and High-Cost Medications. Pharmacotherapy [Internet]. 2016; Available from: http://www.ncbi.nlm.nih.gov/pubmed/27891635 (Fox and Tyler, 2017) • Warkentin J, Flood J, Kanouse J, Shah N, Cronin A. Impact of a Shortage of First-Line Antituberculosis Medication on Tuberculosis Control — United States, 2012–2013. Morb Mortal Wkly Rep - CD [Internet]. 2013;62(20):396–400. Available from: http://www.ncbi.nlm.nih.gov/pubmed/23698603 • Jagsi R., Spence R., Rathmell W.K., Bradbury A., Peppercorn J., et al. Ethical considerations for the clinical oncologist in an era of oncology drug shortages. Oncologist. 2014;19(2):186–92. (Jagsi et al., 2014) • Becker DJ, Talwar S, Levy BP, Thorn M, Roitman J, Blum RH, et al. Impact of oncology drug shortages on patient therapy: unplanned treatment changes. J Oncol Pract. 2013;9(4):122–8. (Becker et al., 2013) • Gupta DK, Huang S-M. Drug Shortages in the United States: A Critical Evaluation of Root Causes and the Need for Action. Clin Pharmacol Ther [Internet]. 2013;93(2):133–5. Available from: http://www.ncbi.nlm.nih.gov/pubmed/23337520 (Gupta and Huang, 2013)	

(Continued)

TABLE 1 | Continued

Region/country	Number	Ref	Total by region
		• Caulder C, Mehta B, Bookstaver P, Sims L, Stevenson B, South Carolina Society of Health-Sy. Impact of Drug Shortages on Health System Pharmacies in the Southeastern United States. Hosp Pharm [Internet]. 2015;50(4):279–86. Available from: https://www.ncbi.nlm.nih.gov/pmc/articles/PMC4589883/pdf/hpj-50-279.pdf (Caulder et al., 2015) • Golembiewski J. Drug shortages in the perioperative setting: causes, impact, and strategies. J Perianesth Nurs [Internet]. 2012 Aug [cited 2013 Mar 7];27(4):286–92. Available from: http://www.ncbi.nlm.nih.gov/pubmed/22828028 (Golembiewski, 2012) • Daley M, Lat I, Kane-Gill S. Applicability of Guideline Recommendations Challenged in the Setting of Drug Shortages. Crit Care Med [Internet]. 2013;41(7):e142–3. Available from: http://content.wkhealth.com/linkback/openurl?sid=WKPTLP:landingpage&an=00003246-201307000-00058 • McLaughlin M, Kotis D, Thomson K, Harrison M, Fennessy G, Postelnick M, et al. Effects on Patient Care Caused by Drug Shortages: A Survey. J Manag Care Pharm [Internet]. 2013;19(9):783–8. Available from: http://www.jmcp.org/doi/10.18553/jmcp.2013.19.9.783 (McLaughlin et al., 2013) • Administra- D, Act I, Hoffman RS. Antidote shortages in the United States: impact and response. Clin Toxicol (Phila) [Internet]. 2014;52(3):157–9. Available from: http://www.ncbi.nlm.nih.gov/pubmed/24397753 (American College of Medical Toxicology, American Academy of Clinical Toxicology, 2015) • Bible JR, Evans DC, Payne B, Mostafavifar L. Impact of Drug Shortages on Patients Receiving Parenteral Nutrition After Laparotomy. J Parenter Enter Nutr [Internet]. 2014;38(2_suppl):65S–71S. Available from: http://journals.sagepub.com/doi/10.1177/0148607114550317	
Oceania			**2**
Australia	1	• The Society of Hospital Pharmacists of Australian, SHPA. Medicine shortages in Australia. A snapshot of shortages in australian hospitals. Victoria; 2017. (The Society of Hospital Pharmacists of Australian, SHPA, 2017)	
Fiji	1	• Walker, J., Chaar, B. B., Vera, N., Pillai, A. S., Lim, J. S., Bero, L., et al. (2017). Medicine shortages in Fiji: a qualitative exploration of stakeholders' views. PLoS ONE 12:e0178429. doi: 10.1371/journal.pone.0178429 (Walker et al., 2017)	
Western Asia			**4**
Iran	1	• Setayesh S, Mackey TK. Addressing the impact of economic sanctions on Iranian drug shortages in the joint comprehensive plan of action: promoting access to medicines and health diplomacy. Global Health [Internet]. 2016;12(1):31. Available from: http://globalizationandhealth.biomedcentral.com/articles/10.1186/s12992-016-0168-6 (Setayesh and Mackey, 2016)	
Iraq	1	• Cousins S. Iraq: staff and medicine shortages are major challenges. Lancet [Internet]. 2014;384(9947):943–4. Available from: http://linkinghub.elsevier.com/retrieve/pii/S0140673614616159 (Cousins, 2014)	
Jordan	1	• Awad, H., Al-Zu'bi, Z.M. F., and Abdallah, A. B. (2016). A quantitative analysis of the causes of drug shortages in Jordan: a supply chain perspective. Int. Bus. Res.9:53. doi: 10.5539/ibr.v9n6p53 (Awad et al., 2016)	
Israel	1	• Schwartzberg E, Ainbinder D, Vishkauzan A, Gamzu R. Drug shortages in Israel: regulatory perspectives, challenges and solutions. Isr J Health Policy Res [Internet]. 2017;6(1):17. Available from: http://ijhpr.biomedcentral.com/articles/10.1186/s13584-017-0140-9%0A http://www.ncbi.nlm.nih.gov/pubmed/28392910%0A http://www.pubmedcentral.nih.gov/articlerender.fcgi?artid=PMC5376685 (Schwartzberg et al., 2017)	
Cross settings comparisons between countries			**1**
The United States and Arabia Saudi – Hospital Setting	1	• Alsheikh, M., Seoane-Vazquez, E., Rittenhouse, B., Fox, E. R., and Fanikos, J. (2016). A comparison of drug shortages in the Hospital Setting in the United States and Saudi Arabia: an exploratory analysis. Hosp. Pharm. 51,370–375. doi: 10.1310/hpj5105-370 (Alsheikh et al., 2016)	

et al., 2015; ISAGS, 2017; Bochenek et al., 2018). One study described the literature review in terms of the characteristics of shortages and country definitions of shortages (De Weerdt et al., 2015a). Another regional study described the shortage situation from the perspective of hospital pharmacists and prescribers (Pauwels et al., 2015).

The United States (US) is the country with more publications in the field (26 references) than many other countries. Many of these publications describe the professionals' perspective of the situation at the health care jurisdictional level (Morrison, 2011; Golembiewski, 2012; Griffith et al., 2012; Becker et al., 2013; McKeever et al., 2013; McLaughlin et al., 2013; Bible et al., 2014; Goldsack et al., 2014; Butterfield et al., 2015; Caulder et al., 2015; McLaughlin and Skoglund, 2015; Gabrielli et al., 2016; Parsons et al., 2016; Setayesh and Mackey, 2016; Bocquet et al., 2017; Fox and Tyler, 2017; Mazer-Amirshahi et al., 2017; Rinaldi et al., 2017; Schwartzberg et al., 2017). Another study performed a comparison of medicines shortages between two hospital settings, one from Arabia Saudi and the other from the US (Alsheikh et al., 2016).

Contexts and Reasons of Medicines Shortage

The description of the shortage situations may be associated with 4 principal causes or determinants, namely: market, supply chain management, manufacturing, and political issues (**Table 2**).

TABLE 2 | Most frequent reasons for medicine shortages.

Category	Cause
Market	Increase in sales (McKeever et al., 2013; Ordre National des Pharmaciens, 2015) Price-related aspects (McKeever et al., 2013; Ordre National des Pharmaciens, 2015; Alevizakos et al., 2016; Yang et al., 2016) Voluntary withdrawal (Griffith et al., 2012; Steers, 2014; Chen et al., 2016; Yang et al., 2016; Rinaldi et al., 2017) Unexpected increases and unexpected changes in clinical practice (Griffith et al., 2012; Yang et al., 2016) Parallel or gray markets (Yang et al., 2016) Loss of market interest (Videau et al., 2019) Relocation of production facilities (Videau et al., 2019) Speculation in international markets (Videau et al., 2019) Mergers of manufacturers and joint purchasing group (Videau et al., 2019)
Supply chain management	Structure of the network or supply chain in the country (Schwartzberg et al., 2017) Supply of raw materials and excipients (Griffith et al., 2012; Ordre National des Pharmaciens, 2015; Chen et al., 2016; Gabrielli et al., 2016; Parsons et al., 2016; Bocquet et al., 2017; Rinaldi et al., 2017; Schwartzberg et al., 2017)
Manufacturing process	Quality concerns (Griffith et al., 2012; Gabrielli et al., 2016; Bocquet et al., 2017; De Weerdt et al., 2017; Rinaldi et al., 2017; Schwartzberg et al., 2017) Changes in the product formulation (Yang et al., 2016; Rinaldi et al., 2017) Industrial development capacities (Steers, 2014; Gabrielli et al., 2016; Yang et al., 2016; Fox and Tyler, 2017) Production problems (Videau et al., 2019)
Political and ethical issues	Regulatory problems (McKeever et al., 2013; Chen et al., 2016; Gabrielli et al., 2016; Parsons et al., 2016; Yang et al., 2016; Bocquet et al., 2017; Schwartzberg et al., 2017). Public policy (Cousins, 2014; Setayesh and Mackey, 2016; French Parliament). Social conflicts (Setayesh and Mackey, 2016; Bochenek et al., 2018). Enhancement of the legal and normative frameworks applicable to the manufacture of medicines (Videau et al., 2019)

Some authors have concluded that these categories are interrelated and have one aspect in common, that is, many cases are related to the availability of safe and effective medicines with low profitability or with low sales making them non-viable commercially (McKeever et al., 2013; Alevizakos et al., 2016; Schwartzberg et al., 2017).

In South American countries, medicine shortages generally occur with mature products without suppliers in the market due to lack of market viability, and correspond mostly to parenteral medicines with low profitability (ISAGS, 2017).

Some countries issue alerts about medicines that are simply not available on the market in their country even if there is enough money to pay for them within their health care systems (Bochenek et al., 2018).

Finally, Bochenek et al. (2018) addressed an increasing amount of evidence where medicines were unavailable in countries even if the products complied with current regulations and were financed within the health care system. As a result, these situations show that ethical and political issues could be affecting the timely availability of first-line therapeutic alternatives. These situations threaten the ability of clinicians and governments to fulfill their moral obligations to patients and society to provide benefit to patients, minimize harm, and promote equity.

Published studies in hospitals allow a better follow up of the health consequences of medicine shortages (Pauwels et al., 2015; de Weerdt et al., 2017); which is more difficult in ambulatory care (Golembiewski, 2012; Becker et al., 2013; Goldsack et al., 2014; Jagsi et al., 2014; Chen et al., 2016). This scoping review identified a number of published articles describing inpatient challenges regarding medicine shortages in the US (Morrison, 2011; Golembiewski, 2012; Griffith et al., 2012; Becker et al., 2013; McKeever et al., 2013; McLaughlin et al., 2013; Bible et al., 2014; Goldsack et al., 2014; Butterfield et al., 2015; Caulder et al., 2015; McLaughlin and Skoglund, 2015; Gabrielli et al., 2016; Parsons et al., 2016; Setayesh and Mackey, 2016; Bocquet et al., 2017; Fox and Tyler, 2017; Mazer-Amirshahi et al., 2017; Rinaldi et al., 2017; Schwartzberg et al., 2017).

Medicines Involved

The characterization of supply shortages, their frequency, and the main groups of medicines affected among countries and regions are described in **Table 3**. The same characterization though is not made for the impact of shortages on patients' health and health care systems. Descriptions in this respect generally correspond to descriptions of cases regarding either the impact of shortages on health conditions or medical specialties, or limitations in obtaining data and estimates made from surveys.

The shortage of essential medicines, including the active ingredients mostly used in injectable chemotherapy medicines, antibiotics, and anesthesia, is causing growing concern across regions including Europe, North America, Asia, and South America. However, the problem is much broader, affecting other classes of medicines - mainly parenteral medicines (Becker et al., 2013; Gulbis et al., 2013; Gupta and Huang, 2013; Jagsi et al., 2014; Caulder et al., 2015; De Weerdt et al., 2015b; De Weerdt et al., 2017; Schwartzberg et al., 2017) including anesthetics, nutrition and electrolyte solutions, enzyme replacement medicines, radiopharmaceuticals and antibiotics. The shortage of medicines has also been observed and documented for instance in Australia, Canada, China and Israel (Gray and Manasse, 2012; Kaposy, 2014; Schwartzberg et al., 2017). Most of the published evidence from countries of South America shows that shortages can occur even with essential medicines and especially injectable forms (ISAGS, 2017) (see **Figure 3**).

The groups of medicines, which were most frequently reported to be in shortage, were the cardiovascular medicines in Canada and Belgium; nervous system medicines in Australia, China, and Israel; and anti-infective medicines for most of the countries in South America (Bogaert et al., 2015; Yang et al., 2016; ISAGS, 2017; Schwartzberg et al., 2017; Videau et al., 2019).

Brazil has reported the national shortage of penicillins (first-line treatment) as a result of the lack of specific raw materials for their production in the international market. This episode

TABLE 3 | Description of medicines classes with shortages in the selected countries.

Region/country*	Nervous system	Cardiovascular system	Anti-infectives systemic use	Cancer	Genitourinary system and sex hormones	Alimentary track and metabolism
South America 2017	17%	9%	21%	10%	7%	Non available
Belgium 2009–2013	23%	21%	11%	9%	Non available	8%
Israel 2013–2015	21%	15%	16%	Non available	8%	7%
US 2013–2017	18%	11%	Non available	9%	Non available	Non available
Canada (Videau et al., 2019)	31.8%	21.9%	8.5%	5.1%	Non available	0.1%
Australia (The Society of Hospital Pharmacists of Australian, SHPA, 2017)	12% (Anaesthetics) 9% (Neurology)	10%	20%	9.5%	10%	Non available
China (Yang et al., 2016)	13%	6%	6%	5.7%	11%	9%

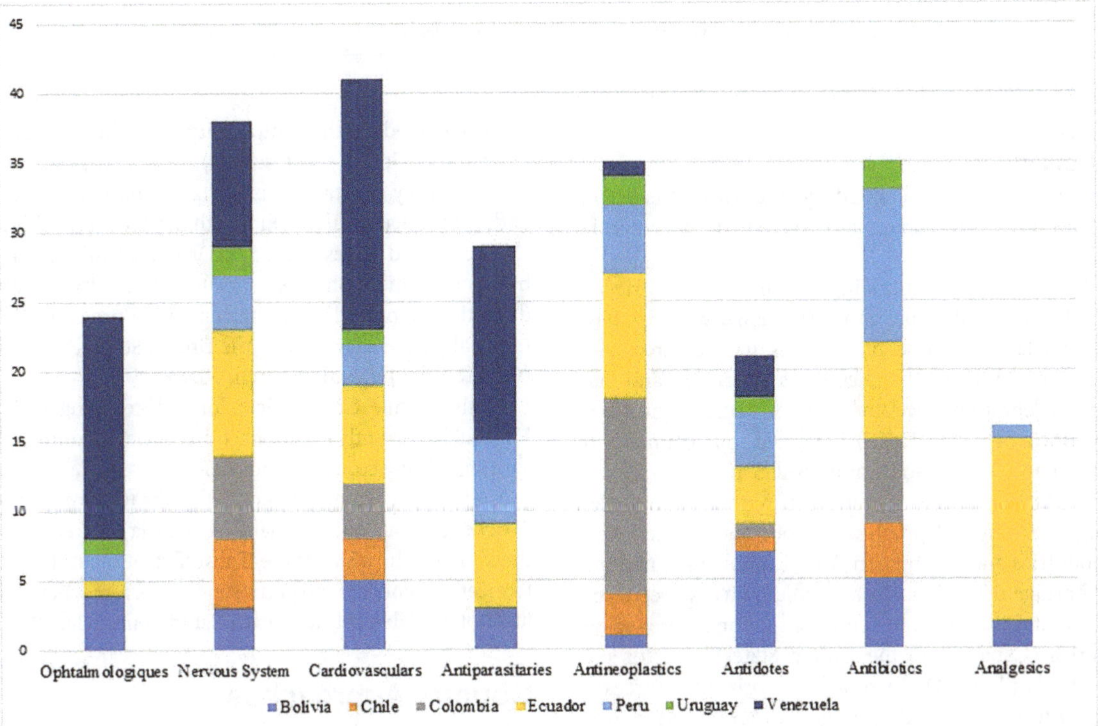

FIGURE 3 | Principal medicine groups experiencing shortages among South American countries.

was described because of the increased incidence of syphilis, including also congenital syphilis, during the last 5 years and the concern this causes (see **Figure 4**). The alternative second-line antibiotics to treat acquired syphilis and the partners of pregnant women in Brazil, i.e., doxycycline and ceftriaxone, have doses of between 8 and 15 days, and there are concerns with adherence in practice (Lazarini and Barbosa, 2017).

In France (Bocquet et al., 2017), supply shortages with 71 types of medicine were identified. According to the ATC classification (Norwegian Institute of Public Nealth, 2018), the most prevalent medicine were antibiotics, oncological medicines, antidepressants, antipsychotics, tuberculosis medicines, vaccines, and immunoglobulins.

In Iran, at least 73 cases of medicine shortages were identified, among which 44% were essential. Potentially, they impacted on successful management of disease areas including HIV, epilepsy, hemophilia, thalassemia, and patients undergoing organ transplants (Setayesh and Mackey, 2016).

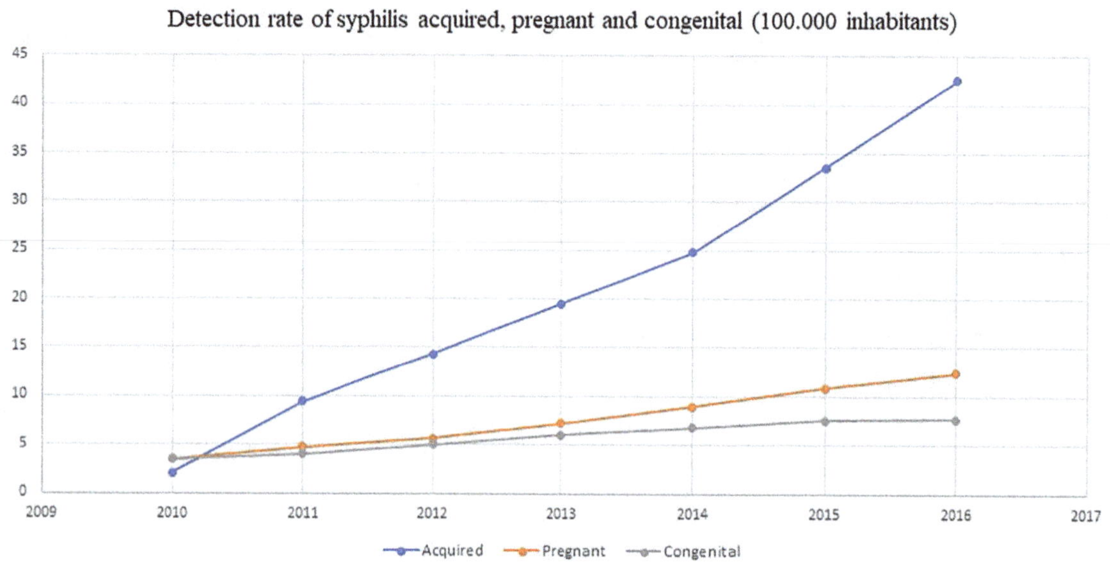

FIGURE 4 | Detection rate of syphilis and congenital syphilis in Brazil. Source: Brazil Ministry of Health.

Definitions

National Definitions

Table 4 contains definitions adopted by countries, considering attributes with the formulation and agreement of potential definitions.

One of the most important findings of this scoping review is that consulted sources, literature and institutional websites, have identified a considerable number of countries that are introducing legislative actions to cope the medicines shortages and had included formal definitions or related terms of medicine shortages.

Recently, Bochenek et al (2018) identified four countries in Europe with specific definitions, and ISAGS in 2017 (ISAGS, 2017) described three definitions for Latin American countries. This scoping review found progress in both regions, i.e., eight European countries and seven Latin America now have national medicines shortage definitions. In addition, by using free terms in the search strategies, we found definitions for one more region, North America (Canada and the United States), and for one country, Australia (**Table 4**). There are two primary sources of definitions: one from health authority agency websites (Argentina, Australia, Brazil, Colombia, Spain, US, Uruguay, Norway), and the other is the published literature for countries including Belgium, Canada, France, Greece, Hungary, and Italy (Bogaert et al., 2015; Bocquet et al., 2017; Bochenek et al., 2018; Videau et al., 2019).

Few countries have currently established a specific definition that includes the term "shortages" alone or in combination with the terms "medicines" or "drugs." These include Belgium, Canada, Colombia, France, Hungary, Greece, Italy, Spain, and the US (**Table 4**).

Some countries have used logistics and market related terms, including Uruguay (declaration of interruption of sale or interruption of marketing), Argentina (medicines lacking), Croatia (disturbance on the medicines' market), Norway (temporary disruption of a medicine's marketing), Brazil, which uses the term "discontinuation" complemented with a term related to the temporality (definitive or unplanned or temporary), Italy (short supply), and Peru, which uses three terms "supply shortage," "unavailable pharmaceutical products," and "pharmaceutical product with limited supply" (**Table 4**).

The United States Food and Drug Administration (US FDA) has focused more on aspects related to scarcity and established a definition: "a period when the demand or projected demand for a medically necessary drug in the United States exceeds its supply" (CDER C for DE and research, 2018).

Bolivia, Chile, Croatia, Ecuador, Greece, Hungary, Norway, and Venezuela currently do not have an official definition of medicine shortage. These countries consider terms associated with medicine shortages but currently do not define the term medicine shortages (Bochenek et al., 2018). Finally, Venezuela differentiates scarcity as the situation in which there is insufficient quantity of a medicine to meet current demand and a supply shortage when the product is just not available (Ministerio de Salud Venezuela, 2017).

Country Approaches

A new website at the European Medicines Agency (EMA) includes information about national legislation and local report mechanisms for 24 of the 30 European countries[1]. In South America, Brazil, Argentina, and Uruguay have regulations that make the reporting of situations that could potentially lead to shortages mandatory. EMA also have a regulation to report these cases.

Two qualitative studies have documented countries' legislation and report mechanisms for three regions: Europe, Western Asia, and South America (ISAGS, 2017; Bochenek et al., 2018). As mentioned, this scoping review described one new region, North America (Center for Drug Evaluation and research C, 2018; Videau et al.,

[1] European Medicines Agency. Medicine shortages. https://www.ema.europa.eu/en/human-regulatory/post-authorisation/medicine-shortages

TABLE 4 | Countries definitions.

Country	Terms/concepts	Definition
Argentina	Medicines lacking	"known circumstances or facts that could jeopardize the supply of products and cause their temporary or definitive discontinuity in the market"[1]
Australia	Shortage of a medicine	"There is a shortage of a medicine in Australia at a particular time if, at any time in the 6 months after that particular time, the supply of that medicine in Australia will not, or will not be likely to, meet the demand for the medicine for all of the patients in Australia who take, or who may need to take, the medicine"[2] (The Society of Hospital Pharmacists of Australian, SHPA, 2017)
Belgium	Unavailability of medicines on the Belgian market	"A drug is unavailable when enterprises that are responsible for the marketing of the drug are unable to deliver that drug for an uninterrupted period of four consecutive days to the community pharmacies, hospital pharmacies or wholesalers in Belgium." (De Weerdt et al., 2015a)
Brazil	"Temporary discontinuation" "Definitive discontinuation" "Unplanned discontinuation of the manufacture or importation of medicines"	of the manufacture or importation of medicines means that the license holder does not intend to cancel or does not intend to require the renewal of the registration of the product. of a product, in its turn, happens when the license holder intends to cancel or not to request the renewal of the registration of the product. Are those cases where quality, efficacy or safety properties of medicines are affected and may lead to a supply shortage in the market. (ISAGS, 2017)
Colombia	Medicines shortage	A situation which there is not enough supply to satisfy the demand of any medicine approved and marketed in at the country. (INVIMA, 2018)
Canada	Drug shortage	A situation in which an authorization holder for a drug is unable to meet the demand for the drug. Drug shortages can include temporary or permanent discontinuances in the production and supply of a drug (Videau et al., 2019)
Croatia	Disturbance on the medicines' market	Not specific.
France	Drug shortage	A drug shortage is defined by law in France as an inability for a community pharmacy or a hospital pharmacy to deliver a drug within 72 h (Ministre des affaires sociales, Ministre de la santè, 2012). Additionally, drug shortages in France have been classified formally into two separate contexts of either stock or supply problems. A stock-related shortage is defined as the lack of possibility to manufacture a medicine, whereas a supply-related shortage is defined as a problem in the distribution chain that makes the supply of a medicine impossible, even if enough of the medicine has been manufactured (De Weerdt et al., 2015a).
Greece	Actual shortages Temporary interruptions in supply	"Pertains to the lack of capability to fulfill the demand and the non-availability of a drug in the whole health care system, without the possibility to obtain that medicine from any source." "It refers to situations when drugs are not commercially available," mainly for commercial reasons, for a limited time duration (Bochenek et al., 2018).
Hungary	"Drug shortage"	As a term is reported to be widely used in the legislation, to report in case they are not able to supply, but without any association with a concrete formal definition (Bochenek et al., 2018).
Italy	Short supply	The Italian Medicines Agency (AIFA) defines medicines in short supply as: "Medicines which are not available or not to be found in the whole Italian market, because the marketing authorization holder (MAH) is unable to guarantee the correct and regular supply to meet patients' needs." (Bochenek et al., 2018).
Norway	Temporary disruption of a medicine's marketing	It is de facto considered to be a shortage as soon as it lasted for at least 2 weeks (Bochenek et al., 2018).
Peru	"Supply shortage" Unavailable Pharmaceutical Products Pharmaceutical product with limited supply	Considered as an operational definition in the management of drug availability indicators employed by the public bodies within the Ministry of Health and Regional Governments. Essential pharmaceutical products not supplied in the national market. Product with limited provision in the pharmaceutical market, which could generate access problems (availability and affordability) for the population
Spain	Supply problem	The Spanish Agency for Medicines and Health Products (Spanish acronym: AEMPS), being part of the Spanish Ministry of Health Care, defined the "supply problem" as a situation in which the number of available units of a drug in the pharmaceutical trade channel is below the level of national or local consumption needs, being often due to problems in the manufacturing or distribution of a drug
United States	Medicines shortages	"A period when the demand or projected demand for a medically necessary drug in the United States exceeds its supply" (Center for Drug Evaluation and research 2018).
Uruguay	Declaration of interruption of sale Interruption of marketing	Interruptions lasting 30 days or more. Due to exceptional interruptions by the manufacturer lasting less than 30 days, which must be communicated to and validated by the Department of Medicines. (ISAGS, 2017)

[1] *Administración Nacional de Medicamentos, Alimentos y Tecnología Médica. https://www.argentina.gob.ar/anmat*

[2] *The Therapeutic Goods Administration. Medicine Shortages Information Initiative Available from: https://apps.tga.gov.au/prod/MSI/search#furtherinformation*

2019). In addition, it was possible to include information from 12 new countries: Australia, Bulgaria, Canada, Czech Republic, Denmark, Finland, Germany, Iceland, Romania, Sweden, United Kingdom (UK), and the US (All-party Pharmacy, 2015; Schwartzberg et al., 2017; The Society of Hospital Pharmacists of Australian, SHPA, 2017; CDER C for DE and research, 2018; Videau et al., 2019).

Information Systems and Vigilance

Countries are taking actions regarding legislation and reporting systems in public websites (**Table 5**). Most of them are at the National Regulatory Agency level (28 countries), whereas others are at the Ministries of Health or National Health System level, including Colombia, Israel, Malta, Poland, Spain, Switzerland,

TABLE 5 | Frequency of update on the publicly available databases to report medicines shortages.

Frequency of updating	Country	Organization in charge of database	Access	Frequency of update	Mandatory Reporting
High	Australia	Therapeutics Goods Administration	https://apps.tga.gov.au/prod/MSI/search	Daily	Yes
	Belgium	Federal Agency of Medicines and Health Products	https://banquededonneesmedicaments.fagg-afmps.be/#/query/supply-problem-history/human	Daily (this is nominal frequency, which may be different)	Yes
	Canada	Bell Canada under contract with Health Canada	www.drugshortagescanada.ca/	Daily	Yes
	Czech Republic	State Institute for drug control	http://www.sukl.eu/dodavky-leciv-se-zamerenim-na-lecive-latky	Daily	Yes
	Latvia	State Agency of Medicines (SAMLV)	https://www.zva.gov.lv//?id=781&lang=&top=334&sa=673	Daily	Yes
	Portugal [1]	Portugal ANF - National Association of Pharmacies (ANF - Associação Nacional de Farmécias)	https://www.anfonline.pt/	Daily	Yes
	Sweden	Swedish medical products agency	https://lakemedelsverket.se/OVRIGA-SIDOR/Restnoteringar/	As soon as posible	Yes
	US	American Society of Health Systems Pharmacist - ASHP	https://www.ashp.org/drug-shortages/current-shortages	Daily	Not
Medium	Austria	Austrian Medicines and Medical Devices Agency (AGES MEA)	www.basg.gv.at/news-center/news/news-detail/article/uebersichtsliste-vertriebseinschraenkungen-986/	Weekly	
	Hungary	National Institute of Pharmacy and Nutrition	https://www.ogyei.gov.hu/temporary_discontinuation_of_sale_/	Weekly	Yes
	Italy	Italian Medicines Agency (AIFA—Agenzia Italiana del ármaco)	http://www.aifa.gov.it/content/carenze-e-indisponibilt%C3%A0	Weekly	Yes
	Malta [1]	Ministry for Health (CPSU—Central Procurement and Supplies Unit)	https://health.gov.mt/en/cpsu/Pages/POYC-OOS.aspx	Weekly	Yes
	Norway	Norwegian Medicines Agency	https://legemiddelverket.no/legemiddelmangel/legemiddelmangel-og-avregistreringer-2017-rad-til-apotek-og-helsepersonell	Weekly	Yes
	Slovakia	The State Institute for Drug Control (SUKL)	http://www.sukl.sk/en/inspection/post-authorization-quality-control/export-of-medicinal-products/list-of-medicinal-products-for-which-they-were-issued-decisions-not-to-allow-the-export-from-slovak-republic?page_id=4006	Weekly	Yes
	Spain [2]	Center for Information on Medicines Supply (in Spanish: Centro de Información sobre el Suministro de Medicamentos; CISMED)	http://www.portalfarma.com/Profesionales/consejoinforma/Paginas/Infarma-2016-CISMED.aspx	Weekly	Yes
	Switzerland [1]	Federal Office of Public Health	https://www.bag.admin.ch/bag/de/home/themen/mensch-gesundheit/biomedizin-forschung/heilmittel/sicherheit-in-der-medikamentenversorgung.html?_organization=317	Weekly	Yes
	Switzerland [2]	Federal Office for national economic supply (FONES)	https://www.bwl.admin.ch/bwl/de/home.html	Weekly	Yes
	Switzerland [3]	Swissmedic (Swiss Agency for Therapeutic Products)	https://www.swissmedic.ch/marktueberwachung/00135/00136/00140/00142/index.html?lang=de	Weekly	Yes
	Switzerland [4]	Martinelli Consulting Switzerland	www.drugshortage.ch	Weekly	Not applicable (private and voluntary but highly effective initiative)

(Continued)

TABLE 5 | Continued

Frequency of updating	Country	Organization in charge of database	Access	Frequency of update	Mandatory Reporting
	Turkey	Turkish Medicines and Medical Devices Agency: TMMDA (in Turkish: Türkiye Ilaç Ve Tibbi Cihaz Kurumu; TİTCK)	http://www.titck.gov.tr/	Weekly	Yes
Low	Argentina	National Administration of Medicines, Food and Medical Technology (ANMAT)	https://www.argentina.gob.ar/faltante-de-medicamentos	Twice a month	Yes
	Croatia	Croatian Health Insurance Fund	http://www.hzzo.hr/zdravstveni-sustav-rh/trazilica-za-lijekove-s-vazecih-lista/	Monthly	Yes
	France [1]	French Agency for Medicines Safety (ANSM – Agence Nationale pour la Sécurité du Medicament)	http://ansm.sante.fr/Mediatheque/Publications/Information-in-English	Yearly	Yes
	France [2]	National Council of the College of Pharmacists (Conseil national de l'ordre national des pharmaciens – CNOP)	http://www.ordre.pharmacien.fr/Le-Dossier-Pharmaceutique/Ruptures-d-approvisionnement-et-DP-Ruptures	Monthly	Yes
	Lithuania	State Medicines Control Agency (SMCA)	www.vvkt.lt	Biweekly	Unspecified
	Greece	National Organization for Medicines (EOF)	http://www.eof.gr/web/guest/eparkeia	Monthly (this is usual frequency)	Yes
	Ireland [1]	Irish Pharmaceutical Union (IPU)	https://ipu.ie/home/ipu-product-file/medicine-shortages/	Minimum monthly, but on demand based on completion of medicines shortages notification form	Yes
	Poland	Ministry of Health	http://www.bip.mz.gov.pl/legislacja/akty-prawne/obwieszczenie-ministra-zdrowia-z-dnia-10-stycznia-2017-r-w-sprawie-wykazu-produktow-leczniczych-srodkow-spozywczych-specjalnego-przeznaczenia-zywieniowego-oraz-wyrobow-medycznych-zagrozonych-brakiem/	At least bimonthly	Yes
Unspecified	Brazil	National Health Surveillance Agency (ANVISA)	http://portal.anvisa.gov.br/descontinuacao-de-medicamentos	As necessary (after every notification by MAH	Yes
	Bulgary	Bulgarian Drug Agency	http://www.bda.bg/bg/	As requiered	Not know
	Colombia [1] (may 2018 until now)	National Institute of Food and Medicines Surveillance (INVIMA)	https://www.invima.gov.co/desabastecimiento-de-medicamentos	As required	Yes
	Colombia [2] (2012 until april 2018)	Ministry of Health	https://www.minsalud.gov.co/salud/MT/Paginas/desabastecimiento.aspx	As required	Yes
	Denmark	Danish Medicines Agency	https://laegemiddelstyrelsen.dk/da/godkendelse/kontrol-og-inspektion/alvorlige-forsyningsvanskeligheder/#	As required	Yes
	Estonia	Estonian State Agency of Medicines	http://www.ravimiamet.ee/ulevaatlik-tabel-humaanravimite-tarneraskustest	As necessary (after every notification by MAH)	Yes
	Finland	The Finnish Medicines Agency - Fimea	https://www.fimea.fi/tietoa_fimeasta/ajankohtaista/saatavuushairiotiedotteet	As required	Yes
	Germany	Instituto Federal de Medicamentos y Dispositivos Médicos	https://www.bfarm.de/DE/BfArM/_node.html	As required	Yesit
	Israel	Ministry of Health	www.health.gov.il	According to the need	Yes
	Ireland [1]	UniPhar	www.uniphar.ie	As required	Yes
	Kosovo	Kosovo Medicines Agency	www.akppm.com	–	No
	Malta [1]	Ministry for Health (CPSU – Central Procurement and Supplies Unit)	https://health.gov.mt/en/cpsu/Pages/Items-Problematic-To-Source.aspx	As required	Yes

(Continued)

TABLE 5 | Continued

Frequency of updating	Country	Organization in charge of database	Access	Frequency of update	Mandatory Reporting
	Republic of Srpska, Bosnia and Herzegovina	The Agency for Medicinal Products and Medical Devices of Bosnia and Herzegovina (ALMBIH)	http://www.almbih.gov.ba/vijesti/	As soon as the ALMBIH is informed by the MAH about shortage of a given medicine	Yes
	Romania	National Agency for Medicines and Medical Devices	https://www.anm.ro/en/	As required	Yes
	Spain [1]	Spanish Agency of Medicines and Health Products (AEMPS), being part of the Spanish Ministry of Health	https://cima.aemps.es/cima/fichasTecnicas.do?metodo=buscarDesabastecidos	As required (whenever a shortage is detected)	Yes
	Slovenia	Agency for Medicinal Products and Medical Devices (JAZMP), and Health Insurance Institute of Slovenia	http://www.jazmp.si/fileadmin/datoteke/seznami/SFE/Prisotnost/Seznam_44_HUM_prenehanja_motnje.pdf www.cbz.si	Irregular	Yes
	United Kingdom	Specialist pharmacy service	https://www.sps.nhs.uk/	As needed	Yes
	Uruguay	Ministry of Public Health	https://tramites.gub.uy/ampliados?id=2659	As needed	Yes
	US [2]	Food and Drug Administration	https://www.accessdata.fda.gov/scripts/drugshortages/	Not specified	Not

UK, and Uruguay). Five countries were documented by Bochenek et al. in 2018 (Gulbis et al., 2013; Bochenek et al., 2018) where pharmacist professional organizations and other stakeholders are involved in medicines shortages reports. Finally, Canada has a website operated by a telecommunication company (**Table 5**).

Some of the main features of these systems include the frequency of updates, the obligation of pharmaceutical companies or marketing authorization holders to notify key stakeholder groups, and public institutions in charge of the database. To enhance our understanding of the characteristics of databases on medicine shortages in selected countries of Europe, Western Asia, North America, and Latin America, all databases have been divided into four groups, depending on frequency of their updating: high (daily), medium (weekly), low (less often than weekly), and unspecified (**Table 5**).

Most of the countries have only a national reporting system, where the Ministry of Health or the National Regulatory Agency manage the database and request mandatory reports. However, other countries have more than one system involved in the gathering of information, such as professional associations in France, Ireland, Malta, Portugal, Spain, and Switzerland (Bochenek et al., 2018). Finally, 12 of 40 countries have not reported databases on medicine shortage, six from Europe (Albania, Cyprus, Lichtenstein, Montenegro, Netherlands, Serbia), seven from South America (Guyana, Suriname, Ecuador, Bolivia, Paraguay, Peru, Venezuela), and Azerbaijan from Western Asia. None of the databases reported affected health conditions, or the possible impact caused by the reported episode.

Although all analyzed European countries have mandatory reporting systems, this scoping review revealed information systems with high frequency of shortages reports in countries, such as Australia, Canada, and the US. Countries of Latin America and Europe have low or unspecified update frequency of their medicines shortages websites on their (**Table 5**).

Networks and Initiatives

In 2014, the South American Council for Health from UNASUR issued a declaration on "Access to medicines and problems of medicines shortage," which stated that medicines shortage is a global and regional problem that manifests itself in diverse and changing ways, with various effects since there is insufficient information to determine the magnitude and features of the problem (ISAGS, 2017).

During 2016, several South American countries proposed to document the shortages situation of essential medicines in the region and to formulate strategies as part of the South American Institute of Government in Health (ISAGS UNASUR) actions for 2017. ISAGS UNASUR, together with the Andean Health Organization (Hipólito Unanue Agreement), undertook a study which described the situation in the member countries of the Andean and South American regions (ISAGS, 2017). An analysis of the medicines shortage situation of essential medicines was developed through the collection of information on decisions related to the problem, types of medicines identified by each country, identified causes, protocols of approach, solutions implemented, management and impact indicators, as well as limitations and experiences both at the country and regional levels that may be relevant to helping overcome the problem.

In 2016, the research collaboration initiative funded by the European Union was started. It is named COST CA15105—European Medicines Shortages Research Network—addressing supply problems to patients (Medicines Shortages) and it aims to stimulate and develop scientific research, as well as to propose solutions by end of 2020 (COST, 2015; COST, 2018). The COST CA15105 network encourages systematic sharing of information and research about shortages of medicines and nutritional products. It also aims to respond to the diverse interests of clinical and financial parties and patients' quality of life, to achieve analytical clarity on the causes of shortages, to simulate appropriate decision making in manufacturing and the trade of medicines, to highlight legal and economic frameworks, to disclose disincentives in the supply chain, as well as to reflect on best coping practices to help ensure patients' health is not compromised by ongoing shortages.

At the EU level, in 2016, the EMA and the Heads of Medicines Agencies (HMA) created an HMA/EMA Task Force on the Availability of Authorized Medicines for Human and Veterinary Use, aiming to provide strategic support and advice to tackle disruptions in the supply of human and veterinary medicines and to ensure their continued availability (EMA, 2019). The key priorities of the HMA/EMA Task Force included i) looking at ways to minimize supply disruptions and avoid shortages; ii) developing strategies to improve prevention and management of shortages caused by disruptions in the supply chain; iii) encouraging best practices within the pharmaceutical industry to prevent shortages; iv) improving sharing of information and best practices among EU regulatory authorities to better coordinate actions across the EU, and v) fostering collaboration with key stakeholders and enhancing communication of supply problems to EU citizens. A set of documents was published by EMA to support regulators involved in coordinating shortage situations due to good manufacturing practice (GMP) non-compliance. A public catalogue for shortages has been established by EMA[2], which is designed to communicate clear information on shortages to patients, health care professionals, and other stakeholders.

DISCUSSION

Studies Description

The studies included in this scoping review describe regional and countries contexts of medicine shortages and current perceptions of stakeholders, as well as their different perspectives. Indexed literature from the last 6 years presents important challenges, such as research on health and economic implications caused by supply disruptions and medicines shortages (Cousins, 2014; Steers, 2014; de Weerdt et al., 2017; Videau et al., 2019). More research efforts are needed to fully estimate the impact of medicine shortages on patients' health especially in ambulatory care.

The descriptive cases reported from the US identified parenteral and hospital medicines with shortages episodes and their implications. Moreover, published studies for countries, including Brazil, help to estimate the health implications of shortages of essential antibiotics (Griffith et al., 2012; Galvao et al., 2013; McKeever et al., 2013; Goldsack et al., 2014; Taylor et al., 2016; Mazer-Amirshahi et al., 2017). Next, efforts are needed to compare the current situation between country and regional levels.

Shortage Definitions and Global Context

Some ministries and health authorities have developed important initiatives to the timely identification of potential medicine shortages alongside initiatives to manage episodes of interruption in the supply chain (Bocquet et al., 2017; Schwartzberg et al., 2017; Administración Nacional de Medicamentos A y TMA, 2018; CDER C for DE and research, 2018; INVIMA, 2018).

De Weerdt et al. (2015a) identified some elements included in the definitions, i.e., "supply," "delivery," "availability," "permanent discontinuation of drugs," and "time frame," to consider a uniform definition for drug shortages among European countries. Definitions from **Table 4** do not involve "delivery" and "availability" as these are not reflected in the current formal definitions. Instead, other common terms are included, such as "market" and "lack."

Other countries, including France, Belgium, Italy, Spain, Brazil, and Colombia, have adopted definitions that include the perspective of shortage and some aspects related to supply chain management and market determinants. However, it is worth mentioning that the US FDA defines the problem of medicines shortage only from the perspective of scarcity and includes also a lead time. In addition, the US FDA, unlike other countries including Brazil and France, states that they will never ask a producer to make medicines or change the amount of medicines to be manufactured as solutions for dealing with drug shortages. They do not see this as their role (CDER C for DE and research, 2018).

A further finding is that a few countries have established a specific period into their definition to confirm the shortage situation: Australia, Belgium, France, Norway, and Uruguay (Bogaert et al., 2015; Bocquet et al., 2017; ISAGS, 2017; The Society of Hospital Pharmacists of Australian, SHPA, 2017; Bochenek et al., 2018). There are though some differences based on the perspective of the definition. Belgium, France, Norway, and Uruguay establish the shortage situation in a specific point of the supply chain, for instance, community pharmacies, or hospital pharmacies, or wholesalers. These countries have included periods for shortages, which varies from 72 h to 30 days (ISAGS, 2017; Bochenek et al., 2018). On the other hand, Australia defined a period of 6 months considering the lack of a medication in the whole country (The Society of Hospital Pharmacists of Australian, SHPA, 2017). Uruguay uses a period less than 30 days as an "interruption of marketing" and more than 30 days as a "declaration of interruption of sale" (ISAGS, 2017).

One main feature of a specific shortage situation is the identity of the involved medicine, e.g., simvastatin (as an individual medicine) or the class of medicines (statins, lipid modulators). Shortages can also refer to a certain pharmaceutical form (e.g., injectable, capsule, or lotion), administration route (e.g., parenteral or oral), or a certain concentration or package size. The way the product episode is defined—broadly or narrowly—depends on the purposes of the analysis and the availability of information.

It should be highlighted that in 2017, a set of two co-existing definitions had been proposed by the WHO. On the supply side: "A 'shortage' occurs when the supply of medicines, health products and vaccines identified as essential by the health system is insufficient to meet public health and patient needs. This definition refers only to products that have already been approved and marketed, to avoid conflicts with research and development agendas." On the demand side: "A 'shortage' will occur when demand exceeds supply at any point in the supply chain and may ultimately create a 'stockout' at the point of appropriate

[2] European Medicines Agency—https://www.ema.europa.eu/en/human-regulatory/post-authorisation/medicine-shortages/shortages-catalogue

service delivery to the patient if the cause of the shortage cannot be resolved in a timely manner relative to the clinical needs of the patient" (WHO, 2017). The needs of patients about essential medicines are an important link in these definitions.

The report of the Director General of the WHO presented at the last Assembly on global shortage of medicines and access to them in 2018 (A71/12) gives considerable relevance to situations that are recognized as a shortage of medicines, which coincide with those recently reported by South American countries (ISAGS, 2017; Organizaciòn Mundial de la Salud O, 2017). They show how different points of the medicines' value chain are affected by concerns with demand, which are caused both by the lack of commercial attractiveness and by logistics, and supply factors that prevent having medicines in a timely manner.

In contrast, the title of the WHO's report refers to the global scarcity of medicines, and throughout the document, the term "shortage" is being used (Organizaciòn Mundial de la Salud O, 2017). In general terms, the difference between the two terms ("scarcity of medicines" and "shortage of medicines") can be minimal. However, it is worth specifying that "scarcity" refers only to those situations in which for a specific need the medication does not exist, whereas "shortage" covers those cases in which it is not possible to obtain the medicine in a timely manner. These latter problems are not solved by activities linked to research, development, and innovation.

Terms, such as "availability" and "affordability," have also to be clearly distinguished to describe the shortage phenomena where these occur to avoid confusion and concentrate on appropriate activities to address the situation.

Regarding "availability," at the jurisdiction/country level, this term usually implies that a medicine has marketing authorization and is marketed (can be bought or obtained from the health system). At the pharmacy level, this usually means that the medicine could be dispensed at demand or within a short period.

To contrast this, the term "affordability" refers to the extent the product is available at a reasonable price/cost for the patient or health care system considering the purchasing capacity of the individuals and/or the health system and does not endanger the financial sustainability of the purchasers. As mentioned earlier, this is particularly important for patients in LMICs where there are currently high co-payments. Affordability is also a growing issue in medium- to high-income countries especially with regard to new cancer medicines and those for orphan diseases with ever increasing prices (Howard et al., 2015; Godman et al., 2017; Godman et al., 2018; Kwon et al., 2018).

The shortage of medicines is related to two main activities planned by the WHO to be implemented between 2019 and 2023. These include i) research and development of medicines, and ii) supply chain management (States, 2019). Previous studies have reported essential medicines that need rapid solutions to address current concerns (ISAGS, 2017), i.e., the penicillins for syphilis and congenital syphilis.

The description of cases, the identified causes, and definitions of medicine shortages typically involve attributes that facilitate the identification of key solutions to address the main challenges of health conditions affected by the shortages. Currently, the specific actions described in the last version of WHO roadmap for 2019 to 2023 (States, 2019) do not discuss ways of approaching this and possible solutions to these cases, which is a concern.

We have highlighted the difficulty of building a simple typology of medicine shortages based on the multiple possible combinations of criteria. It may be more useful to define a checklist of relevant criteria that allows the characterization of the episode and to predict/estimate the potential impact/effects according to the likely magnitude and length of the shortage. This again will be researched further in the future.

Causes and Characteristics of the Context That Determines the Identified Episode

The causes and context that define the shortage episodes or interruptions in the supply chain are different from other areas of policy that affect medicine availability, such as the non-availability of medicines without a marketing license, or those still in the research phase, or issues of affordability, leading to a lack of reimbursement or funding.

Overall, we believe medicine shortages can be defined according to several criteria (**Figure 5**).

In fact, medicine shortages might have multiple causes. Some of the causes might have a sequential cause-effect relationship, such as a reduction of future envisaged demand due to a reduction of the incidence of relevant diseases or reduced use due to the availability of new valued medicines, replacing existing ones, which will negatively impact on future profitability. This might cause the manufacturer to stop investing in the manufacturing process and disregard safety concerns, which may in turn lead to an increase in side effects and subsequent closure of the manufacturing plant.

Beyond an agreed single definition of medicine shortages, the concepts that could be developed must identify precisely the causes and points in the supply chain for which they apply. Topics, such as "shortage episode" could be more related to causes included in the market and policy dimensions (**Table 2**) or "interruption of supply chain episodes" for those situations caused or detected from the dimension of supply chain management.

Global Framework

Once a shortage episode is identified and characterized, including the population and health condition affected, the appropriate pharmaceutical and health policy tools, as well as rational management of medicines and their stocks, could help identify the most effective and efficient available intervention to address the problem. This could include fast tracking authorization and importation of the medicine or an equivalent from another country or recommending physicians to prescribe a substitute medicine; alternatively, potentially increasing reimbursed prices where profitability is a concern. Coordination of national efforts and international cooperation is urgently needed on various levels to address this, including UNASUR, the Andean Health Organization-Hipólito Unanue Agreement, the European Union, and the WHO. We will be following this up in the future as well.

There have been issues in Europe with older cancer medicines when the originator company has sold their molecule to a generic manufacturer, and this was re-launched at a considerably higher price, prompting potential counter measures (Pagliarulo, 2017;

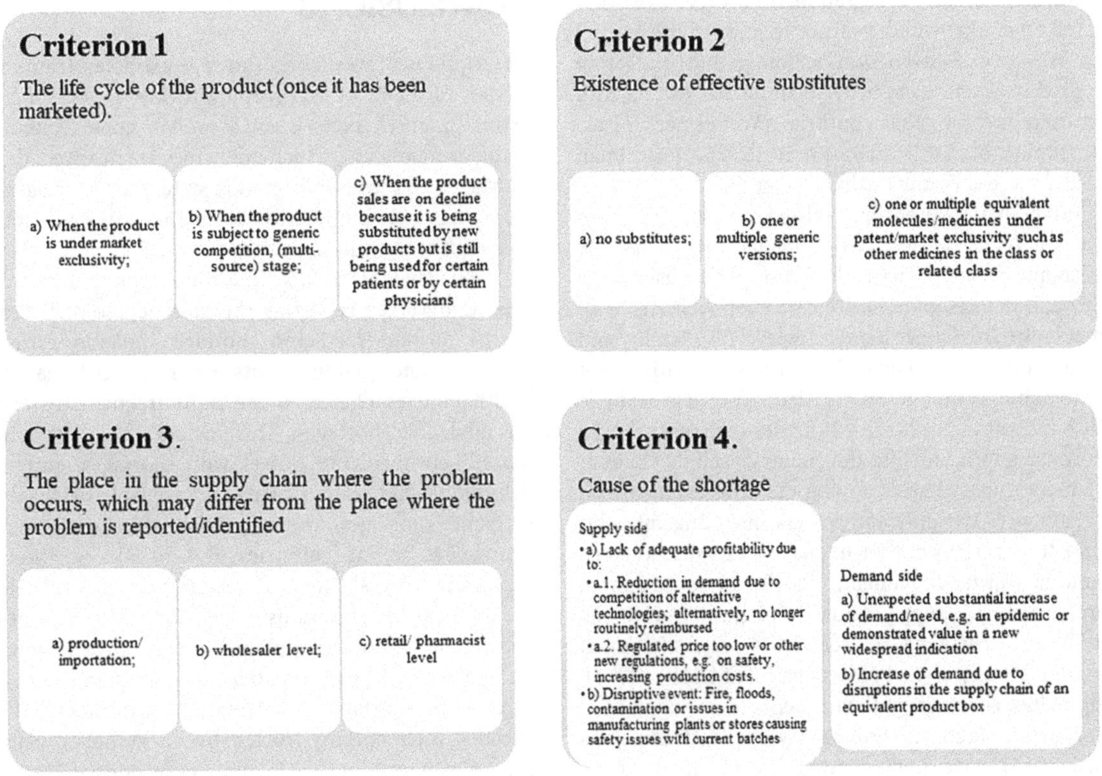

FIGURE 5 | Proposed criteria for different approach on medicines shortage.

Hawkes, 2017; Kahn, 2017; UK Department of Health and Social Care, 2016). Such activities will also be followed up, mindful of the need for manufacturers to make a profit for sustained supply.

Overall, we believe that specific strategies and solutions should be formulated at national and global levels. However, shortages must be clearly distinguished from scarcity. We believe this will lead to improved approaches to address episodes of medicine shortages and interruptions in the supply chain, as well as more pertinent solutions and their implementation to address current concerns.

There is a growing interest in international cooperation in the area of medicine shortages research, its prevention and ways to facilitate actions that provide a timely response. For South American countries, the development of a consensus to build or adapt a definition of medicines shortages demands the compilation of the countries' definitions to generate a glossary related to logistics management and the availability of medicines. Some approaches, such as risk management and a panel of logistical indicators for medicines, can be adapted to each country according to its complexities, including the health system, epidemiological alerts, and geographical peculiarities. At the regional level, it has also been proposed to design a regional platform for horizon scanning and undertaking a pilot project to identify medicines that may be at risk of stock-outs, or possible withdrawals from the market, by reviewing the license status and reviewing databases related to imports and pharmaceutical market. No less important is to develop pilots for those priority medicines that are affecting the population health in the region.

Approaches to Medicine Shortages

The proposed categorization of causes of medicines shortages can be used as a guidance to find potential solutions, as well as considering the supply stage of medicines, market competition, and possible therapeutic substitutes.

The Ministries and Health Authorities must consider which health conditions are affected by the shortage or supply chain interruption. This includes the proposed therapeutic use of the medicine and the availability of other therapeutic options, considering the optimal treatment for the disease or health condition involved within available resources.

Maybe the most critical causes of medicine shortages are those related to market aspects because these situations depend on the will of the producer, seller, or buyer, and the power relationship between each part. Some common situations are when a pharmaceutical company decides to suspend the production of a medicine, or the seller decides to modify the price of a specific pharmaceutical product, affecting its funding and supply. In view of this, possible solutions cannot just be focused on new possible innovations.

Likewise, countries initiatives should not just consist only of designing and implementing systems to compile information about cases of medicine shortages. The specific interventions should be moved forward to address potential shortages, as stated earlier.

Other approaches could include designing and implementing of risk management programs that allow the anticipation of shortage episodes as well as implementing activities, including horizon scanning to identify "programmed obsolescence" of a medicine based on market withdrawals or changes in the pricing of products. We have seen horizon scanning and budgeting successfully used in countries to better plan for the future, with Sweden and exemplar for other countries (Wettermark et al., 2010; Malmström et al., 2013; Eriksson et al., 2017; Godman et al., 2018), and these activities are likely to grow.

On the other hand, problems related to supply chain management are focused on logistics management and the level of the supply chain or network. These problems can be mitigated through the design of health care supply chains, with objectives that look to maximize the service level (availability and accessibility) and optimize the financial component, with recent changes in the public system in South Africa, a recent example among LMICs (Meyer et al., 2017). Ministries of Health should set key performance indicators for the country's supply chain as well as implement improvements among the different agents in the supply chain over the different process including inbound and outbound transportation, fleet management, warehousing, materials handling, order fulfillment, logistics network design, inventory management, supply/demand planning, and the management of third-party logistics services providers (Council of Supply Chain Management Professionals (CSCMP), 2013). This will help reduce shortages in the future.

Some countries, such as France (Ordre National des Pharmaciens, 2015) have implemented actions focused on logistic aspects including defining a dead line to establish supply interruptions and length of shortage episodes. France also established a decree in 2012 to overcome the dysfunctions of the pharmaceutical distribution channel based on supply chain interventions, as well as introducing constraining and coercive measures for the various actors of the distribution channel. The decree defines shortages as the inability for a community or hospital pharmacy to deliver a medicine to a patient within 72 h if the medicine is currently not available, as well as possible therapeutic alternatives if needed, or which supply difficulties may lead to a risk of public health for patients, thereby creating an emergency. France established a procedure whereby all the actors of the medicine's distribution channel should join forces to help address current concerns. The decree also established some regulatory obligations for pharmaceutical companies, including ensuring an appropriate and continuous supply of medicines to wholesalers to meet public and patients' needs, implementing emergency call centers to inform agents about an anticipated or a current medicine shortage, informing the French authorities of emergency supplies, specifying the quantities and addresses, and informing of any risk concerns associated with any medicine shortage. The wholesaler must also declare its distribution territory, meet public obligations, have a selection of medicines at least nine tenths of commercialized pharmaceutical products in France, and ensure to deliver medicines within 8 h from any request (Ordre National des Pharmaciens, 2015; Bocquet et al., 2017). However, there are still challenges especially in the field of medicines with major therapeutic interest, and after 7 years of the introduction of the decree, there are still tensions between the different agents in the supply chain in France due to other causes not related to supply chain management (Biétry, 2018).

CONCLUSIONS

Descriptions of medicines shortage extracted from the multiple studies included in this scoping review allowed the authors to extract main characteristics, as well as contexts and reasons of medicines shortage, which medicines are involved, definitions of shortages, countries information systems on shortage reports and alerts management, and finally any networks between countries and stakeholders' initiatives.

We believe this is first time such a comprehensive study has been undertaken reporting the most representative description of the current medicine shortage situation across multiple countries and giving inputs regarding national and global health policies related to the most frequent reasons reported for medicine shortages. This includes the description of the most likely medicine classes with shortages, current national definitions, and related terms and available databases to report medicine shortages. The study also describes frameworks and approaches among countries to help address these issues in the future. Overall, we believe our findings can help with the development of definitions related to the shortage of medicines that can be universally applied to prevent future confusion.

Signals linked with unattended or affected health conditions because of shortages must also be documented to establish effective interventions from a health authority perspective to ensure patients' health is not compromised. Indeed, policy makers require solutions that prevent those cases in which the population's health is affected by episodes of medicine shortages and/or interruption in the supply chain.

As part of this, we believe it is necessary to develop a consensus to build or adapt definitions of shortage and scarcity, as well as identifying all local definitions, to generate a glossary related to logistics management and the availability of medicines to facilitate aggregation of data from different sources and to better manage future situations. We have started this process with this article.

We also believe it is important to emphasize that for those cases where shortages are due to logistical and supply factors, and it is not possible to have the medicines in a timely manner, that potential ways forward are not related to improving research, development and innovation as some bodies are proposing. This is a very different situation, especially if alternative solutions are available including importation, as well as permitting increased prices if pertinent along with advocating and documenting possible alternatives, and these must be explored first.

Overall, we believe it would also be useful to identify options and best practices on how to address the most common causes of shortages and share these among all countries to provide future direction. These are research topics for the future building on this review across countries.

Our findings show that part of the problem of shortages is focused on provision, especially those cases related to the permanent suspension of production or voluntary suspension, due to, for instance, to the lack of commercial interest, either by low demand, end of the patent, price regulations, use of compulsory licenses and/or the introduction of new medicines. Regarding suspending commercialization, it is important to review specific cases that raise considerable public health concerns, such as antineoplastic and antibiotics, to suggest potential ways to overcome the situation. We have started this process and will continue.

LIMITATIONS

Although the findings presented in this study allows us to make comparisons between countries related with, for instance, national definitions and involved medicines, there are other attributes that may well broaden the situation which we have not discussed. These can be addressed going forward.

RECOMMENDATIONS

Further research is needed to fully assess the clinical and economic impact of medicine shortages at different jurisdictional levels, including both hospital and ambulatory care levels. Additionally, cross-country and regional studies will help to identify current essential medicines supply disruptions and shortages episodes, which need prompt solutions.

AUTHOR CONTRIBUTIONS

AA and EV conducted the study and prepared the first draft of the article and the literature review. JR brought methodologic inputs and assessed preliminary results. JR, BG, and TB commented on and contributed to subsequent iterations on the manuscript.

ACKNOWLEDGMENTS

The work on this article was facilitated by the ISAGS UNASUR institutional program of associate researchers, promoted by Carina Vance, its current Executive Director.

REFERENCES

Administración Nacional de Medicamentos A y TMA (2018). Faltante de medicamentos | Argentina.gob.ar [Internet]. ANMAT. [cited 2019 Jan 19]. Available from: https://www.argentina.gob.ar/faltante-de-medicamentos.

Alevizakos, M., Detsis, M., Grigoras, C. A., Machan, J. T., and Mylonakis, E. (2016). The impact of shortages on medication prices: implications for shortage prevention. *Drugs* 76 (16), 1551–8. doi: 10.1007/s40265-016-0651-7

All-party Pharmacy (2015). Why drug shortages occur. *Drug Ther. Bull.* 53 (3), 33–6. doi: 10.1136/dtb.2015.3.0316

Alsheikh, M., Seoane-Vazquez, E., Rittenhouse, B., Fox, E., and Fanikos, J. (2016). A comparison of drug shortages in the hospital setting in the United States and Saudi Arabia: an exploratory analysis. *Hosp. Pharm.* 51 (5), 370–5. doi: 10.1310/hpj5105-370

American College of Medical Toxicology, American Academy of Clinical Toxicology (2015). Antidote shortages in the USA: Impact and Response. *J. Med. Toxicol.* 11 (1), 144–6. doi: 10.1007/s13181-013-0372-1

Aular de González, Y. (2014). Escasez de medicamentos y su repercusión en la salud. *Salus* 18 (2), 5–6. http://www.redalyc.org/pdf/3759/375939026002.pdf

Awad, H., Al-Zu'bi, Z. M. F., and Abdallah, A. B. (2016). A quantitative analysis of the causes of drug shortages in Jordan: a supply chain perspective. *Int. Bus. Res.* 9 (6), 53. doi: 10.5539/ibr.v9n6p53

Bauters, T., Claus, B. O. M., Norga, K., Huys, I., Simoens, S., and Laureys, G. (2016). Chemotherapy drug shortages in paediatric oncology: a 14-year single-centre experience in Belgium. *J. Oncol. Pharm. Pract.* 22 (6), 766–70. doi: 10.1177/1078155215610915

Becker, D. J., Talwar, S., Levy, B. P., Thorn, M., Roitman, J., Blum, R. H., et al. (2013). Impact of oncology drug shortages on patient therapy: unplanned treatment changes. *J. Oncol. Pract.* 9 (4), e122–8. doi: 10.1200/JOP.2012.000799

Bible, J. R., Evans, D. C., Payne, B., and Mostafavifar, L. (2014). Impact of drug shortages on patients receiving parenteral nutrition after laparotomy. *J. Parenter. Enteral Nutr.* 38 (2_suppl), 65S–71S. doi: 10.1177/0148607114550317

Biétry, G. (2018). Drug shortages causing tension between pharma, wholesalers and pharmacists in France. *APM Health Europe.*

Birgli® ag (2013). An Evaluation of Medicines Shortages in Europe with a more in-depth review of these in France, Greece, Poland, Spain, and the United Kingdom. 68. Available from: http://static.correofarmaceutico.com/docs/2013/10/21/evaluation.pdf.

Bochenek, T., Abilova, V., Alkan, A., Asanin, B., Beriain I de, M., Besovic, Z., et al. (2018). Systemic measures and legislative and organizational frameworks aimed at preventing or mitigating drug shortages in 28 European and Western Asian Countries. *Front. Pharmacol.* 8. doi: 10.3389/fphar.2017.00942

Bocquet, F., Degrassat-Théas, A., Peigné, J., and Paubel, P. (2017). The new regulatory tools of the 2016 Health Law to fight drug shortages in France. *Health Policy (New York).* 121 (5), 471–476. doi: 10.1016/j.healthpol.2017.03.007

Bogaert, P., Bochenek, T., Prokop, A., and Pilc, A. (2015). A Qualitative approach to a better understanding of the problems underlying drug shortages, as viewed from Belgian, French and the European Union's perspectives. Lexchin J, editor. *PLoS One* 10 (5), e0125691. doi: 10.1371/journal.pone.0125691

Bonnanno, V., and Gavril, F. (2011). Seven years of EU Pharmaceutical Regulation in Malta. *WHO Drug Inf.* 25, 343–53.

Butterfield, L., Cash, J., and Pham, K. (2015). Advocacy Committee for the Pediatric Pharmacy Advocacy Group on B of the AC for the PPA. Drug shortages and implications for pediatric patients. *J. Pediatr. Pharmacol. Ther.* 20 (2), 149–52. doi: 10.5863/1551-6776-20.2.149

Cameron, A., Ewen, M., Ross-Degnan, D., Ball, D., and Laing, R. (2009). Medicine prices, availability, and affordability in 36 developing and middle-income countries: a secondary analysis. *Lancet* 373 (9659), 240–9. doi: 10.1016/S0140-6736(08)61762-6

Caulder, C., Mehta, B., Bookstaver, P., Sims, L., and Stevenson, B. (2015). South Carolina Society of Health-Sy. Impact of drug shortages on health system pharmacies in the southeastern United States. *Hosp. Pharm.* 50 (4), 279–86. doi: 10.1310/hpj5004-279

CDER C for DE and research (2018). CDER Conversation: FDA's drug shortages prevention strategies. [cited 2019 Jan 16]; Available from: https://www.fda.gov/drugs/newsevents/ucm432474.htm.

Center for Drug Evaluation and research C (2018). Drug shortages—drug shortages infographic [Internet]. Center for Drug Evaluation and Research; [cited 2019 Jan 26]. Available from: https://www.fda.gov/Drugs/DrugSafety/DrugShortages/ucm441579.htm.

Chen, S. I., Fox, E. R., Kennedy Hall, M., Ross, J. S., Bucholz, E. M., Krumholz, H. M., et al. (2016). Despite federal legislation, shortages of drugs used in acute care settings remain persistent and prolonged. *Health Aff.* 35 (5), 798–804. doi: 10.1377/hlthaff.2015.1157

COST. (2015). CA15105—European Medicines Shortages Research Network—addressing supply problems to patients (Medicines Shortages) [Internet]. Available from: https://www.cost.eu/actions/CA15105/#tabs%7CName:overview.

COST. (2018). European Medicines Shortages Research Network—addressing supply problems to patients (Medicines Shortages) [Internet]. Medicines Shortages in Europe. eCOST Action CA15105. Available from: http://www.medicinesshortages.eu/.

Costelloe, E. M., Guinane, M., Nugent, F., Halley, O., and Parsons, C. (2015). An audit of drug shortages in a community pharmacy practice. *Irish J. Med. Sci.* 184 (2), 435–40. doi: 10.1007/s11845-014-1139-7

Council of Supply Chain Management Professionals (CSCMP) (2013). SCM Definitions and Glossary of Terms [Internet]. [cited 2019 Jan 12]. Available from: https://cscmp.org/CSCMP/Educate/SCM_Definitions_and_Glossary_of_Terms/CSCMP/Educate/SCM_Definitions_and_Glossary_of_Terms.aspx?hkey=60879588-f65f-4ab5-8c4b-6878815ef921.

Cousins, S. (2014). Iraq: staff and medicine shortages are major challenges. *Lancet* 384 (9947), 943–4. doi: 10.1016/S0140-6736(14)61615-9

De Weerdt, E., De Rijdt, T., Simoens, S., Casteels, M., and Huys, I. (2017). Time spent by Belgian hospital pharmacists on supply disruptions and drug shortages: an exploratory study. *PLoS One* 12 (3), 1–15. doi: 10.1371/journal.pone.0174556

De Weerdt, E., Simoens, S., Casteels, M., and Huys, I. (2015a). Toward a European definition for a drug shortage: a qualitative study. *Front. Pharmacol.* 6, 1–9. doi: 10.3389/fphar.2015.00253

de Weerdt, E., Simoens, S., Casteels, M., and Huys, I. (2017). Clinical, economic and policy implications of drug shortages in the European Union. *Appl. Health Econ. Health Policy*, 15 (4), 441–445. doi: 10.1007/s40258-016-0264-z

De Weerdt, E., Simoens, S., Hombroeckx, L., Casteels, M., and Huys, I. (2015b). Causes of drug shortages in the legal pharmaceutical framework. *Regul. Toxicol. Pharmacol.* 71 (2), 251–8. doi: 10.1016/j.yrtph.2015.01.005

EMA. (2019). Medicine shortages [Internet]. Available from: https://www.ema.europa.eu/en/human-regulatory/post-authorisation/medicine-shortages.

Eriksson, I., Wettermark, B., Persson, M., Edström, M., Godman, B., Lindhé, A., et al. (2017). The early awareness and alert system in Sweden: history and current status. *Front. Pharmacol.* 8, 1–8. doi: 10.3389/fphar.2017.00674

Fox, E. R., and Tyler, L. S. (2017). Potential association between drug shortages and high-cost medications. *Pharmacotherapy* 37 (1), 36–42. doi: 10.1002/phar.1861

Ministre des affaires sociales, Ministre de la santè. (2012). Décret n° 2012-1096 du 28 septembre 2012 relatif à l'approvisionnement en médicaments à usage humain [Internet]. Les autres textes législatifs et réglementaires, Décret n° 2012-1096 Version consolidée au 11 septembre 2017 France: Legifrance. Available from: https://www.legifrance.gouv.fr/affichTexte.do?cidTexte=JORFTEXT000026426883&dateTexte=20170911

Gabrielli, A., Layon, N. T., Bones, H. L., and Layon, A. J. (2016). The tragedy of the commons—drug shortages and our patients' health. *Am. J. Med.* 129 (12), 1237–8. doi: 10.1016/j.amjmed.2016.09.007

Galvao, T. F., Silva, M. T., Serruya, S. J., Newman, L. M., Klausner, J. D., Pereira, M. G., et al. (2013). Safety of benzathine penicillin for preventing congenital syphilis: a systematic review. *PLoS One* 8 (2), 1–9. doi: 10.1371/journal.pone.0056463

Godman, B., Bucsics, A., Vella Bonnano, P., Oortwijn, W., Rothe, C., Ferrario, A., et al. (2018). Barriers for access to new medicines: searching for the balance between rising costs and limited budgets. *Front. Public Health* 6, 328. doi: 10.3389/fpubh.2018.00328

Godman, B., Malmström, R. E., Diogene, E., Gray, A., Jayathissa, S., Timoney, A., et al. (2015). Are new models needed to optimize the utilization of new medicines to sustain healthcare systems? *Expert Rev. Clin. Pharmacol.* 8 (1), 77–94. doi: 10.1586/17512433.2015.990380

Godman, B., Petzold, M., Bennett, K., Bennie, M., Bucsics, A., Finlayson, A., et al. (2014). Can authorities appreciably enhance the prescribing of oral generic risperidone to conserve resources? Findings from across Europe and their implications. *BMC Med.* 12, 98. doi: 10.1186/1741-7015-12-98

Godman, B., Shrank, W., Andersen, M., Berg, C., Bishop, I., Burkhardt, T., et al. (2010). Comparing policies to enhance prescribing efficiency in Europe through increasing generic utilization: changes seen and global implications. *Expert Rev. Pharmacoecon. Outcomes Res.* 10 (6), 707–22. doi: 10.1586/erp.10.72

Godman, B., Wild, C., and Haycox, A. (2017). Patent expiry and costs for anticancer medicines for clinical use: expiry and costs anti-cancer medicines. [cited 2019 Jan 27]; Available from: https://strathprints.strath.ac.uk/60241/1/Godman_etal_GABI_2017_Patent_expiry_and_costs_for_anti_cancer_medicines_for_clinical.pdf. doi: 10.5639/gabij.2017.0603.021

Goldsack, J. C., Reilly, C., Bush, C., McElligott, S., Bristol, M. N., Motanya, U. N., et al. (2014). Impact of shortages of injectable oncology drugs on patient care. *Am. J. Health Pharm.* 71 (7), 571–8. doi: 10.2146/ajhp130569

Golembiewski, J. (2012). Drug Shortages in the perioperative setting: causes, impact, and strategies. *J. Perianesth. Nurs.* 27 (4), 286–92. doi: 10.1016/j.jopan.2012.05.005

Gray, A., and Manasse, H. R. (2012). Shortages of medicines: a complex global challenge. *Bull. World Health Organ.* 90 (3), 158–158A. doi: 10.2471/BLT.11.101303

Griffith, M. M., Gross, A. E., Sutton, S. H., Bolon, M. K., Esterly, J. S., Patel, J. A., et al. (2012). The impact of anti-infective drug shortages on hospitals in the United States: trends and causes. *Clin. Infect. Dis.* 54 (5), 684–91. doi: 10.1093/cid/cir954

Gulbis, B. E., Ruiz, M. C., and Denktas, A. E. (2013). The impact of drug shortages on the pharmacy, nursing, and medical staff's ability to effectively care for critically ill patients. *Crit. Care Nurs. Q.* 36 (4), 400–6. doi: 10.1097/CNQ.0b013e3182a10ffe

Gupta, D. K., and Huang, S. M. (2013). Drug shortages in the United States: a critical evaluation of root causes and the need for action. *Clin. Pharmacol. Ther.* 93 (2), 133–5. doi: 10.1038/clpt.2012.229

Hawkes, N. (2017). Drug company Aspen faces probe over hiking generic prices. Available from: https://www.bmj.com/content/357/bmj.j2417. doi: 10.1136/bmj.j2417

Heiskanen, K., Ahonen, R., Kanerva, R., Karttunen, P., and Timonen, J. (2017). The reasons behind medicine shortages from the perspective of pharmaceutical companies and pharmaceutical wholesalers in Finland. *PLoS One* 12 (6), e0179479. doi: 10.1371/journal.pone.0179479

Howard, D. H., Bach, P. B., Berndt, E. R., and Conti, R. M. (2015). Pricing in the Market for Anticancer Drugs. *J. Econ. Perspect.* 29 (1), 139–62. doi: 10.1257/jep.29.1.139

INVIMA (2018). Desabastecimiento de medicamentos-Invima_Instituto Nacional de Vigilancia de Medicamentos y Alimentos [Internet]. [cited 2019 Jan 19]. Available from: https://www.invima.gov.co/desabastecimiento-de-medicamentos.

ISAGS (2017). Situation of Essential Medicines at Risk of Supply Shortage with Emphasis on South American Countries [Internet]. Rio de Janeiro. Available from: http://isags-unasur.org/en/publicacao/situation-of-essential-medicines-at-risk-of-supply-shortage-with-emphasis-on-south-american-countries-2/.

Jagsi, R., Spence, L., Rathmell, W., Bradbury, A., Peppercorn, J., Grubbs, S., et al. (2014). Ethical considerations for the clinical oncologist in an era of oncology drug shortages. *Oncologist* 19 (2), 186–92. doi: 10.1634/theoncologist.2013-0301

Kahn, T. (2017). Aspen loses Italy appeal over cancer drug prices. Available at URL: https://www.businesslive.co.za/bd/companies/healthcare/2017-06-15-aspen-loses-italy-appeal-over-cancer-drug-prices/. Available from: https://www.businesslive.co.za/bd/companies/healthcare/2017-06-15-aspen-loses-italy-appeal-over-cancer-drug-prices/.

Kaposy, C. (2014). Drugs, money, and power: the Canadian drug shortage. *J. Bioeth. Inq.* 11 (1), 85–9. doi: 10.1007/s11673-013-9494-z

Kavanagh, J. (2017). *How Pharmaceutical Supply Chains Can Be Managed to Minimise the Number of Medicines Shortages*. Ireland: College Dublin.

Kwon, H. Y., Kim, H., and Godman, B. (2018). Availability and affordability of drugs with a conditional approval by the European Medicines Agency: comparison of Korea with other countries and the implications. *Front. Pharmacol.* 9, 1–9. doi: 10.3389/fphar.2018.00938

Lazarini, F. M., and Barbosa, D. A. (2017). Educational intervention in Primary Care for the prevention of congenital syphilis. *Rev. Lat. Am. Enfermagem* 25, e2845. doi: 10.1590/1518-8345.1612.2845

Malmström, R. E., Godman, B. B., Diogene, E., Baumgärtel, C., Bennie, M., Bishop, I., et al. (2013). Dabigatran—a case history demonstrating the need for comprehensive approaches to optimize the use of new drugs. *Front. Pharmacol.* 4, 39. doi: 10.3389/fphar.2013.00039

Mazer-Amirshahi, M., Goyal, M., Umar, S. A., Fox, E. R., Zocchi, M., Hawley, K. L., et al. (2017). U.S. drug shortages for medications used in adult critical care (2001–2016). *J. Crit. Care* 41, 283–8. doi: 10.1016/j.jcrc.2017.06.005

McKeever, A. E., Bloch, J. R., and Bratic, A. (2013). Drug shortages and the burden of access to care: a critical issue affecting patients with cancer. *Clin. J. Oncol. Nurs.* 17 (5), 490–495. doi: 10.1188/13.CJON.490-495

McLaughlin, M. M., and Skoglund, E. W. (2015). Drug shortages and patient safety. *J. Infus. Nurs.* 38 (3), 205–8. doi: 10.1097/NAN.0000000000000101

McLaughlin, M., Kotis, D., Thomson, K., Harrison, M., Fennessy, G., Postelnick, M., et al. (2013). Effects on patient care caused by drug shortages: a survey. *J. Manag. Care Pharm.* 19 (9), 783–8. doi: 10.18553/jmcp.2013.19.9.783

Meyer, J. C., Schellack, N., Stokes, J., Lancaster, R., Zeeman, H., Defty, D., et al. (2017). Ongoing initiatives to improve the quality and efficiency of medicine use within the public healthcare system in South Africa; A preliminary study. *Front. Pharmacol.* 8, 1–16. doi: 10.3389/fphar.2017.00751

Ministerio de Salud Venezuela (2017). Comunicación.

Moon, J. C., Godman, B., Petzold, M., Alvarez-Madrazo, S., Bennett, K., Bishop, I., et al. (2014). Different initiatives across Europe to enhance losartan utilisation post generics: impact and implications. *Front. Pharmacol.* 5, 1–10. doi: 10.3389/fphar.2014.00219

Moorkens, E., Vulto, A. G., Huys, I., Dylst, P., Godman, B., Keuerleber, S., et al. (2017). Policies for biosimilar uptake in Europe: an overview. *PLoS One* 12 (12), 1–17. doi: 10.1371/journal.pone.0190147

Morrison, A. (2011). Drug Supply Disruptions [Internet]. [cited 2019 Apr 21]. Available from: https://www.cadth.ca/sites/default/files/pdf/Drug_Supply_Disruptions_es-18_e.pdf.

Norwegian Institute of Public Nealth (2018). WHO—ATC/DDD Index [Internet]. ATC/DDD Index 2019. [cited 2019 Apr 28]. Available from: https://www.whocc.no/atc_ddd_index/.

Nurse-Findlay, S., Taylor, M. M., Savage, M., Mello, M. B., Saliyou, S., Lavayen, M., et al. (2017). Shortages of benzathine penicillin for prevention of mother-to-child transmission of syphilis: an evaluation from multi-country surveys and stakeholder interviews. *PLoS Med.* 14 (12), e1002473. doi: 10.1371/journal.pmed.1002473

Ofori-Asenso, R., and Agyeman, A. (2016). Irrational Use of Medicines—a summary of key concepts. *Pharmacy* 4 (4), 35. doi: 10.3390/pharmacy4040035

Ordre National des Pharmaciens (2015). Ruptures d'approvisionnement de médicaments. *Les cahiers de l'Ordre national des pharmaciens*, 1–29.

Organizaciòn Mundial de la Salud O (2017). La escasez mundial de medicamentos y vacunas y el acceso a ellos. 2016, 9. https://apps.who.int/gb/ebwha/pdf_files/WHA70/A70_20-sp.pdf

Pagliarulo, N. (2017). EU investigating generic drugmaker over cancer drug price hikes. *Biopharmadive.* https://www.biopharmadive.com/news/aspen-pharma-antitrust-generic-drugs-EC-europe-investigation/442722/

Parsons, H. M., Schmidt, S., Karnad, A. B., Liang, Y., Pugh, M. J., Fox, E. R., et al. (2016). ReCAP: Association between the number of suppliers for critical antineoplastics and drug shortages: implications for future drug shortages and treatment. *J. Oncol. Pract.* 12 (3), 249–50. doi: 10.1200/JOP.2015.007237

Pauwels, K., Huys, I., Casteels, M., and Simoens, S. (2014). Drug shortages in European countries: a trade-off between market attractiveness and cost containment? *BMC Health Serv. Res.* 14, 438. doi: 10.1186/1472-6963-14-438

Pauwels, K., Simoens, S., Casteels, M., and Huys, I. (2015). Insights into European drug shortages: a survey of hospital pharmacists. *PLoS One* 10 (3), e0119322. doi: 10.1371/journal.pone.0119322

Pfeffer, K., and Mozoľová, B. (2017). Re-export of drugs in the Slovak Republic Vol 2 The act. Two Birds.

Pham, M. T., Greig, J. D., Sargeant, J. M., and Mcewen, S. A., (2015). A scoping review of scoping reviews: advancing the approach and enhancing the consistency. *Res. Synth. Methods* 5 (4), 371–385.

Rinaldi, F., de Denus, S., Nguyen, A., Nattel, S., and Bussières, J. F. (2017). Drug shortages: patients and health care providers are all drawing the short straw. *Can. J. Cardiol.* 33 (2), 283–6. doi: 10.1016/j.cjca.2016.08.010

Rosa, M. B., Reis, A. M. M., Perini, E., Rosa, M. B., Reis, A. M. M., and Perini, E. (2016). Drug shortage: a public health problem. *Cad. Saude Publica* 32 (10), 1–3. doi: 10.1590/0102-311X00086916

Schwartzberg, E., Ainbinder, D., Vishkauzan, A., and Gamzu, R. (2017). Drug shortages in Israel: regulatory perspectives, challenges and solutions. *Isr. J. Health Policy Res.* 6 (1), 17. doi: 10.1186/s13584-017-0140-9

Schweitzer, S. O. (2013). How the US Food and Drug Administration can solve the prescription drug shortage problem. *Am. J. Public Health* 103 (5), e10–4. doi: 10.2105/AJPH.2013.301239

Servicio Vasco de Salud -Osakidetza (2016). Desabastecimiento De Medicamentos: Un Problema Sin Resolver [Internet]. Vol. 23, INFORMACIÓN FARMACOTERAPÉUTICA DE LA COMARCA. Vitoria - Gasteiz. Available from: http://www.osakidetza.euskadi.eus/contenidos/informacion/cevime_infac/es_cevime/adjuntos/INFAC_Vol_23_N_7_Desabastecimientos.pdf.

Setayesh, S., and Mackey, T. K. (2016). Addressing the impact of economic sanctions on Iranian drug shortages in the joint comprehensive plan of action: promoting access to medicines and health diplomacy. *Global Health* 12 (1), 1–14. doi: 10.1186/s12992-016-0168-6

States, M. (2019), Consultation DFOR. Roadmap for access 2019-2023.

Steers, W. D. (2014). Falling short: causes and implications of drug shortages in the United States. *J. Urol.* 192 (5), 1315–7. doi: 10.1016/j.juro.2014.09.003

Taylor, M. M., Nurse-Findlay, S., Zhang, X., Hedman, L., Kamb, M. L., Broutet, N., et al. (2016). Estimating benzathine penicillin need for the treatment of pregnant women diagnosed with syphilis during antenatal care in high-morbidity countries. *PLoS One* 11 (7), 1–15. doi: 10.1371/journal.pone.0159483

The Society of Hospital Pharmacists of Australian, SHPA (2017). "Medicine Shortages in Australia," in *A snapshot of shortages in Australian hospitals* (Victoria). https://www.shpa.org.au/sites/default/files/uploaded-content/website-content/Fact-sheets-position-statements/medicines_shortages_in_australia-_shpa_snapshot_-_june_2017.pdf

UK Department of Health and Social Care. (2016). Health Service Medical Supplies (Costs) [Internet]. Available from: https://www.gov.uk/government/publications/health-service-medical-supplies-costs/health-service-medical-supplies-costs-bill-factsheet.

UNASUR (2014). Acceso a medicamentos y problemas de desabastecimiento de medicamentos esenciales [Internet]. Surinam. Available from: http://www.isags-unasur.org/uploads/biblioteca/1/bb[503]ling[1]anx[1530].pdf.

Ventola, C. L. (2011). The drug shortage crisis in the United States: causes, impact, and management strategies. *P T* 36 (11), 740–57.

Videau, M., Lebel, D., and Bussières, J. F. (2019). Drug shortages in Canada: Data for 2016–2017 and perspectives on the problem. *Ann. Pharm. Fr.* 77 (3), 205–211. doi: 10.1016/j.pharma.2018.11.007

Walker, J., Chaar, B. B., Vera, N., Pillai, A. S., Lim, J. S., Bero, L., et al. (2017). Medicine shortages in Fiji: A qualitative exploration of stakeholders' views. *PLoS One* 5. doi: 10.1371/journal.pone.0178429

Wettermark, B., Persson, M. E., Wilking, N., Kalin, M., Korkmaz, S., Hjemdahl, P., et al. (2010). Forecasting drug utilization and expenditure in a metropolitan health region. *BMC Health Serv. Res.* 10, 1–14. doi: 10.1186/1472-6963-10-128

WHO 2017. WHO. Meeting Report: Technical Definitions of Shortages and Stockouts of Medicines and Vaccines [Internet]. Geneva; [cited 2019 Jan 31]. Available from: http://www.who.int/about/licensing/copyright_form/en/index.html.

World Health Organization (2018). *Addressing the global shortage of, and access to, medicines and vaccines Report by the Director-General BACKGROUND* Vol. EB142/13. Geneva: World Health Assembly, 50.

Yang, C., Wu, L., Cai, W., Zhu, W., Shen, Q., Li, Z., et al. (2016). Current situation, determinants, and solutions to drug shortages in Shaanxi Province, China: a qualitative study. *PLoS One* 11 (10), 1–16. doi: 10.1371/journal.pone.0165183

14

Where Sepsis and Antimicrobial Resistance Countermeasures Converge

Timothy J. J. Inglis[1,2]* and *Nadia Urosevic*[1,2]

[1] *The Marshall Centre for Infectious Diseases Training and Research, School of Biomedical Sciences, University of Western Australia, Perth, WA, Australia,*
[2] *Department of Microbiology, PathWest Laboratory Medicine WA, Queen Elizabeth II Medical Centre, Nedlands, WA, Australia*

Correspondence:
Timothy J. J. Inglis
tim.inglis@uwa.edu.au

The United Nations General Assembly debate on antimicrobial resistance (AMR) recognizes the global significance of AMR. Much work needs to be done on technology capability and capacity to convert the strategic intent of the debate into operational plans and tangible outcomes. Enhancement of the biomedical science–clinician interface requires better exploitation of systems biology tools for in-laboratory and point of care methods that detect sepsis and characterize AMR. These need to link sepsis and AMR data with responsive, real-time surveillance. We propose an AMR sepsis register, similar in concept to a cancer registry, to aid coordination of AMR countermeasures.

Keywords: antimicrobial resistance, sepsis, integrated systems biology, biocomplexity, microbial forensics, infection control

INTRODUCTION

The United Nations high-level meeting on antimicrobial resistance (AMR) was calculated to thrust the issue of AMR into public view (1) and represents the latest milestone in a global awareness-raising campaign by public health authorities. At first glance, this appears to be the antithesis of precision public health, which places an emphasis on targeted multidisciplinary application of emerging biotechnology to the specific health needs of individuals (2). However, this onslaught against a leading global health challenge is built on a foundation of laboratory AMR surveillance and powered by similar multidisciplinary application of emerging high-throughput biotechnologies (3). The big data outputs obtained in such a way are attractive to public health precisely because they are amenable to mathematical modeling of the ecological and evolutionary processes that lead to AMR (4). These dynamic aspects of infection are complex and have led to a widening comprehension gap. Consequently, the growing public recognition of AMR has yet to acquire a more sophisticated understanding of its personal implications (5, 6). Health professionals who share our concern about escalating AMR support the translation of global policy into action at local, national, and international levels (7). A global campaign to contain and control AMR needs translation from strategic policy into day-to-day health-care practice. Strategy; the practice of the art of war by the *strategos* or general, includes the broader considerations of game theory, complexity, business, and management strategy (8). Biocomplexity provides an attractive framework for placing the cell and molecular biology or biomedical end of the AMR scale in a broader context that includes the clinical pathology of tissues and organs, and ultimately population health including all professional, social, and government regulation (9). So, to understand the mechanistic workings of an emerging public health phenomenon such as the rise in AMR infections, it is necessary to descend the scale of biological organization from population health to the molecular and cellular mechanisms of multiple-drug resistance in different bacterial species (10). A robust assessment of the broad consequences of AMR requires the converse; an ascent from a specific AMR phenotype to multinational surveillance review (11, 12). An unavoidable feature of AMR is its capacity for unpredictable double transmission: the ability to not only enhance case-clusters of transmissible disease, but also for transmission between resistant and previously sensitive bacteria contributing to novel disease case-clusters, as seen in the dissemination and proliferation of multiple mechanisms of carbapenem resistance (13). Both specific mechanisms and means of AMR transmission need consideration, since both the AMR mechanism and its transmission will impact on the ecology and epidemiology of AMR infection and have implications for the measures needed to control AMR (14). New analytical systems biology tools provide scope for evidence-based design of AMR surveillance and control (15). The complex picture that emerges can be used to develop an AMR narrative that covers the wide range of AMR molecular signatures, multiple bacterial species, and AMR mechanism combinations across the broad scale of biological organization (3). However, other emerging systems biology methods such as proteomics, metabolomics, and bacterial cytomics have yet to be integrated in a holistic AMR analysis that forms a more compelling argument for a specific causal effect (16). Practical use of this approach to attribution of causality has been explored in the field of microbial forensics and has wider application in linking the different tiers of analysis up to a strategic level (17). The O'Neill Review identified critical vulnerabilities that could be exploited in control of the global AMR problem and made a series of recommendations (18):

1. A massive global public awareness campaign,
2. Improve hygiene and prevent the spread of infection,
3. Reduce unnecessary use of antimicrobials in agriculture and their dissemination into the environment,
4. Improve global surveillance of drug resistance and antimicrobial consumption in humans and animals,
5. Promote new, rapid diagnostics to cut unnecessary use of antibiotics,
6. Promote development and use of vaccines and alternatives,
7. Improve the numbers, pay and recognition of people working in infectious disease,
8. Establish a Global Innovation Fund for early-stage and non-commercial research,
9. Better incentives to promote investment for new drugs and improving existing ones.

THE CRITICAL DECISION CONTINUUM

The O'Neill Review recognizes that no single measure will solve the problem of AMR and only seeks to lay out a broad agenda. The review's introduction emphasizes the inability of current diagnostic procedures to provide rapid and comprehensive answers, noting that it is

> ...incredible that doctors must still prescribe antibiotics based only on their immediate assessment of a patient's symptoms, just like they used to when antibiotics first entered common use in the 1950s.

Antibiotic prescribers face three major obstacles: (a) AMR is an abstract concept for all but its victims and their physicians; (b) detection of specific forms of AMR does not conclusively determine the best choice of anti-infective therapy; and (c) in severe infections, the wait for laboratory evidence on which to base a choice of antibiotic can have fatal consequences. This last consideration remains a key promoter of emerging AMR and could be described as poorly targeted personal medicine; the antithesis of precision public health. Half a millennium ago, Machiavelli observed that the increase in diagnostic certainty with the passage of time leads to reduced treatment success (19). This makes the physician reluctant to wait for the definitive culture results and subsequent antimicrobial susceptibility before commencing treatment. The clinical laboratory still relies on culture-based methods (20), despite continued interest in sepsis biomarker and other culture-independent technologies. The definition of sepsis has been a point of debate, since it rests on a range of non-specific clinical features and laboratory indicators. The most recent consensus statement on sepsis recognizes only two clinical categories (sepsis and septic shock) and recommends preliminary patient assessment with an easily applied clinical scoring method (qSOFA) (21). The three critical decision steps in the early stages of clinical management of sepsis occur before-, at-, and immediately after hospital admission, which approximate to determination of illness severity, its etiology and the choice of definitive therapy (**Figure 1**). From a precision public health perspective, these correspond to pre-hospital point of care tests that distinguish viral from bacterial infection, rapid hospital biomarker tests for sepsis, or culture-independent tests for severe viral infection and bacteremia and rapid determination of antimicrobial susceptibility. The greatest benefit is most likely to be a pre-hospital, rule-out test that distinguishes possible bacterial from viral infection (22). Improved speed and accuracy of bacterial detection and antimicrobial susceptibility testing has thus become a priority in managing the subsequent stages of sepsis and demands a culture-independent approach (23).

ANTIMICROBIAL SUSCEPTIBILITY TESTS

The mechanisms of AMR are numerous, increasing in variety, prevalence, and geographic distribution (24), but the ecological inevitability of AMR should not have caught us by surprise. Many antimicrobial agents are derivatives of naturally occurring compounds, whose corresponding AMR has its origins in the environment in which the antimicrobial compound evolved (25). However, the global success of a small number of multiresistant species such as *Klebsiella pneumoniae* (26) happened faster than predicted. The invisible, abstract nature of this public health threat is one of the more difficult aspects of the challenge we now face. It is unfortunate that the clinical laboratory markers of AMR do not translate into specific infectious diseases like

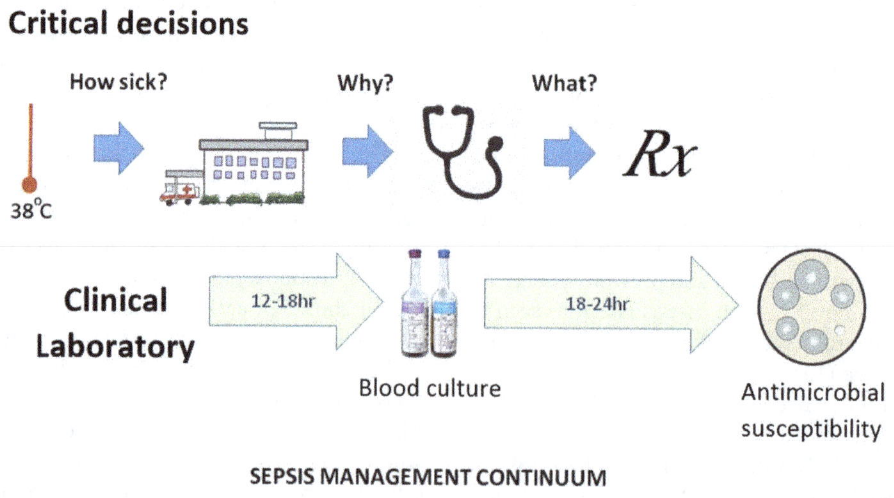

FIGURE 1 | The sepsis management continuum, showing alignment of time-critical clinical decision points with clinical microbiology laboratory data generation.

septicemia, pneumonia, or meningitis. The bacterial species names that appear on public health notification lists are not by themselves notifiable diseases. Despite its limitations, the international standard method of antimicrobial susceptibility testing; broth microdilution minimum inhibitory concentration (MIC), converts the susceptibility of a particular bacterial isolate into a comprehensible measurement (27). The widely performed disc diffusion susceptibility test converts antimicrobial susceptibility into a visible and qualitative approximation to clinical outcome; sensitive or resistant. Disc diffusion and MIC tests, therefore, generate measurable and clinically valuable indicators of the antimicrobial effect against named bacteria, whereas resistance mechanism detection by nucleic acid amplification, gene sequencing, or other molecular means is not a reliable quantitative measure of antimicrobial sensitivity. The guidance these susceptibility tests give the prescriber in their choice of antimicrobial agent relies on a second growth step, which adds a further delay to the clinical laboratory process. Many prescribers are not interested in the specific identity of AMR mechanisms, particularly if the overall AMR phenotype is a combination of multiple molecular mechanisms, with varied *in vivo* expression and an unpredictable impact on clinical outcome. A carbapenem-resistant *K. pneumoniae* septicemia cannot be treated with a carbapenem, whether the mechanism of resistance is NDM-1, OXA-48, VIM, or IMP. The antimicrobial susceptibility phenotype is, therefore, a critical decider in the sepsis management continuum, even if the laboratory result comes 24–48 h after the initial choice of presumptive antimicrobial therapy. The susceptibility phenotype currently determines definitive therapy and ultimately informs the wider public health community. At present, surveillance data on antimicrobial susceptibility vary with laboratory capability, capacity, and locally determined public health priorities. These are all under-resourced, particularly in remote regional settings and in low-income countries (28). Nevertheless, multinational networks such as EARSS and CAESAR collect regional AMR data and interest is growing in standardizing the susceptibility tests on which surveillance relies (29–31). The monitoring task is easier when centers that combine a longstanding interest in sepsis and AMR collect prospective data from invasive infections (32).

EMERGING LABORATORY APPROACHES TO AMR

Rapid, culture-independent phenotypic tests are needed that improve precision in antimicrobial prescribing (17, 18). In particular, tests are needed that measure antimicrobial susceptibility, indicate effective treatment choices and deliver their results closer to the point of care. The wide diversity of molecular mechanisms of AMR limits the value of nucleic acid amplification (PCR assays) as a guide to antibiotic selection in acute clinical settings, particularly for carbapenem-resistant Gram-negative bacteria, which require supplementary tests to improve test sensitivity and overall coverage (33). Much effort has been devoted to detection of AMR mechanisms by rapid whole bacterial genome sequencing (3). Though this approach is not yet feasible as a routine service in the clinical laboratory, bacterial genome sequencing has clear application to public health investigations of AMR infection (3, 11, 26, 34), where decision triggers and task selection procedures can be applied to avoid overloading reference laboratory capacity. Clinical microbiologists who have to cope with the practical scientific challenge of detecting AMR while patients are still under treatment concentrate their effort on standardizing accurate measurement of the AMR phenotype (29). Faster methods of antimicrobial susceptibility testing are now a high priority, as noted in one of the O'Neill Review's technical reports (35). It is here that systems biology applications are beginning to bear fruit (36). However, careful validation is necessary before

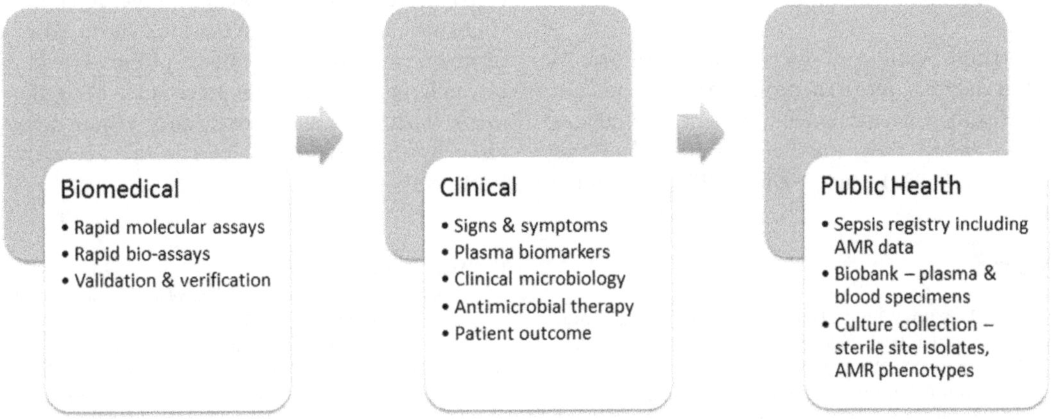

FIGURE 2 | Technical progression in support of AMR/sepsis countermeasures.

emerging technologies can be used in the clinical laboratory. This requires test verification and harmonization to maximize analytical value and avoid poorly coordinated proliferation (29, 30). Systematic validation of new antimicrobial susceptibility test methods against agreed reference standards is a necessary step to delivering sufficient confidence in emerging laboratory methods before they can be used for surveillance and control purposes. High profile incentives such as the UK Longitude Prize are being used to attract new candidate tests for this lengthy development process (37).

A BLEND OF COUNTERMEASURES

Countermeasures need purpose, intent, direction, and evidence for their efficacy. An understanding of the complex intersection of laboratory, clinical, and public health insights will improve their beneficial effect (16). AMR specific countermeasures, therefore, operate at three levels (**Figure 2**) beginning with faster and more accurate phenotypic laboratory assays that use agreed international standards (29, 30, 36). The O'Neill Review expects new laboratory technology to enable recognition of sepsis, its etiology and antimicrobial susceptibility faster than current culture-dependent methods (35). At the clinical level, prescribing physicians need incentives such as faster confirmation of the etiology of infection and its antimicrobial susceptibility to use the evidence-based antimicrobial therapy advocated in the O'Neill Review (18). In addition to the recommended clinical sepsis score (21), prescribing physicians need a bacterial infection rule-out test to support their initial sepsis triage (22) and innovative methods of rapid antimicrobial susceptibility testing to support their decision-making at the point of care. However, a clearer picture of the global burden of AMR and the measures to control it will not emerge until variations in regional AMR notification have been harmonized through introduction of a sepsis/AMR registry (**Figure 2**). Other fields of medicine, such as oncology, use case registries to develop and refine their disease-specific countermeasures (38, 39). A sepsis registry could be used in similar manner as a precision public health tool to stratify sepsis by syndrome, etiology, AMR phenotype, and resistance mechanism, and, therefore, to coordinate AMR countermeasures. The recent consensus definition of sepsis is a helpful starting point for discussion of a sepsis registry (21), but requires a stronger laboratory-based emphasis on bacterial etiology and AMR. Precision is measurable, particularly when supported by archival material in bacterial culture collections and registered clinical biobanks. Claims for the increased accuracy of new methods should thus be verifiable and linked with the clinical laboratory, where the precision of antimicrobial susceptibility tests is already monitored against reference standards and verified by regulatory agencies (29, 30).

CONCLUSION

Antimicrobial resistance has become a global tragedy of the commons, driven by a complex bacterial survival trade-off at a cellular level (40). Now that AMR is recognized as a global priority, it is time to learn to use additional systems biology tools to improve the speed and accuracy of antimicrobial prescribing at an individual patient level and simultaneously increase the precision of AMR sepsis surveillance. Improved confidence in the recognition of early sepsis, faster determination of its etiology, and antimicrobial susceptibility phenotype, and real time surveillance through an AMR sepsis registry will lead to more effective coordination of clinical, laboratory and public health AMR countermeasures. Given the speed with which antimicrobial agents have been compromised by AMR, there is no time to lose introducing these laboratory and surveillance tools into wider use.

AUTHOR CONTRIBUTIONS

The authors are working together on culture-independent pathology test development. TI prepared the initial draft. NU reviewed, edited, and supplemented the first draft with an emphasis on sepsis. Subsequent versions of the manuscript were exchanged between the authors who both approved the final version.

FUNDING

The authors' work on AMR and sepsis countermeasures is supported by translational research project grants from the Department of Health, Government of Western Australia, a Grand Challenges Award from the Bill and Melinda Gates Foundation (OPP 1150984), the NATO SPS Programme (project grant 984835), philanthropic donations from Rotary Clubs and Lab Without Walls Inc., and in-kind contributions from Thermo Fisher Scientific and Biomerieux Australia. This research is conducted in accordance with the Government of Western Australia's governance requirements and supervised by the Department of Health's Research Development Unit.

REFERENCES

1. Boucher HW, Bakken JS, Murray BE. The United Nations and the urgent need for coordinated global action in the fight against antimicrobial resistance. *Ann Intern Med* (2016) 165(11):812–3. doi:10.7326/M16-2079
2. Khoury MJ, Iademarco MF, Riley WT. Precision public health for the era of precision medicine. *Am J Prev Med* (2016) 50(3):398–401. doi:10.1016/j.amepre.2015.08.031
3. Thomsen MC, Ahrenfeld J, Cisneros JL, Jurtz V, Larsen MV, Hasman H, et al. A bacterial analysis platform: an integrated system for analysing bacterial whole genome sequencing data for clinical diagnostics and surveillance. *PLoS One* (2016) 11:e0157718. doi:10.1371/journal.pone.0157718
4. Heesterbeek H, Anderson RM, Andreasen V, Bansal S, De Angelis D, Dye C, et al. Modelling infectious disease dynamics in the complex landscape of global health. *Science* (2015) 347(6227):aaa4339. doi:10.1126/science.aaa4339
5. Carter RR, Sun J, Jump RL. A survey and analysis of the American public's perceptions and knowledge about antibiotic resistance. *Open Forum Infect Dis* (2016) 3(3):ofw112. doi:10.1093/ofid/ofw112
6. Shallcross LJ, Berin M, Roe J, Noursadeghi M. Are the public getting the message about antimicrobial resistance? *Arch Public Health* (2015) 73:55. doi:10.1186/s13690-015-0108-6
7. Premanandh J, Samara BS, Mazen AM. Race against antimicrobial resistance requires coordinated action – an overview. *Front Microbiol* (2016) 6:1536. doi:10.3389/fmicb.2015.01536
8. Freedman L. *Strategy: A History*. Oxford, UK: Oxford University Press (2013).
9. Colwell R. Biocomplexity: an umbrella for many disciplines. *IEEE Eng Med Biol Mag* (2001) 20:13–5.
10. Chang HH, Cohen T, Grad YH, Hanage WP, O'Brien TF, Lipsitch M. Origin and proliferation of multiple drug resistance in bacterial pathogens. *Microbiol Mol Biol Rev* (2015) 79(1):101–16. doi:10.1128/MMBR.00039-14
11. Bradford PA, Kazmierczak KM, Biedenbach DJ, Wise MG, Hackel M, Sahm DF. Correlation of β-lactamase production and colistin resistance among Enterobacteriaceae isolates from a global surveillance program. *Antimicrob Agents Chemother* (2015) 60(3):1385–92. doi:10.1128/AAC.01870-15
12. Hassing RJ, Alsma J, Arcilla MS, van Genderen PJ, Stricker BH, Verbon A. International travel and acquisition of multidrug-resistance Enterobactericeae: a systematic review. *Euro Surveill* (2015) 20(47). doi:10.2807/1560-7917.ES.2015.20.47.30074
13. Lee CR, Lee JH, Park KS, Kim YB, Jeong BC, Lee SH. Global dissemination of carbapenemase-producing *Klebsiella pneumoniae*: epidemiology, genetic context, treatment options, and detection methods. *Front Microbiol* (2016) 7:895. doi:10.3389/fmicb.2016.00895
14. Birger RB, Kouyos RD, Cohen T, Griffiths EC, Huijben S, Mina MJ, et al. The potential impact of coinfection on antimicrobial chemotherapy and drug resistance. *Trends Microbiol* (2015) 23(9):537–44. doi:10.1016/j.tim.2015.05.002
15. Harder T, Takla A, Rehfuess E, Sánchez-Vivar A, Matysiak-Klose D, Eckmanns T, et al. Evidence-based decision-making in infectious diseases epidemiology, prevention and control: matching research questions to study designs and quality appraisal tools. *BMC Med Res Methodol* (2014) 14:69. doi:10.1186/1471-2288-14-69
16. Inglis TJJ. Principia aetiologica: taking causality beyond Koch's postulates. *J Med Microbiol* (2007) 56(Pt 11):1419–22. doi:10.1099/jmm.0.47179-0
17. Inglis TJJ, Eitzen EM, Robertson AG. Forensic investigation of biological weapon use. Ch 2. In: Gall J, Payne-James J, editors. *Current Practice in Forensic Medicine*. Oxford, UK: Wiley-Blackwell (2011). p. 17–42.
18. Anon. Tackling drug-resistant infections globally: final report and recommendations. *The Review on Antimicrobial Resistance*. Westminster, UK: HM Government (2016). p. 1–73.
19. Machiavelli N. *The Prince*. Bull G, trans. London, UK: Penguin (2003).
20. De Santis V, Gresoiu M, Corona A, Wilson AP, Singer M. Bacteraemia incidence, causative organisms and resistance patterns, antibiotic strategies and outcomes in a single university hospital ICU: continuing improvement between 2000 and 2013. *J Antimicrob Chemother* (2015) 70(1):273–8. doi:10.1093/jac/dku338
21. Singer M, Deutschman CS, Seymour CW, Shankar-Hari M, Annane D, Bauer M, et al. The third international consensus definitions for sepsis and septic shock (sepsis-3). *JAMA* (2016) 315(8):801–10. doi:10.1001/jama.2016.0287
22. Sambursky R, Shapiro N. Evaluation of a combined MxA and CRP point-of-care immunoassay to identify viral and/or bacterial immune response in patients with acute febrile respiratory infection. *Eur Clin Respir J* (2015) 2:28245. doi:10.3402/ecrj.v2.28245
23. Inglis TJJ. Culture-independent diagnostic tests. *Annual Scientific Meeting, Perth 3rd July*. Australian Society for Microbiology (2016).
24. Kaye KS, Engemann JJ, Fraimow HS, Abrutyn E. Pathogens resistant to antimicrobial agents. Epidemiology, molecular mechanisms, and clinical management. *Infect Dis Clin North Am* (2004) 18(3):467–511. doi:10.1016/j.idc.2004.04.003
25. Davies J, Davies D. Origins and evolution of antibiotic resistance. *Microbiol Mol Biol Rev* (2010) 74(3):417–33. doi:10.1128/MMBR.00016-10
26. Holt KE, Wertheim H, Zadoks RN, Baker S, Whitehouse CA, Dance D, et al. Genomic analysis of diversity, population structure, virulence, and antimicrobial resistance in *Klebsiella pneumoniae*, an urgent threat to public health. *Proc Natl Acad Sci U S A* (2015) 112(27):E3574–81. doi:10.1073/pnas.1501049112
27. Jorgensen JH, Ferraro MJ. Antimicrobial susceptibility testing: a review of general principles and contemporary practices. *Clin Infect Dis* (2009) 49(11):1749–55. doi:10.1086/647952
28. Ashley EA, Lubell Y, White NJ, Turner P. Antimicrobial susceptibility of bacterial isolates from community acquired infections in Sub-Saharan Africa and Asian low and middle income countries. *Trop Med Int Health* (2011) 16(9):1167–79. doi:10.1111/j.1365-3156.2011.02822.x
29. Kahlmeter G. Defining antibiotic resistance-towards international harmonization. *Ups J Med Sci* (2014) 119(2):78–86. doi:10.3109/03009734.2014.901446
30. Desmet S, Verhaegen J, Glupzcynski Y, Van Eldere J, Melin P, Goossens H, et al. Development of a national EUCAST challenge panel for antimicrobial susceptibility testing. *Clin Microbiol Infect* (2016) 22(8):704–10. doi:10.1016/j.cmi.2016.05.011
31. Brown D, Canton R, Dubreuil L, Gatermann S, Giske C, MacGowan A, et al. Widespread implementation of EUCAST breakpoints for antibacterial susceptibility testing in Europe. *Euro Surveill* (2015) 20(2):21008. doi:10.2807/1560-7917.ES2015.20.2.21008
32. Bell JM, Turnidge JD, Coombs GW, Daley DA, Gottlieb T, Robson J, et al. Australian group on antimicrobial resistance Australian enterobacteriaceae sepsis outcome programme annual report, 2014. *Commun Dis Intell Q Rep* (2016) 40(2):E229–35.
33. Findlay J, Hopkins KL, Meunier D, Woodford N. Evaluation of three commercial assays for rapid detection of genes encoding clinically relevant carbapenemases in cultured bacteria. *J Antimicrob Chemother* (2015) 70(5):1338–42. doi:10.1093/jac/dku571

34. Garvey MI, Pichon B, Bradley CW, Moiemen NS, Oppenheim B, Kearns AM. Improved understanding of an outbreak of methicillin-resistant *Staphylococcus aureus* in a regional burns centre via whole-genome sequencing. *J Hosp Infect* (2016) 94(4):401–4. doi:10.1016/j.jhin.2016.09.013
35. Anon. Rapid diagnostics: stopping unnecessary use of antibiotics. *The Review on Antimicrobial Resistance*. Westminster, UK: HM Government (2015). p. 1–33.
36. VanBelkum A, Dunne WM. Next-generation antimicrobial susceptibility testing. *J Clin Microbiol* (2013) 51(7):2018–24. doi:10.1128/JCM.00313-13
37. Ribbing CG. Awards: longitude prize now an objective decision. *Nature* (2014) 511(7507):31. doi:10.1038/511031e
38. Bellei M, Nabhan C, Pesce EA, Conte L, Vose JM, Foss F, et al. The value and relevance of the T cell lymphoma registries and international collaborations: the case of COMPLETE and the T-cell project. *Curr Hematol Malig Rep* (2015) 10(4):448–55. doi:10.1007/s11899-015-0291-0
39. Rice HE, Englum BR, Gulack BC, Adibe OO, Tracy ET, Kreissman SG, et al. Use of patient registries and administrative datasets for the study of pediatric cancer. *Pediatr Blood Cancer* (2015) 62(9):1495–500. doi:10.1002/pbc.25506
40. MacLean RC. The tragedy of the commons in microbial populations: insights from theoretical, comparative and experimental studies. *Heredity (Edinb)* (2008) 100(5):471–7. doi:10.1038/sj.hdy.6801073

15

Physician's Knowledge of Appropriate Prescribing for the Elderly—A Survey among Family and Internal Medicine Physicians in Nigeria

Joseph O. Fadare[1], Abimbola Margaret Obimakinde[2,3], Okezie O. Enwere[4], Olufemi O. Desalu[5] and Raphael Olasoji Ibidapo[6]*

[1] Department of Pharmacology and Therapeutics, Ekiti State University College of Medicine, Ado-Ekiti, Nigeria, [2] Family Medicine Unit, Department of Community Medicine, College of Medicine, University of Ibadan, Ibadan, Nigeria, [3] Family Medicine Department, University College Hospital, Ibadan, Nigeria, [4] Department of Medicine, Imo State University, Orlu, Nigeria, [5] Department of Medicine, College of Health Sciences, University of Ilorin, Ilorin, Nigeria, [6] Department of Medicine, Ekiti State University Teaching Hospital, Ado-Ekiti, Nigeria

***Correspondence:**
Joseph O. Fadare
joseph.fadare@eksu.edu.ng
jofadare@gmail.com*

Background: Prescription and use of inappropriate medications have been identified as a major cause of morbidity among the elderly. Several screening tools have been developed to identify inappropriate medications prescribed for elderly patients. There is dearth of information about the knowledge of Nigerian physicians regarding these screening tools and appropriate prescribing for the elderly in general. The primary objective of this study was to assess the knowledge of Nigerian physicians about these screening tools and appropriate prescribing of medications for the elderly.

Methods: The study was a cross-sectional questionnaire-based study conducted among physicians working in Family Medicine and Internal Medicine departments of four tertiary health care facilities in Nigeria. The questionnaire consisted of sections on general characteristics of respondents and their knowledge of four selected screening tools for inappropriate medications in the elderly. Ten clinical vignettes representing different therapeutic areas (using the best option type questions) about medicine use in the elderly were included with a score of 1 and 0 for correct and wrong answers, respectively. The knowledge of respondents was classified as (total score, over 10): poor (score, < 5), average (score, 5-6), and good (score, 7-10).

Results: One hundred and five physicians returned completed questionnaires. Twenty percent of respondents knew about Beers criteria, whereas 15.6% were familiar with the STOPP criteria. Majority (83; 84.7%) of the respondents were confident of their ability to prescribeappropriately for elderly patients. The mean knowledge score was 5.3 ± 2.0 with 32 (30.5%), 41 (39%), and 32 (30.5%) having low, average, and good scores, respectively. The association between the knowledge score, duration of practice, and seniority was statistically significant (OR, 3.6, $p = .004$ and OR, 3; $p = .012$), respectively.

Conclusion: There are significant gaps in the knowledge of Nigerian physicians about screening tools for inappropriate medications. There is a need for stakeholders involved in the care of elderly Nigerian patients to develop new strategies to improve services being offered. These may include introduction of modules on appropriate prescribing in the curriculum of undergraduate and postgraduate medical education and the routine use of some screening tools for inappropriate medications in daily clinical practice.

Keywords: inappropriate prescribing, elderly patients, rational prescribing, adverse drug reactions, physicians

INTRODUCTION

Drug treatment of elderly patients is associated with potential adverse drug reactions (ADRs) with prescription and use of inappropriate medications being responsible in many cases (Dormann et al., 2013; Oscanoa et al., 2017). A systematic review on the prevalence and risk factors for ADRs in the elderly found a mean prevalence of 10% (Alhawassi et al., 2014). Patel and Patel (2018) demonstrated a four-fold increase in mortality due to ADR in elderly patients when compared to children. Identified factors for ADR in the elderly include polypharmacy and multiple co-morbidities on the background of declining physiological functions of the liver and kidneys (Joshua et al., 2007; Alhawassi et al., 2014; Sonnerstam et al., 2016). Also, changes in cognitive functions may affect adherence and other medicine-use issues (Wucherer et al., 2017).

Several tools/criteria have been developed over time to address the problem of inappropriate prescribing for elderly patients and these include the Beers criteria, Screening Tool of Older Persons' potentially inappropriate Prescription (STOPP) criteria, Medication Appropriateness Index (MAI), and the Zhan criteria (Beers et al., 1991; Hanlon et al., 1992; Zhan et al., 2001; Gallagher et al., 2008). Other recently developed tools are the European Union list of potentially inappropriate medications (EU(7)-PIM list) (Renom-Guiteras et al., 2015), PRISCUS (developed in Germany) (Holt et al., 2010), and Improved Prescribing in the Elderly Tool (IPET) (Naugler et al., 2000) developed in Canada. Emerging economies like Brazil and Thailand have also developed their own context-specific instruments to screen for inappropriate medications in the elderly building on the foundation of the older instruments (Almeida et al., 2018; Prasert et al., 2018). The Beers list, an explicit criterion initially developed in 1991, has been regularly updated to cater for new scientific findings regarding appropriateness of medications in the elderly. Its latest update was in 2015 by the American Geriatric Society (AGS), and most of the newer tools were developed using it as a model (American Geriatrics Society, 2015). Negative patient outcomes, such as falls and delirium, have been associated with some of the drugs listed in the Beers criteria (Rothberg et al., 2013; Bazargan et al., 2018). The main emphasis of the STOPP criteria is in the area of avoidable adverse drug events (ADEs) and potential drug–drug interactions. Results from a meta-analysis of four randomized control trials (RCTs) showed a reduction in falls and episodes of delirium when STOPP criteria were applied (Hill-Taylor et al., 2016). The MAI is a 10-item question-based implicit criterion that takes into consideration the indication, effectiveness, dose, and direction for use among others (Hanlon and Schmader, 2013). The Zhan criteria, a modification of the Beers criteria, classify into 33 drugs into three categories according to their appropriateness or otherwise (Zhan et al., 2001).

The body of research in the area of prescription of potentially inappropriate medications and its consequences in elderly patients continues to grow in developing countries, like Nigeria and South Africa (Fadare et al., 2013; Fadare et al., 2015; Van Heerden et al., 2016; Akande-Sholabi et al., 2018; Saka et al., 2018). With improvement in the management of communicable diseases, such as HIV/AIDS, malaria, and tuberculosis, people are living longer in many developing countries and as such the proportion of elderly patients is expected to rise significantly in the next decade. Nigeria, the most populous country in Africa, has an estimated population of over 190 million with the elderly comprising just over 5% [Nigerian Demographic and Health Survey (NDHS), 2013]. The health care system is made up of private, faith-based, and public health care facilities. The public health care system of the country currently comprises three levels of care: primary, secondary, and tertiary. The tertiary level facilities, which are made up of Federal Medical Centres and University Teaching Hospitals, are the best equipped and have the most qualified health care personnel in the country. They are also training centers for medical students and postgraduate resident doctors in various specialties of medicine. These centers are the most patronized by the public because of the poor level of functionality of many primary and secondary level facilities in Nigeria. Therefore, there is a need for prescribers to be knowledgeable about potentially inappropriate medications and to actively screen prescriptions written for elderly patients. There are reports from some countries about the knowledge and attitude of physicians toward prescription of potentially inappropriate medications for elderly (Maio et al., 2011; Ramaswamy et al., 2011). There is, however, a dearth of information regarding this important issue in Nigeria and thus is the rationale for this study.

The primary objective of this study was to assess the knowledge of Nigerian physicians working in Family Medicine and Internal Medicine about appropriate prescribing of medications for the elderly. Secondary objectives included familiarity with screening tools for inappropriate medications and identification of barriers limiting appropriate prescription for the elderly.

METHODOLOGY

The study was a cross-sectional questionnaire-based study conducted among physicians working in four tertiary health care facilities in Nigeria.

STUDY SETTING

The study was conducted in the Family and Internal Medicine departments of four tertiary level health care facilities located in the South-Western, South-Eastern, and North-Central regions of Nigeria between January and April 2017. The health care facilities are: Ekiti State University Teaching Hospital, Ado-Ekiti (South-West), University College Hospital, Ibadan (South-West), University of Ilorin Teaching Hospital, Ilorin (North-Central), and the Imo State University Teaching Hospital, Orlu (South-East). The choice of these two specialities is because elderly outpatients are seen mainly in the clinics manned by residents and consultants from the departments. The departments of family and internal medicine in each of these facilities run daily outpatient clinics for ambulatory patients. The participating centers were selected through convenient sampling as some of the co-investigators were based there.

STUDY PARTICIPANTS

Inclusion Criteria

Physicians (residents and consultants) working in the Family and Internal Medicine Departments of the participating health care facilities who consented to the study.

Exclusion Criteria

House physicians working in the Family and Internal Medicine Departments of the participating health care facilities because of their limited knowledge and experience with prescribing.

STUDY INSTRUMENT

The self-administered questionnaire, developed in English language, was adapted from similar studies conducted in Italy and India among primary care physicians (Maio et al., 2011; Ramaswamy et al., 2011) and consisted of two parts: bio-demographics details, prescription experience for the elderly and respondent's perception about factors affecting appropriate prescribing for the elderly are captured in the first section. The second part was made up of 10 clinical vignettes about medication use in the elderly in the form of best option multiple-choice questions with a score of 1 and 0 allocated for a correct and wrong answer, respectively (**Supplementary Material Appendix A**). The scenarios described in the vignettes consisted of therapeutic problems of the central nervous (Nos. 3, 6, 10), endocrine (No. 9), musculoskeletal (No. 5), and cardiovascular systems (Nos. 1, 2, 7, 8). The knowledge of respondents was classified as (total score over 10): poor (score <5), average (score 5–6), and good (score 7–10). The questionnaire was reviewed for reliability and content validity by the principal researcher and two co-authors who are experts in clinical pharmacology and therapeutics, geriatrics and family medicine. Subsequently, it was pilot tested among 10 physicians working in the Family Medicine Department of a tertiary health care facility located within the same region, which was not part of the study. Based on their responses, the questionnaire was revised and necessary adjustments made before administration to study participants.

All physicians working in the departments of Family Medicine and Internal Medicine of the four participating hospitals were approached to participate in the study. The chief residents of the selected departments were asked to distribute the questionnaires to the physicians during mandatory departmental programs such as grand rounds and seminars. A time frame of 30 min was allowed for the completion of the questionnaire.

SAMPLE SIZE

A convenience sampling method that included all 142 physicians working in the Family Medicine and Internal Medicine Departments of four tertiary health care facilities in three geo-political areas of the country was used for this study. All the 142 physicians were invited to participate in the study.

ETHICAL CONSIDERATION

Ethical approval was obtained from the Research and Ethics Committee of the Ekiti State University Teaching Hospital, Ado-Ekiti, Nigeria before commencement of the study. Because the study was questionnaire-based and noninvasive, permission was granted by the other centers based on approval from the primary site.

STATISTICAL ANALYSIS

The information obtained from the questionnaire was coded, entered, and analyzed using IBM SPSS version 19. Analysis was done using descriptive statistics, which was used to obtain the general characteristics of the study participants. Chi-square was used to determine the level of significance of groups of categorical variables. P values < 0.05 were considered significant.

RESULTS

Socio-Demographic Details

One hundred and five physicians returned the completed questionnaires for analysis—a response rate of 73.9%. Majority of respondents (69; 65.7%) were males, senior medical doctors, and worked in internal medicine (65.7%, 52.8%, and 57.3%, respectively). **Table 1** shows the demographic characteristics of respondents. The mean duration of practice was 8.3 ± 6.7 years with 23.8%, 45.7%, and 30.5% of the respondents having practiced for <5 years, 5 to 10 years, and more than 10 years, respectively.

Respondents' Knowledge of Screening Tools for Inappropriate Medications and Sources of Drug Information

The sources of drug information used by respondents were the British National Formulary (BNF), consultations with colleagues, and online sources (**Figure 1**). Regarding respondents' knowledge about screening tools for inappropriate medications, 20.4% and 22.7% of them knew about Beers criteria and MAI, while 15.6% were familiar with the STOPP criteria. **Figure 2** highlights respondents' knowledge of the screening tools. Majority (83; 84.7%) of the respondents were confident of their ability to prescribe rationally for elderly patients.

TABLE 1 | Demographic details of respondents.

Variable	Frequency (%)
Sex	
Male	69 (65.7%)
Female	36 (34.3%)
Position of respondent	
Medical officer	19 (18.1)
Junior resident	31 (29.6)
Senior resident	43 (41)
Consultant	12 (11.4)
Specialty	
Internal medicine	59 (56.2)
Family medicine	46 (43.8)
Duration of practice	
1–5 years	40 (38.1)
>5 years	65 (61.9)

Barriers Against Appropriate Prescribing for the Elderly

Multiple medications (81; 82.6%), potential drug interactions (79; 81.4%), and cost of medicines to the patients (80; 80%) were the most commonly identified barriers against appropriate prescribing for the elderly (**Table 2**).

Respondents' Knowledge of Presented Case Vignettes and Association With Other Study Variables

The mean knowledge score was 5.3 ± 2.0 with 32 (30.5%), 41 (39%), and 32 (30.5%) having low, average, and good scores, respectively. Overall, most respondents had good knowledge of appropriate use of medicines in the elderly in the following therapeutic areas: non-steroidal anti-inflammatory drugs (NSAIDs) (90; 87.6%), centrally acting antihypertensives in the elderly (92; 87.6% and 76; 76.4%), the use of first generation sulfonylureas (81; 77.1%), and the correct use of Nifedipine in hypertensive emergency (80; 76.2%). Poor level of knowledge was demonstrated in therapeutic areas of insomnia (19; 18.1%) and depression (25; 27.2%). The clinical scenario on the effect of NSAIDs on heart failure was answered correctly by 61 (58.1%) respondents.

The variables duration of practice, position, and knowledge score were dichotomized for ease of inferential analysis into the following: younger and older than 5 years, junior (junior residents and medical officers) and senior (senior residents and consultants), and score less than 5 and greater than 5. **Table 3** shows that the association between the knowledge score, duration of practice, and seniority was statistically significant. The strength of this association is further confirmed by the odds ratios (OR) of 3.6 and 3, respectively.

DISCUSSION

This study assessed the knowledge of physicians working in Internal and Family Medicine departments regarding appropriateness of medicines for the elderly and its screening tools. Overall, the knowledge score of respondents was above average with majority of them dealing correctly with clinical scenarios affecting the cardiovascular, endocrine, and gastrointestinal systems.

Screening tools, such as the Beers criteria, STOPP, MAI, and Zhan criteria, are a group of explicit and sometimes implicit classification of medicines used for elderly patients. Medications on these lists have been found to contribute significantly to morbidity in elderly patients (Price et al., 2014; Sarwar et al., 2018). Only about a fifth of respondents in this study knew about the Beers criteria and the MAI with another 15% having information about the STOPP criteria. The knowledge level among respondents in our study is slightly better than that reported in qualitative studies among general practitioners in Australia and Germany (Magin et al., 2015; Pohontsch et al., 2017). In the just-cited studies, respondents showed a high level of confidence in appropriate

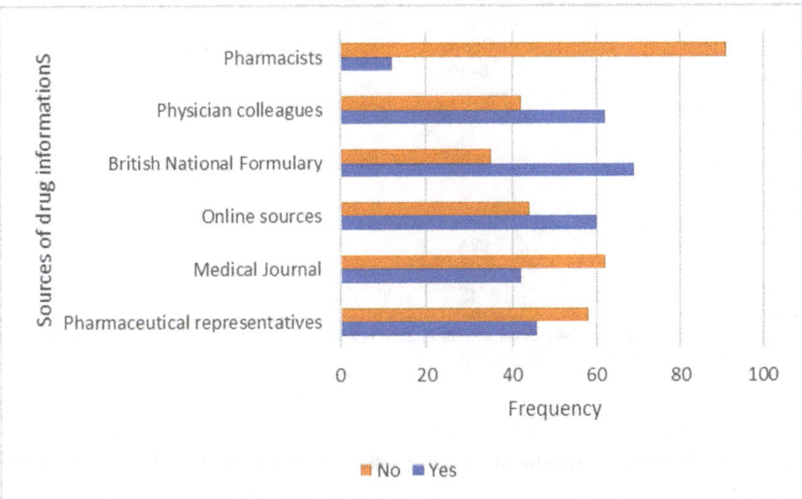

FIGURE 1 | The sources of drug information used by respondents.

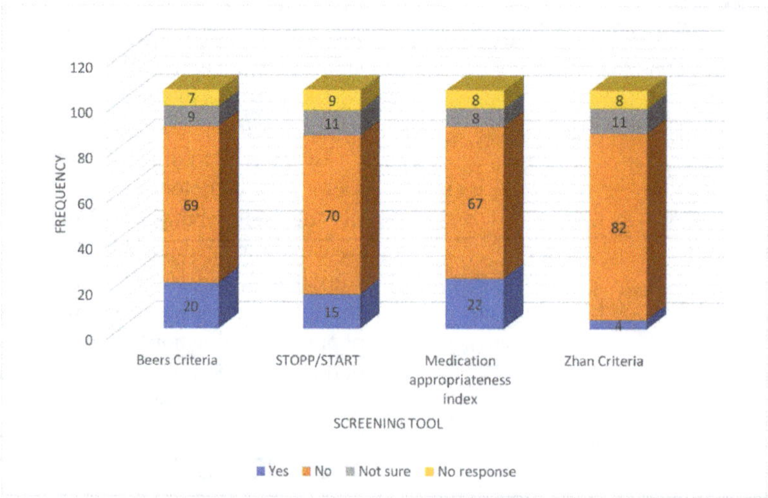

FIGURE 2 | Respondents knowledge of the screening tools.

TABLE 2 | Identified barriers against appropriate prescribing for the elderly.

Factors	Strongly agree (%)	Agree (%)	Neutral (%)	Disagree (%)	Strongly disagree (%)	Missing
Lack of time in the office schedule	12 (12.1)	21 (21.2)	18 (18.2)	35 (35.4)	13 (13.1)	6
Lack of acceptable therapeutic alternatives	5 (5.2)	45 (46.4)	20 (20.6)	21 (21.6)	6 (5.7)	8
Potential drug interactions	24 (24.7)	55 (56.7)	9 (9.3)	7 (7.2)	2 (2.1)	8
Cost of medication to patient	28 (28)	52 (52)	10 (10)	8 (8)	2 (2)	5
Patient request to begin a specific medication	4 (4.1)	29 (29.6)	30 (30.6)	30 (30.6)	4 (4.1)	8
Lack of information about which medications a patient is already taking	5 (5.1)	56 (57.1)	11 (11.2)	24 (24.5)	2 (2)	7
Lack of formal education on prescribing for the elderly	8 (0)	33 (33)	18 (18)	33 (33)	8 (8)	5
Large number of medications a patient is taking	21 (21.2)	61 (61.6)	6 (6.1)	10 (10.1)	1 (1)	6
Unwillingness to discontinue a medication prescribed by another physician	3 (3.1)	34 (34.7)	26 (26.5)	34 (34.7)	1 (1)	7
Difficulty communicating with other physicians who participate in a patient's care	10 10.1)	37 (37.4)	20 (20.2)	30 (30.3)	2 (2)	6
No feedback from the pharmacy	21 (21.4)	34 (34.7)	21 (21.4)	19 (19.4)	3 (3.1)	7

TABLE 3 | Association between the knowledge score and some variables.

Variables	Score 0–4	Score 5–10	Chi-square	OR	95% CI
Junior physician	21	28	.012*	3.0*	1.26–7.16
Senior physician	11	44			
1–5 years practice	19	21	.004*	3.62*	1.52–8.63
>5 years practice	13	52			
Male	20	49	.646	0.82	0.34–1.94
Female	12	24			
Family medicine	15	29	.67	0.78	0.33–1.81
Internal medicine	17	42			

**The variables duration of practice, position, and knowledge score were dichotomized for ease of inferential analysis into the following: less than or greater than 5 years, junior (junior residents and medical officers), and senior (senior residents and consultants).*

prescribing for elderly patients despite their poor knowledge of the screening tools. Similarly, over 80% of our respondents were also confident of appropriate prescribing for the elderly despite their poor knowledge of the screening tools. This might be due to the fact that many physicians may have used their residual knowledge of clinical pharmacology and understanding of the clinical scenarios to address prescribing issues in the elderly.

Respondents in this study identified high cost of medicines, potential drug interactions, and difficulty in communicating with other prescribers as barriers in addition to the ones cited in literature. Barriers to appropriate prescribing for the elderly from literature include limited knowledge of potentially inappropriate medications, extra time needed to consult the criteria, high number of prescribed medications, poor communication, and lack of formal education of prescribing guidelines (Maio et al., 2011; Clyne et al., 2016; Voigt et al., 2016).

Close to 70% of respondents scored above average in the clinical vignettes, indicating a good understanding of therapeutic issues in elderly patients. Our findings are similar to that from an Italian study with seven clinical scenarios where only 17% of respondents had low scores (Maio et al., 2011). Similarly, the mean score in an Indian study among family and internal medicine physicians was above average (3.9/6) (Ramaswamy et al., 2011). Respondents in our study were more knowledgeable in therapeutic areas of hypertension, diabetes mellitus, and osteoarthritis. This is not surprising because these are the most common disease conditions found among Nigerian elderly patients (Fadare et al., 2013, Fadare et al., 2015; Cadmus et al., 2017). This is in contrast to areas like arrhythmias, insomnia, depression, and other central nervous system (CNS) problems where low scores were recorded. The poor knowledge in therapeutic areas of insomnia and depression also resonates with the findings from Nigerian studies on prescription of inappropriate medicines where benzodiazepines (diazepam) and antidepressants (amitriptyline) were among the most common inappropriate medicines identified (Fadare et al., 2013, Fadare et al., 2015; Akande-Sholabi et al., 2018). On the contrary, respondents in the earlier-cited Italian study had better than average knowledge in therapeutic areas of insomnia and depression, whereas a similar poor performance was reported in the clinical vignette on the use of amiodarone in the elderly (Maio et al., 2011). The association between the knowledge score, duration of practice, and position was strong with OR of 3.62 and 3, respectively. In contrast, the study by Maio et al. (2011) reported respondents with low score had been in practice for longer duration. The reported higher score in our study is likely due to the working environment of respondents with many of them at various levels of postgraduate specialist training or were consultant physicians in charge of the training programs.

The BNF, physician colleagues, and the Internet were the most common sources of medicines information used by respondents. Medical textbooks, journals, and physician colleagues were the most identified sources in an earlier study conducted in Italy (Maio et al., 2011). Similarly, report from an earlier Nigerian survey among 163 medical doctors indicated information from colleagues, reference books, and pharmaceutical sales representatives as the main sources (Oshikoya et al., 2011). The rapid growth of information and communication technology (ICT) globally and especially its use in medicine is likely responsible for the change in trend.

STUDY LIMITATIONS

This study is associated with some limitations. The study was conducted in a few tertiary health care facilities and hence may not reflect the reality among physicians working in primary and secondary care facilities worldwide nationwide. Since the questionnaire was also self-administered, there is also the possibility of bias while responding. The lack of similar studies from Nigeria and other African countries with which to compare our findings may also have affected the discussion of this study. However, the use of previously validated questionnaire, relatively high proportion of respondents from the sampling frame, representation from different cadres of physicians and different regions of the country are potential strengths of the study.

CONCLUSION

There are significant gaps in the knowledge of Nigerian physicians about screening tools for inappropriate medications. There is a need for stakeholders involved in the care of elderly Nigerian patients to develop new strategies to improve services being offered. This may include introduction of modules on appropriate prescribing in the curriculum of undergraduate and postgraduate medical education in Nigeria.

IMPLICATIONS FOR PRACTICE (FUTURE DIRECTIONS)

There is a need to incorporate the use of some of the established screening tools, such as the Beers and STOPP criteria in the daily clinical practice of Nigerian physicians. The development of a context-specific screening tool may be the direction to go for stakeholders in geriatric care in Nigeria.

AUTHORS CONTRIBUTIONS

JF conceptualized and designed the study. He also analyzed the data and developed the first draft of the manuscript. AO took active part in conceptualizing the study. She was involved in data acquisition and analysis and reviewed the initial draft of manuscript for critical intellectual content. OE was involved in conducting the literature search for the work and also in data acquisition, and reviewed the initial draft of the manuscript. OD was involved in data acquisition and analysis and reviewed the draft manuscript before final approval. RI was involved in the literature search, data acquisition, and analysis, and also reviewed the draft manuscript. All co-authors approved the final draft of the manuscript.

ACKNOWLEDGMENTS

The authors are grateful to the physicians who took the time to complete the questionnaires.

REFERENCES

Akande-Sholabi, W., Adebusoye, L. A., and Olowookere, O. O. (2018). Potentially inappropriate medication use among older patients attending a geriatric centre in south-west Nigeria. *Pharm. Prac.* 16 (3), 1235. doi: 10.18549/PharmPract.2018.03.1235

Alhawassi, T. M., Krass, I., Bajorek, B. V., and Pont, L. G. (2014). A systematic review of the prevalence and risk factors for adverse drug reactions in the elderly in the acute care setting. *Clin. Interv. Aging* 9, 2079–2086. doi: 10.2147/CIA.S71178

Almeida, T. A., Reis, E. A., Pinto, I. V. L., Ceccato, M., Silveira, M. R., Lima, M. G., et al. (2018). Factors associated with the use of potentially inappropriate medications by older adults in primary health care: an analysis comparing AGS Beers, EU(7)-PIM List, and Brazilian Consensus PIM criteria. *Res. Social Adm. Pharm.* 15 (4), 370–377. doi: 10.1016/j.sapharm.2018.06.002

American Geriatrics Society (2015). Updated Beers Criteria for Potentially Inappropriate Medication Use in Older Adults. *J. Am. Geriatr. Soc.* 63 (11), 2227–2246. doi: 10.1111/jgs.13702

Bazargan, M., Smith, J. L., and King, E. O. (2018). Potentially inappropriate medication use among hypertensive older African-American adults. *BMC Geriatr.* 18 (1), 238. doi: 10.1186/s12877-018-0926-9

Beers, M. H., Ouslander, J. G., Rollingher, I., Reuben, D. B., Brooks, J., and Beck, J. C. (1991). Explicit criteria for determining inappropriate medication use in nursing home residents. UCLA Division of Geriatric Medicine. *Arch. Intern. Med.* 151 (9), 1825–1832. doi: 10.1001/archinte.1991.00400090107019

Cadmus, E. O., Adebusoye, L. A., Olowookere, O. O., Oluwatosin, O. G., Owoaje, E. T., and Alonge, T. O. (2017). A descriptive study of the morbidity pattern of older persons presenting at a Geriatric Centre in Southwestern Nigeria. *Niger. J. Clin. Pract.* 20 (7), 873–878. doi: 10.4103/njcp.njcp_362_16

Clyne, B., Cooper, J. A., Hughes, C. M., Fahey, T., and Smith, S. M. (2016). 'Potentially inappropriate or specifically appropriate?' Qualitative evaluation of general practitioners views on prescribing, polypharmacy and potentially inappropriate prescribing in older people. *BMC Fam. Pract.* 17 (1), 109. doi: 10.1186/s12875-016-0507-y

Dormann, H., Sonst, A., Muller, F., Vogler, R., Patapovas, A., Pfistermeister, B., et al. (2013). Adverse drug events in older patients admitted as an emergency: the role of potentially inappropriate medication in elderly people (PRISCUS). *Dtsch Arztebl. Int.* 110 (13), 213–219. doi: 10.3238/arztebl.2013.0213

Fadare, J. O., Agboola, S. M., Opeke, O. A., and Alabi, R. A. (2013). Prescription pattern and prevalence of potentially inappropriate medications among elderly patients in a Nigerian rural tertiary hospital. *Ther. Clin. Risk. Manag.* 9, 115–120. doi: 10.2147/TCRM.S40120

Fadare, J. O., Desalu, O. O., Obimakinde, A. M., Adeoti, A. O., Agboola, S. M., and Aina, F. O. (2015). Prevalence of inappropriate medication prescription in the elderly in Nigeria: a comparison of Beers and STOPP criteria. *Int. J. Risk Asses. Saf. Med.* 27 (4), 177–189. doi: 10.3233/JRS-150660

Gallagher, P., Ryan, C., Byrne, S., Kennedy, J., and O'Mahony, D. (2008). STOPP (Screening Tool of Older Person's Prescriptions) and START (Screening Tool to Alert doctors to Right Treatment). Consensus validation. *Int. J. Clin. Pharmacol. Ther.* 46 (2), 72–83. doi: 10.5414/CPP46072

Hanlon, J. T., and Schmader, K. E. (2013). The medication appropriateness index at 20: where it started, where it has been, and where it may be going. *Drugs Aging* 30 (11), 893–900. doi: 10.1007/s40266-013-0118-4

Hanlon, J. T., Schmader, K. E., Samsa, G. P., Weinberger, M., Uttech, K. M., Lewis, I. K., et al. (1992). A method for assessing drug therapy appropriateness. *J. Clin. Epidemiol.* 45 (10), 1045–1051. doi: 10.1016/0895-4356(92)90144-C

Hill-Taylor, B., Walsh, K. A., Stewart, S., Hayden, J., Byrne, S., and Sketris, I. S. (2016). Effectiveness of the STOPP/START (Screening Tool of Older Persons' potentially inappropriate Prescriptions/Screening Tool to Alert doctors to the Right Treatment) criteria: systematic review and meta-analysis of randomized controlled studies. *J. Clin. Pharm. Ther.* 41 (2), 158–169. doi: 10.1111/jcpt.12372

Holt, S., Schmiedl, S., and Thurmann, P. A. (2010). Potentially inappropriate medications in the elderly: the PRISCUS list. *Dtsch. Arztebl. Int.* 107 (31–32), 543–551. doi: 10.3238/arztebl.2010.0543

Joshua, L., Devi, P. D., and Guido, S. (2007). Adverse drug reactions in nephrology ward inpatients of a tertiary care hospital. *Indian J. Med. Res.* 61 (10), 562–569. doi: 10.4103/0019-5359.35806

Magin, P., Goode, S., and Pond, D. (2015). GPs, medications and older people: a qualitative study of general practitioners' approaches to potentially inappropriate medications in older people. *Aust. J. Ageing* 34 (2), 134–139. doi: 10.1111/ajag.12150

Maio, V., Jutkowitz, E., Herrera, K., Abouzaid, S., Negri, G., and Del Canale, S. (2011). Appropriate medication prescribing in elderly patients: how knowledgeable are primary care physicians? A survey study in Parma, Italy. *J. Clin. Pharm. Ther.* 36 (4), 468–480. doi: 10.1111/j.1365-2710.2010.01195.x

Naugler, C. T., Brymer, C., Stolee, P., and Arcese, Z. A. (2000). Development and validation of an improving prescribing in the elderly tool. *Can. J Clin. Pharmacol.* 7 (2), 103–107.

Nigerian Demographic and Health Survey (NDHS). (2013). In: Macro NPCaI, editor. Abuja, Nigeria: National Population Commission and ICF Macro, 2013.

Oscanoa, T. J., Lizaraso, F., and Carvajal, A. (2017). Hospital admissions due to adverse drug reactions in the elderly. A meta-analysis. *Eur. J. Clin. Pharmacol.* 73 (6), 759–770. doi: 10.1007/s00228-017-2225-3

Oshikoya, K. A., Oreagba, I., and Adeyemi, O. (2011). Sources of drug information and their influence on the prescribing behaviour of doctors in a teaching hospital in Ibadan, Nigeria. *Pan Afr. Med. J.* 9, 13. doi: 10.4314/pamj.v9i1.71188

Patel, T. K., and Patel, P. B. (2018). Mortality among patients due to adverse drug reactions that lead to hospitalization: a meta-analysis. *Eur. J. Clin. Pharmacol.* 74 (6), 819–832. doi: 10.1007/s00228-018-2441-5

Pohontsch, N. J., Heser, K., Loffler, A., Haenisch, B., Parker, D., Luck, T., et al. (2017). General practitioners' views on (long-term) prescription and use of problematic and potentially inappropriate medication for oldest-old patients-A qualitative interview study with GPs (CIM-TRIAD study). *BMC Fam. Pract.* 18 (1), 22. doi: 10.1186/s12875-017-0595-3

Prasert, V., Akazawa, M., Shono, A., Chanjaruporn, F., Ploylearmsang, C., Muangyim, K., et al. (2018). Applying the Lists of Risk Drugs for Thai Elderly (LRDTE) as a mechanism to account for patient age and medicine severity in assessing potentially inappropriate medication use. *Res. Social Adm. Pharm.* 14 (5), 451–458. doi: 10.1016/j.sapharm.2017.05.012

Price, S. D., Holman, C. D., Sanfilippo, F. M., and Emery, J. D. (2014). Association between potentially inappropriate medications from the Beers criteria and the risk of unplanned hospitalization in elderly patients. *Ann. Pharmacother.* 48 (1), 6–16. doi: 10.1177/1060028013504904

Ramaswamy, R., Maio, V., Diamond, J. J., Talati, A. R., Hartmann, C. W., Arenson, C., et al. (2011). Potentially inappropriate prescribing in elderly: assessing doctor knowledge, confidence and barriers. *J. Eval. Clin. Pract.* 17 (6), 1153–1159. doi: 10.1111/j.1365-2753.2010.01494.x

Renom-Guiteras, A., Meyer, G., and Thurmann, P. A. (2015). The EU(7)-PIM list: a list of potentially inappropriate medications for older people consented by experts from seven European countries. *Eur. J. Clin. Pharmacol.* 71 (7), 861–875. doi: 10.1007/s00228-015-1860-9

Rothberg, M. B., Herzig, S. J., Pekow, P. S., Avrunin, J., Lagu, T., and Lindenauer, P. K. (2013). Association between sedating medications and delirium in older inpatients. *J. Am. Geriatr. Soc.* 61 (6), 923–930. doi: 10.1111/jgs.12253

Saka, S. A., Nlooto, M., and Oosthuizen, F. (2018). American Geriatrics Society-Beers Criteria and adverse drug reactions: a comparative cross-sectional study of Nigerian and South African older inpatients. *Clin. Interv. Aging* 13, 2375–2387. doi: 10.2147/CIA.S176899

Sarwar, M. R., Dar, A. R., Mahar, S. Y., Riaz, T., Danish, U., and Iftikhar, S. (2018). Assessment of prescribing potentially inappropriate medications listed in Beers criteria and its association with the unplanned hospitalization: a cross-sectional study in Lahore, Pakistan. *Clin. Interv. Aging* 13, 1485–1495. doi: 10.2147/CIA.S173942

Sonnerstam, E., Sjolander, M., and Gustafsson, M. (2016). Inappropriate prescription and renal function among older patients with cognitive impairment. *Drugs Aging* 33 (12), 889–899. doi: 10.1007/s40266-016-0408-8

Van Heerden, J. A., Burger, J. R., and Gerber, J. J. (2016). Inappropriate medicine prescribing in older South Africans: a cross-sectional analysis of medicine claims data. *S. Afr. Med. J.* 106 (10), 1010–1016. doi: 10.7196/SAMJ.2016.v106i10.10627

Voigt, K., Gottschall, M., Koberlein-Neu, J., Schubel, J., Quint, N., and Bergmann, A. (2016). Why do family doctors prescribe potentially inappropriate medication to elderly patients? *BMC Fam. Pract.* 17, 93. doi: 10.1186/s12875-016-0482-3

Wucherer, D., Thyrian, J. R., Eichler, T., Hertel, J., Kilimann, I., Richter, S., et al. (2017). Drug-related problems in community-dwelling primary care patients screened positive for dementia. *Int. Psychogeriatr.* 29 (11), 1857–1868. doi: 10.1017/S1041610217001442

Zhan, C., Sangl, J., Bierman, A. S., Miller, M. R., Friedman, B., Wickizer, S. W., et al. (2001). Potentially inappropriate medication use in the community-dwelling elderly: findings from the 1996 Medical Expenditure Panel Survey. *JAMA* 286 (22), 2823–2829. doi: 10.1001/jama.286.22.2823

16

Precision in Setting Cancer Prevention Priorities: Synthesis of Data, Literature and Expert Opinion

Jennifer Girschik [1], Laura Jean Miller [1], Tony Addiscott [2], Mike Daube [3], Paul Katris [4], David Ransom [5], Terry Slevin [6], Tim Threlfall [7] and Tarun Stephen Weeramanthri [1]*

[1] Public Health Division, Department of Health Western Australia, Perth, WA, Australia, [2] Health Consumers Council, Perth, WA, Australia, [3] Faculty of Health Sciences, Curtin University, Perth, WA, Australia, [4] Western Australian Clinical Oncology Group, Perth, WA, Australia, [5] Cancer and Palliative Care Network, Department of Health Western Australia, Perth, WA, Australia, [6] Cancer Council Western Australia, Perth, WA, Australia, [7] Western Australian Cancer Registry, Department of Health Western Australia, Perth, WA, Australia

Correspondence:
Jennifer Girschik
jennifer.girschik@health.wa.gov.au

Cancer will continue to be a leading cause of ill health and death unless we can capitalize on the potential for 30–40% of these cancers to be prevented. In this light, cancer prevention represents an enormous opportunity for public health, potentially saving much of the pain, anguish, and cost associated with treating cancer. However, there is a challenge for governments, and the wider community, in prioritizing cancer prevention activities, especially given increasing financial constraints. This paper describes a method for identifying cancer prevention priorities. This method synthesizes detailed cancer statistics, expert opinion, and the published literature for the priority setting process. The process contains four steps: assessing the impact of cancer types; identifying cancers with the greatest impact; considering opportunities for prevention; and combining information on impact and preventability. The strength of our approach is that it is straightforward, transparent and reproducible for other settings. Applying this method in Western Australia produced a priority list of seven adult cancers which were identified as having not only the biggest impact on the community but also the best opportunities for prevention. Work conducted in an additional project phase went on to present data on these priority cancers to a public consultation and develop an agenda for action in cancer prevention.

Keywords: cancer prevention, cancer control, preventability, prioritization, policy, public health

INTRODUCTION

Cancer is a major cause of ill health and death in Western Australia (WA). Almost 12,000 Western Australians are diagnosed with cancer and around 4,000 lose their lives to the disease every year (1). In addition, approximately 85,000 non-melanoma skin cancers are treated each year in WA (2). Consequently, cancer is also a major source of government expenditure. The most recent national report estimates that total health system expenditure on cancer (excluding population screening programs) was $4.5 billion in 2009 (3). Recent studies have estimated that 30–40% of cancers could be prevented (4, 5), which, if achieved, would save much of the pain, anguish, and cost associated with treating cancer.

The Western Australian State Health Department is responsible for establishing policies for cancer prevention in the state. As in most government departments, this responsibility is being enacted in an environment that demands a robust evidence base along with collaboration, transparency, and accountability in decision-making, all within increasing fiscal constraints. This can be a difficult undertaking in any area, but can be uniquely complicated for cancer prevention.

Specifically, the evidence base for prioritizing between cancer prevention targets is not always obvious. Determining the relative impact of the different types of cancer would, in theory, highlight the areas where resources are most needed. However, cancer impact can be measured across a range of domains including incidence, morbidity, duration, mortality, years of potential life lost and cost, and the choice of domain can impact significantly on the relative priority of different cancers. In addition, impact alone is not sufficient to drive public health expenditure if scientifically proven prevention strategies are not available (6). Additionally, cancer prevention involves a range of organizations, services, and expertise, all of which have their own perspectives, priorities, and funding constraints, and may not easily sit together. Moreover, public preferences and community values play a role in the allocation of public resources, for both practical reasons around policy effectiveness and ethical reasons around civic participation and democratic legitimacy (7). In some instances, public opinion and behavior can be at odds with the available evidence on cancer prevention (8–11). For example, screening programs regularly report participation rates well below the target rate, despite the programs being publicly funded and having well-documented population benefits (12–14). Above all, there is significant pressure to ensure the best return for investment.

In this context, how do policy makers appropriately appraise and balance these complex and sometimes competing demands to ensure policy development that will maximize public good and ensure the best return for the limited cancer prevention dollar?

This was a challenge faced in the Western Australian Department of Health (WA DoH); the solution was to develop a method for, and undertake a process of, priority setting through a project called *Priorities and Preferences for Cancer Control in Western Australia*. The project was conducted by the Public Health Division under the auspices of the Chief Health Officer. The ultimate aim of the project was to develop a list of cancer prevention priority areas in WA informed by evidence, expert opinion, and public priorities and preferences. This list could then serve as the basis for more technical discussions around appropriate prevention/health promotion strategies, including issues of cost-effectiveness, delivery, and evaluation. To achieve this aim, the project was conducted in two phases. The first phase identified a priority list of cancers with both the biggest impact on the WA community and the best opportunities for prevention. The second phase involved using evidence of the impact and preventability of our priority cancers to engage the public in a discussion around their preferences for cancer control in the state.

This paper describes the first phase of the project, the process of identifying and prioritizing cancers. It is hoped that our perspective paper will inform others who may also be challenged by the process of priority setting in cancer prevention.

ESTABLISHING AN EXPERT ADVISORY GROUP

The initial step in this project was the establishment of an expert advisory group to provide oversight and review of the analysis and interpretation undertaken by the project staff. The expert advisory group consisted of eight local cancer experts representing a range of relevant disciplines, including prevention, health promotion, clinical oncology, cancer registration, epidemiology, consumer advocacy, and policy development. The advisory group met regularly and reviewed all aspects of the project from analysis through community consultation and finally to dissemination of the project findings.

ACCESSING AND ANALYZING DATA

The second task involved intensive data review and analysis in an attempt to describe the impact of cancer on the WA community. WA, like most Australian states, has a dedicated population-based cancer registry whose legislative mandate is to collect and collate information on diagnoses and deaths from cancer in WA (1). De-identified data provided by the WA Cancer Registry (WACR) was central to much of the analysis describing the impact of cancer in WA. Approval for the project and access to the de-identified data were granted by the WACR Data Custodian, in accordance with our institutional ethics committee terms of reference (15).

Statistics for 55 different cancer types recorded in the WACR were generated by the project team including age-standardized incidence and mortality rates, person years of life lost, and hospital length of stay for 2012 (data extracted December 2013). In addition, relative 5-year survival was calculated for three 5-year time periods: 1986–1990, 1996–2000, and 2006–2010. These statistics were calculated for males and females combined and separately. In addition, trends over time were calculated for incidence, mortality, and survival.

Data from outside the scope of the WACR was also sought, including Burden of Disease and costing information. Disability-adjusted life years for 2012 for WA were available as projections from the 2006 WA Burden of Disease study (16). Burden of Disease data were extracted for men and women combined and separately. Estimated lifetime treatment cost per case and total health system cost were also extracted from a national report produced by the Australian Institute for Health and Welfare for males and females combined (17). However, there were limitations to both Burden of Disease and cost data as information was not available for all the cancer types recorded in WACR and some classifications of cancer types were different (17, 18).

International data were also sought to place the WA results in a global context. For this purpose, data from the International Agency for Research on Cancer project Globocan 2012 was used, as it is the global source with the most reliable data (19). This World Health Organization initiative produces estimates with the most recent data available at the time. Using the Globocan 2012 project's age-standardized incidence and mortality rates for Organisation for Economic Cooperation and Development countries, of which Australia is a member, the complement of the mortality to incidence ratio (MIR) was calculated. The MIR is the best available method for international comparisons of cancer survival. Again, however, Globocan did not have information available for all the cancer types recorded in the WACR (19).

While an extensive number of data analyses were conducted, they all used standard methods and therefore can easily be replicated. The more difficult phase was determining how to compare and prioritize the varied analysis to define the cancers that have the biggest effect on the community. Should we prioritize a cancer with a high number of new cases but a low death rate above or below a cancer with a low number of cases but a high death rate? Should we prioritize a cancer with a small number of cases but a high treatment cost above or below a cancer with a short hospital length of stay but a large number of cases? And who should be making this decision—an epidemiologist, a policy maker, or the community?

ASSESSING CANCER IMPACT

As a first step in assessing the impact of individual cancers, the expert advisory group reviewed the cancer types recorded in the WACR. From this review, the classification of esophageal and stomach cancer was changed. Whereas the WACR classified esophageal and stomach cancer separately (ICD-O codes C15 and C16 respectively), expert opinion from the advisory group argued for their amalgamation on the grounds that in Western Societies they most commonly occur at the gastroesophageal junction making the classification of "esophageal" or "gastric" somewhat arbitrary. Statistics were then recalculated for esophageal and stomach cancer combined.

As the second step in assessing the impact of individual cancers, the expert advisory group reviewed the available data to decide which variables might best reflect the overall impact of each cancer on the general population. There was consensus among the advisory group that, in general, incidence and mortality were the strongest indicators of the impact of cancer on people in the community, which is consistent with the conclusions of earlier studies that had similar aims (6, 20). In addition, the incidence and mortality datasets were derived from the WACR and we were confident in the accuracy and completeness of these datasets for the full scope of cancers. Furthermore, it was felt that incidence and mortality would be the easiest to interpret for a general audience. This was important as the second phase of this project was to present the data to the general public and facilitate a discussion around setting priorities and preferences for cancer prevention in the state. Although Burden of Disease data are considered a very good tool for priority setting, in this case, the age of the source data and the reliance on projections made it less than ideal, and there was also some concern that it would not be easily understood by a general audience.

IDENTIFYING THE CANCERS WITH THE GREATEST IMPACT

Using incidence and mortality data, the list of 55 cancers was refined based on meeting at least two of four possible criteria (**Figure 1**):

- Top 12 for incidence rate (2012).
- Top 12 for mortality rate (2012).
- Statistically significant change in incidence trend (1992–2012).
- Statistically significant change in mortality trend (1992–2012).

For non-sex-specific cancers (excluding breast cancer), the cancer had to meet the minimum criteria in both males and females to be considered for inclusion.

Applying these criteria reduced the list of 55 cancers to 12 cancers considered to have a large impact on the WA community: breast, cervical, ovarian, uterine, prostate, colorectal, leukemia, lung, lymphoma, melanoma, pancreatic, and esophageal/stomach cancer. The unknown primary site category also met the criteria, but this category was excluded from the list due to a lack of specificity regarding these cancers (21).

CONSIDERING OPPORTUNITIES FOR PREVENTION

The project then considered the cancers in terms of their potential preventability. However, operationalizing the concept of preventability also proved challenging. What was meant by a "preventable" cancer? Did this mean completely preventable, mostly preventable or just partially preventable? Should it be preventable in the whole population or only in specific high-risk groups? How would population-based screening and early detection as forms of secondary prevention fit into any "preventability" definition? And importantly, at what level of "preventability" should public health action be triggered?

The scientific literature was reviewed for paradigms of preventability. Although a body of literature is available, only one paper was located that attempted to operationalize the concept (8, 22–24). Smith et al. (8) defined three categories of preventability: "*all or mostly preventable*" if 50% or more of cases were considered preventable, "*sometimes preventable*" for 20–49% and "*rarely preventable*" for less than 20%, although it is not clear what data were used to estimate the proportion of preventability. No papers were identified that provided a recommendation for the level of preventability that should trigger public health action. The resulting discussion among the expert advisory group and project staff led to the development of three categories:

1. Clearly established strategies for primary or secondary prevention (defined as known modifiable risk factors accounting for more than half of cases and/or a viable and recommended population-based screening program exists).
2. No clearly established strategies for primary or secondary prevention, but potential for targeted primary or secondary prevention in population subgroups.
3. No clearly established strategies for primary or secondary prevention.

COMBINING INFORMATION ON IMPACT AND PREVENTABILITY

For the 12 high impact cancers, the literature was reviewed to identify: (i) strong evidence and/or scientific consensus regarding modifiable risk factors; (ii) data on population attributable fractions

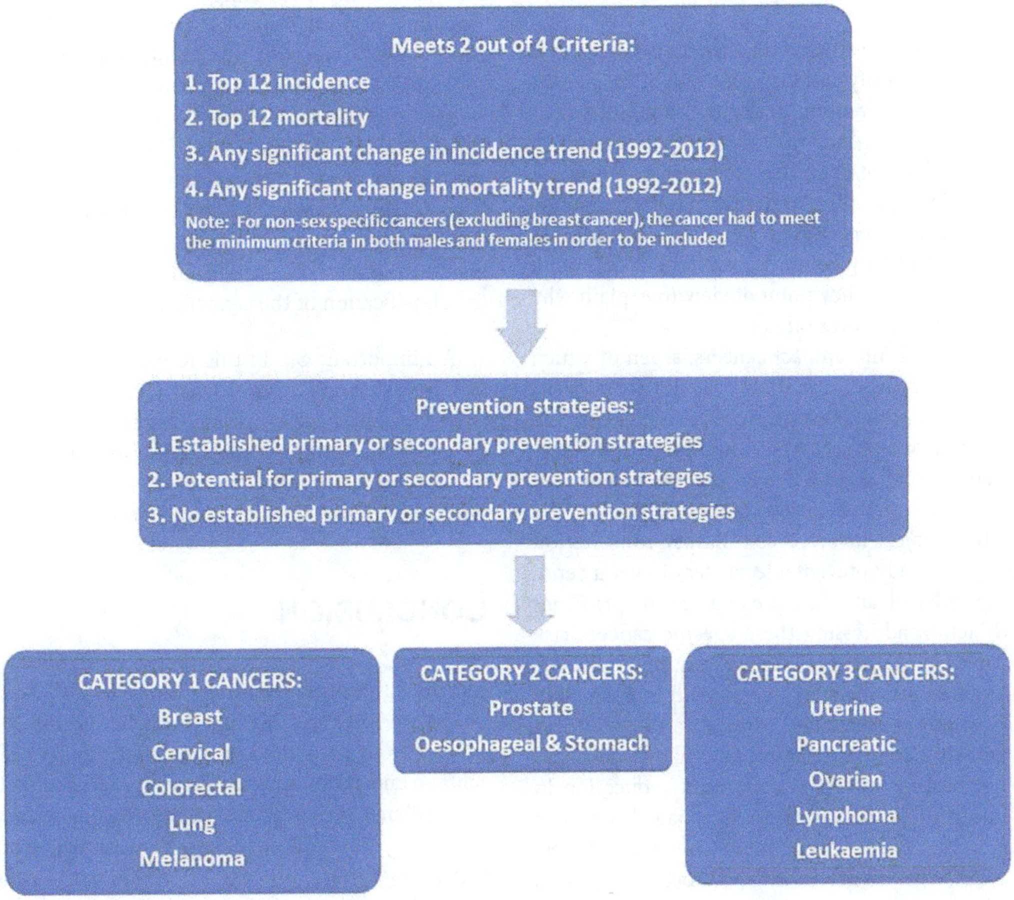

FIGURE 1 | Flowchart of the process for prioritizing cancers with both the biggest impact and the best opportunities for prevention in Western Australia.

for the risk factors that might be relevant to the WA context; (iii) information on population-based screening programs that were currently operating or proposed for WA; and (iv) any evidence to support specific screening programs in particular populations and/or high-risk groups.

The International Agency for Research on Cancer was the source for much of the information on risk factors (25–28), while data for the population attributable fractions came primarily from one large study conducted in the UK (5). Population-based screening programs for bowel, breast, and cervical cancer are operating in WA (12–14). Evidence was found to suggest possible screening strategies for three cancers, lung (in heavy smokers), prostate, and esophageal/stomach (among certain Asian populations and/or groups with high consumption of salt-preserved foods) (29, 30).

This literature review process was used to classify the 12 cancers in terms of the three categories of preventability for the WA context. Cancers with clearly established strategies for primary or secondary prevention (category 1) included breast, cervical, colorectal, lung, and melanoma. Cancers with potential for targeted primary or secondary prevention in population subgroups (category 2) included prostate and esophageal/stomach. Cancers with no clearly established strategies for primary or secondary prevention (category 3) included uterine, pancreatic, ovarian, and leukemia. The seven cancers that were determined to have both a high impact and also some potential for prevention (category 1 and 2 cancers) became our priority cancers for phase two of the project.

The source data behind identifying the cancers with the greatest impact and combining impact and preventability is summarized in two publically available reports called "Choosing Cancers for Your Say on Cancer in WA" and "The data behind Your Say on Cancer in WA" which are both available from: http://www.healthywa.wa.gov.au/yoursayoncancerwa.

FURTHER WORK

The second phase of the project went on to present data on our seven priority cancers to a public consultation on preferences for cancer control. The results of this consultation and the agenda for action that arose out of it were published as the Chief Health Officer's Report, "*Priorities and Preferences for Cancer Control in Western Australia*" (31) and are available online at: http://www.healthywa.wa.gov.au/yoursayoncancerwa.

DISCUSSION

The value of this paper lies in describing a method for priority setting that attempts to identify and unravel some of the factors that contribute to cancer prevention policy-making, but which are rarely made explicit. For example, this project examined a wide range of statistics that could be used to determine the relative impact of different cancers and attempted to explicitly justify why certain statistics were chosen over others. In addition, the project sought to explicitly define what might constitute a "preventable" cancer from a policy point of view to explain why some cancers were prioritized over others.

The result is a list of 12 high impact cancers, seven of which have been identified as having at least some potential for prevention (categories 1 and 2) in the Western Australian context. The collaborative nature of our project has ensured that the selection of these seven cancers as priority cancers has widespread acceptance among the cancer prevention community in WA. The second phase of this project involved community consultation around the seven potentially preventable cancers to get a sense of the public's knowledge of, and their preferences and priorities for, public health action addressing these specific cancers/risk factors. This process found that respondents were generally surprised by the preventability of cancer overall, and in particular, the preventability of bowel cancer and cervical cancer. Red and processed meat intake, alcohol consumption, and salt were also identified as clear areas for increased community education in the immediate future (31). We have already engaged with our health promotion partners in reviewing the evidence-based messages for these areas. Work to determine the most efficient and cost-effective prevention strategies in these areas is an important next step and the process of developing, delivering, and evaluating programs will be ongoing.

The strength of this project is that the methods can be readily replicated by others who seek to identify cancer prevention priorities in different settings. In addition, the involvement of an expert advisory group at every stage was beneficial in providing context and perspective to cancer-related data, as well as building relationships across the relevant disciplines. Access to high-quality data that were specific to the WA community for a large range of cancer types was a strength of our assessment of cancer impact.

Limitations included the following: first, a lack of certain types of information, in particular up-to-date Burden of Disease information and costings for some of the less common cancers. Second, the arbitrary cutoff of including only the top 12 for incidence and mortality rate, however the ranking of the top 25 cancers (mortality and incidence, male and female separately) was documented for transparency and is available from http://www.healthywa.wa.gov.au/yoursayoncancerwa. Third, the absence of any clear definition of preventability in cancer prevention. The use of a 50% cutoff for known modifiable risk factors in defining a preventable cancer was based on limited evidence, and the heavy reliance on UK data sources for the population attributable fractions was suboptimal. The subsequent publication of a study estimating Australian population attributable fractions supports some, but not all, of the UK study's findings. Most notably, the Australian study estimated that only 63% of Melanomas were due to exposure to UV radiation, as opposed to 86% of melanomas in the UK (4, 5). However, even the lower population attributable fraction of 63% would not have changed the classification of melanoma in this study as a category 1 "preventable" cancer. Differences also occurred in population attributable fractions for ovarian cancer and leukemia, but these were of a smaller magnitude, and again would not have changed the classification of the cancers in this study (4, 5).

An important gap in this research topic more broadly is the lack of discussion around what level of "preventability" should trigger public health action for cancer. This is in contrast to other areas within public health, for example, infectious diseases management, where there are published guidelines for the level of public health threat which stimulates action (32, 33).

CONCLUSION

Cancer will continue to be a leading cause of ill health and death, unless we can capitalize on the potential for 30–40% of these cancers to be prevented. In this light, cancer prevention represents an enormous opportunity for public health. However, there is a challenge for governments in prioritizing cancer prevention targets, especially in financially constrained environments. This paper describes a process for synthesizing information from detailed cancer statistics, expert opinion, and the published literature to help identify cancer prevention priorities. The strength of our approach is that it is transparent, reproducible, and applicable to other settings. The result is a list of 12 high impact cancers in adults, 7 of which have been identified as having at least some potential for prevention in the Western Australian context. This list has been used to justify and drive further work around cancer prevention opportunities and priorities in WA. Broader discussion around defining preventability and initiating prevention actions for cancer would contribute to international efforts to reduce the incidence and impact of these diseases globally.

AUTHOR CONTRIBUTIONS

JG and LM assisted with study design, conducted the study including data extraction and analysis, reviewed the literature, and wrote the manuscript. TW conceptualized the project, chaired the expert advisory group, and reviewed the manuscript. TA, MD, PK, DR, TS and TT constituted the expert membership of the advisory group and provided advice and supervision on study design and analysis, data interpretation, and reviewed the manuscript.

ACKNOWLEDGMENTS

The contribution of staff who contributed to all aspects of the project throughout its duration is greatly appreciated especially: Bridget Egan, David Gibson, Andrew Jardine, Colleen Koh, Stacey-Mae Prokopyszyn, Peter Somerford, Wendy Sun, and Marcia Van Zeller. In addition, we acknowledge the contribution of Professors Lin Fritschi and Simone Pettigrew as members of the expert advisory group.

FUNDING

This project was conducted within Western Australian Department of Health operational resources.

REFERENCES

1. Threlfall TJ, Thompson JR. *Cancer Incidence and Mortality in Western Australia, 2013*. Perth, WA: Department of Health (2015). Statistical Series Number 101.
2. Australian Institute of Health and Welfare. *Skin Cancer in Australia*. Canberra: AIHW (2016). Report No: CAN 96.
3. Australian Institute of Health and Welfare. *Health System Expenditures on Cancer and Other Neoplasms in Australia, 2008–09*. Canberra: AIHW (2013). Report No: CAN 78.
4. Whiteman DC, Webb PM, Green AC, Neale RE, Fritschi L, Bain CJ, et al. Cancers in Australia in 2010 attributable to modifiable factors: summary and conclusions. *Aust N Z J Public Health* (2015) 39(5):477–84. doi:10.1111/1753-6405.12468
5. Parkin DM, Boyd L, Walker LC. 16. The fraction of cancer attributable to lifestyle and environmental factors in the UK in 2010. *Br J Cancer* (2011) 105(S2):S77–81. doi:10.1038/bjc.2011.489
6. Lillquist PP, Alciati MH, Baptiste MS, Nasca PC, Kerner JF, Mettlin C. Cancer control planning and establishment of priorities for intervention by a state health department. *Public Health Rep* (1994) 109(6):791–803.
7. Head BW. Australian experience: civic engagement as symbol and substance. *Public Adm Dev* (2011) 31(2):102–12. doi:10.1002/pad.599
8. Smith B, Sullivan E, Bauman A, Powell-Davies G, Mitchell J. Lay beliefs about the preventability of major health conditions. *Health Educ Res* (1999) 14(3):315–25. doi:10.1093/her/14.3.315
9. American Institute for Cancer Research. *The AICR 2015 Cancer Risk Awareness Survey*. Washington, DC: American Institute for Cancer Research (2015).
10. Sullivan HW, Finney Rutten LJ, Hesse BW, Moser RP, Rothman AJ, McCaul KD. Lay representations of cancer prevention and early detection: associations with prevention behaviors. *Prev Chronic Dis* (2010) 7(1):A14.
11. Jalleh G, Donovan RJ, Lin C, Slevin T, Clayforth C, Pratt IS, et al. Beliefs about bowel cancer among the target group for the National Bowel Cancer Screening Program in Australia. *Aust N Z J Public Health* (2010) 34(2):187–92. doi:10.1111/j.1753-6405.2010.00505.x
12. Australian Institute of Health and Welfare. *National Bowel Cancer Screening Program Monitoring Report 2013–2014*. Canberra: AIHW (2015). Report No: CAN 92.
13. Australian Institute of Health and Welfare. *BreastScreen Australia Monitoring Report 2012–2013*. Canberra: AIHW (2015). Report No: CAN 93.
14. Australian Institute of Health and Welfare. *Cervical Screening in Australia 2012–2013*. Canberra: AIHW (2015). Report No: CAN 91.
15. Department of Health WA Human Research Ethics Comittee. *When Is Department of Health WA Human Research Ethics Committee Approval Required?* Perth, WA: Department of Health (2012). Available from: http://www.health.wa.gov.au/healthdata/docs/HREC_terms_of_reference.pdf
16. Epidemiology Branch. *Burden of Disease in Western Australia. WA Burden of Disease Study*. Perth, WA: Department of Health (2010).
17. Australian Institute of Health and Welfare. *Health System Expenditures on Cancer and Other Neoplasms in Australia, 2000–01*. Canberra: AIHW (2005). Report No: HWE 29.
18. Somerford P, Katzenellenbogen J. *Western Australian Burden of Disease Study: Disability-Adjusted Life Years: Technical Overview*. Perth, WA: Department of Health (2004).
19. Ferlay J, Soerjomataram I, Ervik M, Dikshit R, Eser S, Mathers C, et al. *GLOBOCAN 2012 v1.0, Cancer Incidence and Mortality Worldwide: IARC CancerBase No. 11*. Lyon, France: International Agency for Research on Cancer (2013). Available from: http://globocan.iarc.fr
20. Boss LP, Suarez L. Uses of data to plan cancer prevention and control programs. *Public Health Rep* (1990) 105(4):354–60.
21. Hemminki K, Bevier M, Hemminki A, Sundquist J. Survival in cancer of unknown primary site: population-based analysis by site and histology. *Ann Oncol* (2012) 23(7):1854–63. doi:10.1093/annonc/mdr536
22. Colditz GA, Sellers TA, Trapido E. Epidemiology – identifying the causes and preventability of cancer? *Nat Rev Cancer* (2006) 6(1):75–83. doi:10.1038/nrc1784
23. Dart H, Wolin KY, Colditz GA. Commentary: eight ways to prevent cancer: a framework for effective prevention messages for the public. *Cancer Causes Control* (2012) 23(4):601–8. doi:10.1007/s10552-012-9924-y
24. Colditz GA, Wei EK. Preventability of cancer: the relative contributions of biologic and social and physical environmental determinants of cancer mortality. *Annu Rev Public Health* (2012) 33:137–56. doi:10.1146/annurev-publhealth-031811-124627
25. International Agency for Research on Cancer. Personal habits and indoor combustion. Volume 100E. A review of human carcinogens. *IARC Monographs on the Evaluation of Carcinogenic Risks to Humans*. (Vol. 100), Lyon: World Health Organization, International Agency for Research on Cancer (2012). p. 1–441.
26. International Agency for Research on Cancer. Biological agents. Volume 100B. A review of human carcinogens. *IARC Monographs on the Evaluation of Carcinogenic Risks to Humans* (Vol. 100), Lyon: World Health Organization, International Agency for Research on Cancer (2012). p. 1–441.
27. International Agency for Research on Cancer. Radiation. Volume 100D. A review of human carcinogens. *IARC Monographs on the Evaluation of Carcinogenic Risks to Humans* (Vol. 100), Lyon: World Health Organization, International Agency for Research on Cancer (2012). p. 1–437.
28. International Agency for Research on Cancer. Pharmaceuticals. Volume 100A. A review of human carcinogens. *IARC Monographs on the Evaluation of Carcinogenic Risks to Humans* (Vol. 100), Lyon: World Health Organization, International Agency for Research on Cancer (2012). p. 1–463.
29. International Agency for Research on Cancer. *World Cancer Report 2014*. Lyon, France: IARC (2014).
30. National Health and Medical Research Council. *Prostate-Specific Antigen (PSA) Testing in Asymptomatic Men: Evidence Evaluation Report*. Canberra: NHMRC (2013).
31. Girschik J, Miller LJ, Sun W, Jardine A, Weeramanthri TS. *Priorities and Preferences for Cancer Control in Western Australia*. Perth, WA: Government of Western Australia (2016). Available from: http://healthywa.wa.gov.au/~/media/Files/HealthyWA/Original/Your-say-on-cancer-wa/13009-chief-health-officer-report.ashx
32. Australian Government Department of Health. *Communicable Diseases Network Australia Series of National Guidelines (SoNGs)*. Canberra: Australian Government Department of Health (2016).
33. Department of Health Western Australia. *State Hazard Plan for Human Epidemic*. Perth, WA: Government of Western Australia (2016). Available from: https://www.semc.wa.gov.au/Documents/Resources/Legislation%2c%20Policy%2c%20Plans%2c%20Procedure%20and%20Guidelines/Plans/Westplans2016/WestplanHumanEpidemicSEMCapproved24052016.pdf

17

Suspected Adverse Drug Reactions Related to Breast Cancer Chemotherapy: Disproportionality Analysis of the Brazilian Spontaneous Reporting System

Flávia Campos Barcelos[1], Guacira Corrêa de Matos[2], Mario Jorge Sobreira da Silva[1]*, Fabrício Alves Barbosa da Silva[3] and Elisangela da Costa Lima[2]**

[1] Brazilian National Cancer Institute (INCA), Rio de Janeiro, Brazil, [2] Faculty of Pharmacy, Federal University of Rio de Janeiro, Rio de Janeiro, Brazil, [3] Oswaldo Cruz Foundation (Fiocruz), Rio de Janeiro, Brazil

***Correspondence:**
Flávia Campos Barcelos
fbarcelos1979@gmail.com
Mario Jorge Sobreira da Silva
mjsobreira@yahoo.com.br
Elisangela da Costa Lima
eclima.ufrj@gmail.com

Spontaneous reporting systems may generate a large volume of information in real world conditions with a relatively low cost. Disproportionality measures are useful to indicate and quantify unexpected safety issues associated with a given drug-event pair (signals of disproportionality), based upon differences compared to the background reporting frequency. This cross-sectional study (2008 to 2013) aimed to analyse the feasibility of detecting such signals in the Brazilian Pharmacovigilance Database comprising suspected adverse drug reactions related to the use of doxorubicin, cyclophosphamide, carboplatin, trastuzumab, docetaxel, and paclitaxel for breast cancer chemotherapy. We first accessed overall database features (patient information and suspected adverse drug reactions) and further conducted a disproportionality analysis based on Reporting Odds Ratios with a confidence interval of 95% in order to identify possible signals of disproportionate reporting, only among serious suspected adverse drug reactions. Of all data reports of adverse reactions (n = 2603), 83% were classified as serious, with the highest prevalence with docetaxel (78.1%). The final analysis was performed using 1,309 reports with 3,139 drug-reaction pairs. The following signals of disproportionate reporting, some rare or not mentioned on labels, were observed: tachypnea with docetaxel; bronchospasm, syncope, cyanosis, and anaphylactic reaction with paclitaxel; and anaphylactic shock with trastuzumab. Structured management of spontaneous adverse drug reaction reporting is essential for monitoring the safe use of drugs and detecting early safety signals. Disproportionality signal analysis represents a viable and applicable strategy for oncology signal screening in the Brazilian Pharmacovigilance Database.

Keywords: pharmacovigilance, oncology, disproportionatily analysis, spontaneous reporting system, adverse drug reaction

INTRODUCTION

Pharmacovigilance activities—aimed at monitoring the safe use of medicines—are particularly important in oncology due to the inherent toxicity of antineoplastic agents (Baldo and De Paoli, 2014). Given the high incidence, prevalence and mortality of breast cancer in the worldwide female population (International Agency for Research on Cancer., 2014), knowledge of the toxicity profile of the main drugs used in its treatment is important strategically for prevention, detection and early management of suspected adverse drugs reactions (ADRs) related to chemotherapy.

Spontaneous reporting of ADRs contributes substantially to signal detection in drug safety surveillance, especially for rare and acute reactions (Arnaud et al., 2017). In pharmacovigilance, a signal is reported information on a possible causal relationship between an adverse event and a drug exposure, which was previously unknown or incompletely documented. It also refers to an increased number adverse events compared to the frequency of reactions normally expected with the use of a given product (U.S. Department of Health and Human Services et al., 2005; World Health Organization (WHO)., 2018).

Reports of ADR screening from the national surveillance system may offer data pertaining to different drug-event combinations (or drug-event pairs). These include methods of disproportionality analysis (DPA) that represent the main class of analytical methods for spontaneous report systems (SRS) data analysis in pharmacovigilance (Harpaz et al., 2012; European Medicines Agency., 2016)

Such methods, aimed at drawing attention to unexpected associations by generating hypothesis, have been guiding pharmacovigilance experts from health agencies worldwide in their investigations to draw definitive conclusions (Courtois et al., 2018).

Quantitative signal detection methods for spontaneously reported data include Proportional Reporting Ratio (PRR), Reporting Odds Ratio (ROR), and Empirical Bayes Geometric Mean (EBGM). These methods may identify relevant associations in SRS databases, focusing on projections of lower data dimensionality, more specifically two-dimensional contingency tables. Frequentist approaches are usually accompanied by independence hypothesis tests (Bate and Evans, 2009).

Brazilian Reporting System in Health Surveillance (Notivisa) was created in 2008. Since then, no evaluations of signal detection through disproportionality analysis have been made using this national database (Mota et al., 2018).

This study aimed to analyse serious ADRs associated with the most commonly used drugs in first-line adjuvant chemotherapy for breast cancer, reported from the Brazilian Surveillance System, in order to verify the feasibility of identifying potential signals through DPA using this database.

MATERIALS AND METHODS

We carried out a cross-sectional study related exclusively to spontaneous ADRs reported in Notivisa from 2008 to 2013 during breast cancer treatment with doxorubicin, cyclophosphamide, carboplatin, trastuzumab, docetaxel, and paclitaxel—which are the preferred regimens according to National Comprehensive Cancer Network and Brazilian guidelines (National Comprehensive Cancer Network., 2017; Brasil, 2018).

Notivisa is a computerized system developed by the National Health Surveillance Agency (Anvisa) to receive notifications of incidents, adverse events and technical complaints related to the use of products and services under sanitary surveillance (Mota et al., 2018; National Health System Surveillance (Anvisa)., 2018). Anvisa supplied data on the Notivisa website reports (Pharmacovigilance Module) as a Microsoft Excel® file, which was made available by collaboration research. The database provided did not allow patient identification. The study was approved by the Research Ethics Committee of the Federal University of Rio de Janeiro.

Suspected ADRs were analyzed for their origin (geographical location), the patient's age (in years) and suspected drug (Anatomical Therapeutic Chemical Classification System), and were also classified according to severity and System Organ Class (SOC/MedDRA). The findings were also compared to the information contained in drug labels (MedDRA, 2018).

We accessed only serious ADR reports by using the signals of disproportionate reporting (SDR) method and thresholds recommended by the European Medicines Agency (EMA), namely Reporting Odds Ratio (ROR) and thresholds based on the 95% confidence interval and number of individual cases (European Medicines Agency., 2016).

DPA methodologies use frequency analysis of two-dimensional contingency tables to estimate surrogate measures of statistical association between specific drug-event combinations mentioned in databases of spontaneous reports. For instance, the Reporting Odds Ratio (ROR) measure is defined by the formula below:

$$ROR = (a.d)/(c.b)$$

Where:

- The value "a" indicates the number of individual cases that list the target drug **P** and the target ADR **R**;
- The value "b" indicates the number of individual cases that list the target drug **P** but not the target ADR **R**;
- The value "c" indicates the number of individual cases that list the target ADR **R** but not the target drug **P**;
- The value "d" indicates the number of individual cases that do not list the target ADR **R** or the target drug **P**

Eudravigilance adopts the following criteria to define an SDR (European Medicines Agency., 2016):

- The lower bound of the 95% confidence interval of the ROR measure is >1;
- The number of individual cases (value "a") is greater than or equal to 3 for active substances contained in medicinal products, included in an additional monitoring list defined by the European Medicines Agency;
- The number of individual cases is greater than or equal to 5 for the other active substances;

- The event belongs to the Important Medical Event Terms (IME) list, as defined by EudraVigilance.

In this work, we adopted a conservative approach: ROR calculations were performed for all drugs with $\boldsymbol{a} \geq 3$, and defined the concept of *SDR intensity* as a measure directly related to the value 'a'. Therefore, we differentiated between drug-event pairs with $\boldsymbol{a} \geq 5$ (higher intensity) and pairs with $3 \leq \boldsymbol{a} < 5$ (lower intensity).

A situation occurs when $\boldsymbol{c} = 0$, i.e., when all database reports containing a specific suspected ADR are associated to only one drug. In this case, the ROR cannot be computed and the value of the ROR is arbitrarily set at 99.9 to reflect the presence of a possible SDR, according to EudraVigilance (European Medicines Agency., 2016).

We adopted the same approach in this work. The observed signals were listed and further classified according to their intensity and ADR frequency, described in drug labels as: very common, not common, rare or very rare.

RESULTS

Overall analysis was performed on 1,309 reports with 3,139 drug-event pairs (4% of total Brazilian reports for all medicines in the study period).

All reports came exclusively from nine out of the 27 Brazilian States (Rio de Janeiro, São Paulo, Minas Gerais, Rio Grande do Sul, Santa Catarina, Paraná, Mato Grosso, Mato Grosso do Sul e Bahia). Most (64.7%) were from hospitals located in the state of Rio de Janeiro. The median age of the female patients was 51.7 years (range: 25–87 years).

Around 83% (n=2603) of total suspected ADR (drug-reaction pairs) were classified as serious, for causing: death ($n = 6$), life-threatening conditions ($n = 79$), hospitalizations ($n = 57$), permanent disabilities (n=19) and medically important events ($n = 2472$). Of all serious ADRs, the majority (78.1%) were associated with docetaxel, with the greatest prevalence of those classified as general disorders (**Table 1**).

Disproportionality Analysis

SDRs of higher intensity ($a \geq 5$) and lower intensity ($a \geq 3$ and $a < 5$; $a \geq 3$ and $c = 0$*) were observed for docetaxel, paclitaxel, trastuzumab, doxorubicin and cyclophosphamide. The disproportionality analysis did not identify any SDR for carboplatin.

Unexpected events considered rare, not common or not even mentioned on their respective drug labels and also known as acute and life-threatening were identified. The following are noteworthy: tachypnea with docetaxel, bronchospasm, anaphylactic reaction, cyanosis and syncope with paclitaxel and anaphylactic shock with trastuzumab (**Table 2**).

DISCUSSION

The overall analysis in Notivisa has identified the reported prevalence of serious suspected ADRs with docetaxel and paclitaxel, mostly due to infusion-related reactions (IRR) that usually present with: flushing, rash, pruritus, fever, tremor, rigor, dyspnea, chest/back pain, nausea, light hypotension and tachycardia. Nevertheless, these sets of reactions tend to be mild to moderate and also common, occurring during the first few minutes of a first or a second drug infusion (Picard and Castells, 2015).

In fact, severe hypersensitivity reactions with taxanes are considered rare (incidence 3–5%) but have the potential to evolve rapidly toward a high risk scenario, characterized by a significant drop in blood pressure (systolic ≤ 90 mmHg) and/or syncope, bronchospasm, oxygen desaturation and anaphylaxis, which requires immediate therapeutic intervention (Brown, 2004; Picard, 2017).

The analyzed data indicated that careful monitoring of such reactions likely should have been done in Brazilian breast cancer patients, in the view of the large number of suspected ADRs related to docetaxel reported to the Notivisa. However, such high prevalence must be observed with caution due to the fact that the study time frame (2008–2013) corresponds exactly to the period immediately after the Sanofi-Aventis patent of Taxotere (docetaxel) expired in Brazil. This scenario might have influenced many health professionals and also pharmaceutical companies toward notification of suspected ADRs, due to the entrance of new generic brands of docetaxel into the Brazilian market. In addition, patients and health professionals often believe that generic cancer drugs have less quality, effectiveness and safety than branded-name drugs, leading to continuous attention and

TABLE 1 | Serious ADRs related to breast cancer chemotherapy by system organ groups (Brazilian Health System Surveillance, 2008–2013).

Drugs	Serious ADRs (%)	Main ADR reporting groups- SOC/MedDRA (n)				
		General disorders	Vascular disorders	Respiratory disorders	Muscular disorders	GI disorders
Docetaxel	2032 (78, 1)	750	480	395	289	147
Paclitaxel	240 (9, 2)	37	51	45	21	8
Doxorubicin	136 (5, 2)	36	22	8	0	14
Cyclophosphamide	43 (1, 6)	3	4	12	0	2
Trastuzumab	137 (5, 3)	65	18	7	11	7
Carboplatin	15 (0, 6)	3	1	3	0	4
Total	2603 (100)	894	576	470	321	182

ADRs, suspected adverse drug reactions; SOC, System Organ Class; MedDRA, Medical Dictionary for Regulatory Activities; GI, gastrointestinal.

TABLE 2 | Disproportionality analysis conducted on Notivisa (Brazil) data according to the methods recommended by EudraVigilance for routine signal detection.

Drug	ADR	ROR (lower bound of the 95% CI)	SDR Intensity	ADR frequency on drug labels
Docetaxel	Dyspnea	2.15	a ≥ 5	Very common
	Abdominal pain	2.39		Common
	Back pain	7.97		Common
	Thoracic pain	5.39		Common
	Flushing	4.94		Common
	Oral Discomfort	–	a ≥ 3 and c = 0*	Not Mentioned
	Throat pain	–		Not Mentioned
	Dry throat	–		Not Mentioned
	Bone pain	–		Common
	Scintillating scotomas	–		Rare#
	Blurred vision	–		Rare#
	Lipothymia	–		Not Mentioned
	Mouth paresthesia	–		Not Mentioned
	Tachypnea	–		Not Mentioned
	Somnolence	–		Not Mentioned
Paclitaxel	Allergy (unspecific)	15.11	a ≥ 5	Common
	Hypersensitivity	45.27		Common
	Hypertension	5.44		Common
	Hypotension	30.25		Very Common
	General discomfort	6.70		Rare
	Bronchospasm	14.94	a ≥ 3 and a<5	Not Mentioned
	Anaphylactic reaction	14.94		Rare
	Cyanosis	9.95		Not Mentioned
	Myalgia	7.99		Very Common
	Syncope	4.97		Not Mentioned
Trastuzumab	Chills	102.69	a ≥ 5	Very Common
	Hypertension	2.24		Common
	Rash	4.63		Very Common
	Tremor	49.40		Not Mentioned
	Headache	4.09	a ≥ 3 and a < 5	Very Common
	Anaphylactic shock	–	a ≥ 3 and c = 0*	Not Common
Doxorubicin	Neutropenia	10.77	a ≥ 5	Very Common
	Nausea	4.50		Very Common
	Erythema	17.27		Common
	Pruritus	16.95		Common
	Phlebitis	–		Common
Cyclophosphamide	Neutropenia	47.03	a ≥ 5	Common
	Nasal discomfort	191.85	a ≥ 3 and a < 5	Not Mentioned
	Successive sneezing	–	a ≥ 3 and c = 0*	Not Mentioned

SDR, Signals of Disproportionate Reporting (lower bound of the ROR 95% confidence interval >1); ROR, Reporting Odds Ratio (with 95% confidence interval calculated for each drug-reaction pair of serious ADRs in comparison to drug labels information).
**ROR measure for a≥3 and c = 0 defined arbitrarily as 99.9 in order to reflect the presence of a possible SDR.*
#Included in post-marketing period.

a higher tendency to report ADRs (Yang et al., 2016). It is also common to note that ADRs and therapeutic failure reports significantly increase after the entry of generic oncology drug into the marketplace (Pitts et al., 2016).

As trastuzumab, a monoclonal antibody, is also highly associated with IRR, symptoms such as fever, chills and tremor that were observed in Notivisa are considered common and may affect up to 40% of patients. However, urticaria, angioedema, anaphylaxis and anaphylactic shock resulting in hospitalization or death are quite infrequent (Lenz, 2007).

We also noticed that serious ADRs (cardiovascular, gastrointestinal and neurologic events) have been scarcely reported in Notivisa, despite being widely observed among patients undergoing chemotherapy for breast cancer with the studied drugs, both in the literature and in VigiAcces®–the free access platform of the UMC/WHO database VigiBase (Barbour, 2008; De Lullis et al., 2015; Frise et al., 2017; Martel et al., 2017).

Despite its importance in terms of drug safety monitoring, pharmacovigilance activities remain a challenge, mostly due to under-reporting. This common problem especially impacts the field of oncology due to the fact that ADRs are often considered "normal" (or inevitable) in cancer treatment. Additionally, the sensitivity and availability toward spontaneously reporting suspected ADRs can also vary between different kinds of health professionals and health systems all around the world (Baldo and De Paoli, 2014).

Therefore, using disproportionality measures, a quick, inexpensive and sensitive method of signal screening, has benefits and strengths in that it can provide valuable information on ADRs of greater clinical importance and higher risk in oncology (Montastruc et al., 2011; Dias et al., 2014; Tuccori et al., 2015).

In our study we managed to identify SDRs for docetaxel, paclitaxel, trastuzumab, and less frequently, for doxorubicin and cyclophosphamide, but not for carboplatin. The following drug-event pairs should be highlighted: allergy/ hypersensitivity, anaphylactic reaction and bronchospasm with paclitaxel and classical IRRs with docetaxel and trastuzumab.

In addition, DPA analysis could also identify some important drug-event pairs, whose ADRs were not clearly mentioned on labels or were considered uncommon in clinical trials, such as: docetaxel and tachypnea; paclitaxel and bronchospasm (not mentioned in label, but related to severe RRI); paclitaxel and anaphylactic reaction; paclitaxel and cyanosis; paclitaxel and syncope (not mentioned in label, but related to severe IRR); trastuzumab and tremor and trastuzumab and anaphylactic shock (both related to IRR).

However, such results should be interpreted with caution due to specific limitations of reporting system databases, with which it is not possible to ascertain causality. Thus, a relative increase in the proportion of notifications of a given drug-event pair may in fact be a false positive without any kind of causal relationship, particularly in cases with low report numbers, where the statistical disproportionality may reflect one or more biases (Dias et al., 2014; Hauben et al., 2017).

In addition, it is relevant to mention that some external factors, such as: (i) time on the market (new or old drugs); (ii) tendency to report only severe adverse events and (iii) selective reporting for a given drug may affect the reliability of detected disproportionality signals (Bate and Evans, 2009; Arora et al., 2017). These important points seem also to justify the great number of docetaxel reports in Notivisa (2008–2013).

Based on our findings, and in accordance with the literature, it would be possible to select specific events identified and investigate their relationship to all drugs (event-based approach) or to select specific drugs to monitor and their relationship with all possible events (drug-based approach) (Bate and Evans, 2009; Trifirò et al., 2009; Dias et al., 2014).

The study limitations result from characteristics related to the Brazilian Surveillance System Database (Notivisa) and other SRSs (biases of under-reporting, heterogeneity and selectivity), limits of DPA itself and the fact that the majority of suspected ADRs originated from only one Brazilian State. This last limitation seems to be due to the fact that one of the most important cancer treatment centers (National Cancer Institute/INCA—considered a reference standard in the treatment of breast cancer in Brazil) is located in the Rio de Janeiro State.

Finally, it must be said that data mining methods in pharmacovigilance are considered complementary and not substitutes for traditional signal identification strategies. It is necessary to evaluate, in advance, the accuracy of the signaling criteria used, the nature and the number of drugs and warning events to monitor, the potential impact of false positives or false negatives and the availability of resources (Bate and Evans, 2009; Montastruc et al., 2011; Hauben et al., 2017).

Nevertheless, our analysis indicates a potential use of Notivisa for signal detection in regards to clinical or regulatory applications, as it was able to identify relevant disproportionate signals considered severe and rare, and not mentioned on drug labels.

To our knowledge, this was the first study to apply DPA methods to the Brazilian surveillance database system (Notivisa).

CONCLUSION

Our analysis using Notivisa showed a predominance of serious ADRs in regards to docetaxel and paclitaxel, as well as a greater tendency to report general, vascular and respiratory disorders, mostly related to IRR.

The DPA applied was able to identify some interesting signals worthy of further investigation related to antineoplastic agents in Notivisa, suggesting that such a method might be useful for other drug classes.

Despite its inherent limitations, SRS seems to benefit from this kind of approach, as it can potentially contribute to research, surveillance and the ever safer use of medicines in low and medium-income countries such as Brazil.

AUTHOR CONTRIBUTIONS

FCB, ECL, and GCM conceived and designed the study. FABS contributed to the disproportionality analysis. GCM and ECL contributed to the acquisition and the interpretation of data for the work. FCB, ECL, and MJSS discussed the results. FCB drafted the manuscript with support from ECL and MJSS. All authors critically revised the work and approved the final manuscript.

ACKNOWLEDGMENTS

The authors thank the National Council for Scientific and Technological Development (CNPQ) for the funding support and National Health Surveillance Agency (ANVISA) for providing access to Notivisa data.

REFERENCES

Arnaud, M., Bégaud, B., Thurin, N., Morre, N., Pariente, A., and Salvo, F. (2017). Methods for safety signal detection in healthcare databases: a literature review. *Expert Opin. Drug Saf.* 16, 721–732. doi: 10.1080/14740338.2017.1325463

Arora, A., Jalali, R.K., and Vohora, D. (2017). Relevance of the Weber effect in contemporary pharmacovigilance of oncology drugs. *Ther. Clin. Risk Manag.* 13, 1195–1203. doi: 10.2147/TCRM.S137144

Baldo, P., and De Paoli, P. (2014). Pharmacovigilance in oncology: evaluation of current practice and future perspectives. *J. Eval. Clin. Pract.* 20, 559–569. doi: 10.111/jep.12184

Barbour, S. Y. (2008). Caring for the treatment-experienced breast cancer patient: the phrmacist's role. *Am. J. Health Syst. Pharm.* 65 (10 Suppl. *3)*, 16–22. doi: 10.2146/ajhp080090

Bate, A., and Evans, S. J. W. (2009). Quantitative signal detection using spontaneous ADR reporting. *Pharmacoedidemiol. Drug Saf.* 18, 427–436. doi: 10.1102/pds.1742

Brasil (2018). Health Ministry. *Therapeutic Guidelines for Breast Carcinoma.* Available online at: http://portalarquivos2.saude.gov.br/images/pdf/2018/fevereiro/07/PORTARIA-no-04-PCDT.carcinoma.mama.2018.pdf (accessed July 30, 2018).

Brown, S. G. (2004). Clinical features and severity grading of anaphylaxis. *J. Allerg. Clin. Immunol.* 114, 371–376. doi: 10.1016/j.jaci.2004.04.029

Courtois, É., Pariente, A., Salvo, F., Volatier, É., Tubert-Bitter, P., and Ahmed, I. (2018). Propensity score-based approaches in high dimension for pharmacovigilance signal detection: an empirical comparison on the French spontaneous reporting database. *Front Pharmacol.* 9:1010. doi: 10.3389/fphar.2018.01010

De Lullis, F., Taglieri, L., Salerno, G., Lanza, R., and Scarpa, S. (2015). Taxane induced-neuropathy in patients affected by breast cancer: Literature review. *Crit. Rev. Oncol. Hematol.* 96, 34–45. doi: 10.1016/j.critrevonc.2015.04.011

Dias, P., Ribeiro, C. F., and Marques, F. B. (2014). Medidas de desproporcionalidade na detecção de sinal em farmacovigilância. *Rev. Port. Farmacoter.* 6, 31–35. doi: 10.25756/rpf.v6il.36

European Medicines Agency. (2016). *Screening for Adverse Reactions in EudraVigilance.* Available online at: http://www.ema.europa.eu/docs/en_GB/document_library/Other/2016/12/WC500218606.pdf (accessed August 10, 2018).

Frise, C. R., Harrison, J. M., Janz, N. K., Jagsi, R., Morrow, M., Li, Y., et al. (2017). Treatment-associated toxicities reported by patients with early stage invasive breast cancer. *Cancer* 123, 1925–1934. doi: 10.1002/cncr.30547

Harpaz, R., DuMouchel, W., Shah, N. H., Madigan, D., Ryan, P., and Friedman, C. (2012). Novel data-mining methodologies for adverse drug event discovery and analysis. *Clin. Pharmacol. Therapeut.* 91, 1010–1021. doi: 10.1038/clpt.2012.50

Hauben, M., Hung, E., Wood, J., Soitkar, A., and Reshef, D. (2017). The impact of database restriction on pharmacovigilance signal detection of selected cancer therapies. *Ther. Adv. Drug Saf.* 8, 145–156. doi: 10.1177/2042098916685010

International Agency for Research on Cancer. (2014). *World Cancer Report 2014.* Available online at: https://www.iarc.fr/ (accessed November 16, 2018).

Lenz, H. J. (2007). Management and preparedness for infusion and hypersensitivity reactions. *Oncologist* 12, 601–609. doi: 10.1634/theoncologist.12-5-601

Martel, S., Maurer, C., Lambertini, M., Pondé, N., and Azambuja, E. (2017). Breast cancer treatment-induced cardiotoxicity. *Expert Opin. Drug Saf.* 16, 1021–1038. doi: 10.1080/14740338.2017.1351541

MedDRA (2018). *Medical Dictionary for Regulatory Activities.* Available online at: https://www.meddra.org/ (accessed August 16, 2018).

Montastruc, J. L., Sommet, A., Bagheri, H., and Lapevre-Mestre, M. (2011). Benefits and stengths of the disproportionality analysis for identification of adverse drug reactions in a pharmacovigilance database. *Brit. J. Clin. Pharmacol.* 72, 905–908. doi: 10.1111/j.1365-2125.2011.04037.x

Mota, D. M., Vigo, A., and Kuchenbecker, R. S. (2018). Evolution and key elements of the Brazilian pharmacovigilance system: a escoping review beginning with the creation of the Brazilian Health Regulatory Agency. *Cad. Saúde Públ.* 34:e00000218. doi: 10.1590/0102-311x00000218

National Comprehensive Cancer Network. (2017). *Guidelines NCCN Evidence Blocks.* Available online at: https://www.nccn.org/evidenceblocks/default.aspx (accessed September 28, 2017).

National Health System Surveillance (Anvisa). (2018). *Sistema de Notificação em Vigilância Sanitária (Notivisa).* Available online at: http://portal.anvisa.gov.br/notivisa/ (accessed July 13, 2018).

Picard, M. (2017). Management of hypersentivity reactions to taxanes. *Immunol. Allerg. Clin. North Am.* 37, 679–693. doi: 10.1016/j.iac.2017.004

Picard, M., and Castells, M. C. (2015). Re-visiting hypersensitivity reactions to taxanes: a comprehensive review. *Clin. Rev. Allerg. Immunol.* 49, 177–191. doi: 10.1007/s12016-014-8416-0

Pitts, P. J., Louet, H. L., Moride, Y., and Conto, R. M. (2016). 21st Century pharmacovigilance: efforts, roles and responsabilities. *Lancet Oncol.* 17, 486–492. doi: 10.1016/s1470-2015(16)30312-6

Trifirò, G., Pariente, A., Coloma, P. M., Kors, J. A., Polimeni, G., Miremont-Salamé, G., et al. (2009). Data mining on eletronic health record databases for signal detection in pharmacovigilance: which events to monitor? *Pharmacoepidemiol. Drug Saf.* 18, 1176–1184. doi: 10.1002/pds.1836

Tuccori, M., Montagnani, S., Capogrosso-Sansone, A., Mantarro, S., Antonioli, L., Fornai, M., et al. (2015). Adverse reactions to oncologic drugs: spontaneous reporting and signal detection. *Expert Rev. Clin. Pharmacol.* 8, 61–75. doi: 10.1586/17512433.2015.974555

U.S. Department of Health and Human Services, Food and Drug Administration, Center for Drug Evaluation and Research, and Center for Biologics Evaluation and Research (2005). *Guidance for industry. Good Pharmacovigilance Practices and Pharmacoepidemiologic Assessment.* Rockville, MD. Available online at: https://www.fda.gov/downloads/Drugs/GuidanceComplianceRegulatoryInformation/Guidances/UCM071696.pdf (accessed January 21, 2019).

World Health Organization (WHO). (2018). *Uppsala Monitoring Centre.* Available online at: https://www.who-umc.org/research-scientific-development/signal-detection/what-is-a-signal/ (accessed December 28, 2018).

Yang, Y. T., Nagai, S., Chen, B. K., Qureshi, Z. P., Lebby, A. A., Kessler, S., et al. (2016). Generic oncology drugs: are they all safe? *Lancet Oncol.* 17, e493–e501. doi: 10.1016/s1470-2015(16)30384-9

18

Policy Making in Newborn Screening Needs a Structured and Transparent Approach

Marleen E. Jansen[1,2], Karla J. Lister[3], Henk J. van Kranen[2,4] and Martina C. Cornel[1]*

[1] *Section Community Genetics, Department of Clinical Genetics, Amsterdam Public Health Research Institute, Amsterdam, Netherlands,* [2] *Institute for Public Health Genomics, School for Oncology and Developmental Biology (GROW), Faculty of Health, Medicine, and Life Sciences, Maastricht University, Maastricht, Netherlands,* [3] *Screening Policy Section, Office of Population Health Genomics, Department of Health, Government of Western Australia, Perth, WA, Australia,* [4] *Center for Nutrition, Prevention and Health Services, National Institute for Public Health and the Environment, Bilthoven, Netherlands*

Correspondence:
Marleen E. Jansen
m.jansen5@vumc.nl

Purpose: Newborn bloodspot screening (NBS) programs have expanded significantly in the past years and are expected to expand further with the emergence of genetic technologies. Historically, NBS expansion has often occurred following *ad hoc* consideration of conditions, instead of a structured and transparent approach. In this review, we explore issues pertinent to NBS policy making, through the lens of the policy cycle: (a) agenda setting, (b) policy advice, (c) policy decision, (d) implementation, and (e) evaluation.

Methods: A literature search was conducted to gather information on the elements specific to NBS and its policy making process.

Results: The review highlighted two approaches to nominate a condition: a structured approach through horizon scanning; and an *ad hoc* process. For assessment of a condition, there was unanimous support for a robust process based on criteria. While the need to assess harms and benefits was a repeated theme in the articles, there is no agreed-upon threshold for benefit in decision-making. Furthermore, the literature was consistent in its recommendation for an overarching, independent, multidisciplinary group providing recommendations to government. An implementation plan focusing on the different levels on which NBS operates and the information needed on each level is essential for successful implementation. Continuously monitoring, and improving a program is vital, particularly following the implementation of screening for a new condition. An advisory committee could advise on implementation, development, review, modification, and cessation of (parts of) NBS.

Conclusion: The results highlight that there are a wave of issues facing NBS programs that policy makers must take into account when developing policy processes. What conditions to screen, and the technologies used in NBS, are both up for debate.

Keywords: decision making, newborn screening, public health policy, genomic screening, genetic testing

INTRODUCTION

Newborn bloodspot screening (NBS) is the longest running and most successful population screening program worldwide (1). NBS tests newborns within the first days of life for multiple serious conditions (2). The traditional aim of NBS is to prevent serious consequences for the newborn by enabling timely diagnoses and treatment for early onset childhood conditions (3). In recent years, technological developments, changes in understanding of conditions, and new treatments, have fueled the expansion of NBS (4, 5). The aim of this study is to explore issues influencing each phase of the policy cycle. In doing so, this study provides policy makers insight in the pressures facing NBS to inform them on approaches to successfully guide programs into the future.

An archetypal example of the policy pressures facing NBS was the advent of tandem mass spectrometry (MS/MS), and the resultant impact it had upon programs worldwide. This technology emerged in the 1990s and made it possible to test for several conditions at once in a cost-effective manner (4, 5). Correspondingly, several programs adopted the technology and significantly increased the number of conditions screened. Programs using these technologies regularly screen from 9 to over 50 conditions (1, 6–9). Even more than MS/MS, genetic technologies may enable screening for a larger number of conditions (3, 10, 11). Debate abounds in the academic literature on the appropriateness of expanding NBS (4, 10, 12): some authors advocate for targeted approaches (13, 14); while elsewhere next generation sequencing is being applied in the research setting to study it's potential for NBS (15, 16).

Previous expansions and the divergent programs that have evolved, suggest that the emergence of genetic technologies is likely to be a significant turning point for NBS. Given the reach of NBS, that NBS tests our most vulnerable population, and the potential to increasingly expand programs, it is essential that decisions on what to screen are carefully considered. Thus policy approaches are needed which can successfully navigate in the changing environment (14). It can be expected that an expansion occurring in some countries will become an example of what is possible for other countries (17). At a minimum, further debate will emerge on the pros and cons of expanded screening, and experts, consumers, and advocacy groups are likely to increase calls for screening for specific conditions (17). The emergence of debates on further expanding NBS presents decision makers worldwide with the challenge of weighing the benefits and harms of screening in the changing landscape of NBS. Policy frameworks, which are developed in light of the range of policy issues, will be essential for policy makers to ensure their programs can effectively respond to the pressures facing the program, now and in the future.

Given the pressures for NBS, the current study aims to identify what the scientific literature outlines are the key policy considerations currently facing NBS. This is achieved by exploring issues pertinent to NBS policy making, through the lens of the policy cycle (10): (a) agenda setting, (b) policy advice, (c) policy decision, (d) implementation, and (e) evaluation. Without detailing current developments in genomic technologies, we aim to explore issues influencing each phase of the policy cycle. In doing so, this study will enable policy makers responsible for existing or emerging NBS programs to consider the best policy structure to respond to the changing environment in which NBS operates.

METHODS

We explored academic literature to summarize relevant factors pertinent to policy making for NBS. International policy making processes have been recently reviewed elsewhere (1, 12). The current study builds upon what is known about the tangible policy making process, by highlighting issues facing NBS identified in academic literature. This then provides policy makers an outline of the issues that should be considered in the development of policies. To be included in the review an article needed to discuss one or more of the following topics: nomination of a condition (agenda setting); consideration of a condition (policy advice); deciding on a condition (policy decision); addition of a condition (implementation); or quality assurance and improvement (evaluation). Articles were also included if they discussed all elements of the policy cycle, such as mention of a comprehensive policy framework for NBS policy making.

We searched PubMed for articles regarding *newborn screening* and *policy*. We combined the two key search terms with the following search terms: 1. *program development*, 2. *decision-making*, 3. *governance*, 4. *management*, 5. *perspective*, 6. *future*, and 7. *disease* or *condition*. Only English publications on dried bloodspot screening were included. Articles concerning other types of newborn screening (e.g., hearing, hip dysplasia) were excluded, because we wanted to focus on the complex policy making specific to bloodspot screening.

RESULTS

The initial literature search identified 59 articles. Twenty-seven articles discussed one or more of the elements of the policy cycle (Table S1 in Supplementary Material). Most literature originated from western societies, predominantly the USA (13 of 27 articles, Table S1 in Supplementary Material) and was initiated from a clinical background rather than a public health background (Figure S1 in Supplementary Material). The main technology discussed in the articles shows a shift through time from MS/MS toward discussing genetic technologies as the challenge for NBS: 3 of 13 articles until 2008 discuss mainly genetic technologies and 6 of 14 published since 2009 (Table S1 in Supplementary Material). Recent articles discussing MS/MS report on results from current screening programs or previous decision-making processes (18). The following outlines the results, stepping through the policy cycle.

Agenda Setting: Nominating a Condition

The review highlighted two approaches to nominating a condition. The first is a structured approach focused on horizon scanning;

the second approach is much more *ad hoc* and influenced by external drivers, such as advocacy (18–20).

The structured, horizon scanning approach generally includes an independent body that undertakes horizon scanning to identify a range of relevant conditions to evaluate for NBS and support expansion through an evidence-based process (10, 21, 22). Such an approach has been successfully used by several countries in agenda setting based on an objective threshold of criteria (18, 22). In horizon scanning, potential conditions are identified and recommended for further in-depth review, through initial assessment of criteria. Contrary to the organized horizon scanning approach, the majority of the literature focused on an *ad hoc* approach. In this approach, conditions became the focus of an assessment for NBS in response to new technologies, broader disease definition, insight into pathophysiology, and advocacy (5, 23–26). In the past, NBS policy direction and program expansion have been strongly influenced by technological drivers, often evaluated *ad hoc* (18–20).

Advocacy is a key driver for change within NBS. Pressure by consumers, clinicians, and scientists to screen for a condition dates back to the very first condition screened in NBS, phenylketonuria (PKU). NBS for PKU was advocated by Dr Guthrie, whose son was born mentally handicapped and whose niece experienced intellectual disability due to undiagnosed and unmanaged PKU (5). Dr Guthrie developed a test to identify the condition and advocated for mass screening of PKU through community support groups (5). Recent examples of advocate pressure leading to the introduction of a condition include in the instance of X-linked adrenoleukodystrophy and Krabbe disease in the USA (5, 10, 27). However, the benefits of screening, for Krabbe are disputed in literature and referred to as "dangerous and expensive" (27).

Policy Advice: Assessment of a Condition

Within the literature reviewed, there was unanimous support for a robust assessment process based on criteria. However, a key issue relating to the assessment of nominated conditions centered on the appropriateness of using criteria originating from the Wilson and Jungner principles (10, 28, 29). Criticisms are voiced that the Wilson and Jungner principles are developed to evaluate individual conditions, while modern day technology pushes toward the possibility and sometimes the need to evaluate groups of conditions at once (30, 31). Furthermore, there is no objective tool developed from the Wilson and Jungner principles, which leaves them open to interpretation into different criteria between programs (31).

While the need to assess harms and benefits was a repeated theme in the articles, there is no agreed-upon threshold for benefit (10, 22, 29). This is essential to effectively explore the benefits and harms of screening, to ensure that the former outweighs the latter. The benefit of screening is intrinsically related to the primary aim of screening, which is predominantly to avoid preventable harm in newborns. The aim and beneficiary screening should both be specified in policies, as they are open to interpretation (9, 32, 33). That is, to support assessing the appropriateness of a condition, there needs to a clear understanding of who will benefit from screening, what is the perceived benefit, and how should it be weighed in decisions (10, 22). In general, three groups were mentioned as potential beneficiaries of NBS: the child, the family, and/or society (34). In the recent report from the Health Council of the Netherlands, the beneficiary of screening was specifically defined as the child. Consequently, this lead to conditions without clear clinical benefits to the child to be assessed as inappropriate for inclusion within NBS (12).

Policy Decision: Deciding on a Condition

The literature focused on two key areas when deciding whether to screen a condition. The first focused on who makes the decision, and the second focused on the evidence on which the decision is made. The literature was consistent in its recommendation for an overarching, independent, multidisciplinary group providing recommendations to government (18, 24, 28).

In terms of evidence, authors of the reviewed literature identified that decisions in NBS often need to be made based on incomplete information (22). A main concern identified in several articles, is the lack of data to support evidence-based decisions. There is the need for interoperable databases to collect sufficient data on the diseases considered and included in NBS (10, 23, 35). Alternatively, authors suggested that innovations in NBS should be implemented in a research paradigm, to facilitate data collection for policy decisions, and gain informed consent from parents participating with their child(ren) in the study (22, 30, 33, 35). Pilot studies are vital to the development of a strong evidence base to support decision-making regarding the addition of new conditions. As shown in Denmark, the Faroe Island, and Greenland, a pilot program of 7 years eventually provided information for evaluation and the subsequent decision to not include 11 conditions in the routine screening program in 2009 (36).

Implementation: Addition of a Condition

Once a condition is approved for implementation in a NBS program, an implementation plan focusing on the different levels on which NBS operates and the information needed at each level should be developed (21, 37, 38). Issues across programs are similar when looking at implementation and relate to five fields: education, finances, logistics, politics, and culture (5, 24). These fields extend beyond "public health" to also include follow-up in the clinical setting. Key issues include the need for work flow across these fields to be coordinated, and ensuring professionals have the relevant skills and knowledge for the new condition(s) (24, 39). Issues to ensure skills and knowledge are particularly challenging where conditions are being identified in the pre-symptomatic phase, and there may be a lack of evidence or consensus in clinical guidelines. This will be further challenged if the preferred technology moves toward genome-based technologies, which can identify genetic variations that have implications for family members. These technologies will lead to issues relating to privacy and confidentiality, residual specimen storage and usage policies, and educational material to become even more pressing (40).

Evaluation: Quality Assurance and Improvement

Continuously monitoring, and improving a program is vital, particularly following the implementation of screening for a new condition (30). It is possible that a condition assessed as being appropriate to screen, will not meet the parameters upon which this decision was based. For example, the false positives or negatives recorded for a test within a trial period might not align with those that occur in the real world setting. Thus quality assurance (QA) is required to monitor the program's performance against defined targets to ensure it aligns with the anticipated outcomes (22, 29, 34).

QA provides essential ongoing assessment of feasibility, cost, and equitable delivery of testing (10, 32, 37). Some authors suggest principles for QA, such as clear guidelines on responsibilities throughout the chain of NBS; standards on aspects regarding confidentiality; and protocols for storage of blood spot specimens (21). Importantly, QA should be complemented by quality improvement (QI). QI builds upon QA, to drive improvements and achieve success. Issues for QI within NBS include managing the improvement process across the NBS system: from health-care professionals to laboratory experts. Ways to overcome fragmentation of providing information on the key indicators while gaining data on them from all parts of NBS can be providing training, develop written educational materials for parents and health-care professionals, and redesign laboratory slips for blood collection (21).

Policy Cycle in General

Authors advocated a transparent, structured, and evidence-based process (22, 25, 41). Policy making for NBS can be governed both locally and nationally (38, 42). Governance is a process that focuses on balancing competing influences and demands (43). The need for harmonization of national policies is often referred to in literature: to ensure a national balance in competing interests and equity in access to early interventions (29, 31). A central body like a national or federal government should play a core role in overseeing NBS. In addition, consultation and engagement is a key theme, which some authors highlight should be managed through a multidisciplinary advisory committee providing advice through the policy cycle (28). An advisory committee could advise them on implementation, development, review, modification, and cessation of (parts of) NBS (21, 29, 38).

DISCUSSION

Stepping through the policy cycle illustrated that NBS is on the precipice of great change. Programs are facing a wave of pressures, including in response to new treatments and new technologies. The history of NBS suggests the programs are flexible in responding to a continually changing environment. However, the historical *ad hoc* approach to adding conditions to NBS is recognized as potentially problematic in the light of future developments. Current NBS programs might contain conditions that have not been robustly evaluated through an agreed policy advice process. Future developments and challenges highlight that policy makers need to take stock of the issues facing the programs, and develop policies that will ensure safe and appropriate growth of programs (22, 25, 41).

The growing number of conditions that could be screened is a key issue for NBS programs, particularly in the face of pressures from next generation sequencing (13, 44). Moreover, the potentially growing number of conditions extends beyond what is technologically possible, to challenge the fundamental purpose of the programs. Internationally, there are increasing calls to move further beyond the traditional aim of NBS, and screen for "untreatable" conditions (33, 34). Untreatable conditions do not always have a certain treatment benefit or treatment is not urgently needed in the newborn period. For untreatable conditions to be implemented in NBS, some argue that the aim has to shift from clinical benefits solely for the child, to include family benefits (24, 29). Such a shift in the focus of beneficiary beyond the newborn, will lead to a vast increase in the number and type of conditions eligible for screening (3, 22): a great number of conditions may have family benefit through information on relevant reproductive options compared to a limited amount of conditions that have direct clinical benefit for the newborn (34).

The above issues overwhelmingly outline the need for robust and considered policy making for NBS. However, it is unclear whether such policy making can fully combat the pressures facing the program. Many nomination processes can still be considered passive where a nomination is awaited, instead of active horizon scanning for relevant conditions. Further, should there be a shift in focus or a push for more conditions to be screened, it is recommended that this be accompanied with consideration as to whether NBS is the right place to screen for such conditions. Specifically, in order to protect the programs and ensure they stay true to their aim, consideration should be given to preconception, prenatal, or screening during early childhood.

Our study has several limitations, data from the USA were overrepresented (13 of the 27 articles) and a sample of 27 articles might not be representative for international policy making in NBS. Further, the policy cycle is theoretical. As such, the recommendations from academic literature are prone to interpretational disparity between theory and practice. Nonetheless, this review shows relevant aspects in policy making and addresses gaps in the current processes. Our results suggests that there is the need for a structured and timely approach that responds to the changing environment.

Through a systematic, continuous policy process, NBS programs will be able to anticipate developments, as opposed to being reactive and heavily influenced by external drivers. A policy process that is developed in light of the issues raised here will help the programs to anticipate challenges and progress in a safe and effective way. A framework to facilitate this approach should be strived for. Only by making careful and considered decisions, can we ensure that NBS of the future is as successful as the existing programs we know today.

AUTHOR CONTRIBUTIONS

MJ contributed to the conception and design of the work, analysis and interpretation of data, drafted the work, and revised it. KL contributed to the interpretation of data and critically revised the work. HK contributed to the design of the work and critically revised it. MC contributed to the conception and design of the work, interpretation of data, and critically revised the work. All authors approved the version to be published, and agreed to be accountable for all aspects of the work in ensuring that questions related to the accuracy or integrity of any part of the work are appropriately investigated and resolved.

SUPPLEMENTARY MATERIAL

FIGURE S1 | Proportion of the affiliations of the first authors of the articles included in the review.

TABLE S1 | Articles included in the review (*n* = 26) with a short summary of each article, as well as the main stakeholder groups discussed, articles are sorted based on publication date to illustrate the shift in the technologies discussed

REFERENCES

1. Therrell BL, Padilla CD, Loeber JG, Kneisser I, Saadallah A, Borrajo GJC, et al. Current status of newborn screening worldwide: 2015. *Semin Perinatol* (2015) 39:171–87. doi:10.1053/j.semperi.2015.03.002
2. Health Council of the Netherlands. *Neonatal Screening: New Recommendations*. The Hague: Health Council of the Netherlands (2015).
3. Bombard Y, Miller FA, Hayeems RZ, Avard D, Knoppers BM. Reconsidering reproductive benefit through newborn screening: a systematic review of guidelines on preconception, prenatal and newborn screening. *Eur J Hum Genet* (2010) 18:751–60. doi:10.1038/ejhg.2010.13
4. Moyer VA, Calonge N, Teutsch SM, Botkin JR. Expanding newborn screening: process, policy, and priorities. *Hastings Cent Rep* (2008) 38(3):32–9. doi:10.1353/hcr.0.0011
5. Therrell BL. U.S. newborn screening policy dilemmas for the twenty-first century. *Mol Genet Metab* (2001) 74:64–74. doi:10.1006/mgme.2001.3238
6. Dezateux C. Evaluating newborn screening programmes based on dried blood spots: future challenges. *Br Med Bull* (1998) 54(4):877–90. doi:10.1093/oxfordjournals.bmb.a011735
7. Pollitt RJ. Introducing new screens: why are we all doing different things? *J Inherit Metab Dis* (2007) 360:423–9. doi:10.1007/s10545-007-0647-2
8. Pollitt RJ. Newborn blood spot screening: new opportunities, old problems. *J Inherit Metab Dis* (2009) 32:395–9. doi:10.1007/s10545-009-9962-0
9. Potter BK, Avard D, Wilson BJ. Newborn blood spot screening in four countries: stakeholder involvement. *J Public Health Policy* (2008) 29(1):121–42. doi:10.1057/palgrave.jphp.3200161
10. Bailey DB, Beskow LM, Davis AM, Skinner D. Changing perspectives on the benefits of newborn screening. *Ment Retard Dev Disabil Res Rev* (2006) 12:270–9. doi:10.1002/mrdd.20119
11. Topol EJ. Individualized medicine from prewomb to tomb. *Cell* (2014) 157(1):241–53. doi:10.1016/j.cell.2014.02.012
12. Jansen ME, Metternick-Jones SC, Lister KJ. International differences in the evaluation of conditions for newborn bloodspot screening: a review of scientific literature and policy documents. *Eur J Hum Genet* (2016) 25(1):10–6. doi:10.1038/ejhg.2016.126
13. Howard HC, Knoppers BM, Cornel MC, Wright Clayton E, Senecal K, Borry P, et al. Whole-genome sequencing in newborn screening? A statement on the continued importance of targeted approaches in newborn screening programmes. *Eur J Hum Genet* (2015) 23(12):1593–600. doi:10.1038/ejhg.2014.289
14. Knoppers BM, Sénécal K, Borry P, Avard D. Whole-genome sequencing in newborn screening programs. *Sci Transl Med* (2014) 6(229):229cm2. doi:10.1126/scitranslmed.3008494
15. Roberts JS, Dolinoy DC, Tarini BA. Emerging issues in public health genomics. *Annu Rev Genomics Hum Genet* (2014) 15:461–80. doi:10.1146/annurev-genom-090413-025514
16. Nowogrodzki A. *Should Babies Have Their Genomes Sequenced?* (2015). Available from: http://www.technologyreview.com/news/538931/should-babies-have-their-genomes-sequenced/
17. Metternick-Jones SC, Lister KJ, Dawkins HJS, White CA, Weeramanthri TS. Review of current international decision-making processes for newborn screening: lessons for Australia. *Front Public Health* (2015) 3:214. doi:10.3389/fpubh.2015.00214
18. Fischer KE, Grosse SD, Rogowski WH. The role of health technology assessment in coverage decisions on newborn screening. *Int J Technol Assess Health Care* (2011) 27(4):313–21. doi:10.1017/S0266462311000468
19. Avard D, Stanton Jean M, Grégoire G, Page M. Public involvement in health genomics: the reality behind the policies. *Int J Consum Stud* (2010) 34(5):508–24. doi:10.1111/j.1470-6431.2010.00914.x
20. EURORDIS. *The Voice of Rare Disease Patients in Europe*. (2015). Available from: http://www.eurordis.org/
21. Atkinson K, Zuckerman B, Sharfstein JM, Levin D, Blatt RJR, Koh HK. A public health response to emerging technology: expansion of the Massachusetts newborn screening program. *Public Health Rep* (2001) 116:122–31. doi:10.1016/S0033-3549(04)50004-3
22. Grosse SD, Boyle CA, Kenneson A, Khoury MJ, Wilfond BS. From public health emergency to public health service, the implications of evolving criteria for newborn screening panels. *Pediatrics* (2006) 117(3):923–9. doi:10.1542/peds.2005-0553
23. Bailey DB, Skinner D, Davis AM, Withmarsh I, Powell C. Ethical, legal, and social concerns about expanded newborn screening: fragile X syndrome as a prototype for emerging issues. *Pediatrics* (2008) 121:e693–704. doi:10.1542/peds.2007-0820
24. Dhondt J. Expanded newborn screening: social and ethical issues. *J Inherit Metab Dis* (2010) 33(Suppl 2):S211–7. doi:10.1007/s10545-010-9138-y
25. Hayeems RZ, Miller FA, Bombard Y, Avard D, Carroll J, Wilson B, et al. Expectations and values about expanded newborn screening: a public engagement study. *Health Expect* (2013) 18(3):419–29. doi:10.1111/hex.12047
26. Therrell BL Jr. Considerations in choosing screening conditions: one (US) approach. *Ann Acad Med Singapore* (2008) 37(12 Suppl):22–5.
27. Dees RH, Kwon JM. The ethics of Krabbe newborn screening. *Public Health Ethics* (2013) 6(1):114–28. doi:10.1093/phe/phs033
28. Plass AMC, van El CG, Pieters T, Cornel MC. Neonatal screening for treatable and untreatable disorders: prospective parents' opinions. *Pediatrics* (2009) 125:e99–106. doi:10.1542/peds.2009-0269
29. Elliman DAC, Dezateux C, Bedford HE. Newborn and childhood screening programmes: criteria, evidence, and current policy. *Arch Dis Child* (2002) 87:6–9. doi:10.1136/adc.87.1.6
30. Arn PH. Newborn screening: current status. *Health Aff* (2007) 26(2):559–66. doi:10.1377/hlthaff.26.2.559
31. Petros M. Revisiting the Wilson-Jungner criteria: how can supplemental criteria guide public health in the era of genetic testing? *Genet Med* (2012) 14(1):129–34. doi:10.1038/gim.0b013e31823331d0
32. Burke W, Laberge A-M, Press N. Debating clinical utility. *Public Health Genomics* (2010) 13:215–23. doi:10.1159/000279623
33. Clayton EW. What should be the role of public health in newborn screening and prenatal diagnosis? *Am J Prev Med* (1999) 16(2):111–5. doi:10.1016/S0749-3797(98)00142-1
34. Bailey DB. The blurred distinction between treatable and untreatable conditions in newborn screening. *Health Matrix* (2009) 19(1):141–53.
35. Botkin JR, Lewis MH, Watson MS, Swoboda KJ, Anderson R, Berry SA, et al. Parental permission for pilot newborn screening research: guidelines from the NBSTRN. *Pediatrics* (2014) 133:e410–7. doi:10.1542/peds.2013-2271

36. Lund AM, Hougaard DM, Simonsen H, Andresen BS, Christensen M, Dunø M, et al. Biochemical screening of 504,049 newborns in Denmark, the Faroe Islands and Greenland—experience and development of a routine program for expanded newborn screening. *Mol Genet Metab* (2012) 107(3):281–93. doi:10.1016/j.ymgme.2012.06.006
37. Comeau AM, Parad R, Gerstle R, O'Sullivan BP, Dorkin HL, Dovey M, et al. Challenges in implementing a successful newborn cystic fibrosis screening program. *J Pediatr* (2005) 147:S89–93. doi:10.1016/j.jpeds.2005.08.006
38. Cornejo V, Raimann E, Cabello JF, Valiente A, Becerra C, Opazo M, et al. Past, present and future of newborn screening in Chile. *J Inherit Metab Dis* (2010) 33(Suppl 3):S301–6. doi:10.1007/s10545-010-9165-8
39. Kasper DC, Ratschmann R, Metz TF, Mechtler TP, Moslinger D, Konstantopoulou V, et al. The national Austrian newborn screening program – eight years experience with mass spectrometry. Past, present, and future goals. *Wien Klin Wochenschr* (2010) 122:607–13. doi:10.1007/s00508-010-1457-3
40. Bombard Y, Miller FA, Hayeems RZ, Barg C, Cressman C, Carroll JC, et al. Public views on participating in newborn screening using genome sequencing. *Eur J Hum Genet* (2014) 22(11):1248–54. doi:10.1038/ejhg.2014.22
41. Benkendorf J, Goodspeed T, Watson MS. Newborn screening residual dried blood spot use for newborn screening quality improvement. *Genet Med* (2010) 12:S269–72. doi:10.1097/GIM.0b013e3181fea489
42. Hiller EH, Landenburger G, Natowicz MR. Public participation in medical policy-making and the status of consumer autonomy: the example of newborn screening programs in the United States. *Am J Public Health* (1997) 87(8):1280–8. doi:10.2105/AJPH.87.8.1280
43. WHO. *Governance: World Health Organization.* (2015). Available from: http://www.who.int/healthsystems/topics/stewardship/en/
44. Chen R, Shi L, Hakenberg J, Naughton B, Sklar P, Zhang J, et al. Analysis of 589,306 genomes identifies individuals resilient to severe Mendelian childhood diseases. *Nat Biotechnol* (2016) 34(5):531–8. doi:10.1038/nbt.3514

19

Development of a Complex Intervention to Improve Adherence to Antidiabetic Medication in Older People Using an Anthropomorphic Virtual Assistant Software

Isa Brito Félix[1], Mara Pereira Guerreiro[1,2], Afonso Cavaco[3], Ana Paula Cláudio[4], Anabela Mendes[1], João Balsa[4], Maria Beatriz Carmo[4], Nuno Pimenta[5] and Adriana Henriques[1]*

[1] Unidade de Investigação e Desenvolvimento em Enfermagem (UI&DE), Lisbon Nursing School, Lisbon, Portugal, [2] Centro de Investigação Interdisciplinar Egas Moniz (CiiEM), Instituto Universitário Egas Moniz, Monte de Caparica, Portugal, [3] iMed. ULisboa, Faculty of Pharmacy, University of Lisbon, Lisbon, Portugal, [4] Biosystems & Integrative Sciences Institute (BioISI), Faculty of Sciences, University of Lisbon, Lisbon, Portugal, [5] Sport Sciences School of Rio Maior, Polytechnic Institute of Santarém, Santarém, Portugal

***Correspondence:**
Mara Pereira Guerreiro
mara.guerreiro@esel.pt

Introduction: Improving adherence to antidiabetic medication is crucial, resulting in improved health outcomes, cost reduction, and minimization of waste. A lack of underlying theory in existing interventions may explain the limited success in sustaining behavior change. This paper describes the development of a theory and evidence-based complex intervention to improve adherence to oral antidiabetics in older people *via* a software prototype with an anthropomorphic virtual assistant.

Methods: The Behavior Change Wheel (BCW) was used to develop a theoretical understanding of the change process, corresponding to the first phase of the Medical Research Council Framework for developing and evaluating complex interventions. At the BCW core is a model of human behavior (COM-B), which posits that human behavior (B) results from the interaction between capabilities (C), opportunities (O), and motivation (M). Literature-derived medication adherence determinants were mapped onto COM-B components. Then, intervention functions (IFs) were selected employing the APEASE criteria. Finally, standardized behavior change techniques (BCTs) were chosen based on their suitability and their effectiveness on medication adherence trials. The prototype was developed for android devices; its core was implemented in Unity3D, using a female 3D virtual assistant, named Vitória.

Results: Two COM-B components were identified as main targets for behavior change—psychological capability and reflective motivation; these were linked with four IFs—education, persuasion, enablement, and environmental restructuring. Eleven BCTs were, in turn, linked with the IFs. An example of a BCT is "problem solving"; it requires users to pinpoint factors influencing non-adherence and subsequently offers strategies to achieve the desired behavior. BCTs were operationalized into the dialogues with Vitória and into supplementary software features. Vitória communicates with users verbally and non-verbally, expressing emotions. Input options consist of buttons or recording values, such as medication taken.

Conclusion: The present approach enabled us to derive the most appropriate BCTs for our intervention. The use of an explicit bundle of BCTs, often overlooked in interventions promoting medication adherence, is expected to maximize effectiveness and facilitates replication. The first prototype is being refined with users and health professionals' contributions. Future work includes subjecting the prototype to usability tests and a feasibility trial.

Keywords: relational agent, older adult, type 2 diabetes, medication adherence, virtual assistant, behavior change wheel, intervention development, complex intervention

INTRODUCTION

Globally, diabetes affects more than 425 million people, of which one-third is older than 65 years (International Diabetes Federation, 2017). Type 2 diabetes (T2D) is the most prevalent form around the world, affecting 90% of the diabetic adults (Zheng et al., 2018). Glycemic control, which is key to prevent complications, requires sustained adherence to an appropriate diet, adequate physical activity, and, frequently, antidiabetic medication.

A systematic review including 27 studies found that adherence to antidiabetic medication can be as low as 38.5% (Krass et al., 2015). A recent study reported an overall antidiabetics adherence in older people of 72.4% (Juste et al., 2018). Additionally, Spanish elderly patients receiving oral antidiabetics showed rates of discontinuation for oral antidiabetics of 46.8% (Menditto et al., 2018).

Poor medication adherence in T2D is associated with negative outcomes, including increased morbidity and mortality, increased costs of ambulatory and hospital care, as well as loss of quality of life (Iuga and McGuire, 2014).

A wide array of factors associated with non-adherence has been described, which may differ according to study designs. For example, key nonpatient factors (e.g., healthcare systems limitations), non-modifiable patient factors (e.g., young age, low income level), and modifiable patient factors (e.g., beliefs about perceived treatment efficacy and medication burden) may be associated with non-adherence (Polonsky and Henry, 2016). Capoccia et al. (2016) mentioned lower adherence when medications were not tolerated or were taken more than twice daily.

Strategies to overcome poor medication adherence should consider the reduction of the medication burden, not only from a drug perspective (e.g., using fixed combinations) but also tools for an easier therapy management, plus responding to negative medication beliefs (Polonsky and Henry, 2016; Capoccia et al., 2016). Modifiable psychosocial factors belong to the overarching domains of knowledge, beliefs (and related cognitive constructs), behavioral skills, and coping (Gonzalez et al., 2016); thus, interventions targeting these aspects are expected to improve antidiabetic medication adherence.

Until recently, very few interventions to improve medication adherence were technology-based. Williams et al. (2014) reported a systematic review on effective interventions to improve medication adherence in T2D, in which the literature was searched from 2000 to 2013. The authors only found five studies using mobile phones or the Internet.

The advantages of technology-based interventions include automation and convenience of access. While simple electronic reminders, such as SMS, have shown improvement in medication adherence in chronic diseases (Vervloet et al., 2012), they are not without caveats. These reminders target essentially unintentional non-adherence and their long-term effects are uncertain (Vervloet et al., 2012). Technological development brought supplementary approaches, such as web-based interfaces, mobile applications, or smartwatches.

Currently, one of the most used technologies is referred to as mHealth apps (mobile health applications, typically for iOS or android devices). The rapid growth of these apps occurs in the context of aging population. The mHealth advances align well with the growing interest of older adults to integrate technology in the self-management of chronic conditions (Gilbert et al., 2015; Kim and Lee, 2017).

Concerning medication adherence, Anglada-Martinez et al. (2015) concluded that 65% of the mHealth application trials reported positive results. Virtual humans, designed to build long-term socioemotional relationships with users, can be incorporated in mHealth applications. Such virtual humans are commonly referred to as relational agents, although the term is often used interchangeably with virtual agent or assistant. There is a considerable body of knowledge on the effect or acceptability of relational agents in different populations. The acceptability to older people, including those with low literacy, has been studied (Bickmore et al., 2010). These authors found that individuals with inadequate literacy generally report higher levels of satisfaction with the relational agent and ask more questions than those with adequate health literacy. This has implications for our project, as the health literacy of older people in Portugal is limited (Mota-Pinto et al., 2010; Paiva et al., 2017).

Additionally, research suggests that a relational agent software is effective in promoting medication adherence and accepted by people with schizophrenia (Bickmore et al., 2010). Recently, the effect of an embodied conversional agent on antiretroviral therapy adherence was researched, using a 3-month pre-post design (Dworkin et al., 2019). This study demonstrated a positive effect on pill count, which improved from 62% at baseline to 88% at follow-up. The use of these agents to support diabetes self-care, including medication adherence, seems to have received less attention. Exceptions are papers describing coaching interventions for diabetes patients, which focus on medication adherence (op den Akker et al., 2011; Monkaresi et al., 2013). However, these papers lack data on usability or the effect on endpoints of interest.

The present paper aims to describe the development of a theory and evidence-based complex intervention to improve adherence to oral antidiabetics in older people *via* a software prototype with an anthropomorphic virtual assistant (VASelfCare). This is part of a wider intervention, targeting also lifestyle change of elderly T2D patients.

MATERIALS AND METHODS

Complex interventions include several interacting components that impact on the length and complexity of the causal chain and are influenced by features of the local context (Craig et al., 2008). The components usually include behaviors, characteristics of behavior (e.g., timing) and methods of organizing, and delivering those behaviors (e.g., setting and location). Many healthcare interventions are considered complex. The Medical Research Council (MRC) framework for developing and evaluating complex interventions has been widely employed (Bleijenberg et al., 2018); it provides guidance on the methodological and practical decision-making on healthcare interventions. The rationale for resorting to this framework is that interventions carefully designed and tested in an early stage are more likely to prevent negative or inconclusive trials (Craig et al., 2008).

Figure 1 depicts the MRC framework phases. Phase 1 encompasses three elements (Craig et al., 2008), two of which are focused in the present paper: "identifying the existing evidence" and "identifying or developing theory." Identifying the existing evidence included a mapping review on the effectiveness of relational agents, on the design of these interventions and on successful medication adherence interventions. We followed guidelines for self-management of people with T2D, focusing on key dimensions of lifestyle (diet and physical activity) plus medication adherence (Powers et al., 2015). It has been suggested that interventions targeting behaviors in a stepwise approach are more effective in promoting change than targeting multi-behaviors simultaneously (Sweet and Fortier, 2010).

The mapping review informed the intervention components. One of the intervention components is the nurse interaction with older people upon referral from the software prototype, in predefined circumstances. Moreover, the experience of Bleijenberg and colleagues (2018) with the MRC framework indicates that it is important to consider the elements of context, e.g., how the receiver (older people with T2D) and the provider (nurse) interact within the intervention. In Portugal, diabetes nursing consultations in primary care have been formally established as supplementary to medical consultations.

Another key task in phase 1 (**Figure 1**) is to develop a theoretical understanding of the underlying processes of change. The section Deriving the Active Ingredients of the Intervention describes the use of theory for deriving the active ingredients of the intervention. Then the section Development of the VASelfCare Software Prototype provides a brief description of how the software prototype was developed.

Deriving the Active Ingredients of the Intervention

We chose the Behavior Change Wheel (BCW) (Michie et al., 2014) as the theoretical framework underpinning the intervention. The BCW is a recent approach to design research of behavior change interventions through a systematic and structured process (Michie et al., 2011; Cane et al., 2012). This process enables the evidence-based selection of intervention components, ensuring that the intervention targets the underlying determinants of behavior.

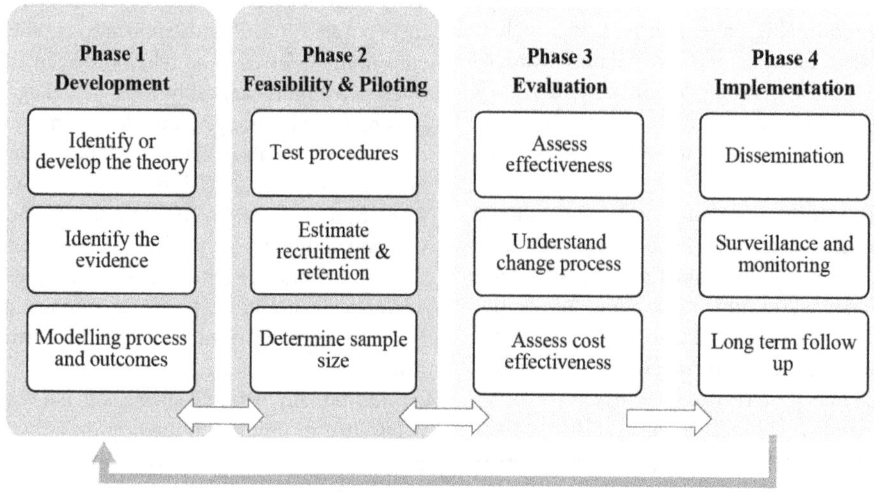

FIGURE 1 | Medical Research Council framework (Craig et al., 2008).

At the BCW core is a model of human behavior—the COM-B—which posits that human behavior (B) results from the interaction between physical and psychological capabilities (C), opportunities provided by the physical and social environment (O) and reflective and automatic motivation (M) (Michie et al., 2014). The COM-B is supported by the Theoretical Domains Framework (TDF), which describes 14 factors derived from 33 theories of behavior change. These factors fall under the categories of capability, opportunity, and motivation (Cane et al., 2012).

In the next sections, we will describe the stepwise approach to derive behavior change techniques (BCTs) for improving medication adherence based on the BCW.

Stage 1: Understanding the Behavior

We tackled this stage by reviewing the evidence on adherence and its determinants, which includes both barriers and facilitators to medication use. Several recent systematic literature reviews on determinants of adherence have been published. In particular, we draw on the seminal WHO on adherence determinants (Sabaté, 2003) and on systematic reviews and literature with the same scope to understand influences to medication use (Gellad et al., 2011; Kardas et al., 2013; Zeber et al., 2013; Capoccia et al., 2016; Yap et al., 2016; Choi and Smaldone, 2018). Subsequently, we mapped these determinants into the COM-B and identified key domains more influential to behavior change, through a multidisciplinary consensus discussion within the research team. This team has expertise in nursing, medication adherence, clinical pharmacology, and clinical communication.

Stage 2: Identifying Intervention Functions

Intervention functions (IFs) are defined as "broad categories of means by which an intervention can change behavior" (Michie et al., 2014, 192). Based on a systematic review of frameworks of behavior change interventions, Michie et al. (2011) put forward nine IFs. The BCW links COM-B domains to IFs and subsequent policy categories most likely to achieve behavioral change (Michie et al., 2011, 2014). Policy categories represent "types of decisions made by authorities that help to support and enact the intervention" (Michie et al., 2014, 235). We did not address these categories as they fell outside the scope of our intervention.

The IFs and their relation to the COM-B domains were organized in a mapping matrix (Michie et al., 2014). The former were selected based on their links to COM-B domains, as prescribed by the authors (Michie et al., 2014). The same IF can be linked to different COM-B domains. IFs most likely to affect behavior change were selected in a multidisciplinary consensus discussion within the research team, using the APEASE criteria: 1) affordability, 2) practicality, 3) effectiveness and cost-effectiveness, 4) acceptability, 5) side-effects/safety, and 6) equity (Michie et al., 2014).

Stage 3: Identifying Behavior Change Techniques

A BCT is an observable, replicable, and irreducible component of an intervention designed to change behavior (Michie et al., 2013). BCTs are known as the active ingredients of the intervention. They have been organized in a taxonomy, designated in brief by BCTTv1 (Michie et al., 2013; Cane et al., 2015), which provides a definition for each of the 93 techniques, enabling a consistent application.

There is guidance on the BCTs better suited to certain IFs and their underlying theoretical domains (Michie et al., 2008; Cane et al., 2015). From the list of 93 BCTs, the most appropriate for our intervention were selected based on:

- The most common BCTs under each IF (Michie et al., 2014).
- Effective medication adherence interventions from which BCTs could be derived (Nieuwlaat et al., 2014; Williams et al., 2014; Sapkota et al., 2015).
- A multidisciplinary discussion informed by the APEASE criteria, in particular on the practicality of including the BCT in light of the automated nature of the intervention.

Development of the VASelfCare Software Prototype

We decided that the application would run in tablets with android system without requiring Internet connection. This decision was grounded on the need to secure inclusive access, considering that presently a significant percentage of older adults' homes do not have Internet available (INE, 2014). Such decision, in turn, influenced software development options.

The overall development of the application was guided by usability principles for older people with T2D (Arnhold et al., 2014). For example, redundancy of both audio and written information may help reduce any communication shortcomings, such as lower eyesight accuracy and hearing deficits.

The core of VASelfCare solution was implemented in Unity3D (https://unity3d.com/pt), a software for the development of video games.

The virtual assistant chosen for this first prototype was a female 3D model with a realistic look, obtained from Daz3D (https://www.daz3d.com/). The choice for a 3D character is supported by studies that concluded that realistic-looking virtual agents are more appropriate for medical tasks (Ring et al., 2014; van Wissen et al., 2016). Other applications have also employed female figures as relational agents, for example (Bickmore et al., 2005a; Bickmore et al., 2005b).

Body animations and facial expressions are activated by the software that controls the virtual assistant behavior and verifies the context of the on-going interaction. Conveying emotions to users, beyond messages content, intends to establish an affective and effective communication. Furthermore, this has been acknowledged as the cornerstone for engagement and long-term use (Bickmore et al., 2010).

To support the virtual assistant speech, first dialogues had to be created, then the corresponding sound is generated and mouth animations that simulate the articulation of the sound were provided.

Dialogues were iteratively created by team members with a nursing and pharmacy background. Quality of the output was ensured by agreeing on principles at the outset of the process, by discussing dialogue structured regularly and through independent double-checking of scripts. To streamline this creative process, we adopted Yarn (https://github.com/InfiniteAmmoInc/Yarn), a graphical dialogue editor simple to use and compatible with the other software tools that were being used. Yarn provides an interface where the speech lines of the virtual assistant and the options that the user may choose (i.e., buttons in the interface) are inserted in text boxes. These are sequentially connected in a way that expresses the possible progressions of the dialogue during the interaction between the user and the virtual assistant.

General principles were deployed to write a comprehensive and optimal dialogue for each individual user (Migneault et al., 2006). One principle was tailoring content, which has been defined as "any combination of information and behavior change strategies intended to reach one specific person based on characteristics that are unique to that person related to the outcome of interest and derived from an individual assessment" (Kreuter et al., 2000). A meta-analysis showed that tailored web-based interventions have a significantly greater effect in health behavior outcomes than non-tailored counterparts (Lustria et al., 2013). Another principle was personalization, which broadly involves giving an indication that the software "knows who is talking to" (Migneault et al., 2006). A non-judgmental approach was employed to create the dialogues, resorting to a helpful-cooperative communication style (Niess and Diefenbach, 2016). Such an approach aims at creating rapport and a trust-bond, so that effectiveness of BCTs may be enhanced, along with other psychological benefits, as reported in the literature on virtual assistant-based interventions (Velicer et al., 2015).

A rule-based component was implemented to control the dialogue flow of the interaction. This component corresponds to the definition of a set of if–then rules (rules of the form "if *some conditions hold* then *execute some action*"), where the *conditions* may include context information regarding the interaction (e.g., user characteristics, such as age, or the date when interaction takes place) and the *action* represents the subsequent locutionary act performed by the virtual assistant. This approach allows greater flexibility in the dialogue definition and in the generation of diversified interactions.

Speech2Go from Harpo (https://harposoftware.com) was used to generate the audio files. This is a text-to-speech (TTS) software, which converts the written dialogues to audio speech. Since the virtual assistant is currently represented by a female character, the female voice of Inês, a European Portuguese voice, has been used. The speech rate has been slowed down, taking into consideration the target population.

Visemes describe the animations of the virtual assistant's mouth that simulate phonemes' articulation. Conversion of written dialogues to the viseme files is performed by a software developed in a previous project (Cláudio et al., 2015).

SQLite (https://www.sqlite.org/index.html) was the database engine chosen to control all the information stored locally in each tablet as it encompasses a secure storage mechanism. The local database, initially empty, will store clinical data registered by the care nurse, such as the prescribed antidiabetic medication, weight, and HbA1c. It will then be filled with data inserted during user interactions, including clinical data such as blood glucose levels, medication taken, and number of daily steps. These data are deployed in future interactions with the user and enable analysis at a later stage, contributing to the further development of the software prototype. Periodically, the database in each tablet is copied to an institutional computer using a secure connection and the access to this repository is reserved for credentialed personal. Privacy is further ensured by restricting access to this repository only to the researcher responsible for data analysis; data will be extracted omitting any reference that could identify the user.

RESULTS

Deriving the Active Ingredients of the Intervention

Stage 1: Understanding the Behavior

The target behavior of this intervention is medication adherence, defined briefly as the behavioral response to an agreed medical recommendation (Sabaté, 2003). Recently, medication adherence has been defined as a process consisting of three stages: initiation, implementation, and discontinuation (Vrijens et al., 2012). The target behavior for this intervention was further defined as taking between 80% and 100% of the prescribed antidiabetic doses. The 80% cut-off point is underpinned by previous research that stratified adherent and non-adherent individuals based on predicting subsequent hospital admission across prevalent chronic conditions, including diabetes (Karve et al., 2009). The clinical implications of non-adherence to antidiabetic agents have been discussed earlier in the Introduction section.

To be effective the software prototype should target modifiable determinants of adherence (Allemann et al., 2016). Therefore, determinants with a negative effect on adherence, amenable of change by the prototype or other intervention components, were extracted from the literature (Gellad et al., 2011; Kardas et al., 2013; Zeber et al., 2013; Capoccia et al., 2016; Yap et al., 2016; Choi and Smaldone, 2018). For example, medication cost is not directly modifiable by the software prototype, but can be addressed *via* referral to the primary care nurse. The same applies to suspected adverse drug reactions, which the prototype cannot manage on its own. **Table 1** depicts the determinants influential on behavior change mapped into key domains of the COM-B.

Stage 2: Identifying Intervention Functions

Table 2 presents the IFs selected and the reasons for their inclusion or exclusion. Overall, two IFs—"modeling" and "training"—were excluded because they were deemed impracticable to be applied *via* the software.

TABLE 1 | Adherence determinants mapped into the COM-B model.

Adherence determinants	COM-B components
Comprehension of disease and treatment	Psychological capability
Cognitive functioning (e.g., memory)	
Perception of illness	Reflective motivation
Concerns about medication	
Beliefs about medication necessity	
Outcome expectancies about treatment	
Self-efficacy	

TABLE 2 | Links between the COM-B model and relevant intervention functions.

COM-B components	Intervention function	Intervention function definition	Reasons for inclusion/exclusion (APEASE criteria)	Included/excluded from the next stage
Psychological capability	Education	Increasing knowledge or understanding	Considered affordable, practical, potentially effective, potentially acceptable, safe, and equative.	Included
	Training	Imparting skills	Not practical to delivery through the software prototype.	Excluded
	Enablement	Increasing means/reducing barriers to increase capability (beyond education/training) or opportunity (beyond environmental restructuring)	Considered affordable, practical, potentially effective, acceptable, safe, and equative.	Included
	Environmental restructuring	Changing the physical or social context	Considered affordable, practical, potentially effective, potentially acceptable, safe, and equative.	Included
Reflective motivation	Education	Increasing knowledge or understanding	Considered affordable, practical, potentially effective, potentially acceptable, safe, and equative.	Included
	Persuasion	Using communication to induce positive or negative feelings or stimulate action	Considered affordable, practical, potentially effective, potentially acceptable, safe, and equative.	Included
	Modelling	Providing an example for people to aspire to or imitate	Not practical to delivery through the software prototype.	Excluded
	Education	Increasing knowledge or understanding	Considered affordable, practical, potentially effective, potentially acceptable, safe, and equative.	Included
	Persuasion	Using communication to induce positive or negative feelings or stimulate action	Considered affordable, practical, potentially effective, potentially acceptable, safe, and equative.	Included
	Modelling	Providing an example for people to aspire to or imitate	Not practical to delivery through the software prototype.	Excluded
	Enablement	Increasing means/reducing barriers to increase capability (beyond education/training) or opportunity (beyond environmental restructuring)	Considered affordable, practical, potentially effective, potentially acceptable, safe, and equative.	Included

Stage 3: Identifying Behavior Change Techniques

Eleven BCTs were selected to be included in the software prototype (**Table 3**).

The selected BCTs can serve more than one IF. For example, "feedback on behavior" could be linked to the "education" and "persuasion" functions. This BCT was operationalized by providing information on medication-taking behavior *via* a chart (**Figure 2**), described by the virtual assistant, plus giving supportive messages about the user's abilities to perform the desired behavior. **Figures 3**, **4**, and **5** depict software interfaces representing "biofeedback," "self-monitoring of behavior," and "problem-solving," respectively. While the software prototype is in Portuguese, we present figures in English to facilitate readers' understanding.

Development of the Medication Adherence Component of the VASelfCare Prototype

Prior to the user's first interaction with the prototype, registration by a nurse providing care in diabetes consultations is required. There is a specific interface for this purpose that includes mandatory clinical information, such as the prescribed antidiabetic medication and the last HbA1c level.

When a user interacts with the prototype for the first time, a number of features are available. A key feature, described in the next section, is the dialogue view, in which the user interacts with Vitória, an anthropomorphic virtual assistant. Supplementary features are offered in other views. The prototype is designed to allow no more than one full interaction with Vitória per day. Access to the other views is unrestricted.

Interaction With the Dialogue View

Vitória is capable of speaking, by means of a synthetic voice, and features also text subtitles, reproducing the verbal content. Furthermore, Vitória expresses herself non-verbally with users, providing emotions through facial and body animations, depending on the user's response. The user communicates with Vitória using buttons or by recording values, such as medication taken.

To attain a more convincing experience, the 3D scenario where Vitória is displayed changes, for example, according to the time of the day and season of the year.

Initially, the user is prompted to select a component to start with (medication adherence or lifestyle changes—diet or physical activity). Assuming the medication component is selected, the first 3 days are devoted to evaluation. The main purpose of this phase is to collect data on user's knowledge about antidiabetic agents, current behavior on medication-taking and perceived self-efficacy in medication management, for future tailoring of the intervention.

The evaluation phase was structured as a six-step interaction: opening; social talk; assessment; feedback; pre-closing; and closing. This structure has been adapted from the literature (Bickmore et al., 2005b). The "opening" step consists of greeting the user and it is followed by the "social talk," which includes inquiries about the user's general emotional and physical state (e.g., "how are you feeling today?"). "Assessment" is the step in which questions about the aforementioned constructs are posed. In the "feedback" step, brief information on the answers is provided. Finally, the contents of the next interaction are described ("pre-closing") and a farewell is delivered ("closing").

TABLE 3 | BCTs selected for the VASelfCare software prototype (antidiabetics adherence).

Intervention functions	BCTs	Definition (Michie et al., 2014)
Education / Persuasion	Feedback on behavior (2.2)	Monitor and provide informative or evaluative feedback on performance of the behavior (e.g., form, frequency, duration, intensity)
Education / Persuasion	Information about health consequences (5.1)	Provide information (e.g., written, verbal, visual) about health consequences of performing the behavior
Education / Persuasion	Biofeedback (2.6)	Provide feedback about the body (e.g., physiological or biochemical state) using an external monitoring device as part of a behavior change strategy
Education	Self-monitoring of behavior (2.3) Prompts/cues (7.1)	Establish a method for the person to monitor and record their behavior(s) as part of a behavior change strategy Introduce or define environmental or social stimulus with the purpose of prompting or cueing the behavior. The prompt or cue would normally occur at the time or place of performance.
Enablement	Action planning (1.4)	Prompt detailed planning of performance of the behavior (must include at least one of context, frequency, duration, and intensity). Context may be environmental (physical or social) or internal (physical, emotional or cognitive) (includes "implementation intentions")
Enablement	Social support (unspecified) (3.1)	Advise on, arrange or provide social support (e.g., from friends, relatives, colleagues, "buddies," or staff) or non-contingent praise or reward for performance of the behavior. It includes encouragement and counseling, but only when it is directed at the behavior
Enablement	Social support (practical) (3.2)	Advise on, arrange, or provide practical help (e.g., from friends, relatives, colleagues, "buddies," or staff) for performance of the behavior
Enablement	Goal setting (behavior) (1.1)	Set or agree on a goal defined in terms of the behavior to be achieved Note: only code goal-setting if there is sufficient evidence that goal set as part of intervention; if goal unspecified or a behavioral outcome, code 1.3, goal setting (outcome); if the goal defines a specific context, frequency, duration, or intensity for the behavior, also code 1.4, action planning
Enablement	Problem solving (1.2)	Analyze, or prompt the person to analyze, factors influencing the behavior and generate, or select strategies that include overcoming barriers and/or increasing facilitators (includes "relapse prevention" and "coping planning")
Environmental restructuring	Restructuring the physical environmental (12.1)	Change, or advise to change the physical environment in order to facilitate performance of the wanted behavior or create barriers to the unwanted behavior (other than prompts/cues, rewards, and punishments)

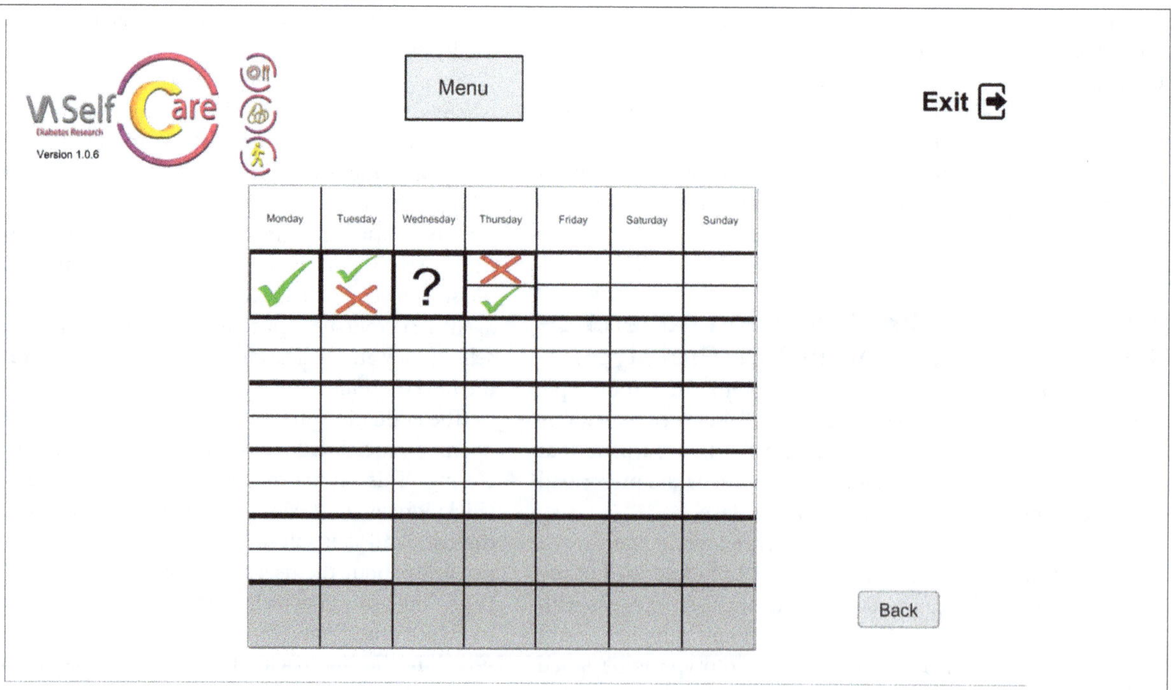

FIGURE 2 | Calendar depicting antidiabetics-taking for one oral antidiabetic, two daily doses; question mark means no self-reported data ("feedback on behavior").

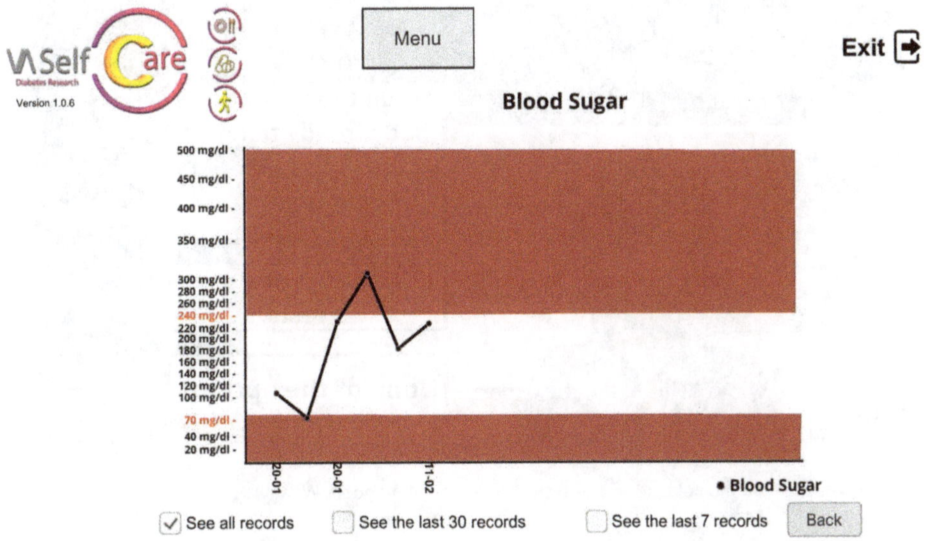

FIGURE 3 | Chart to present blood glucose levels ("biofeedback").

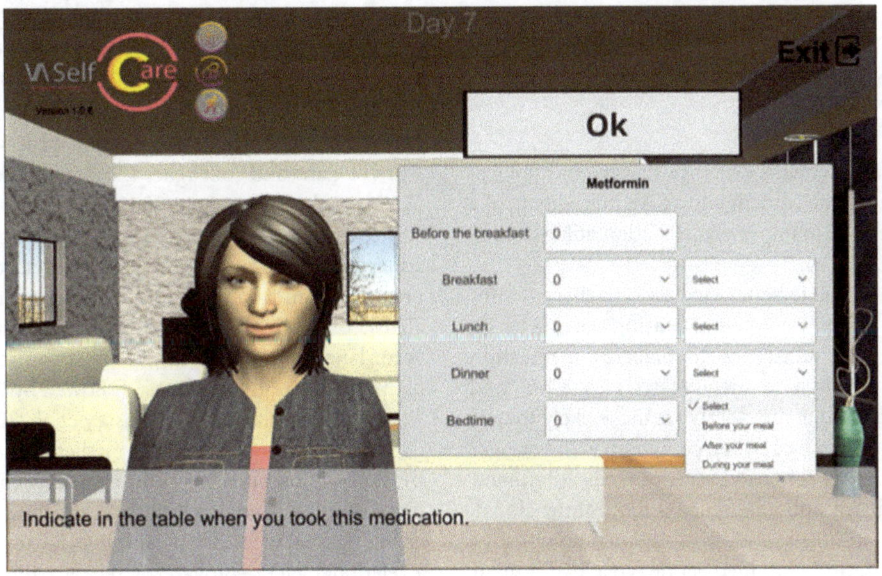

FIGURE 4 | Virtual assistant collecting information on antidiabetics-taking ("self-monitoring of behavior").

The second phase, designated by follow-up, has a main purpose of promoting the desired behavior or to maintaining it. The dialogues in this phase are also structured in repeated sequential steps, described in the literature (Bickmore et al., 2005b). The first two (opening and social talk) and the last two steps (pre-closing and closing) correspond to those described in the evaluation phase. In the "review tasks" step, information is collected about previously agreed tasks or behaviors. Then, feedback is provided and behavior determinants are discussed where pertinent ("assess"). The "counseling" step has a twofold end. Firstly, it offers strategies to overcome previously identified adherence barriers, if applicable. Secondly, it provides tailored educational contents to users. This is exemplified by information about adverse drug reactions, according to knowledge gaps identified in the evaluation phase. In the "assign tasks" step, the user negotiate new behavioral goals and tasks with Vitória.

The selected BCTs are incorporated into different steps of the dialogues, as shown in **Table 4**.

Tailoring was applied not only at the information level, but also in what concerns specific BCTs. For instance, social support

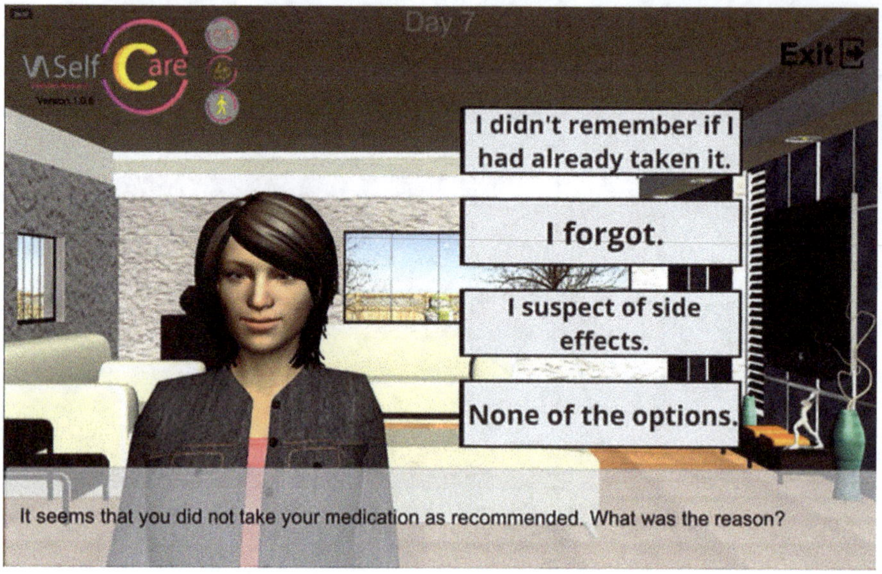
Day 7
VASelf Care
Exit
I didn't remember if I had already taken it.
I forgot.
I suspect of side effects.
None of the options.
It seems that you did not take your medication as recommended. What was the reason?

FIGURE 5 | Virtual assistant listing factors that influence antidiabetics adherence ("problem-solving").

(**Table 4**) is only employed when non-adherence determinants cannot be addressed by the software prototype.

DISCUSSION

This article illustrates a systematic, evidence-driven, and theory-based approach to specify the content and active ingredients of a software prototype, devised to improve medication adherence in older adults with T2D.

Older age has been related to better medication adherence; for example, a systematic review identified increasing age as a factor positively associated with adherence to diabetes medication (Krass et al., 2015). Likewise, a meta-analysis by Choi and Smaldone (2018) indicates that the elderly are more likely to take diabetes medication as prescribed, when compared with younger adults. While *per se* older age seems to affect positively adherence, it is widely recognized that non-adherence is multidimensional. Other factors such as multiple morbidities, regimen complexity, cognitive decline, dexterity, and medication cost can impair adherence (Gellad et al., 2011). This case is illustrated by recent Portuguese data on medication adherence in type 2 diabetic patients measured by the Morisky Medication Adherence Scale (MMAS-4), which categorizes adherence in good, median, and bad (Pinto et al., 2019). The 60 to 79 years group presented both a higher proportion of good and bad medication adherence in relation to lower age groups. The fact that adherence interventions in older people merit research efforts is illustrated by the plethora of trials addressing this population group (Marcum et al., 2017).

We departed from published literature on potential determinants of medication adherence to ensure that the intervention targets known modifiable factors. Four IFs associated with psychological capability and reflective motivation in the COM-B model were subsequently selected—education, persuasion, enablement, and environmental restructuring—resorting to structured criteria (APEASE). Finally, 11 standardized BCTs were chosen from the BCTTv1, based on their suitability to the selected IFs and their effectiveness on medication adherence research trials. This developmental process was guided by the work of Cane and colleagues (2015) and the mapping work from Michie and collaborators (2008).

Morrissey et al. (2016) surveyed 166 smartphone medication adherence applications on the market to identify the BCTs present. From a range of 93 possible techniques (Michie et al., 2013), only 12 were found in the evaluated applications. In accordance with our work, the most common ones were "action planning" and "prompt/cues," followed by "self-monitoring" and "feedback on behavior" (Morrissey et al., 2016).

Interventions to improve medication adherence often use BCTs combinations. Future research could examine which particular BCTs or combinations of BCTs are most effective in changing the medication-taking behavior in older people *via* a relational agent software. A recent study based on a different BCTs taxonomy found that specific BCTs configurations were effective in promoting medication adherence in the context of non-digital interventions (Kahwati et al., 2016). Overall, there is paucity of evidence on this topic, in particular concerning BCTTv1, maybe related to its novelty.

From the software standpoint, we have obtained a first prototype of a multi-behavior intervention, designed in light of usability requirements of older adults. It features an anthropomorphic virtual assistant, designed as a relational agent, able to communicate verbally and non-verbally in an empathic fashion. The agent tailors information to users' level of knowledge, self-reported adherence, and perceived self-efficacy in managing medication. Moreover, it personalizes the

TABLE 4 | Description of the operationalization of each BCT.

BCTs	Strategies	
	Dialogue view	Other views
Feedback on behavior (2.2)	Verbal and visual information on antidiabetics-taking, *via* Vitória's speech, using a helpful-cooperative communication style, and *via* a calendar ("assess" step).	Calendar depicting antidiabetics-taking (the same used by the virtual assistant)
Information about health consequences (5.1)	Verbal explanation on the consequences of not taking antidiabetic agents, *via* Vitória's speech, using a helpful-cooperative communication style. ("counseling" step)	Not applicable
Biofeedback (2.6)	Not applicable	Charts with HbA1C levels on baseline, 3 and 6 months and with self-monitoring of blood glucose levels (if conducted)
Self-monitoring of behavior (2.3)	Information on antidiabetics-taking is collected by the virtual assistant *via* a self-completed form ("review tasks" step)	Record of antidiabetics-taking (available only if not asked by the virtual assistant; depends on the stage of the intervention)
Prompts/cues (7.1)	The virtual assistant offers the possibility of setting up a customizable medication reminder if forgetfulness is identified as a determinant of non-adherence ("counseling")	Setting up a customizable medication reminder
Action planning (1.4)	The virtual assistant offers the possibility of setting up a plan, depending on the determinants of non-adherence ("counseling" step)	Not applicable
Social support (unspecified) (3.1)	The virtual assistant suggests resorting to a friend, relative or health professional, depending on the determinants of non-adherence ("counseling" step). Vitória's helpful-cooperative communication style throughout several dialogue steps provides occasionally non-contingent encouragement.	Not applicable
Social support (practical) (3.2)	Referral to a health professional when non-adherence determinants cannot be addressed by the application ("counseling" step)	Not applicable
Goal setting (behavior) (1.1)	The virtual assistant asks whether the user intends to take oral antidiabetics as prescribed ("assign tasks" step)	Not applicable
Problem solving (1.2)	The virtual assistant lists the factors influencing antidiabetics adherence and generate strategies that include overcoming barriers or increasing facilitators ("assess" and "counseling" steps)	Not applicable
Restructuring the physical environmental (12.1)	The user is advised to change the physical environment according to the barriers that influence medication adherence ("counseling" step)	Not applicable

interaction by, for example, mentioning the user's name and referring to a relative or friend. The prototype offers several features in addition to the dialogue with the virtual assistant, such as a calendar depicting antidiabetics-taking behavior and a chart with HbA1C levels.

The question of whether applications to promote medication adherence using anthropomorphic virtual agents are advantageous when compared to their simpler, text-only counterparts, remains essentially unanswered. The few studies published present limitations, such as relatively small and younger non-clinical populations, which raises generalizability issues for older populations with prevalent chronic diseases. For instance, one study compared an application for behavior change in healthy eating using a female virtual agent versus simple text messages in a sample of 60 higher education students (Mazzotta et al., 2009); information quality and persuasion strength were better rated for the virtual agent modality. By contrast, a study comparing a virtual coach for healthy lifestyle versus text messages in a sample of 43 office workers was unable to demonstrate the virtual agent superiority (op den Akker et al., 2016). Once our intervention is matured, it can get trialed, contributing to answer this question.

Strengths and Limitations

One of the strong points of our work is the theory-driven approach we pursued to the development of the medication adherence intervention. Absence of a theoretical underpinning has been associated with limited effectiveness in these interventions in older people and other patient groups (Nieuwlaat et al., 2014; Patton et al., 2017). Resorting to theory enables a better understanding of the behavior change process (Patton et al., 2017) and tends to have a significant effect on outcomes (Webb et al., 2010).

Another strength is providing a detailed description of the chosen BCTs. Published work on the development of behavior change interventions does not always offer such a description (Wells et al., 2012; Glasziou et al., 2014), which is critical to tout reproducibility. Portraying the content used in an intervention is crucial for reporting, replication, and synthesizing evidence (Proctor et al., 2013; Hoffmann et al., 2014).

However, this work presents also limitations. One of the limitations is whether the behavior change strategies devised by us truly represents a particular BCT. For instance, we were of the understanding that monitoring and recording blood glucose levels did not represent "self-monitoring of outcomes of behavior (2.4)", as we did not provide a method for that purpose, indicating timing and frequency, as others did (Goyal et al., 2016). We attempted to overcome this uncertainty by in-depth discussion within the research team, aided by examples of BCTs in the scientific literature.

Another drawback is the fact that evidence on the effect of BCTs in medication adherence is limited. For instance, while a Cochrane review reported that education, counseling, daily treatment support, and additional support from family or peers were effective for improving adherence (Nieuwlaat et al., 2014), the interventions description may be insufficient to allow coding with a taxonomy. Furthermore, there are cases in which no standardized description of the active components is provided, nor referenced to a taxonomy. This is exemplified by a systematic review on effective interventions to improve medication adherence in T2D (Williams et al., 2014). Problem-solving emerged as effective in improving medication adherence and HbA1c levels (Williams et al., 2014), but it is arguable what it actually means. In other studies interventions addressed problem-solving through action plans and goal setting (Walker et al., 2011; Bogner et al., 2012; Sapkota et al., 2015); it is unclear whether these techniques are identical to their counterparts in BCTTv1. Describing interventions using a comprehensive taxonomy with agreed definitions could promote a better integration of research findings into practice and consequently to building a cumulative knowledge of intervention effectiveness (Presseau et al., 2015).

From an operational standpoint, one of the limitations of the current prototype is that medication adherence and tolerability is assessed only in respect to oral antidiabetics. Future efforts should be directed to the full medication regimen of users and not only blood glucose lowering medication.

The virtual assistant was designed to establish rapport and trust and to provide automated, long-term support to older adults with T2D, supplementing nursing and other health consultations. As previously mentioned, the virtual assistant is able to discuss nonadherence determinants and, according to the adherence barrier identified, provides strategies to overcome them. For example, beliefs about medicines may be tackled by providing information about antidiabetics medication and the disease. This represents a step ahead of many currently available applications. However, it is unlikely that the relational agent is able to manage all instances of non-adherence. The prototype is programed to refer to the primary care nurse or other healthcare professional if problems persist, potentially preventing sustained lack of adherence.

Future Work

We have obtained a first prototype of a software application with an anthropomorphic virtual assistant, which has been used to elicit informed opinions on pre-requisites from nine older people with T2D and 19 health professionals' in five primary care units of the Portuguese national health service (ethical approval 6104/CES/2018/ARSLVT). Results were overall positive and highlighted opportunities for improvement. These were prioritized and actioned.

In parallel with the software development, we are conducting a cross-sectional study in three primary care units to characterize the study population in respect to variables of interest, such as functional and cognitive status, HbA1c levels, and medication adherence. These results will inform the feasibility trial.

The next step is subjecting the prototype to usability tests in a purposive sample of around 10 older patients with T2D, employing the Portuguese version of the System Usability Scale (SUS) (Martins et al., 2015). Usability will also be evaluated by up to five experts, chosen by their experience in aspects such as interface design and diabetes management. This iteration will contribute to further fine-tune the prototype.

Subsequently, the software prototype will be tested in a non-randomized, non-controlled feasibility trial in participating primary care units. For this trial, we envisage to recruit about 20 end users enrolled in nursing consultations. Inclusion and exclusion criteria will be informed by the aforementioned cross-sectional study. Acceptability to users will be researched by focus groups, conducted at the end of the feasibility trial. This represents the second phase of the MRC framework.

CONCLUSIONS

The BCW enabled the identification of the most appropriate BCTs for a novel intervention to promote adherence to antidiabetic medication in older people *via* an anthropomorphic virtual assistant. This stepwise approach involved the identification of four IFs, linked to two key COM-B categories (psychological capability and reflective motivation). Subsequently, 11 BCTs were considered potentially effective. The process outlined here can be used by researchers to guide a comprehensive intervention development, maximizing effectiveness, and facilitating replication.

AUTHOR CONTRIBUTIONS

IF, MG, and AH conceived the idea for the paper. IF guided the team through the behavior change wheel theoretical framework. All authors contributed to the first draft of the manuscript. IF and MG performed a first critical review, which was then commented by all authors. All authors approved the manuscript in its final version for submission and agreed to be accountable for the work presented.

FUNDING

This project is supported by FCT and Compete 2020 (grant number LISBOA-01-0145-FEDER-024250, 02/SAICT/2016). It is also supported by UID/MULTI/04046/2019 Research Unit grant from FCT, Portugal (to BioISI).

ACKNOWLEDGMENTS

The authors are indebted to other VASelfCare team members for their contribution to the software development (http://vaselfcare.rd.ciencias.ulisboa.pt/index-en.html).

REFERENCES

Allemann, S. S., Nieuwlaat, R., van den Bemt, B. J., Hersberger, K. E., and Arnet, I. (2016). Matching adherence interventions to patient determinants using the theoretical domains framework. *Front. Pharmacol.* 7, 429. doi: 10.3389/fphar.2016.00429

Anglada-Martinez, H., Riu-Viladoms, G., Martin-Conde, M., Rovira-Illamola, M., Sotoca-Momblona, J. M., and Codina-Jane, C. (2015). Does MHealth Increase adherence to medication? Results of a systematic review. *Int. J. Clin. Pract.* 69 (1), 9–32. doi: 10.1111/ijcp.12582

Arnhold, M., Quade, M., and Kirch, W. (2014). Mobile applications for diabetics: a systematic review and expert-based usability evaluation considering the special requirements of diabetes patients age 50 years or older. *J. Med. Internet Res.* 16 (4), 1–185. doi: 10.2196/jmir.2968

Bickmore, T. W., Caruso, L., and Clough-Gorr, K. (2005a). Acceptance and usability of a relational agent interface by urban older adults. *CHI '05 Extended Abstracts on Human Factors in Computing Systems - CHI '05*, 1212. doi: 10.1145/1056808.1056879

Bickmore, T. W., Caruso, L., Clough-Gorr K., and Heeren, T. (2005b). 'It's just like you talk to a friend' relational agents for older adults. *Interact. Comput.* 17 (6), 711–735. doi: 10.1016/j.intcom.2005.09.002

Bickmore, T. W., Mitchell, S. E., Jack, B. W., Paasche-Orlow, M. K., Pfeifer, L. M., and O'Donnell, J. (2010). Response to a relational agent by hospital patients with depressive symptoms. *Interact. Comput.* 22 (4), 289–298. doi: 10.1016/j.intcom.2009.12.001

Bickmore, T. W., Pfeifer, L. M., Byron, D., Forsythe, S., Henault, L. E., Jack, B. W., et al. (2010). Usability of conversational agents by patients with inadequate health literacy: evidence from two clinical trials. *J. Health Commun.* 15 (S2), 197–210. doi: 10.1080/10810730.2010.499991

Bickmore, T. W., Puskar, K., Schlenk, E. A., Pfeifer, L. M., and Sereika, S. M. (2010). Maintaining reality: relational agents for antipsychotic medication adherence. *Interact. Comput.* 22, 276–288. doi: 10.1016/j.intcom.2010.02.001

Bleijenberg, N., de Man-van Ginkel, J. M., Trappenburg, J. C. A., Ettema, R. G. A., Sino, C. G., Heim, N., et al. (2018). Increasing value and reducing waste by optimizing the development of complex interventions: enriching the development phase of the Medical Research Council (MRC) framework. *Int. J. Nurs. Stud.* 79, 86–93. doi: 10.1016/j.ijnurstu.2017.12.001

Bogner, H. R., Morales, K. H., de Vries, H. F., and Cappola, A. R. (2012). Integrated management of type 2 diabetes mellitus and depression treatment to improve medication adherence: a randomized controlled trial. *Ann. Fam. Med.* 10 (1), 15–22. doi: 10.1370/afm.1344

Cane, J., O'Connor, D., and Michie, S. (2012). Validation of the theoretical domains framework for use in behaviour change and implementation research. *Implement. Sci.* 7 (37), 1–17. doi: 10.1186/1748-5908-7-37

Cane, J., Richardson, M., Johnston, M., Ladha, R., and Michie, S. (2015). From lists of behaviour change techniques (BCTs) to structured hierarchies: comparison of two methods of developing a hierarchy of BCTs. *Br. J. Health Psychol.* 20 (1), 130–150. doi: 10.1111/bjhp.12102

Capoccia, K., Odegard, P. S., and Letassy, N. (2016). Medication adherence with diabetes medication: a systematic review of the literature. *Diabetes Educ.* 42 (1), 34–71. doi: 10.1177/0145721715619038

Choi, Y. J., and Smaldone, A. M. (2018). Factors associated with medication engagement among older adults with diabetes: systematic review and meta-analysis. *Diabetes Educ.* 44 (1), 15–30. doi: 10.1177/0145721717747880

Cláudio, A. P., Carmo, M. B., Pinto, V., Cavaco, A., and Guerreiro, M. P., (2015). Virtual humans for training and assessment of self-medication consultation skills in pharmacy students, in *10th International Conference on Computer Science and Education*, vol. no. ICCSE, Cambridge, UK: IEEE, 175–180. doi: 10.1109/ICCSE.2015.7250238

Craig, P., Dieppe, P., Macintyre, S., Michie, S., Nazareth, I., and Petticrew, M. (2008). Developing and evaluating complex interventions: the new medical research council guidance. *BMJ* 337 (a1655), 979–983. doi: 10.1136/bmj.a1655

Dworkin, M. S., Lee, S., Chakraborty, A., Monahan, C., Hightow-Weidman, L., Garofalo, R., et al. (2019). Acceptability, feasibility, and preliminary efficacy of a theory-based relational embodied conversational agent mobile phone intervention to promote hiv medication adherence in young hiv-positive african american msm. *AIDS Educ. Prev.* 31 (1), 17–37. doi: 10.1521/aeap.2019.31.1.17

Gellad, W. F., Grenard, J. L., and Marcum, Z. A. (2011). A systematic review of barriers to medication adherence in the elderly: looking beyond cost and regimen complexity. *Am. J. Geriatr. Pharmacother.* 9 (1), 11–23. doi: 10.1016/j.amjopharm.2011.02.004

Gilbert, B. J., Goodman, E., Chadda, A., Hatfield, D., Forman, D. E., and Panch, T. (2015). The role of mobile health in elderly populations. *Curr. Geriatr. Rep.* 4 (4), 347–352. doi: 10.1007/s13670-015-0145-6

Glasziou, P., Altman, D. G., Bossuyt, P., Boutron, I., Clarke, M., Julious, S., et al. (2014). Reducing waste from incomplete or unusable reports of biomedical research. *The Lancet* 383 (9913), 267–276. doi: 10.1016/S0140-6736(13)62228-X

Gonzalez, J. S., Tanenbaum, M. L., and Commissariat, P. V. (2016). Psychosocial factors in medication adherence and diabetes self-management: implications for research and practice. *Am. Psychol.* 71 (7), 539–551. doi: 10.1037/a0040388

Goyal, S., Morita, P., Lewis, G. F., Yu, C., Seto, E., and Cafazzo, J. A. (2016). The systematic design of a behavioural mobile health application for the self-management of type 2 diabetes. *Can. J. Diabetes* 40 (1), 95–104. doi: 10.1016/j.jcjd.2015.06.007

Hoffmann, T. C., Glasziou, P. P., Boutron, I., Milne, R., Perera, R., Moher, D., et al. (2014). better reporting of interventions: template for intervention description and replication (TIDieR) checklist and guide. *BMJ (Online)* 348, 1–12. doi: 10.1136/bmj.g1687

INE (2014). *Sociedade Da Informação e Do Conhecimento - Inquérito à Utilização de Tecnologias Da Informação e Da Comunicação Pelas Famílias.* Lisboa.

International Diabetes Federation (2017). *IDF Diabetes Atlas.* 8th ed. Brussels, Belgium: International Diabetes Federation.

Iuga, A. O., and McGuire, M. J. (2014). Adherence and health care costs. *Risk Manag. Healthc. Policy* 7, 35–44. doi: 10.2147/RMHP.S19801

Juste, A. M., Gimeno Miguel, A., Poblador Plou, B., González Rubio, F., Aza Pascual-Salcedo, M. M., Menditto, E., et al. (2018). Adherence to treatment of hypertension, hypercholesterolaemia and diabetes in an elderly population of a spanish cohort. *Medicina Clínica* 29. doi: 10.1016/j.medcli.2018.10.023

Kahwati, L., Viswanathan, M., Golin, C. E., Kane, H., Lewis, M., and Jacobs, S. (2016). Identifying configurations of behavior change techniques in effective medication adherence interventions: a qualitative comparative analysis. *Syst. Rev.* 5 (83), 1–9. doi: 10.1186/s13643-016-0255-z

Kardas, P., Lewek, P., and Matyjaszczyk, M. (2013). Determinants of patient adherence: a review of systematic reviews. *Front. Pharmacol.* 4, 1–16. doi: 10.3389/fphar.2013.00091

Karve, S., Cleves, M. A., Helm, M., Hudson, T. J., West, D. S., and Martin, B. C. (2009). Good and poor adherence: optimal cut-point for adherence measures using administrative claims data. *Curr. Med. Res. Opin.* 25 (9), 2303–2310. doi: 10.1185/03007990903126833

Kim, B. Y. B., and Lee, J. (2017). Smart devices for older adults managing chronic disease: a scoping review. *JMIR Mhealth Uhealth* 5 (5), e69. doi: 10.2196/mhealth.7141

Krass, I., Schieback, P., and Dhippayom, T. (2015). Adherence to diabetes medication: a systematic review. *Diabet. Med.* 32, 725–737. doi: 10.1111/dme.12651

Kreuter, M., Farrell, D., Olevitch, L., and Brennan, L., (2000). *Tailoring Health Messages: Customizing Communication with Computer Technology.* Mahwah New Jersey: Lawrence Erlbaum Associates. https://www.popline.org/node/174671.

Lustria, M. L. A., Noar, S. M., Cortese, J., Van Stee, S. K., Glueckauf, R. L., and Lee, J. (2013). A meta-analysis of web-delivered tailored health behavior change interventions. *J. Health Commun.* 18 (9), 1039–1069. doi: 10.1080/10810730.2013.768727

Marcum, Z. A., Hanlon, J. T., and Murray, M. D. (2017). Improving medication adherence and health outcomes in older adults: an evidence-based review of randomized controlled trials. *Drugs Aging* 34 (3), 191–201. doi: 10.1007/s40266-016-0433-7

Martins, A. I., Rosa, A. F., Queirós, A., Silva, A., and Rocha, N. P. (2015). European Portuguese Validation of the System Usability Scale (SUS). *Procedia Comput. Sci.* 67 (Dsai), 293–300. doi: 10.1016/j.procs.2015.09.273

Mazzotta, I., Novielli, N., and De Carolis, B., (2009). "Are ECAs more persuasive than textual messages?," in *Lecture Notes in Computer Science*, vol. 5773. Eds. Z. Ruttkay, M. Kipp, A. Nijholt, and H. H. Vilhjálmsson (Berlin, Heidelberg: Springer), 527–528. doi: 10.1007/978-3-642-04380-2_75

Menditto, E., Cahir, C., Aza-Pascual-Salcedo, M., Bruzzese, D., Poblador-Plou, B., Malo, S., et al. (2018). Adherence to chronic medication in older populations: application of a common protocol among three european cohorts. *Patient Prefer. Adherence* 12, 1975–1978. doi: 10.2147/PPA.S164819

Michie, S., Atkins, L., and West, R. (2014). *The Behavior Change Wheel: A Guide To Designing Interventions*. First edit. London: Silverback Publishing.

Michie, S., Johnston, M., Francis, J., Hardeman, W., and Eccles, M. (2008). From theory to intervention: mapping theoretically derived behavioural determinants to behaviour change techniques. *App. Psychol.* 57 (4), 660–680. doi: 10.1111/j.1464-0597.2008.00341.x

Michie, S., Richardson, M., Johnston, M., Abraham, C., Francis, J., Hardeman, W., et al. (2013). The behavior change technique taxonomy (v1) of 93 hierarchically clustered techniques: building an international consensus for the reporting of behavior change interventions. *Ann. Behav. Med.* 46, 81–95. doi: 10.1007/s12160-013-9486-6

Michie, S., M van Stralen, M., and West, R. (2011). The behaviour change wheel: a new method for characterising and designing behaviour change interventions. *Implement. Sci.* 6 (42), 1–11. doi: 10.1186/1748-5908-6-42

Migneault, J. P., Farzanfar, R., Wright, J. A., and Friedman, R. H. (2006). How to write health dialog for a talking computer. *J. Biomed. Inform.* 39, 468–481. doi: 10.1016/j.jbi.2006.02.009

Monkaresi, H., Calvo, R. A., Pardo, A., Chow, K., Mullan, B., Lam, M., et al. (2013). "Intelligent diabetes lifestyle coach," in *Fifth International Workshop on Smart Healthcare and Wellness Applications (SmartHealth'13)*, Adelaide, Australia: OzCHI, 1–4.

Morrissey, E. C., Corbett, T. K., Walsh, J. C., and Molloy, G. J. (2016). Behavior change techniques in apps for medication adherence: a content analysis. *Am. J. Prev. Med.* 50 (5), e143–e146. doi: 10.1016/j.amepre.2015.09.034

Mota-Pinto, A., Rodrigues, V., Botelho, A., Veríssimo, M. T., Morais, A., Alves, C., et al. (2010). A socio-demographic study of aging in the portuguese population: The EPEPP Study. *Arch. Gerontol. Geriatr.* 52 (3), 304–308. doi: 10.1016/j.archger.2010.04.019

Niess, J., and Diefenbach, S. (2016). Communication styles of interactive tools for self-improvement. *Psychol. Well Being* 6 (1), 3. doi: 10.1186/s13612-016-0040-8

Nieuwlaat, R., Wilczynski, N., Navarro, T., Hobson, N., Jeffery, R., Keepanasseril, A., et al. (2014). Interventions for enhancingmedication adherence (review). *Cochrane Database Syst. Rev.* 11, 1–730. doi: 10.1002/14651858.CD000011.pub4

op den Akker, R., Klaassen, R., and Nijholt, A. (2016). "Virtual Coaches for Healthy Lifestyle," in *Toward Robotic Socially Believable Behaving Systems - Volume II. Modeling Social Signals*, vol. 106. Eds. A. L. Esposito and C. Jain (Switzerland: Springer International Publishing).

op den Akker, R., Klaassen, R., Lavrysen, T., Geleijnse, G., van Halteren, A., Schwietert, H., et al. (2011). "A Personal Context-Aware Multi-Device Coaching Service That Supports a Healthy Lifestyle," in *BCS-HCI'11 Proceedings of the 25th BCS Conference on Human-Computer Interaction*, Swinton, UK: British Computer Society, 443–448.

Paiva, D., Silva, S., Severo, M., Moura-Ferreira, P., Lunet, N., and Azevedo, A. (2017). Limited health literacy in portugal assessed with the newest vital sign prevalência de literacia em saúde inadequada em portugal medida com o newest vital sign. *Acta Med. Port.* 30 (12), 861–869. doi: 10.20344/amp.9135

Patton, D. E., Hughes, C. M., Cadogan, C. A., and Ryan, C. A. (2017). Theory-based interventions to improve medication adherence in older adults prescribed polypharmacy: a systematic review. *Drugs Aging* 34 (2), 97–113. doi: 10.1007/s40266-016-0426-6

Pinto, D. M., Santiago, L. M., Maurício, K., and Silva, I. R. (2019). Health profile and medication adherence of diabetic patients in the portuguese population. *Prim. Care Diabetes* doi: 10.1016/j.pcd.2019.02.004

Polonsky, W. H., and Henry, R. R. (2016). Poor medication adherence in type 2 diabetes: recognizing the scope of the problem and its key contributors. *Patient Prefer. Adherence* 10, 1299–1307. doi: 10.2147/PPA.S106821

Powers, M. A., Bardsley, J., Cypress, M., Duker, P., Funnell, M. M., Fischl, A. H., et al. (2015). Diabetes self-management education and support in type 2 diabetes: a joint position statement of the american diabetes association, the american association of diabetes educators, and the academy of nutrition and dietetics. *J. Acad. Nutr. Diet.* 115 (8), 1323–1334. doi: 10.2337/diaclin.34.2.70

Presseau, J., Ivers, N. M., Newham, J. J., Knittle, K., Danko, K. J., and Grimshaw, J. M. (2015). Using a behaviour change techniques taxonomy to identify active ingredients within trials of implementation interventions for diabetes care. *Implement. Sci.* 10 (55), 1–10. doi: 10.1186/s13012-015-0248-7

Proctor, E. K., Powell, B. J., and McMillen, J. C. (2013). Implementation strategies: recommendations for specifying and reporting. *Implement. Sci.* 8 (139), 1–11. doi: 10.1186/1748-5908-8-139

Ring, L., Utami, D., and Bickmore, T. (2014). The right agent for the job? The effects of agent visual appearance on task domain, in *Lecture Notes in Computer Science*, vol. 8637. Eds Bickmore, T., Marsella, S., and Sidner, C. (Switzerland: Springer, Cham), 374–384. doi: 10.1007/978-3-319-09767-1_49

Sabaté, E. (2003). *Adherence to Long-Term Therapies*. Switzerland: World Health Organization. doi: 10.1016/S1474-5151(03)00091-4

Sapkota, S., Brien, J. A. E., Greenfield, J. R., and Aslani, P. (2015). A systematic review of interventions addressing adherence to anti-diabetic medications in patients with type 2 diabetes - components of interventions. *PLoS ONE* 10 (2), 1–17. doi: 10.1371/journal.pone.0128626

Sweet, S. N., and Fortier, M. S. (2010). Improving physical activity and dietary behaviours with single or multiple health behaviour interventions? A synthesis of meta-analyses and reviews. *Int. J. Environ. Res. Public Health* 7 (4), 1720–1743. doi: 10.3390/ijerph7041720

van Wissen, A., Vinkers, C., and van Halteren, A. (2016). "Developing a Virtual coach for chronic patients: a user study on the impact of similarity, familiarity and realism," in *Persuasive Technology*. Eds. A. Meschtscherjakov, B. De Ruyter, V. Fuchsberger, M. Murer, and M. Tscheligi (Cham: Springer International Publishing), 263–275. doi: 10.1007/978-3-319-31510-2_23

Velicer, W., Redding, C., Blissmer, B., Babbin, S., Paiva, A., Bickmore, T., et al. (2015). Using relational agents to increase engagement in computer-based interventions: preliminary outcomes. *Eur. Health Psychol.* 17 (S), 451.

Vervloet, M., Linn, A. J., van Weert, J. C. M., de Bakker, D. H., Bouvy, M. L., and van Dijk, L. (2012). The effectiveness of interventions using electronic reminders to improve adherence to chronic medication: a systematic review of the literature. *J. Am. Med. Inform. Assoc.* 19 (5), 696–704. doi: 10.1136/amiajnl-2011-000748

Vrijens, B., De Geest, S., Hughes, D. A., Przemyslaw, K., Demonceau, J., Ruppar, T., et al. (2012). A new taxonomy for describing and defining adherence to medications. *Br. J. Clin. Pharmacol.* 73 (5), 691–705. doi: 10.1111/j.1365-2125.2012.04167.x

Walker, E. A., Shmukler, C., Ullman, R., Blanco, E., Scollan-Koliopoulus, M., and Cohen, H. W. (2011). Results of a successful telephonic intervention to improve diabetes control in urban adults. A randomized trial. *Diabetes Care* 34 (1), 2–7. doi: 10.2337/dc10-1005

Webb, T. L., Joseph, J., Yardley, L., and Michie, S. (2010). Using the internet to promote health behavior change: a systematic review and meta-analysis of the impact of theoretical basis, use of behavior change techniques, and mode of delivery on efficacy. *J. Med. Internet Res.* 12 (1), 1–18. doi: 10.2196/jmir.1376

Wells, M., Williams, B., Treweek, S., Coyle, J., and Taylor, J. (2012). Intervention description is not enough: evidence from an in-depth multiple case study on the untold role and impact of context in randomised controlled trials of seven complex interventions. *Trials* 13 (1), 1. doi: 10.1186/1745-6215-13-95

Williams, J. L. S., Walker, R. J., Smalls, B. L., Campbell, J. A., and Egede, L. E. (2014). Effective interventions to improve medication adherence in type 2 diabetes: a systematic review. *Diabetes Manag.* 4 (1), 29–48. doi: 10.2217/dmt.13.62

Yap, A. F., Thirumoorthy, T., and Kwan, Y. H. (2016). Systematic review of the barriers affecting medication adherence in older adults. *Geriatr. Gerontol. Int.* 16, 1093–1101. doi: 10.1111/ggi.12616

Zeber, J. E., Manias, E., Williams, A. F., Hutchins, D., Udezi, W. A., Roberts, C. S., et al. (2013). A systematic literature review of psychosocial and behavioral factors associated with initial medication adherence: a report of the ispor medication adherence & persistence special interest group. *Value Health* 16, 891–900. doi: 10.1016/j.jval.2013.04.014

Zheng, Y., Ley, S. H., and Hu, F. B. (2018). Global aetiology and epidemiology of type 2 diabetes mellitus and its complications. *Nat. Rev. Endocrinol.* 14 (2), 88–98. doi: 10.1038/nrendo.2017.151

20

Applying Precision Public Health to Prevent Preterm Birth

John P. Newnham[1,2]*, Matthew W. Kemp[1], Scott W. White[1,2], Catherine A. Arrese[1], Roger J. Hart[1] and Jeffrey A. Keelan[1]

[1] School of Women's and Infants' Health, The University of Western Australia, Crawley, WA, Australia,
[2] Department of Maternal Fetal Medicine, King Edward Memorial Hospital, Subiaco, WA, Australia

****Correspondence:***
John P. Newnham
john.newnham@uwa.edu.au

Preterm birth (PTB) is one of the major health-care challenges of our time. Being born too early is associated with major risks to the child with potential for serious consequences in terms of life-long disability and health-care costs. Discovering how to prevent PTB needs to be one of our greatest priorities. Recent advances have provided hope that a percentage of cases known to be related to risk factors may be amenable to prevention; but the majority of cases remain of unknown cause, and there is little chance of prevention. Applying the principle of precision public health may offer opportunities previously unavailable. Presented in this article are ideas that may improve our abilities in the fields of studying the effects of migration and of populations in transition, public health programs, tobacco control, routine measurement of length of the cervix in mid-pregnancy by ultrasound imaging, prevention of non-medically indicated late PTB, identification of pregnant women for whom treatment of vaginal infection may be of benefit, and screening by genetics and other "omics." Opening new research in these fields, and viewing these clinical problems through a prism of precision public health, may produce benefits that will affect the lives of large numbers of people.

Keywords: preterm birth, cervix length, progesterone, smoking, genomics, proteomics, transcriptomics, screening

INTRODUCTION

Preterm birth (PTB) is the single major cause of death in children up to 5 years of age in the developed world (1–3). In low-resource countries, early birth is the second greatest cause of death in young children, second only to pneumonia. Most children born too early will survive and go on to lead a normal and healthy life, but for many there will be life-long disability. Health issues may include neurodevelopmental delay, hearing and visual loss, cerebral palsy, and learning and behavioral problems. The potential impact on individuals, families, and society are considerable (4, 5).

Providing optimal care for very preterm infants in dedicated neonatal intensive care units is vital to minimize any potential for life-long harm, but such care comes at considerable financial cost. The potential costs to society in terms of lost productivity throughout the lifespan may be even greater (6). Considerable benefit has arisen from the discovery in 1972 that administration of corticosteroids to the mother at risk of early birth will halve the rate of death and respiratory distress syndrome in the preterm newborn, but the treatment does not in itself delay the age at birth (7, 8).

Preterm birth is defined as birth before 37 and after 20 completed weeks of gestation. There are many potential pathways to this complication of pregnancy (9). At all gestational ages, and especially the very early ages, inflammation in the pregnant uterus, either due to infectious or non-infectious causes, is commonly associated with preterm deliveries (10). For cases where the age is closer to term, a major concern is medical intervention which at times may not be medically indicated. In other cases, the delivery may be expedited to prevent stillbirth or maternal morbidity, such as for preeclampsia, fetal growth restriction, or diabetes. In half of all cases of PTB, labor commences spontaneously for no known reason or the membranes rupture unexpectedly leading later to the birth. These various phenotypes are diverse and poorly classified, reflecting our incomplete understanding of their various causal pathways and mechanisms.

The impetus to discover strategies by which PTB rates may be lowered has been driven at least in part by advances in neonatal care resulting in more babies surviving at lower gestational ages at birth, but often at high cost in human and financial terms. Starting in the 1960s, much attention was given to developing and refining tocolytic drugs, which are therapeutic agents aiming to inhibit uterine contractions and hence prevent early birth. These drugs may have some usefulness in delaying PTB by hours or a few days, but do not extend pregnancies to gestational ages that will lower the rate of PTB (11).

SUCCESS SO FAR

There has been success in lowering PTB rates to some extent in some environments (5). In USA, the rising rates of non-medically indicated late preterm and early-term birth, peaking in 2007, led to the launch of several quality assurance programs aiming to prevent unnecessary early births (6). These programs have resulted in successfully lowering the rates of late PTB in those hospitals and regions that were targeted. In part, as a result of these programs, the rate of PTB in USA fell for 8 years in a row, but has now been reported in late 2016 to have increased again from 9.57 to 9.63% (12).

The first whole of population and whole of geographic region PTB prevention initiative was recently reported for the state of Western Australia (13). Six strategies were applied: administration of progesterone based on prior history of a PTB or the finding of a shortened cervix measured routinely in mid-pregnancy on ultrasound examination, appropriate use of cervical cerclage, avoidance of non-medically indicated induction of labor or Cesarean section, avoidance of exposure to cigarette smoke, judicious use of fertility treatments, and a dedicated PTB prevention clinic at the state's sole tertiary level perinatal center for referral of cases at highest risk. Implementation involved a state-wide outreach program aiming to ensure that all obstetricians, general practitioners, midwives, and ultrasound imaging specialists had training and expertise in the various aspects of the program. Women and their families were made aware of the strategies through print and social media. The program overall was badged as thewholeninemonths™. After the first full 12 months of implementation, the state-wide rate of PTB had reduced by 7.6% when compared with the years prior to initiation. Statistical modeling estimated that approximately 200 preterm births had been prevented with avoidance of more than 40 in the <32-week gestational age group. Analysis by run charts indicated the rate of late PTB had decreased rapidly, suggesting an effect of educational programs aiming to discourage practitioners and women from unnecessary early intervention. A more delayed effect was observed in reducing births in the 28–31 week category, possibly reflecting use of cervix length screening, administration of progesterone, and surgical cerclage. The benefits extended across the gestational age spectrum from 28–31 weeks onward, although any effect at ages before that time was not statistically significant possibly due to low numbers. An even greater effect in reducing the overall PTB rate was observed within the tertiary level center itself, where awareness among practitioners and pregnant women may have been greater. Together, these results indicate that a comprehensive and multi-faceted geographic-based PTB prevention program in a relatively high resource setting can significantly reduce the rate of PTB using existing knowledge, with an effect of 7–8%.

The magnitude of this reduction in PTB rates recently observed in the Western Australian program is generally consistent with a previous estimate of the effect that could result from effective implementation of known strategies. In an analysis of the potential reduction in preterm births for countries with a very high human development index conducted by the Boston Consulting Group and published in 2013, it was estimated conservatively that the combined impact of implementing known strategies may be a reduction in rate of 5% (14).

We are now left with two great challenges. First is to explore how the array of known strategies can be applied effectively across other population groups. Second is to discover new strategies by which our modest success so far can be expanded. One possibility may be to apply the principles of Precision Public Health to the field of PTB prevention.

PRECISION PUBLIC HEALTH

Precision public health has arisen from the emerging field of precision medicine (15, 16). Contemporary clinical practice is built upon practice guidelines that are developed and refined by the principles of evidence-based medicine. Typically, such guidelines are applied to individuals with specified symptoms or signs or abnormalities in laboratory or imaging tests. There is much greater potential benefit if the case selection could be refined by tests predicting that a given treatment is likely to be most effective for a given individual with a given disease. As an example, the drug crizotinib has been shown to be much more effective for the treatment of non-small cell lung cancer if the patient has a particular chromosomal translocation involving the gene encoding ALK that drives tumor growth (17).

But there is far more potential to the concept of precision medicine than just "drugs, genes, and disease." Rather than merely targeting individuals by identifying specific phenotypic or genotypic characteristics, a population approach is possibly the next logical step. Identifying population groups rather than just individuals may yield great benefits. With such an approach, development of precision public health may enable us to benefit the right population at the right time.

Using a population-level approach, the massive amount of data currently being generated from multiple sources could be harnessed for the purpose. Such data collection systems include genomic, transcriptomic and microbiome analysis, and lifestyle characteristics measurable by electronic machines worn or carried by individuals. We also need to expand our capabilities in harnessing data that describe the social and environmental determinants of our health. Clinicians have traditionally incorporated informal information on these determinants into their clinical decision-making, but never before have we had access to data that can provide an accurate description of such factors. We are no longer lacking in information. Our challenge is how to embrace these massive data sources and use the information to identify the right populations at the right time for the right treatment.

The purpose of this article is to explore ways in which the principles of precision public health could be applied to the field of PTB prevention. Different scenarios will be discussed covering some of the strategies that are currently being employed for this task, and we will explore some of the possible avenues by which the principles of precision public health may be incorporated. The concept and examples are illustrated diagrammatically in **Figure 1**.

NATIONAL DIFFERENCES, POPULATIONS IN TRANSITION AND HEALTH INEQUALITIES

There are many lessons to be learnt from studying the rates of PTB in various nations, how these rates change with time, and the effects of migration.

The PTB rate varies markedly between different countries. In a study of national estimates of PTB rates in 2010 and published in 2013, rates ranged from 5.3 per 100 live births in Latvia to 14.7 per 100 live births in Cyprus (14). Northern European countries had very low rates ranging from 5.5 per 100 live births in Finland to 5.9 in Sweden and 6.0 in Norway. More southern European nations had slightly higher rates with 6.5 in Italy, 6.7 in France, and 8.0 in the Netherlands. In contrast, the rate in USA was 12.0 per 100 live births.

Different migrant subgroups have different reproductive responses to migration (18). Black and Hispanic migrant women are less likely to deliver preterm than US-born Blacks and Hispanics, but the effect does not extend to White and Asian migrants. The duration of residence in the new country also contributes greatly. In a study of migrants to Canada, recent immigrants of less than 5 years had a lower risk of PTB than non-immigrants; but after 15 years or more, the protective effect was reversed and a higher

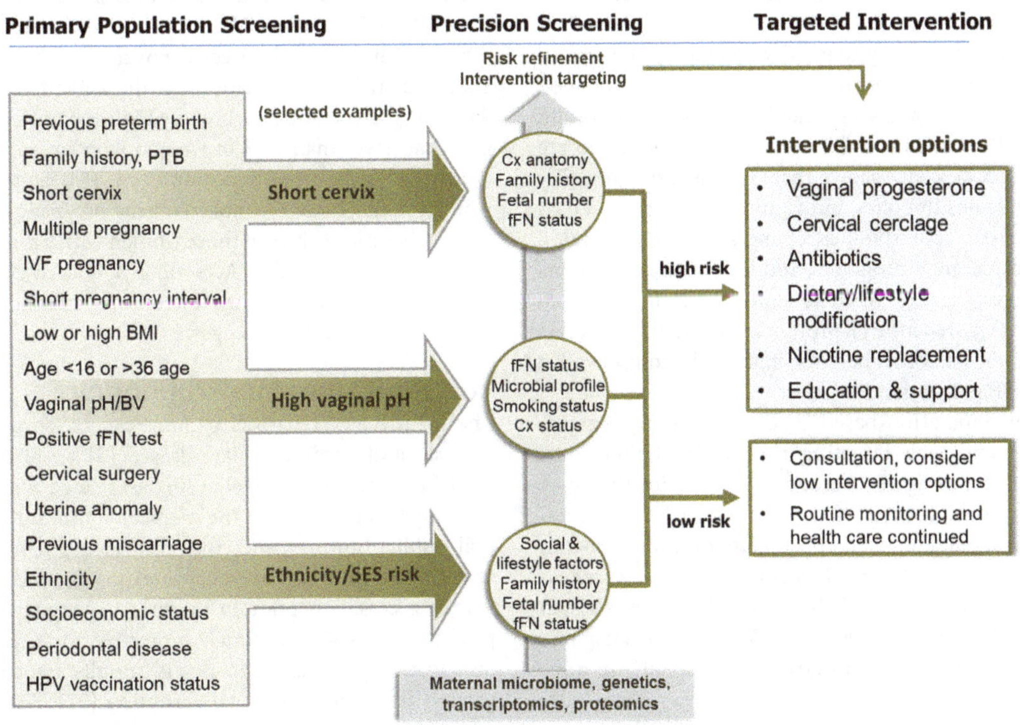

FIGURE 1 | The application of precision population health principles to preterm birth (PTB) prevention. Primary population screening using a number of known epidemiological, social, and obstetric factors can identify women with increased risk of PTB but has poor predictive value. In the three examples illustrated, women identified with a specific risk factor are then further evaluated using precision screening, aided by the application of various "omic" technologies, to identify those at greater risk of PTB associated with specific etiologies. This precision risk profile is then used to target treatment and prevention strategies to those who are most likely to benefit. Women who are unlikely to benefit from treatment are also identified through this process. This approach will enhance efficacy, reduce unnecessary interventions, and make optimal use of clinical resources. Abbreviations: BMI, body mass index; BV, bacterial vaginosis; Cx, cervix; fFN, fetal fibronectin; PTB, preterm birth.

risk of PTB than in non-immigrants was observed. No such effect was found on birth weight relative to gestational age (19). Chinese women living in Jiangsu Province were found to have a much lower rate of PTB than China-born women living in Hong Kong and Western Australia (20). In China-born women living in Western Australia, the ability to be fluent in English and no longer need a translator was associated with a doubling in risk of the pregnancy ending preterm, suggesting that environment was overriding genetics in terms of PTB risk.

The wide variation in PTB rates between countries, and the changes observed with migration, provides strong evidence for environmental contributors and clues to the magnitude of effect that may be amenable to change in any prevention strategy. But what factors associated with migration are operating to decrease and increase PTB rates, and how might this information be exploited in a precision public health approach? Large amounts of data are now available in various government agencies on people as they either reside in their country of origin or migrate. Details are also available on when they moved, at what age, and the circumstances under which they re-located. It seems likely that harnessing these databases would add greatly to our ability to identify women at risk of PTB and enable us to devise public health strategies that may mitigate this risk. Much of the information of course is collected for other purposes and the challenge now is to bridge the gap with the many government and private agencies that generate and control such data bases.

Geographic information systems (GIS) employ sophisticated software and hardware platforms to analyze and collate data on geospatial distribution of disease incidence, risks, and health outcomes (21–23). While the technology and its applications are in their infancy, studies have shown that GIS is a useful modality for guiding public health policy and gaining high precision data on population risks, comorbidities, changes in incidence rates, effectiveness of treatment programs, and socioeconomic factors associated with risk (24–26). As far as we are aware, this approach has not yet been explored for PTB prevention, but there are clearly opportunities to be exploited here for improved and innovative public health PTB prevention initiatives.

A variety of population-based PTB prevention programs are now underway, each targeting the needs of their own communities and aiming to overcome deficiencies that may be contributing to high rates of early birth. In USA, several programs have been launched aiming to overcome health inequalities. Much of this work has resulted from awareness of the very different rates of PTB among the various racial groups. In 2014, the rates ranged from 13.2% in non-Hispanic Black women through to 9.4% in Hispanics and 8.9% in non-Hispanic Whites (27, 28).

In Kentucky, one such program named "Healthy Babies Are Worth The Wait" has focused on improving access to antenatal care by incorporating a range of modifiable factors including group care (6, 28). When compared with surrounding states, there has been evidence of improved rates of PTB.

Central to the high rates of PTB in women of poor socio-economic and educational standards may be factors operating in their neighborhoods and lifestyles that produce chronic stress and a sense of alienation (6, 28). Living in environments of high crime rates, low wages, lack of employment opportunities, sub-standard services, and feeling excluded from society is associated with higher rates of PTB. Understanding the pathways by which these multiple factors lead to pregnancy complications and other adverse health outcomes will require a much broader view of an individual's life than we have previously appreciated. Tackling these considerable challenges may be assisted by access to large data bases and an understanding of the importance of the entire life-course in health and disease, as well as gaining a better understanding of how inter-generational effects, such as history of slavery and disempowerment may leave enduring effects on people and their communities. Much work is left to be done, but applying the principles of Precision public health may enable progress that has so far remained elusive.

TOBACCO EXPOSURE AND PTB

Exposure to tobacco products, either directly or from environmental sources, is recognized as a significant threat to human health and a significant cause of PTB. The importance of controlling tobacco exposure during pregnancy is underscored by tobacco exposure being designated the single largest preventable risk factor for non-communicable human disease (29). Data published by the World Health Organization show that some 6% of all female and 12% of all male deaths are attributable to tobacco use (30). By 2020, the WHO projects that 7.5 million people will die from direct and indirect exposure to tobacco smoke (30). Data drawn from populations in the United States, Denmark, Sweden, and Canada (i.e., broadly high-income economies) suggest that fewer than 50% of women who smoke cease smoking during pregnancy; Swedish data from 2000 suggest that 13% of women in that country smoked during pregnancy, with smoking persistence more likely in those women with a lower level of educational attainment (31). Accordingly, tobacco control and PTB prevention constitute tightly intertwined and hugely important global public health challenges.

Tobacco Use and Pregnancy

The greatly elevated risks of lung cancer, chronic respiratory disease, and cardiovascular disease [71%, 42%, and 10% of total incidence, respectively (30)] associated with smoking are well appreciated by both the medical community and the general public; however, the risk of adverse pregnancy outcomes associated with maternal tobacco exposure, and the benefits of smoking cessation prior to or early in pregnancy, are equally profound (32–34). Although protective for preeclampsia (35, 36), smoking during pregnancy is causally associated with fetal growth restriction, placental abruption (37), PTB (38, 39), and sudden infant death syndrome (40). At least one-third of all cases of fetal growth restriction in developed countries is attributable to the effects of maternal tobacco use (41). There are also data to suggest that fetal exposure to many chemicals in tobacco smoke is associated with a host of childhood developmental abnormalities, including subnormal weight gain (42) and neuro-behavioral disorders, such as attention deficit hyperactivity disorder and deficits in auditory and cognitive ability (43).

A 1990 report by the US Surgeon General concluded that "women who stop smoking before pregnancy or during the first 3–4 months of pregnancy reduce their risk of having a low birth weight baby to that of a woman who never smoked" (44). Perhaps, the most important element of this report, in keeping with seminal studies into smoking-related mortality among UK doctors by Doll and colleagues, is that the adverse effects of tobacco exposure on pregnancy are not immutable and can be reduced or even entirely abrogated by timely smoking cessation (45). Numerous subsequent studies, both experimental (46) and epidemiological (47–49), have demonstrated both the significant potential harm to pregnancy and the developing fetus caused by maternal tobacco smoke exposure and, promisingly, the profound benefits to both that may be gained from effective tobacco control.

It is now well established that PTB is a complex syndrome, in many cases likely patient and/or population specific, and a syndrome for which very few preventative interventions exist (9). Of the limited armamentarium presently available to the medical and public health communities, tobacco control is among the most uniformly effective interventions. A meta-analysis of the effects of implementing smoke-free legislation in North America and Europe reported a statistically significant 10% reduction in PTB [1,366,862 cases; −10.4% (95% CI −18.8 to −2.0); $p = 0.016$] (48). Similar benefits have been reported in response to tobacco control measures adopted in Switzerland, with benefits to population pregnancy health correlating with the extent of tobacco control achieved in a particular canton (50). Recent modeling by Levy and colleagues identified that a $2/pack cost increase in cigarette excise tax, combined with cessation programs, health warnings, and public smoking bans would deliver a 33.5% reduction in smoking prevalence among US women aged 15–49 by 2065; relative to maintaining the *status quo*, such policy measures would deliver 227,300 fewer (132,600–302,300) low birth weight infants and 351,000 (137,100–501,300) fewer preterm births over the same period (51).

Controlling Tobacco Exposure to Prevent PTB *via* Precision Public Health: A Nuanced, Multilevel Approach

Reducing the adverse impact of tobacco exposure on pregnancy outcomes likely requires a combination of national-level initiatives, supported by complementary, culturally, and contextually appropriate programs targeted at specific communities and individual patients. Given the substantial body of data linking tobacco exposure to human disease generally (29, 45), preventive programs based around national public education and legislative control (52) (high levels of tobacco excise tax, comprehensive advertising bans, prohibition of tobacco use in public places, public education campaigns) are clearly warranted and, when well-executed, demonstrate marked reductions in population-level tobacco use coincident with significant reductions in population PTB rates (47, 48, 50). Such programs, targeting both males and females, are important as there is very good evidence that both direct maternal tobacco use and environmental exposure in the home, workplace, or public transport, convey sizeable risks to pregnancy health. In addition to the risks of second-hand smoke, data from the Generation R study in the Netherlands also suggest that, in a number of communities, partner smoking is associated with smoking during pregnancy (53).

Unfortunately, countries employing comprehensive, multifaceted tobacco control measures at a national level remain in the minority. Many of the countries with sub-optimal tobacco control measures are the same low- and middle-income countries that are home to 80% of the world's smokers (31) and report some of the highest rates of PTB in the world (2, 4, 54). Even in countries with effective national-level controls, there are marked differences in the effectiveness of national-level tobacco control measures between communities (53, 55), seemingly contingent on a host of socioeconomic factors. In addition to determining maternal tobacco use history and environmental exposure (especially in the home), a precision public health approach to preventing tobacco-associated PTB would likely require assessment of maternal and/or community factors, including (but not limited to), ethnicity, education, poverty, the ability to access social support networks, and the ability to access health-care services.

Ethnicity should be accounted for when designing pregnancy smoking risk assessments and interventions. An analysis of smoking habits in the Netherlands as part of the Generation R study showed significant differences in smoking rates between women of Turkish (43.7%), Dutch (24.1%), and Moroccan (7.0%) ethnicities; moreover, women of Turkish and Moroccan ethnicity were more likely to continue smoking during pregnancy (72.0 and 70.6%, respectively) than women of Dutch ethnicity (58.6%) (53). In South Australia, data collected during the 1990s revealed a marked difference in smoking rates between Aboriginal and non-Aboriginal women (57.8 vs. 24.0%) at their first antenatal visit (56). A similar disparity is evident in more recent data collected in Queensland between 2005 and 2006, with 54% of Indigenous and 19% of non-Indigenous women reporting smoking during pregnancy (55). In the study, adjusted pregnancy outcomes in non-smoking Indigenous and non-Indigenous women were almost equivalent, underscoring the profound impact of smoking on pregnancy and the potential benefits to be gained from effective cessation support (55).

A mother's level of educational attainment and financial situation are known to be important predictors of peri-conceptual smoking habits and the ability to quit smoking once pregnancy is established (31, 57). Hibbs and colleagues undertook a cross-sectional study of PTB rates among women residing in low-income urban areas in Illinois; the findings of this study showed that impoverished African-American women who smoked exhibited a pattern of "weathering" with advanced maternal age associated with increased rate of PTB [25.2% among 30- to 35-year-old women vs. 17.9% for teenagers; RR = 1.5 (1.1–2.0)]. Interestingly, the authors reported that impoverished White mothers (irrespective of smoking status) and non-smoking African-American mothers did not exhibit a similar pattern of increased rates of PTB with increasing maternal age. The authors concluded that their findings underscore the "potential public health benefit of cigarette smoking cessation programs aimed at the most economically disadvantaged African-American women" (57).

The level of social support and community integration available to a mother is believed to play an important role in pregnancy outcomes and may impact behaviors, such as smoking, during pregnancy. Indeed, smoking has been reported as one means by which women cope with stress in adverse domestic situations, including poverty and disadvantage. In a Turkish study, Ergin et al. reported that young age (<20), low education level, and migrant status were associated with smoking during pregnancy (58). Similarly, in a German cohort, Elsenbruch and colleagues reported that a lack of social support in pregnancy is a key risk-factor for adverse outcomes and that women categorized as having low social support during pregnancy were far more likely (34 vs. 17%) to self-report smoking during the first trimester of pregnancy than women categorized as having high levels of social support (59). These findings mirror earlier findings summarized by Dejin-Karlsson and colleagues, wherein women with strong social support networks are more successful at successfully quitting smoking, and that an absence of support networks is one reason why some pregnant women continue to smoke (60).

Given the relationships between PTB and inadequate antenatal care, economic disadvantage, low-educational attainment, and ethnicity, a number of investigators have recommended the use of community outreach programs or clinics involving multiple disciplines sensitive to the particular needs of the community in question (61). Interventions based on nuanced patient risk assessments that consider individual and community-level factors may thus benefit attempts to reduce the rate of tobacco-associated PTB, and should be considered in any precision public health approach to PTB prevention. Risk assessments could be used to design and deliver targeted, culturally and contextually appropriate interventions at community (i.e., comprehensive anti-smoking programs and cessation support through community, religious, sporting and cultural groups, supported by community leaders) and individual (psychotherapy and pharmacotherapy for smoking cessation, midwife outreach programs, access to social support and mental health services, assisted transport to access health-care services) levels.

POPULATION-BASED CERVIX LENGTH SCREENING

While there are many pathways leading to PTB, some cases may be predicted by measurement of the length of the cervix in mid-pregnancy (62–64). This measurement may be done as a component of the standard mid-pregnancy morphology scan typically conducted between 18 and 24 weeks gestation.

If the cervix appears shortened on trans-abdominal scan, a transvaginal scan is then recommended. For pregnancies where the risk of PTB is perceived to be increased, the standard of practice is generally to proceed to transvaginal scan to measure the cervix length.

The finding of a shortened cervix in mid-pregnancy is predictive of PTB, and there are treatments that reduce that risk, at least for singleton pregnancies. Administration of natural progesterone vaginally as a single evening dose has been shown to nearly halve the risk of PTB in such circumstances. This benefit has been shown in large randomized controlled trials and also by meta-analysis of individual patient data (65–67).

So, we now have strong evidence that the risk of PTB can be reduced dramatically, perhaps by about half, in women found in mid-pregnancy to have a short cervix and then using that information to prescribe natural vaginal progesterone which is a relatively simple and safe treatment. Should the test and its subsequent treatment be applied to the entire population of pregnant women?

In the largest American randomized controlled trial, Hassan and colleagues screened 32,091 women by transvaginal scan to identify 733 with a cervix shortened and measuring between 10 and 20 mm (65). Two hundred thirty-six were randomized to the vaginal progesterone treatment group, 229 to placebo and 268 declined to participate further. The effect was to nearly halve the rate of early PTB in those found to be at risk; the number of births <33 weeks was 21 cases in the treatment group (8.9%) and 36 cases in the placebo group (16.1%). Thus, if the findings of this trial were to be replicated in general clinical practice with no women receiving a placebo and all women participating in the treatment, then screening 32,000 women would identify 2.3% of women requiring treatment and would result in the prevention of 47 cases of births <33 weeks (5).

More recently, the largest randomized controlled trial to have been conducted so far, based in UK, observed a non-significant effect on three primary outcomes—fetal death or birth <34 weeks gestation, a composite of neonatal outcomes, and a standardized cognitive score at 2 years of age (68). There were multiple entry criteria and the treatment consisted of vaginal progesterone from 22–24 to 34 weeks. When the data from the various trials are included in an updated meta-analysis, the beneficial effect of vaginal progesterone treatment for prevention of PTB in women with a singleton pregnancy and shortened cervix in mid-pregnancy remains statistically significant (67).

A cohort study assessing the introduction of routine cervix length screening in mid-pregnancy at a single tertiary level center in Chicago, IL, USA, observed a reduction in preterm births that appeared to be spread across the preterm gestational age spectrum when compared with outcomes prior to introduction of the program (69). The reductions were from 6.7 to 6.0% for births <37 weeks, 1.9 to 1.7% for <34 weeks, and 1.1 to 1.0% for <32 weeks gestation. In this population, the frequency of cervix length less than 25 mm in mid-pregnancy was 0.89%.

But would it be cost-effective to introduce this protocol into clinical practice across the entire population? In a USA-based decision analysis model of a single cervix length measurement in mid-pregnancy compared with no such measurement, with treatment with vaginal progesterone if the cervix were found to be shortened, it was estimated the program would save $12 million/year and gain 424 quality-adjusted life years (70).

A more recent USA-based analysis asked if risk-based screening would be more or less effective than universal screening of all pregnancies (71). Results of the decision analytic model indicated that both risk-based and universal screening would be more cost-effective than no screening. Of the two approaches, universal screening of cervix length measurement of all pregnancies was superior to risk-based screening and would result in a higher cost-effectiveness ratio.

Despite the evidence presented above, there remain as many unknowns as knowns. What is the prevalence of shortened cervix in mid-pregnancy in the various populations of the world? Even within the USA there is considerable variation, ranging from 0.89% <25 mm in the Chicago study (69) to 2.3% <20 mm in the multicentered trial reported by Hassan and colleagues (65). Regions such as northern Europe where the rate of PTB is much lower are likely to have even lower prevalence of shortened cervix in mid-pregnancy. Further, we have few data describing the phenotypic and genotypic variables that influence mid-pregnancy cervix length and the response to treatment, and we have little understanding how to monitor and manage cases undergoing treatment and the drivers of treatment success and failure. This is a key issue in the context of precision public health (**Figure 1**). Interestingly, a small USA study found that progesterone and cerclage therapies were only effective in women with biomarkers of inflammation in the amniotic fluid and that without inflammation the risk of PTB was actually increased (72). This preliminary evidence suggests that the inclusion of additional screening parameters, such as inflammation, might improve precision and response to targeted therapies.

To achieve improvements in precision, we need to progress beyond case studies and randomized controlled trials. In the first instance, we need sound and reliable population-based data. Most high resource nations have perinatal collection systems collecting basic information on demographics, the birth, and the newborn. To fully understand and maximize the benefit from mid-pregnancy cervix length measurement and treatment, such data collection systems will require much greater complexity and capability. The expansion will be complicated by the fact that many health-care systems are fragmented, with antenatal investigations and treatments often being dislocated from hospital-based birthing processes. Prevention of PTB is of great benefit to individuals and the community, and development of cost-effective models of health-care delivery using this intervention should be entirely feasible. At this time, it would seem reasonable to expect that the most effective solution will come from population-based screening, but followed by further precision analysis to best understand the most appropriate treatment for each case and the manner by which that treatment should then be monitored for effectiveness.

AVOIDANCE OF NON-MEDICALLY INDICATED LATE PRETERM AND EARLY-TERM BIRTH

The rates of late preterm, and early-term, birth have been increasing over recent decades in many countries (73, 74). These trends have been underpinned by a general assumption held by many people that birth close to term will not be associated with any enduring compromise for the offspring. A wealth of data, from multiple societies, now suggest otherwise.

Being born late preterm, defined as birth between 34 and 36 weeks and 6 days gestation, places the infant at risk of neonatal and childhood consequences (75). For the neonate, complications may include the need to be admitted to a neonatal intensive special care unit, and special support to maintain respiratory function, temperature control, prevention of infection, and maintenance of normal glucose levels, and much more (75, 76). For the child, there are increased risks of death, re-admission to hospital, cerebral palsy, developmental delay, and behavioral and learning problems at school age (77, 78). In recent years, the findings of potential compromise from prematurity for the child have been extended to birth in the early-term period, ranging from 37 weeks and 0 days to 38 weeks and 6 days.

For those cases in which early birth is required for maternal or fetal reasons, the benefits may outweigh any risks of prematurity. But, we now have strong evidence that there are many cases where such a benefit is not the case, and steps need to be taken to ensure that any elective early births can be fully justified.

Population-based study of the factors involved in rising rates of early births has shown clear demographic differences (2, 14, 79). In a USA study of early births between 1992 and 2002, the major increase in rate was observed in non-Hispanic White births (80). During the decade of study, rates of early births in Hispanic and Black women had remained relatively constant. The factors underpinning these observations are uncertain, but suggest that socioeconomic factors are involved and that both medical and patient contributions need to be considered.

Reducing the rate of early intervention is particularly challenging, but progress has been made by some health-care systems. In a study of 27 health-care facilities in USA, each organization was invited to choose one of three protocols to reduce their rate of non-medically indicated late preterm and early-term birth (81). The options ranged from just education of staff through to complete prohibition of early birth. The gestational age below which non-medically indicated birth was to be discouraged was 39 completed weeks. Outcome data revealed that the most interventionist protocols produced the greatest benefit, with significant reductions in early birth rates and admissions to neonatal intensive care units. The still birth rate did not change during the time of the study. Education alone did not improve outcomes, but of importance, the program only involved the medical staff and did not include education of other health-care practitioners or the patients themselves.

At a national level, there has been considerable public advocacy across USA led by the March of Dimes though a campaign called "Healthy Babies are Worth the Wait," coupled with quality improvement initiatives (6). These programs have been aimed primarily at health-care providers and pregnant women to discourage unnecessary early intervention. The results of these and other programs suggest that the rates of non-medically indicated late preterm and early-term birth rates can be reduced, but there are many confounding factors.

First, the effect is entirely dependent on the extent to which unnecessary early intervention is prevalent in a particular health-care environment. Further, it is clear that individual health-care practitioners and their pregnant patients actively choose to make such decisions. Understanding when preventative policies should be introduced requires detailed understanding of not just health-care outcomes but also the practices of individual practitioners and the attitudes of women and families who access such care.

Second, are the health-care workforce implications of discouraging elective birth before 39 weeks gestation. Such a policy will inevitably increase the number of cases of spontaneous labor, and there are clear implications for the work–life balance of busy practitioners, especially those in solo or small group practices. In a secondary analysis of a randomized controlled trial in Denmark comparing planned elective Cesarean births at 38 or 39 weeks gestation, delaying the surgery by 1 week resulted in a 60% increase in unscheduled Cesarean sections and a 70% increase in births out-of-hours (82). Imposing health-care guidelines that potentially compromise the daily activities of practitioners and hospitals requires considerable justification and a thorough understanding of the issues involved in each health-care environment.

Third, is the potential for stillbirth or fetal compromise by delaying birth. There is no convincing evidence at a population level that earlier delivery is associated with lesser rates of stillbirth but it is logical to assume that a background risk of fetal death must remain present by continuing the pregnancy, even in the absence of any known risk factors. Any such risk would need to be weighed against any potential risk of death or morbidity resulting from late preterm or early-term birth. Reassuringly, the American trial of three management options in 27 hospitals significantly reduced early birth rates and there was no evidence of any increase in risk to the child. In the Danish RCT of elective Cesarean delivery at 38 or 39 weeks gestation, there was a small reduction in rate of delivery to the NICU in the delayed delivery group, but no other signs of danger (82, 83).

It is clear, therefore, that the challenge to prevent non-medically indicated late preterm/early-term births is scientifically justified, but confounded by regional differences, possible benefits and risks to the child by continuing the pregnancy, and potential adverse effects on the practitioners and their health-care facilities. For each health-care environment, detailed and ongoing data availability and analysis are vital if preventative strategies are to be introduced and be maintained. So far, in USA and Western Australia, there has been success in lowering the rates of late preterm/early-term births, but continuing success and translation into other environments where the baseline PTB rates are already lower may be more challenging. The principles of precision public health may offer the solution to this major problem. By applying precision analysis using factors such as genetic predisposition, prior history, and lifestyle variables, we may better understand which pregnancies can safely be left until after 39 weeks gestation and which cases require earlier intervention.

PREVENTION OF INFECTION-DRIVEN PTB

It is well established that microbial infection of the extra-placental membranes, amniotic cavity, and fetus is an important driver of PTB, particularly in the deliveries at the earliest gestational ages (9, 84, 85). Animal models and clinical studies demonstrate a causal relationship between infection and PTB, while the immune-pathophysiological pathways responsible for triggering preterm labor in response to infection have been studied, replicated and characterized in a variety of models (86–88). The most common pathway *via* which bacteria trigger PTB is the so-called ascending infection route: microorganisms residing in cervico-vaginal fluid in pregnancy ascend through the cervical barrier and colonize the fetal membranes, passing through in some cases to colonize the amniotic fluid and from there infect the fetus (86, 89). The severity of the infection and the ensuing inflammatory response determines, to a large part, the obstetric and neonatal outcomes, including the timing and onset of preterm labor, the effectiveness of tocolytic therapy, and the risk of serious neonatal morbidities.

While the majority of preterm deliveries occur in the 32- to 36-week period, the costs and risks of serious perinatal morbidities are highest in deliveries <32-week gestation, the majority of which are infection-associated (9, 84, 85). Hence, preventing PTB as a result of intrauterine infection has the largest potential gains in terms of reducing major morbidity and death and reducing perinatal and lifetime health-care costs (90, 91).

Unfortunately, identifying women at risk of infection-driven PTB and treating them to prevent the infection is challenging, both from an individual patient and public health perspective (92–94). Gestational tissues exposed at different times in pregnancy to different bacteria exhibit variable immune responses depending on dose, duration, distribution, maternal and fetal genetics, ethnicity, lifestyle, and anatomical factors (such as previous cervical surgery). This level of heterogeneity makes identification and risk prediction particularly difficult. There are several well-documented approaches which can identify women at increased risk of infection-related PTB, yet their prognostic value is generally too weak to alter clinical decision-making and treatment. Many of the trials of prophylactic antibiotic therapy given to pregnant women to prevent PTB have failed to employ robust inclusion criteria or delivered poorly effective antibiotic regimens (95, 96). Identifying women who will benefit from treatment is a key requirement for primary prevention: prescribing antibiotics to large numbers of women in pregnancy in order to prevent PTB in a small percentage of recipients is not justifiable in light of the emerging recognition of the potential developmental effects of disrupting the maternal and neonatal microbiomes with antibiotics in pregnancy (97–100).

To date, primary prevention research has focused on identifying and treating women with abnormal vaginal microbiota in early pregnancy prior to the onset of preterm labor (101, 102). This strategy is based on the assumption that women with vaginal dysbiosis have increased risk of ascending infection and that antibiotic treatment will eradicate the pathogens, prevent infection, and thus prevent PTB. The odds ratio of women delivering preterm with bacterial vaginosis (BV) or aerobic vaginitis (AV) is approximately 2–7, and even higher if diagnosed before 16-week gestation (103–105). The presence of *Ureaplasma* in the vagina is also associated with an approximately twofold increased risk of PTB (106–108). However, due to its high prevalence in pregnant women (~50%) (109), detection of *Ureaplasma* alone is not sufficiently diagnostic to warrant prophylactic treatment. The prognostic significance of the presence of specific *Ureaplasma* serovars is currently under investigation (109).

A large number of trials have employed standard microbiological or clinical approaches to identify women with vaginal dysbiosis and treated them with antibiotics (with or without probiotics) to prevent PTB (84, 110, 111). Many of these studies failed to significantly lower the rate of PTB (111–114), although a few studies employing clindamycin treatment before 22 weeks of pregnancy have shown significant maternal and neonatal benefits (95, 96). The negative findings are, in part, due to lack of effective antimicrobial interventions (95) and the failure to treat the dysbiosis or address recurrence (115–117). However, the major impediment to therapeutic progress is the poor prognostic precision of current identification methods. Most women with vaginal dysbiosis or urogenital tract pathogens do not deliver preterm, and our ability to identify those at sufficiently high risk to warrant treatment (OR > 10) is poor (102). Primary prevention studies have focused on defining clinical vaginal microbial disorders and recruiting patients based on these definitions, rather than identifying subgroups of women who are at particularly high risk of delivering preterm as a result of microbial profile and/or other risk factors and targeting them for appropriate and effective treatment. Currently, although rapid molecular tests for diagnosing BV and AV are being developed (118, 119), we lack an accurate, rapid, and affordable test to identify women at high risk of infection-related PTB (120, 121).

Nevertheless, despite these uncertainties and qualifications, there is encouraging evidence that public health screening for BV or other forms of abnormal vaginal microbiota using traditional techniques can be an effective primary prevention strategy in reducing PTB rates. A recently published Austrian study, implemented following the results of a randomized clinical trial, retrospectively analyzed the pregnancy outcome data of over 17,000 women at high risk of PTB (based on general, family, and obstetric risk factors) across a 10-year timespan following introduction of a voluntary antenatal infection "screen and treat" program (122). All women received standard antenatal care; 49.5% entered the screen and treat program, which consisted of testing of vaginal swabs at 10- to 16-week gestation for detection of BV and presence of *Candida* spp. or *Trichomonas vaginalis*, followed by antimicrobial treatment with either clindamycin, clotrimazole, or metronidazole as appropriate. Recurrent infections were retreated and women with BV were given probiotics after treatment to prevent recurrence. Women in the treated group had a significantly lower rate of stillbirth (0.4 vs. 2.0%), miscarriage (0.5 vs. 1.4%), PTB <37 weeks (9.7 vs. 22.3%), and PTB <32 weeks gestation (1.9 vs. 8.3%). The effect of the program on the rates of early/extreme PTB was particularly impressive, with a more than 77% reduction observed; this is consistent with the known role of intrauterine infection in the majority of deliveries <32 weeks. The major weakness in this study is its retrospective, non-randomized design, although confounding is minimal and unlikely to alter the findings (122).

These data are similar to the achievements of an earlier public health program implemented in Germany in late 1997 (123). The program consisted of a free self-test vaginal pH kit offered to 2,722 women in obstetric care (>12-week gestation), with optional follow-up with obstetricians if the test was positive. Elevated vaginal fluid pH is a weak surrogate marker of BV and AV, typically associated with a lack of *Lactobacillus* spp. Treatment with antibiotics (clindamycin) was indicated if clinical symptoms of BV were present following obstetric examination. The program resulted in much lower rates of PTB <32 weeks in the women who participated (14% of the cohort) compared to women under the same care who did not engage in the pH testing program (0.3 vs. 4.1%). Subsequently, a large prospective trial was conducted, enrolling 8,000 women in the state of Thuringia over a 6-month period. Women who self-tested their vaginal pH and sought medical treatment based on the result (8% of the cohort) had lower rates of PTB at <32 weeks (0.3 vs. 1.6%) and at <37 weeks of gestation (5.3 vs. 8.5%). After discontinuation of the program, PTB rates returned to historical levels in the state (123).

In order to obtain greater precision, we need to refine our ability to identify women at high risk of infection-driven PTB (OR > 10) and target them with appropriate follow-up and treatment. Many of the bacteria found in the amniotic cavity of preterm deliveries are normal commensals of the urogenital tract (124, 125), so vaginal microbiological profiling alone is unlikely to have a high positive predictive value. It remains to be determined whether more refined and selective molecular techniques may help to improve diagnostic discrimination (109). It is likely that a combination of clinical risk factors (e.g., prior PTB, cervical imaging, and abnormality detection), high-resolution microbial profiling (possibly including bacterial strain identification), and immunological/inflammatory biomarker assessment will be needed, in combination with a highly effective antimicrobial regimen (97, 126), to enable a truly effective maternal "screen and treat" program to achieve the desired level of precision and effectiveness required for a primary prevention public health program (127–133).

"OMICS" AND PRECISION PUBLIC HEALTH

Identification of At-Risk Individuals: Genomic Approach

The contribution of genomic variation to the etiology of PTB is thought to be in the order of 40% by twin and family studies (134). Women who were born preterm, or who have close family members with a PTB, have a significantly higher risk of PTB. Rates of prematurity are influenced by ethnicity (135): studies have shown that the rates of PTB in African-Americans is significantly higher than other racial groups in similar socioeconomic settings, and that women married to African-American men have higher prevalence of PTB. Determining the precise nature of the genomic variants responsible for determining risk of PTB is hampered by the complex biology of preterm labor (135). From an evolutionary perspective, PTB is detrimental to the survival of the species, and there are multiple levels of redundancy in the biological process of labor initiation, which combine to reduce the incidence of PTB. The genetic basis of PTB is, therefore, unlikely to be monogenic. Rather, in all but the most extreme of phenotypes, multiple changes with gene pathways are required to overcome physiological redundancy and culminate in PTB.

The advantage of genome-based screening tests is that they may be applied prior to pregnancy and allow ample time to initiate primary prevention, rather than attempting to slow or reverse the premature activation of parturition which leads to spontaneous preterm labor. Many gene-targeted analyses and genome-wide association studies (GWAS) have been carried out in an attempt to identify genetic variants associated with PTB (135). Sheikh et al., in a recent review of the literature, identified 119 candidate genes with SNPs that had potential association with PTB in an evaluation of 92 different studies. Many studies have found association between SNPs in parturition-associated genes such as the progesterone receptor, oxytocin receptor, relaxin, the prostaglandin EP3 receptor, and the CRH receptor 1, although the level of risk associated with these polymorphisms is not sufficiently high to be useful clinically (136). Other target genes have yielded more promising SNPs, in particular heat-shock protein 47 (SERPINH1), which is involved in the maturation of collagen molecules and is enriched in African and African-American populations. Polymorphism in other tissue remodeling-related genes like metallopeptidase inhibitor-1 and 2, COL1A2, COL5A2, and COL5A1 also significantly increase the risk of PTB (136). Overall, many of the SNPs significantly associated with PTB are related in some way to inflammation. Lack of replication and population-based heterogeneity remain major hurdles to be overcome.

Identification of combinations of multiple subtle genomic contributors are now feasible with advances in high-throughput genomic sequencing and bioinformatics. In a recent study of women with 2–3 generations of PTB using a meta-genomic, bi-clustering algorithm, Uzun et al. (137) identified variations in 33 genes within five genetic pathways associated with altered PTB risk. Brubaker et al. employed protein network analysis with tissue-specific gene expression data to identify functionally important candidate genes that would be overlooked by standard GWAS techniques. Their analysis identified significant sub-networks and genes not previously associated with PTB, including sub-networks associated with inflammation, muscle function, and ion channels (138). It is likely that extensions of such work will ultimately permit the characterization of an individual's overall genomic risk of PTB as a screening test to identify those at risk, with the molecular consequences of the variation being used to guide preventive interventions.

Further advances are likely to originate from advances in the use of phenotypic data from rare genetic diseases to identify variants associated with common pathways shared by multiple disorders (139). To this end, the recently expanded Human Phenotype Ontology (www.http://human-phenotype-ontology.github.io) now contains 250,000 phenotypic annotations for over 10,000 rare and common diseases (140, 141), which can be used to examine the phenotypic overlap among common diseases with shared risk alleles or those linked by genomic location. Other databases and platforms have been developed to allow accurate assessment of the causal relationship between genetic variants and phenotype; these are becoming critical tools in clinical genetic diagnostics (140), for comparing phenotypes between patient cohorts (142) and for identifying new disease genes *via* the linkage of novel variants with well-defined phenotypes (141, 143). Application of such approaches to understanding the genetic causes of PTB and identifying populations at risk remains to be explored. However, several examples have already been identified. Insights may be expected from analyzing the links between PTB and Prader–Willi Syndrome (144, 145) or by studying Beckwith–Wiedemann Syndrome, which is associated with increased rates of PTB, gestational diabetes, polyhydramnios, and intrauterine bleeding (146). Advances in this area may lead to improved knowledge regarding genetic variants and pathways to PTB which can be exploited to enhance screening programs and develop and target interventions.

Identification of At-Risk Individuals: Transcriptomic Approach

Transcriptomic methods assess RNA in tissue and quantify the extent to which genes are functioning, rather than inferring variations in function related to variations in sequence. By examining expression of genes related to inflammation, for example, one can find evidence of inflammation prior to the development of clinical manifestations. In PTB, a screening test could be developed to identify individuals with premature activation of parturition at a stage where treatment can reverse such activation prior to the tipping point to inevitable preterm labor (147).

As was the case for genomic methods, alterations in the transcriptome in the lead up to PTB are likely to arise from multiple pathways. Heng et al. (148) described a method considering the expression levels of multiple genes from multiple pathways in maternal whole blood and their relationship to subsequent PTB. Applied to asymptomatic pregnant women at 28-week gestation and including clinical factors, their model predicted PTB with sensitivity of 65%, specificity of 88%, and false positive rate of 11%; their birth cohort had been enriched, with a PTB rate of 31%. This method requires further validation in average-risk populations before being considered for clinical application. Alternative methods may employ samples other than maternal blood such as cervico-vaginal fluid, or analysis of micro RNAs and other related molecules which may give insights into placental pathologies and associated risk factors. With refinement, this approach could be useful in the identification of the woman heading toward PTB in whom interventions could arrest this course and allow safe delivery at term.

Identification of At-Risk Individuals: Proteomic Approach

As transcriptomics looks at the actual expression of genes rather than the sequence, proteomics goes a step further in examining the protein end products of gene function, giving insight into the physiological alterations related to gene sequence and expression. High-throughput proteomic assessments allow the identification of differentially produced proteins in association with clinically relevant phenotypes. From a PTB perspective, proteomic variation may herald early delivery prior to the development of clinically apparent symptoms.

The most commonly employed protein assessment is fetal fibronectin in women who present with symptoms suggestive of preterm labor. This protein is found in greater quantities in the cervico-vaginal fluid in women who will deliver preterm than in those women whose pregnancy will continue to term (149). Quantitative or qualitative assessment of fetal fibronectin levels permit the rationalization of therapies aimed at delaying delivery or reducing the adverse sequelae of prematurity.

A natural extension of the use of fetal fibronectin testing to stratify risk of PTB in symptomatic women is its application to asymptomatic women. To date, there is little evidence to support the adoption of such screening into routine clinical practice in low-risk pregnant women (150). It may have greater utility in the screening of women with other established risk factors (151–153).

Kim et al. (154) assessed the utility of amniotic fluid MMP-8 as a screening test for subsequent PTB in women undergoing diagnostic amniocentesis in the mid-trimester. The test was highly specific (100%) for subsequent PTB, albeit with relatively low sensitivity (42%). The major limitation of this approach is the invasive nature of the test which is unlikely to be acceptable to the majority of women due to the low but significant risk of pregnancy loss. Several other studies of amniotic fluid proteome have been carried out, with a number of candidate biomarkers identified for predicting PTB and neonatal adverse outcomes secondary to intrauterine inflammation (155, 156), but these have not been clinically exploited (157).

A more acceptable, less invasive testing strategy based on analysis of cervico-vaginal fluids may have greater prognostic potential and acceptance. Gravett et al. (158) undertook a proteomic study of the cervico-vaginal fluid in a non-human primate model of iatrogenic intra-amniotic infection, a major contributor to PTB, with the aim of identifying a non-invasive biomarker for this condition. Twenty-six proteins were found to be differentially expressed in the presence of intra-amniotic infection compared to controls, with a preponderance of proteins involved in inflammatory regulation. Of these, IGFBP1 was increased 16-fold in the presence of intra-amniotic infection, and this is a potential biomarker for clinical application. Many other studies have investigated levels of inflammatory cytokines and proteins in cervico-vaginal fluids, and candidate proteins such as IL-6 have been consistently identified (159, 160), but these have not yielded biomarkers with sufficient prognostic utility to be useful clinically. Georgiou and colleagues employed proteomic analysis of cervico-vaginal fluid samples in at-risk asymptomatic women to identify candidate biomarkers of impending preterm delivery (161). They found that thioredoxin and interleukin 1 receptor antagonist levels were significantly reduced up to 90 days prior to preterm labor compared with women who delivered at term. Both proteins had a positive predictive value of >72% and negative predictive value of >95%. The prognostic value of these biomarkers has yet to be demonstrated in independent studies and populations; however, and to date, proteomic approaches have not yet yielded clinically useful tests that have been commercialized and widely adopted (162).

PRECISION REFINEMENT USING NEW TECHNOLOGIES

"Omic" approaches may be suitable for both primary screening, as well as precision refinement in women previously identified as being at risk of PTB by other screening modalities (**Figure 1**). Gene–environment interactions underlie almost all responses of complex organisms to external stimuli. This principle is the basis of pharmacogenomics, whereby an individual's genetic susceptibility to the effects of a drug determines whether or not that drug is used. However, this may be used on a larger scale than is currently employed in order to direct interventions in those who screen at increased risk of PTB. For example, women who are genetically more likely to succeed in smoking cessation with nicotine replacement therapy may be offered this intervention, while those genetically likely to fail may avoid the potential adverse outcomes of this therapy (163).

As high-throughput genomic sequencing technology becomes more affordable and rapid and point-of-care devices are developed, future technological advances may provide exciting new avenues for further refinement of risk. Other risk factors likely to be amenable to "omic" precision refinement include bacterial dysbiosis, previous inflammatory and infection-related PTB, as well as cervical dysfunction (**Figure 1**).

Other technological advances are likely to be able to be exploited in the near future to gain greater precision in PTB prevention strategies. Wearable mobile sensor technologies have been developed for a number of applications requiring real-time monitoring of physiological parameters that allow monitoring of health status/responses and identification of individuals at risk. Examples include remote monitoring of the elderly after transfer to a community care setting (164, 165). Sophisticated systems have been developed and trialed for measuring multiple physiological parameters (166), and it could be envisaged that such systems could be adapted and used in high-risk women to identify changes in uterine activity, for example, suggestive of early onset of labor (164).

In addition, E-registries and web-based surveillance systems are exciting developments in health information systems that have applications in monitoring maternal health trends and outcomes together with changes in population characteristics and risks (167, 168). A simple example that illustrates the potential is the use of a mobile SMS-based system for monitoring maternal health in low-resource settings (169).

AUTHOR CONTRIBUTIONS

JN: first draft of introduction, populations in transition, cervix length screening and non-medically indicated preterm birth, and responsible for overall manuscript. MK: first draft of smoking section and review of entire manuscript. SW: first draft of genetics and -omic section and review of entire manuscript. CA: coordination of authors and review and submission of manuscript. RH: contributed to writing of overall manuscript and review. JK: first draft of infection-associated preterm birth, preparation of figure, and review of overall manuscript.

FUNDING

This work was funded in part by the Australian National Health and Medical Research Council grant number APP1077931.

REFERENCES

1. Chang HH, Larson J, Blencowe H, Spong CY, Simpson JL, Lawn JE. Preterm births in countries with a very high human development index – authors' reply. *Lancet* (2013) 381:1356–7. doi:10.1016/S0140-6736(13)60878-8
2. Blencowe H, Cousens S, Oestergaard MZ, Chou D, Moller AB, Narwal R, et al. National, regional, and worldwide estimates of preterm birth rates in the year 2010 with time trends since 1990 for selected countries: a systematic analysis and implications. *Lancet* (2012) 379:2162–72. doi:10.1016/S0140-6736(12)60820-4
3. Liu L, Oza S, Hogan D, Perin J, Rudan I, Lawn JE, et al. Global, regional, and national causes of child mortality in 2000-13, with projections to inform post-2015 priorities: an updated systematic analysis. *Lancet* (2015) 385:430–40. doi:10.1016/S0140-6736(14)61698-6
4. Lawn JE, Cousens S, Zupan J; Lancet Neonatal Survival Steering Team. 4 million neonatal deaths: when? Where? Why? *Lancet* (2005) 365:891–900. doi:10.1016/S0140-6736(05)71048-5
5. Newnham JP, Dickinson JE, Hart RJ, Pennell CE, Arrese CA, Keelan JA. Strategies to prevent preterm birth. *Front Immunol* (2014) 5:584. doi:10.3389/fimmu.2014.00584
6. McCabe ER, Carrino GE, Russell RB, Howse JL. Fighting for the next generation: US prematurity in 2030. *Pediatrics* (2014) 134:1193–9. doi:10.1542/peds.2014-2541
7. Liggins GC, Howie RN. A controlled trial of antepartum glucocorticoid treatment for prevention of the respiratory distress syndrome in premature infants. *Pediatrics* (1972) 50:515–25.
8. Vogel JP, Oladapo OT, Manu A, Gulmezoglu AM, Bahl R. New WHO recommendations to improve the outcomes of preterm birth. *Lancet Glob Health* (2015) 3:e589–90. doi:10.1016/S2214-109X(15)00183-7
9. Romero R, Dey SK, Fisher SJ. Preterm labor: one syndrome, many causes. *Science* (2014) 345:760–5. doi:10.1126/science.1251816
10. Goldenberg RL, Hauth JC, Andrews WW. Intrauterine infection and preterm delivery. *N Engl J Med* (2000) 342:1500–7. doi:10.1056/NEJM200005183422007
11. Haas DM, Caldwell DM, Kirkpatrick P, McIntosh JJ, Welton NJ. Tocolytic therapy for preterm delivery: systematic review and network meta-analysis. *BMJ* (2012) 345:e6226. doi:10.1136/bmj.e6226
12. The L. The unfinished agenda of preterm births. *Lancet* (2016) 388:2323. doi:10.1016/S0140-6736(16)32170-5
13. Newnham JP, White SW, Meharry S, Lee HS, Pedretti MK, Arrese CA, et al. Reducing preterm birth by a state-wide multifaceted program: an implementation study. *Am J Obstet Gynecol* (2016) 1.e1–1.e9. doi:10.1016/j.ajog.2016.11.1037
14. Chang HH, Larson J, Blencowe H, Spong CY, Howson CP, Cairns-Smith S, et al. Preventing preterm births: analysis of trends and potential reductions with interventions in 39 countries with very high human development index. *Lancet* (2013) 381:223–34. doi:10.1016/S0140-6736(12)61856-X
15. Collins FS, Varmus H. A new initiative on precision medicine. *N Engl J Med* (2015) 372:793–5. doi:10.1056/NEJMp1500523
16. Khoury MJ, Iademarco MF, Riley WT. Precision public health for the era of precision medicine. *Am J Prev Med* (2016) 50:398–401. doi:10.1016/j.amepre.2015.08.031
17. Soda M, Choi YL, Enomoto M, Takada S, Yamashita Y, Ishikawa S, et al. Identification of the transforming EML4-ALK fusion gene in non-small-cell lung cancer. *Nature* (2007) 448:561–6. doi:10.1038/nature05945
18. Urquia ML, Glazier RH, Blondel B, Zeitlin J, Gissler M, Macfarlane A, et al. International migration and adverse birth outcomes: role of ethnicity, region of origin and destination. *J Epidemiol Community Health* (2010) 64:243–51. doi:10.1136/jech.2008.083535
19. Urquia ML, Frank JW, Moineddin R, Glazier RH. Immigrants' duration of residence and adverse birth outcomes: a population-based study. *BJOG* (2010) 117:591–601. doi:10.1111/j.1471-0528.2010.02523.x
20. Newnham JP, Sahota DS, Zhang CY, Xu B, Zheng M, Doherty DA, et al. Preterm birth rates in Chinese women in China, Hong Kong and Australia – the price of Westernisation. *Aust N Z J Obstet Gynaecol* (2011) 51:426–31. doi:10.1111/j.1479-828X.2011.01327.x
21. Jia P, Cheng X, Xue H, Wang Y. Applications of geographic information systems (GIS) data and methods in obesity-related research. *Obes Rev* (2017) 18(4):400–11. doi:10.1111/obr.12495
22. Ebener S, Guerra-Arias M, Campbell J, Tatem AJ, Moran AC, Amoako Johnson F, et al. The geography of maternal and newborn health: the state of the art. *Int J Health Geogr* (2015) 14:19. doi:10.1186/s12942-015-0012-x
23. Makanga PT, Schuurman N, von Dadelszen P, Firoz T. A scoping review of geographic information systems in maternal health. *Int J Gynaecol Obstet* (2016) 134:13–7. doi:10.1016/j.ijgo.2015.11.022
24. Fleisch AF, Rifas-Shiman SL, Koutrakis P, Schwartz JD, Kloog I, Melly S, et al. Prenatal exposure to traffic pollution: associations with reduced fetal growth and rapid infant weight gain. *Epidemiology* (2015) 26:43–50. doi:10.1097/EDE.0000000000000203
25. MacQuillan EL, Curtis AB, Baker KM, Paul R, Back YO. Using GIS mapping to target public health interventions: examining birth outcomes across GIS techniques. *J Community Health* (2016). doi:10.1007/s10900-016-0298-z
26. Yazdy MM, Werler MM, Feldkamp ML, Shaw GM, Mosley BS, Vieira VM, et al. Spatial analysis of gastroschisis in the National Birth Defects Prevention Study. *Birth Defects Res A Clin Mol Teratol* (2015) 103:544–53. doi:10.1002/bdra.23375
27. Hamilton BE, Martin JA, Osterman MJ. Births: preliminary data for 2015. *Natl Vital Stat Rep* (2016) 65:1–15.
28. Shapiro-Mendoza CK, Barfield WD, Henderson Z, James A, Howse JL, Iskander J, et al. CDC grand rounds: public health strategies to prevent preterm birth. *MMWR Morb Mortal Wkly Rep* (2016) 65:826–30. doi:10.15585/mmwr.mm6532a4
29. WHO. *WHO Global Report: Mortality Attributable to Tobacco*. Geneva: WHO (2012).
30. WHO. *Global Status Report on Noncommunicable Diseases 2010*. Geneva: WHO (2010).
31. Cnattingius S. The epidemiology of smoking during pregnancy: smoking prevalence, maternal characteristics, and pregnancy outcomes. *Nicotine Tob Res* (2004) 6:S125–40. doi:10.1080/14622200410001669187
32. Banderali G, Martelli A, Landi M, Moretti F, Betti F, Radaelli G, et al. Short and long term health effects of parental tobacco smoking during pregnancy and lactation: a descriptive review. *J Transl Med* (2015) 13:327. doi:10.1186/s12967-015-0690-y
33. Mei-Dan E, Walfisch A, Weisz B, Hallak M, Brown R, Shrim A. The unborn smoker: association between smoking during pregnancy and adverse perinatal outcomes. *J Perinat Med* (2015) 43:553–8. doi:10.1515/jpm-2014-0299
34. Wagijo MA, Sheikh A, Duijts L, Been JV. Reducing tobacco smoking and smoke exposure to prevent preterm birth and its complications. *Paediatr Respir Rev* (2017) 22:3–10. doi:10.1016/j.prrv.2015.09.002
35. Karumanchi SA, Levine RJ. How does smoking reduce the risk of preeclampsia? *Hypertension* (2010) 55:1100. doi:10.1161/HYPERTENSIONAHA.109.148973
36. Wikström A-K, Stephansson O, Cnattingius S. Tobacco use during pregnancy and preeclampsia risk: effects of cigarette smoking and snuff. *Hypertension* (2010) 55:1254–9. doi:10.1161/HYPERTENSIONAHA.109.147082
37. Salihu HM, Wilson RE. Epidemiology of prenatal smoking and perinatal outcomes. *Early Hum Dev* (2007) 83:713–20. doi:10.1016/j.earlhumdev.2007.08.002
38. Iams JD, Berghella V. Care for women with prior preterm birth. *Am J Obstet Gynecol* (2010) 203:89–100. doi:10.1016/j.ajog.2010.02.004
39. Simmons LE, Rubens CE, Darmstadt GL, Gravett MG. Preventing preterm birth and neonatal mortality: exploring the epidemiology, causes, and interventions. *Semin Perinatol* (2010) 34:408–15. doi:10.1053/j.semperi.2010.09.005
40. Mitchell EA, Milerad J. Smoking and the sudden infant death syndrome. *Rev Environ Health* (2006) 21:81–103. doi:10.1515/REVEH.2006.21.2.81
41. Benowitz N, Dempsey D, Goldenberg R, Hughes J, Dolan-Mullen P, Ogburn P, et al. The use of pharmacotherapies for smoking cessation during pregnancy. *Tob Control* (2000) 9:iii91–4. doi:10.1136/tc.9.suppl_3.iii91
42. Oken E, Levitan EB, Gillman MW. Maternal smoking during pregnancy and child overweight: systematic review and meta-analysis. *Int J Obes* (2008) 32:201–10. doi:10.1038/sj.ijo.0803760
43. Pauly JR, Slotkin TA. Maternal tobacco smoking, nicotine replacement and neurobehavioural development. *Acta Paediatr* (2008) 97:1331–7. doi:10.1111/j.1651-2227.2008.00852.x

44. Services UDoHaH. *The Health Benefits of Smoking Cessation*. Washington, DC: Services UDoHaH (1990).
45. Doll R, Peto R, Boreham J, Sutherland I. Mortality in relation to smoking: 50 years' observations on male British doctors. *BMJ* (2004) 328:1519. doi:10.1136/bmj.38142.554479.AE
46. Abbott LC, Winzer-Serhan UH. Smoking during pregnancy: lessons learned from epidemiological studies and experimental studies using animal models. *Crit Rev Toxicol* (2012) 42:279–303. doi:10.3109/10408444.2012.658506
47. Bartholomew KS, Abouk R. The effect of local smokefree regulations on birth outcomes and prenatal smoking. *Matern Child Health J* (2016) 20:1526–38. doi:10.1007/s10995-016-1952-x
48. Been JV, Nurmatov UB, Cox B, Nawrot TS, Van Schayck CP, Sheikh A. Effect of smoke-free legislation on perinatal and child health: a systematic review and meta-analysis. *Lancet* (2014) 383:1549–60. doi:10.1016/S0140-6736(14)60082-9
49. Jaddoe VW, Troe EJ, Hofman A, Mackenbach JP, Moll HA, Steegers EA, et al. Active and passive maternal smoking during pregnancy and the risks of low birthweight and preterm birth: the Generation R study. *Paediatr Perinat Epidemiol* (2008) 22:162–71. doi:10.1111/j.1365-3016.2007.00916.x
50. Vicedo-Cabrera AM, Schindler C, Radovanovic D, Grize L, Witassek F, Dratva J, et al. Benefits of smoking bans on preterm and early-term births: a natural experimental design in Switzerland. *Tob Control* (2016) 25(e2):e135–41. doi:10.1136/tobaccocontrol-2015-052739
51. Levy D, Mohlman MK, Zhang Y. Estimating the potential impact of tobacco control policies on adverse maternal and child health outcomes in the United States using the SimSmoke tobacco control policy simulation model. *Nicotine Tob Res* (2016) 18:1240–9. doi:10.1093/ntr/ntv178
52. WHO. *WHO Report on the Global Tobacco Epidemic, 2015; Raising Taxes on Tobacco*. Geneva: WHO (2015).
53. Troe EJ, Raat H, Jaddoe VW, Hofman A, Steegers EA, Verhulst FC, et al. Smoking during pregnancy in ethnic populations: the Generation R study. *Nicotine Tob Res* (2008) 10:1373–84. doi:10.1080/14622200802238944
54. Jha P, Chaloupka FJ. The economics of global tobacco control. *BMJ* (2000) 321:358–61. doi:10.1136/bmj.321.7257.358
55. Wills RA, Coory MD. Effect of smoking among Indigenous and non-Indigenous mothers on preterm birth and full-term low birthweight. *Med J Aust* (2008) 189:490–4.
56. Chan A, Keane RJ, Robinson JS. The contribution of maternal smoking to preterm birth, small for gestational age and low birthweight among Aboriginal and non-Aboriginal births in South Australia. *Med J Aust* (2001) 174:389–93.
57. Hibbs S, Rankin KM, David RJ, Collins JW. The relation of neighborhood income to the age-related patterns of preterm birth among white and African-American Women: the effect of cigarette smoking. *Matern Child Health J* (2016) 20:1432–40. doi:10.1007/s10995-016-1941-0
58. Ergin I, Hassoy H, Tanik FA, Aslan G. Maternal age, education level and migration: socioeconomic determinants for smoking during pregnancy in a field study from Turkey. *BMC Public Health* (2010) 10:325. doi:10.1186/1471-2458-10-325
59. Elsenbruch S, Benson S, Rucke M, Rose M, Dudenhausen J, Pincus-Knackstedt MK, et al. Social support during pregnancy: effects on maternal depressive symptoms, smoking and pregnancy outcome. *Hum Reprod* (2007) 22:869–77. doi:10.1093/humrep/del432
60. Dejin-Karlsson E, Hanson BS, Ostergren PO, Ranstam J, Isacsson SO, Sjoberg NO. Psychosocial resources and persistent smoking in early pregnancy – a population study of women in their first pregnancy in Sweden. *J Epidemiol Community Health* (1996) 50:33–9. doi:10.1136/jech.50.1.33
61. Heaman MI, Gupton AL, Moffatt ME. Prevalence and predictors of inadequate prenatal care: a comparison of aboriginal and non-aboriginal women in Manitoba. *J Obstet Gynaecol Can* (2005) 27:237–46. doi:10.1016/S1701-2163(16)30516-3
62. Andersen HF, Nugent CE, Wanty SD, Hayashi RH. Prediction of risk for preterm delivery by ultrasonographic measurement of cervical length. *Am J Obstet Gynecol* (1990) 163:859–67. doi:10.1016/0002-9378(90)91084-P
63. Iams JD, Goldenberg RL, Meis PJ, Mercer BM, Moawad A, Das A, et al. The length of the cervix and the risk of spontaneous premature delivery. National Institute of Child Health and Human Development Maternal Fetal Medicine Unit Network. *N Engl J Med* (1996) 334:567–72. doi:10.1056/NEJM199602293340904
64. Hassan SS, Romero R, Berry SM, Dang K, Blackwell SC, Treadwell MC, et al. Patients with an ultrasonographic cervical length < or =15 mm have nearly a 50% risk of early spontaneous preterm delivery. *Am J Obstet Gynecol* (2000) 182:1458–67. doi:10.1067/mob.2000.106851
65. Hassan SS, Romero R, Vidyadhari D, Fusey S, Baxter JK, Khandelwal M, et al. Vaginal progesterone reduces the rate of preterm birth in women with a sonographic short cervix: a multicenter, randomized, double-blind, placebo-controlled trial. *Ultrasound Obstet Gynecol* (2011) 38:18–31. doi:10.1002/uog.9017
66. da Fonseca EB, Bittar RE, Carvalho MH, Zugaib M. Prophylactic administration of progesterone by vaginal suppository to reduce the incidence of spontaneous preterm birth in women at increased risk: a randomized placebo-controlled double-blind study. *Am J Obstet Gynecol* (2003) 188:419–24. doi:10.1067/mob.2003.41
67. Romero R, Nicolaides KH, Conde-Agudelo A, O'Brien JM, Cetingoz E, Da Fonseca E, et al. Vaginal progesterone decreases preterm birth ≤34 weeks of gestation in women with a singleton pregnancy and a short cervix: an updated meta-analysis including data from the OPPTIMUM study. *Ultrasound Obstet Gynecol* (2016) 48:308–17. doi:10.1002/uog.15953
68. Norman JE, Marlow N, Messow CM, Shennan A, Bennett PR, Thornton S, et al. Vaginal progesterone prophylaxis for preterm birth (the OPPTIMUM study): a multicentre, randomised, double-blind trial. *Lancet* (2016) 387:2106–16. doi:10.1016/S0140-6736(16)00350-0
69. Son M, Grobman WA, Ayala NK, Miller ES. A universal mid-trimester transvaginal cervical length screening program and its associated reduced preterm birth rate. *Am J Obstet Gynecol* (2016) 214:.e1–5. doi:10.1016/j.ajog.2015.12.020
70. Werner EF, Han CS, Pettker CM, Buhimschi CS, Copel JA, Funai EF, et al. Universal cervical-length screening to prevent preterm birth: a cost-effectiveness analysis. *Ultrasound Obstet Gynecol* (2011) 38:32–7. doi:10.1002/uog.8911
71. Einerson BD, Grobman WA, Miller ES. Cost-effectiveness of risk-based screening for cervical length to prevent preterm birth. *Am J Obstet Gynecol* (2016) 215:.e1–7. doi:10.1016/j.ajog.2016.01.192
72. Kiefer DG, Peltier MR, Keeler SM, Rust O, Ananth CV, Vintzileos AM, et al. Efficacy of midtrimester short cervix interventions is conditional on intraamniotic inflammation. *Am J Obstet Gynecol* (2016) 214:.e1–6. doi:10.1016/j.ajog.2015.09.006
73. Shapiro-Mendoza CK, Lackritz EM. Epidemiology of late and moderate preterm birth. *Semin Fetal Neonatal Med* (2012) 17:120–5. doi:10.1016/j.siny.2012.01.007
74. Morris JM, Algert CS, Falster MO, Ford JB, Kinnear A, Nicholl MC, et al. Trends in planned early birth: a population-based study. *Am J Obstet Gynecol* (2012) 207:.e1–8. doi:10.1016/j.ajog.2012.06.082
75. Engle WA, Tomashek KM, Wallman C. "Late-preterm" infants: a population at risk. *Pediatrics* (2007) 120:1390–401. doi:10.1542/peds.2007-2952
76. Spong CY. Defining "term" pregnancy: recommendations from the Defining "Term" Pregnancy Workgroup. *JAMA* (2013) 309:2445–6. doi:10.1001/jama.2013.6235
77. Gray RF, Indurkhya A, McCormick MC. Prevalence, stability, and predictors of clinically significant behavior problems in low birth weight children at 3, 5, and 8 years of age. *Pediatrics* (2004) 114:736–43. doi:10.1542/peds.2003-1150-L
78. Robinson M, Whitehouse AJ, Zubrick SR, Pennell CE, Jacoby P, McLean NJ, et al. Delivery at 37 weeks' gestation is associated with a higher risk for child behavioural problems. *Aust N Z J Obstet Gynaecol* (2013) 53:143–51. doi:10.1111/ajo.12012
79. Brown HK, Speechley KN, Macnab J, Natale R, Campbell MK. Neonatal morbidity associated with late preterm and early term birth: the roles of gestational age and biological determinants of preterm birth. *Int J Epidemiol* (2014) 43:802–14. doi:10.1093/ije/dyt251
80. Davidoff MJ, Dias T, Damus K, Russell R, Bettegowda VR, Dolan S, et al. Changes in the gestational age distribution among U.S. singleton births: impact on rates of late preterm birth, 1992 to 2002. *Semin Perinatol* (2006) 30:8–15. doi:10.1053/j.semperi.2006.01.009
81. Clark SL, Frye DR, Meyers JA, Belfort MA, Dildy GA, Kofford S, et al. Reduction in elective delivery at <39 weeks of gestation: comparative

effectiveness of 3 approaches to change and the impact on neonatal intensive care admission and stillbirth. *Am J Obstet Gynecol* (2010) 203:.e1–6. doi:10.1016/j.ajog.2010.05.036

82. Glavind J, Henriksen TB, Kindberg SF, Uldbjerg N. Randomised trial of planned caesarean section prior to versus after 39 weeks: unscheduled deliveries and facility logistics – a secondary analysis. *PLoS One* (2013) 8:e84744. doi:10.1371/journal.pone.0084744
83. Nicholson JM, Kellar LC, Ahmad S, Abid A, Woloski J, Hewamudalige N, et al. US term stillbirth rates and the 39-week rule: a cause for concern? *Am J Obstet Gynecol* (2016) 214:.e1–9. doi:10.1016/j.ajog.2016.02.019
84. Goldenberg RL, Culhane JF, Iams JD, Romero R. Epidemiology and causes of preterm birth. *Lancet* (2008) 371:75–84. doi:10.1016/S0140-6736(08)60074-4
85. Romero R, Miranda J, Chaiworapongsa T, Korzeniewski SJ, Chaemsaithong P, Gotsch F, et al. Prevalence and clinical significance of sterile intra-amniotic inflammation in patients with preterm labor and intact membranes. *Am J Reprod Immunol* (2014) 72:458–74. doi:10.1111/aji.12296
86. Romero R, Gotsch F, Pineles B, Kusanovic JP. Inflammation in pregnancy: its roles in reproductive physiology, obstetrical complications, and fetal injury. *Nutr Rev* (2007) 65:S194–202. doi:10.1301/nr.2007.dec.S194-S202
87. Kemp MW. Preterm birth, intrauterine infection, and fetal inflammation. *Front Immunol* (2014) 5:574. doi:10.3389/fimmu.2014.00574
88. Combs CA, Gravett M, Garite TJ, Hickok DE, Lapidus J, Porreco R, et al. Amniotic fluid infection, inflammation, and colonization in preterm labor with intact membranes. *Am J Obstet Gynecol* (2014) 210(125):e1–15. doi:10.1016/j.ajog.2013.11.032
89. Kim SM, Romero R, Lee J, Mi Lee S, Park CW, Shin Park J, et al. The frequency and clinical significance of intra-amniotic inflammation in women with preterm uterine contractility but without cervical change: do the diagnostic criteria for preterm labor need to be changed? *J Matern Fetal Neonatal Med* (2012) 25:1212–21. doi:10.3109/14767058.2011.629256
90. Soilly AL, Lejeune C, Quantin C, Bejean S, Gouyon JB. Economic analysis of the costs associated with prematurity from a literature review. *Public Health* (2014) 128:43–62. doi:10.1016/j.puhe.2013.09.014
91. Mangham LJ, Petrou S, Doyle LW, Draper ES, Marlow N. The cost of preterm birth throughout childhood in England and Wales. *Pediatrics* (2009) 123:e312–27. doi:10.1542/peds.2008-1827
92. Morken NH, Kallen K, Jacobsson B. Predicting risk of spontaneous preterm delivery in women with a singleton pregnancy. *Paediatr Perinat Epidemiol* (2014) 28:11–22. doi:10.1111/ppe.12087
93. Iams JD. Clinical practice. Prevention of preterm parturition. *N Engl J Med* (2014) 370:254–61. doi:10.1056/NEJMcp1103640
94. Donders GG. Reducing infection-related preterm birth. *BJOG* (2015) 122:219. doi:10.1111/1471-0528.13109
95. Lamont RF. Advances in the prevention of infection-related preterm birth. *Front Immunol* (2015) 6:566. doi:10.3389/fimmu.2015.00566
96. Oliver RS, Lamont RF. Infection and antibiotics in the aetiology, prediction and prevention of preterm birth. *J Obstet Gynaecol* (2013) 33:768–75. doi:10.3109/01443615.2013.842963
97. Keelan JA, Payne MS, Kemp MW, Ireland DJ, Newnham JP. A new, potent, and placenta-permeable macrolide antibiotic, solithromycin, for the prevention and treatment of bacterial infections in pregnancy. *Front Immunol* (2016) 7:111. doi:10.3389/fimmu.2016.00111
98. Walker WA. Initial intestinal colonization in the human infant and immune homeostasis. *Ann Nutr Metab* (2013) 63(Suppl 2):8–15. doi:10.1159/000354907
99. Metsala J, Lundqvist A, Virta LJ, Kaila M, Gissler M, Virtanen SM. Prenatal and post-natal exposure to antibiotics and risk of asthma in childhood. *Clin Exp Allergy* (2015) 45:137–45. doi:10.1111/cea.12356
100. Mueller NT, Whyatt R, Hoepner L, Oberfield S, Dominguez-Bello MG, Widen EM, et al. Prenatal exposure to antibiotics, cesarean section and risk of childhood obesity. *Int J Obes* (2005) 2015(39):665–70. doi:10.1038/ijo.2014.180
101. Honest H, Forbes CA, Duree KH, Norman G, Duffy SB, Tsourapas A, et al. Screening to prevent spontaneous preterm birth: systematic reviews of accuracy and effectiveness literature with economic modelling. *Health Technol Assess* (2009) 13:1–627. doi:10.3310/hta13430
102. Witkin S. The vaginal microbiome, vaginal anti-microbial defence mechanisms and the clinical challenge of reducing infection-related preterm birth. *BJOG* (2015) 122(2):213–8. doi:10.1111/1471-0528.13115
103. McDonald HM, Brocklehurst P, Gordon A. Antibiotics for treating bacterial vaginosis in pregnancy. *Cochrane Database Syst Rev* (2007) 1:CD000262. doi:10.1002/14651858.CD000262.pub3
104. Cunnington M, Kortsalioudaki C, Heath P. Genitourinary pathogens and preterm birth. *Curr Opin Infect Dis* (2013) 26:219–30. doi:10.1097/QCO.0b013e328360dc31
105. Donders GG, Van Calsteren K, Bellen G, Reybrouck R, Van den Bosch T, Riphagen I, et al. Predictive value for preterm birth of abnormal vaginal flora, bacterial vaginosis and aerobic vaginitis during the first trimester of pregnancy. *BJOG* (2009) 116:1315–24. doi:10.1111/j.1471-0528.2009.02237.x
106. Capoccia R, Greub G, Baud D. *Ureaplasma urealyticum, Mycoplasma hominis* and adverse pregnancy outcomes. *Curr Opin Infect Dis* (2013) 26:231–40. doi:10.1097/QCO.0b013e328360db58
107. Kataoka S, Yamada T, Chou K, Nishida R, Morikawa M, Minami M, et al. Association between preterm birth and vaginal colonization by mycoplasmas in early pregnancy. *J Clin Microbiol* (2006) 44:51–5. doi:10.1128/JCM.44.1.51-55.2006
108. Breugelmans M, Vancutsem E, Naessens A, Laubach M, Foulon W. Association of abnormal vaginal flora and *Ureaplasma* species as risk factors for preterm birth: a cohort study. *Acta Obstet Gynecol Scand* (2010) 89:256–60. doi:10.3109/00016340903418769
109. Payne MS, Ireland DJ, Watts R, Nathan EA, Furfaro LL, Kemp MW, et al. *Ureaplasma parvum* genotype, combined vaginal colonisation with *Candida albicans*, and spontaneous preterm birth in an Australian cohort of pregnant women. *BMC Pregnancy Childbirth* (2016) 16:312. doi:10.1186/s12884-016-1110-x
110. Simcox R, Sin WT, Seed PT, Briley A, Shennan AH. Prophylactic antibiotics for the prevention of preterm birth in women at risk: a meta-analysis. *Aust N Z J Obstet Gynaecol* (2007) 47:368–77. doi:10.1111/j.1479-828X.2007.00759.x
111. Thinkhamrop J, Hofmeyr GJ, Adetoro O, Lumbiganon P, Ota E. Antibiotic prophylaxis during the second and third trimester to reduce adverse pregnancy outcomes and morbidity. *Cochrane Database Syst Rev* (2015) 6:CD002250. doi:10.1002/14651858.CD002250.pub3
112. Brocklehurst P, Gordon A, Heatley E, Milan SJ. Antibiotics for treating bacterial vaginosis in pregnancy. *Cochrane Database Syst Rev* (2013) 1:CD000262. doi:10.1002/14651858.CD000262.pub4
113. Subramaniam A, Abramovici A, Andrews WW, Tita AT. Antimicrobials for preterm birth prevention: an overview. *Infect Dis Obstet Gynecol* (2012) 2012:157159. doi:10.1155/2012/157159
114. Mercer B. Antibiotics in the management of PROM and preterm labor. *Obstet Gynecol Clin North Am* (2012) 39:65–76. doi:10.1016/j.ogc.2011.12.007
115. Macklaim JM, Clemente JC, Knight R, Gloor GB, Reid G. Changes in vaginal microbiota following antimicrobial and probiotic therapy. *Microb Ecol Health Dis* (2015) 26:27799. doi:10.3402/mehd.v26.27799
116. Pendharkar S, Brandsborg E, Hammarstrom L, Marcotte H, Larsson PG. Vaginal colonisation by probiotic lactobacilli and clinical outcome in women conventionally treated for bacterial vaginosis and yeast infection. *BMC Infect Dis* (2015) 15:255. doi:10.1186/s12879-015-0971-3
117. Mayer BT, Srinivasan S, Fiedler TL, Marrazzo JM, Fredricks DN, Schiffer JT. Rapid and profound shifts in the vaginal microbiota following antibiotic treatment for bacterial vaginosis. *J Infect Dis* (2015) 212:793–802. doi:10.1093/infdis/jiv079
118. Abramovici A, Lobashevsky E, Cliver SP, Edwards RK, Hauth JC, Biggio JR. Quantitative polymerase chain reaction to assess response to treatment of bacterial vaginosis and risk of preterm birth. *Am J Perinatol* (2015) 32:1119–25. doi:10.1055/s-0035-1549294
119. Blankenstein T, Lytton SD, Leidl B, Atweh E, Friese K, Mylonas I. Point-of-care (POC) diagnosis of bacterial vaginosis (BV) using VGTest™ ion mobility spectrometry (IMS) in a routine ambulatory care gynecology clinic. *Arch Gynecol Obstet* (2015) 292:355–62. doi:10.1007/s00404-014-3613-x
120. Romero R, Hassan SS, Gajer P, Tarca AL, Fadrosh DW, Bieda J, et al. The vaginal microbiota of pregnant women who subsequently have spontaneous

preterm labor and delivery and those with a normal delivery at term. *Microbiome* (2014) 2:18. doi:10.1186/2049-2618-2-18
121. Mysorekar IU, Cao B. Microbiome in parturition and preterm birth. *Semin Reprod Med* (2014) 32:50–5. doi:10.1055/s-0033-1361830
122. Farr A, Kiss H, Hagmann M, Marschalek J, Husslein P, Petricevic L. Routine use of an antenatal infection screen-and-treat program to prevent preterm birth: long-term experience at a tertiary referral center. *Birth* (2015) 42:173–80. doi:10.1111/birt.12154
123. Hoyme UB, Huebner J. Prevention of preterm birth is possible by vaginal pH screening, early diagnosis of bacterial vaginosis or abnormal vaginal flora and treatment. *Gynecol Obstet Invest* (2010) 70:286–90. doi:10.1159/000314019
124. DiGiulio DB. Diversity of microbes in amniotic fluid. *Semin Fetal Neonatal Med* (2012) 17:2–11. doi:10.1016/j.siny.2011.10.001
125. Mendz GL, Kaakoush NO, Quinlivan JA. Bacterial aetiological agents of intra-amniotic infections and preterm birth in pregnant women. *Front Cell Infect Microbiol* (2013) 3:58. doi:10.3389/fcimb.2013.00058
126. Griffin C. Probiotics in obstetrics and gynaecology. *Aust N Z J Obstet Gynaecol* (2015) 55:201–9. doi:10.1111/ajo.12303
127. Sananes N, Langer B, Gaudineau A, Kutnahorsky R, Aissi G, Fritz G, et al. Prediction of spontaneous preterm delivery in singleton pregnancies: where are we and where are we going? A review of literature. *J Obstet Gynaecol* (2014) 34:457–61. doi:10.3109/01443615.2014.896325
128. Shahshahan Z, Hashemi L. Maternal serum cytokines in the prediction of preterm labor and response to tocolytic therapy in preterm labor women. *Adv Biomed Res* (2014) 3:126. doi:10.4103/2277-9175.133243
129. Ireland DJ, Keelan JA. The maternal serological response to intrauterine *Ureaplasma* sp. infection and prediction of risk of pre-term birth. *Front Immunol* (2014) 5:624. doi:10.3389/fimmu.2014.00624
130. Liong S, Di Quinzio MK, Fleming G, Permezel M, Rice GE, Georgiou HM. New biomarkers for the prediction of spontaneous preterm labour in symptomatic pregnant women: a comparison with fetal fibronectin. *BJOG* (2015) 122:370–9. doi:10.1111/1471-0528.12993
131. Kuhrt K, Hezelgrave N, Foster C, Seed PT, Shennan AH. Development and validation of a predictive tool for spontaneous preterm birth, incorporating quantitative fetal fibronectin, in symptomatic women. *Ultrasound Obstet Gynecol* (2015) 47(2):210–6. doi:10.1002/uog.14894
132. von Schoning D, Fischer T, von Tucher E, Slowinski T, Weichert A, Henrich W, et al. Cervical sonoelastography for improving prediction of preterm birth compared with cervical length measurement and fetal fibronectin test. *J Perinat Med* (2015) 43(5):531–6. doi:10.1515/jpm-2014-0356
133. van de Mheen L, Schuit E, Lim AC, Porath MM, Papatsonis D, Erwich JJ, et al. Prediction of preterm birth in multiple pregnancies: development of a multivariable model including cervical length measurement at 16 to 21 weeks' gestation. *J Obstet Gynaecol Can* (2014) 36:309–19. doi:10.1016/S1701-2163(15)30606-X
134. Clausson B, Lichtenstein P, Cnattingius S. Genetic influence on birthweight and gestational length determined by studies in offspring of twins. *BJOG* (2000) 107:375–81. doi:10.1111/j.1471-0528.2000.tb13234.x
135. Parets SE, Knight AK, Smith AK. Insights into genetic susceptibility in the etiology of spontaneous preterm birth. *Appl Clin Genet* (2015) 8:283–90. doi:10.2147/TACG.S58612
136. Sheikh IA, Ahmad E, Jamal MS, Rehan M, Assidi M, Tayubi IA, et al. Spontaneous preterm birth and single nucleotide gene polymorphisms: a recent update. *BMC Genomics* (2016) 17:759. doi:10.1186/s12864-016-3089-0
137. Uzun A, Schuster J, McGonnigal B, Schorl C, Dewan A, Padbury J. Targeted sequencing and meta-analysis of preterm birth. *PLoS One* (2016) 11:e0155021. doi:10.1371/journal.pone.0155021
138. Brubaker D, Liu Y, Wang J, Tan H, Zhang G, Jacobsson B, et al. Finding lost genes in GWAS via integrative-omics analysis reveals novel sub-networks associated with preterm birth. *Hum Mol Genet* (2016) 25:5254–64. doi:10.1093/hmg/ddw325
139. Gahl WA. The battlefield of rare diseases: where uncommon insights are common. *Sci Transl Med* (2012) 4:154ed7. doi:10.1126/scitranslmed.3004980
140. Groza T, Kohler S, Moldenhauer D, Vasilevsky N, Baynam G, Zemojtel T, et al. The human phenotype ontology: semantic unification of common and rare disease. *Am J Hum Genet* (2015) 97:111–24. doi:10.1016/j.ajhg.2015.05.020
141. Trujillano D, Oprea GE, Schmitz Y, Bertoli-Avella AM, Abou Jamra R, Rolfs A. A comprehensive global genotype-phenotype database for rare diseases. *Mol Genet Genomic Med* (2017) 5:66–75. doi:10.1002/mgg3.262
142. Glueck M, Gvozdik A, Chevalier F, Khan A, Brudno M, Wigdor D. PhenoStacks: cross-sectional cohort phenotype comparison visualizations. *IEEE Trans Vis Comput Graph* (2017) 23:191–200. doi:10.1109/TVCG.2016.2598469
143. Hu Y, Zhou W, Ren J, Dong L, Wang Y, Jin S, et al. Annotating the function of the human genome with gene ontology and disease ontology. *Biomed Res Int* (2016) 2016:4130861. doi:10.1155/2016/4130861
144. Dudley O, Muscatelli F. Clinical evidence of intrauterine disturbance in Prader-Willi syndrome, a genetically imprinted neurodevelopmental disorder. *Early Hum Dev* (2007) 83:471–8. doi:10.1016/j.earlhumdev.2006.09.002
145. Lionti T, Reid SM, White SM, Rowell MM. A population-based profile of 160 Australians with Prader-Willi syndrome: trends in diagnosis, birth prevalence and birth characteristics. *Am J Med Genet A* (2015) 167A:371–8. doi:10.1002/ajmg.a.36845
146. Wangler MF, Chang AS, Moley KH, Feinberg AP, Debaun MR. Factors associated with preterm delivery in mothers of children with Beckwith-Wiedemann syndrome: a case cohort study from the BWS registry. *Am J Med Genet A* (2005) 134A:187–91. doi:10.1002/ajmg.a.30595
147. Eidem HR, Ackerman WE, McGary KL, Abbot P, Rokas A. Gestational tissue transcriptomics in term and preterm human pregnancies: a systematic review and meta-analysis. *BMC Med Genomics* (2015) 8:27. doi:10.1186/s12920-015-0099-8
148. Heng YJ, Pennell CE, McDonald SW, Vinturache AE, Xu J, Lee MW, et al. Maternal whole blood gene expression at 18 and 28 weeks of gestation associated with spontaneous preterm birth in asymptomatic women. *PLoS One* (2016) 11:e0155191. doi:10.1371/journal.pone.0155191
149. Malak TM, Sizmur F, Bell SC, Taylor DJ. Fetal fibronectin in cervicovaginal secretions as a predictor of preterm birth. *Br J Obstet Gynaecol* (1996) 103:648–53. doi:10.1111/j.1471-0528.1996.tb09832.x
150. Jwala S, Tran TL, Terenna C, McGregor A, Andrel J, Leiby BE, et al. Evaluation of additive effect of quantitative fetal fibronectin to cervical length for prediction of spontaneous preterm birth among asymptomatic low-risk women. *Acta Obstet Gynecol Scand* (2016) 95:948–55. doi:10.1111/aogs.12907
151. Vandermolen BI, Hezelgrave NL, Smout EM, Abbott DS, Seed PT, Shennan AH. Quantitative fetal fibronectin and cervical length to predict preterm birth in asymptomatic women with previous cervical surgery. *Am J Obstet Gynecol* (2016) 215:.e1–10. doi:10.1016/j.ajog.2016.05.020
152. Hezelgrave NL, Abbott DS, Radford SK, Seed PT, Girling JC, Filmer J, et al. Quantitative fetal fibronectin at 18 weeks of gestation to predict preterm birth in asymptomatic high-risk women. *Obstet Gynecol* (2016) 127:255–63. doi:10.1097/AOG.0000000000001240
153. Abbott DS, Hezelgrave NL, Seed PT, Norman JE, David AL, Bennett PR, et al. Quantitative fetal fibronectin to predict preterm birth in asymptomatic women at high risk. *Obstet Gynecol* (2015) 125:1168–76. doi:10.1097/AOG.0000000000000754
154. Kim SM, Romero R, Lee J, Chaemsaithong P, Lee MW, Chaiyasit N, et al. About one-half of early spontaneous preterm deliveries can be identified by a rapid matrix metalloproteinase-8 (MMP-8) bedside test at the time of mid-trimester genetic amniocentesis. *J Matern Fetal Neonatal Med* (2016) 29:2414–22. doi:10.3109/14767058.2015.1094049
155. Buhimschi CS, Bhandari V, Hamar BD, Bahtiyar MO, Zhao G, Sfakianaki AK, et al. Proteomic profiling of the amniotic fluid to detect inflammation, infection, and neonatal sepsis. *PLoS Med* (2007) 4:e18. doi:10.1371/journal.pmed.0040018
156. Chaemsaithong P, Romero R, Korzeniewski SJ, Martinez-Varea A, Dong Z, Yoon BH, et al. A rapid interleukin-6 bedside test for the identification of intra-amniotic inflammation in preterm labor with intact membranes. *J Matern Fetal Neonatal Med* (2016) 29:349–59. doi:10.3109/14767058.2015.1006620
157. Cobo T, Palacio M, Navarro-Sastre A, Ribes A, Bosch J, Filella X, et al. Predictive value of combined amniotic fluid proteomic biomarkers and interleukin-6 in preterm labor with intact membranes. *Am J Obstet Gynecol* (2009) 200:.e1–6. doi:10.1016/j.ajog.2008.12.036
158. Gravett MG, Thomas A, Schneider KA, Reddy AP, Dasari S, Jacob T, et al. Proteomic analysis of cervical-vaginal fluid: identification of novel biomarkers for detection of intra-amniotic infection. *J Proteome Res* (2007) 6:89–96. doi:10.1021/pr060149v

159. Taylor BD, Holzman CB, Fichorova RN, Tian Y, Jones NM, Fu W, et al. Inflammation biomarkers in vaginal fluid and preterm delivery. *Hum Reprod* (2013) 28:942–52. doi:10.1093/humrep/det019
160. Hadzi-Lega M, Markova AD, Stefanovic M, Tanturovski M. Correlation of cervical length, fetal fibronectin, phIGFBP-1, and cytokines in spontaneous preterm birth up to 14 days from sampling. *J Perinat Med* (2015) 43(5):545–51. doi:10.1515/jpm-2014-0275
161. Liong S, Di Quinzio MK, Fleming G, Permezel M, Rice GE, Georgiou HM. Prediction of spontaneous preterm labour in at-risk pregnant women. *Reproduction* (2013) 146:335–45. doi:10.1530/REP-13-0175
162. Hernandez-Nunez J, Valdes-Yong M. Utility of proteomics in obstetric disorders: a review. *Int J Womens Health* (2015) 7:385–91. doi:10.2147/IJWH.S79577
163. Bergen AW, Javitz HS, Krasnow R, Nishita D, Michel M, Conti DV, et al. Nicotinic acetylcholine receptor variation and response to smoking cessation therapies. *Pharmacogenet Genomics* (2013) 23:94–103. doi:10.1097/FPC.0b013e32835cdabd
164. Majumder S, Mondal T, Deen MJ. Wearable sensors for remote health monitoring. *Sensors (Basel)* (2017) 17:E130. doi:10.3390/s17010130
165. Pigini L, Bovi G, Panzarino C, Gower V, Ferratini M, Andreoni G, et al. Pilot test of a new personal health system integrating environmental and wearable sensors for telemonitoring and care of elderly people at home (SMARTA Project). *Gerontology* (2017). doi:10.1159/000455168
166. Miramontes R, Aquino R, Flores A, Rodriguez G, Anguiano R, Rios A, et al. PlaIMoS: a remote mobile healthcare platform to monitor cardiovascular and respiratory variables. *Sensors (Basel)* (2017) 17:E176. doi:10.3390/s17010176
167. Froen JF, Myhre SL, Frost MJ, Chou D, Mehl G, Say L, et al. eRegistries: electronic registries for maternal and child health. *BMC Pregnancy Childbirth* (2016) 16:11. doi:10.1186/s12884-016-0801-7
168. Liabsuetrakul T, Prappre T, Pairot P, Oumudee N, Islam M. Development of a web-based epidemiological surveillance system with health system response for improving maternal and newborn health: field-testing in Thailand. *Health Informatics J* (2016) 1–15. doi:10.1177/1460458216628312
169. Ngabo F, Nguimfack J, Nwaigwe F, Mugeni C, Muhoza D, Wilson DR, et al. Designing and implementing an innovative SMS-based alert system (RapidSMS-MCH) to monitor pregnancy and reduce maternal and child deaths in Rwanda. *Pan Afr Med J* (2012) 13:31. doi:10.11604/pamj.2012.13.31.1864

21

Pharmacokinetic Aspects of Nanoparticle-in-Matrix Drug Delivery Systems for Oral/Buccal Delivery

*Renata Carvalho Feitosa[1,2], Danilo Costa Geraldes[1,2], Viviane Lucia Beraldo-de-Araújo[1], Juliana Souza Ribeiro Costa[1,2] and Laura Oliveira-Nascimento[1]**

[1] *Laboratory of Pharmaceutical Technology (Latef), Faculty of Pharmaceutical Sciences, State University of Campinas, Campinas, Brazil,*

[2] *Institute of Biology, State University of Campinas, Campinas, Brazil*

Correspondence:
Laura Oliveira-Nascimento
lauraon@unicamp.br

Oral route maintains its predominance among the ones used for drug delivery, especially when medicines are self-administered. If the dosage form is solid, therapy gains in dose precision and drug stability. Yet, some active pharmaceutical substances do not present the required solubility, permeability, or release profile for incorporation into traditional matrices. The combination of nanostructured drugs (nanoparticle [NP]) with these matrices is a new and little-explored alternative, which could bring several benefits. Therefore, this review focused on combined delivery systems based on nanostructures to administer drugs by the oral cavity, intended for buccal, sublingual, gastric, or intestinal absorption. We analyzed published NP-in-matrix systems and compared main formulation characteristics, pharmacokinetics, release profiles, and physicochemical stability improvements. The reported formulations are mainly semisolid or solid polymers, with polymeric or lipid NPs and one active pharmaceutical ingredient. Regarding drug specifics, most of them are poorly permeable or greatly metabolized. The few studies with pharmacokinetics showed increased drug bioavailability and, sometimes, a controlled release rate. From our knowledge, the gathered data make up the first focused review of these trendy systems, which we believe will help to gain scientific deepness and future advancements in the field.

Keywords: nanoparticle, oral delivery, buccal delivery, matrix delivery, drug absorption

INTRODUCTION

Medicines administered by the oral cavity have different fates, according to their varied processes: (i) immediate delivery and absorption, (ii) slow delivery from an adherent drug delivery system (DDS), followed by absorption or local action; and (iii) transport to the gastrointestinal region for absorption or local action. The latter is the gold standard for medicines and the most common process used for self-administered drug intake. Recently, buccal permeation (items i and ii) strategies increased in number of developments; this route bypasses hepatic and gastrointestinal effects, which is advantageous to sensitive drugs (Barua et al., 2016).

Regardless of the process, drug solubility can impair efficient release from DDS and subsequent mucosal crossing. Therefore, several solubilization strategies are available, such as salt forms of active molecules, pH modifiers, cosolvents, amorphization, solid dispersions, inclusion complexes, microemulsions, and nanotechnology (Kalepu and Nekkanti, 2015). The latter represents a large portion of published research but a few marketed products and no buccal-based options.

In addition to the solubility enhancement, nanoparticles (NPs) aid drug efficacy in at least four different ways (**Figure 1**). The simpler way relates to transport throughout the gastrointestinal lumen and local release (mode 1). Another possibility consists of carrier adherence to the mucosal surface/mucus to enhance drug absorption, but without carrier crossing (mode 2). Nanoparticles may also be absorbed and transport the drug systemically, enhancing its plasma half-life (mode 3). Absorbed NPs can then perform passive targeting due to charge, size, morphology, and constituents. For a detailed review on mechanisms of NP/absorption and uptake, see Griffin et al. (2016). Mode 4 happens when specific surface molecules or pH-responsive mechanisms allow the carrier to perform an active targeting after absorption. Modes 3 and 4 can still avoid first-pass metabolism if absorption happens in the buccal mucosa or lymphatic vessels. However, like other delivery strategies, NPs can fail to liberate drugs at an expected rate or target, as described in the following paragraphs.

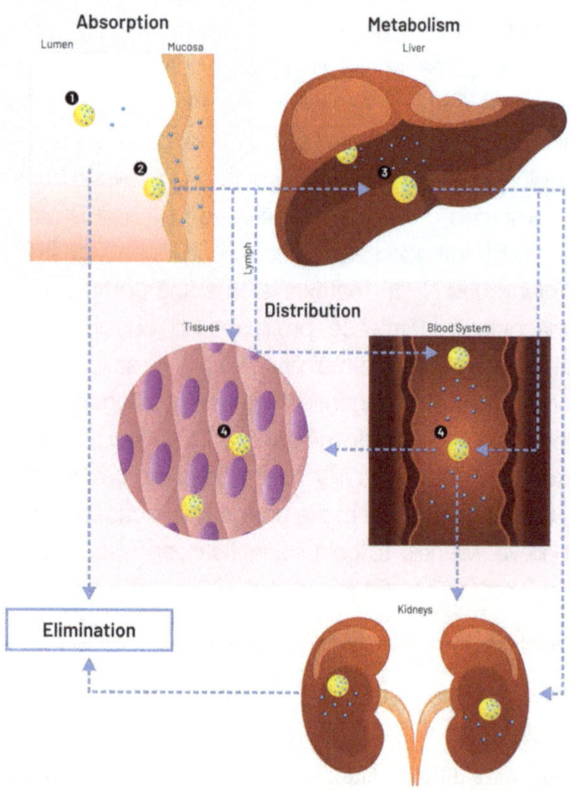

FIGURE 1 | Scheme (not to scale) of drug (blue circles) loaded nanoparticles (NPs, yellow circles) interacting with physiological environments. Nanoparticle modes to enhance drug systemic delivery through the oral or buccal routes. 1: Lumen release (solubility enhancement), followed by NP excretion or degradation. 2: Adherence to mucus or mucosal surface for enhanced drug absorption (no NP permeation), followed by NP excretion or degradation. 3: NP absorption for enhanced plasma half-life, followed by NP liver degradation or lymphatic drainage. 4: Tissue or cell targeting. Figure created for this review in CorelDRAW Graphics Suite X7.

For drug uptake enhancement, NPs need to interact with the respective mucosal surface/mucus during an adequate amount of time. Some particles do stick to mucosa under continuous rinsing, such as thiolated chitosan NPs. But, in this case, NPs were freeze dried and applied on top of the mucosa in an *ex vivo* test (Bernkop-Schnürch et al., 2006). Since powder formulations require specific devices or encapsulation for a precise dosage, they generally require an additional delivery strategy to be administered.

A noteworthy NP disadvantage is the burst effect: a rapid initial drug release followed by a sustained or controlled release. Rapid plasma peaks or local drug concentration are desirable in some therapies; however, burst behavior is frequently uncontrollable and irreproducible. The phenomenon occurs due to several reasons, including weakly bound drugs, molecule migration to the particle surface, and nanomatrix heterogeneity (Kamaly et al., 2016). Strategies to prevent it include coating or nanomatrix reformulation (Kamaly et al., 2016), not always straightforward because both processes change NP physicochemical characteristics.

The majority of oral DDSs are biodegradable, so they will erode or degrade at some point. In fact, some systems rely on both properties as a release mechanism. If the carrier liberates as desired, it may not be resistant to pH/enzymes during traffic or at the action site. An earlier instability may interfere with the desired drug liberation profile, such as for regular gelatin NPs: their degradation in the stomach requires coating, chemical modification or an outermatrix embedment to allow intestinal release (Imperiale and Sosnik, 2013).

Apart from degradation, NPs can change their fate, uptake, or release rate due to *in vitro* or *in vivo* aggregation. The *in vitro* facet shows that cell media for cell culture is quite different from lumen or saliva environments, which makes it hard to predict aggregation during *in vivo* absorption (Moore et al., 2015).

All failure modes described above can be solved or attenuated with NP dispersion in micromatrices and macromatrices (**Figure 2**), reasons why this technique became important for buccal and oral delivery. As opposed to coating and core modifications, matrix embedment brings an extra added value: it can be applied to several kinds of NPs, with a better general prediction of the release behavior.

Considering all points above, this review intends to analyze pharmacokinetic improvements with the use of NPs incorporated in matrices for drug delivery (NP-in-matrix). Therefore, we focused here on pharmacokinetic data from animal and humans (when available). Several NP-in-matrix systems were tested only with *in vitro* assays. However, correlation of *in vivo* behavior is not guaranteed, and an extensive array of protocols impairs model comparisons (discussed in the following topic). Combined systems resulting in nanosized carriers (NP-in-NP) were not included in this work. Based on the theoretical analysis, we intend to verify and clarify matrix role on permeation and bioavailability of nanocarriers.

PHARMACOKINETICS AND EVALUATION MODES FOR ORAL AND BUCCAL ADMINISTRATION

Pharmacokinetics describes absorption, distribution, metabolism, and excretion processes after drug intake. This knowledge remains essential for safety and efficacy assessments of the therapy in

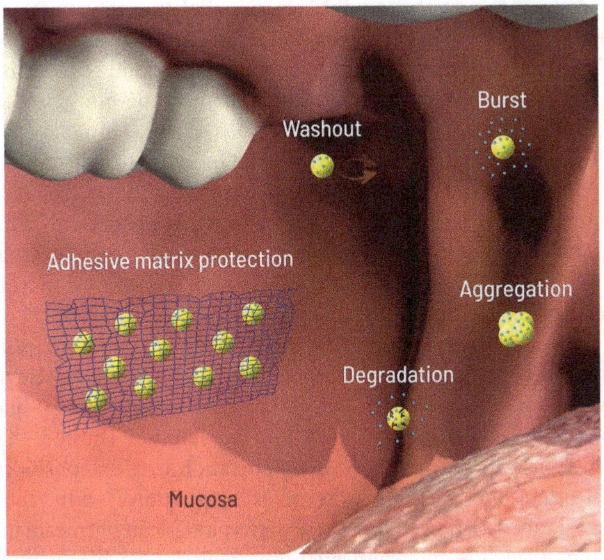

FIGURE 2 | Scheme (not to scale) of the failure modes of nanoparticles (NPs, yellow circles) loaded with drug (blue circles) after oral/buccal administration: early washout in mouth or intestinal cavities; early degradation due to pH or enzymes; burst release upon contact with aqueous media (saliva, stomach acid); aggregation due to pH, osmotic environment, and protein binding. The network on the left shows matrix protection through adhesion (wash out elimination), shielding (degradation and burst elimination/decrease), and physical separation (aggregation elimination). Figure created for this review in CorelDRAW Graphics Suite X7 and Adobe Photoshop CS6.

the search for the optimal DDS. However, *in vivo* tests must be a final step toward product development. It should succeed an extensive physicochemical characterization, together with promising *in vitro* data assessing biorelevant properties. **Table 1** lists the most common assays used to evaluate and predict *in vivo* parameters related to pharmacokinetics, together with drug and NP predictors. Because matrix-based formulations aid mainly in absorption, this process will be discussed in more detail below.

Nanoparticle permeation happens only after mucus barrier crossing (gastrointestinal) and subsequent cellular uptake for transcytosis (M cells, enterocytes) or paracellular transport. *In vivo* absorption is generally better predicted by *ex vivo* mucosal permeation than *in vitro* tests with synthetic membranes; the extracted tissue offers a biochemical, anatomical, and structural resemblance to its *in vivo* counterpart that is difficult to replicate (Berben et al., 2018).

When it comes to gastrointestinal absorption, Caco-2 cell model stands out among the options, joining cell layer with synthetic membrane permeation. This system is frequently used to classify drugs in a permeation rank to direct dosage form development. However, a review covering Caco-2 correlation with *in vivo* intestinal permeability stressed the test fragility. Based on several studies, the authors concluded that the model is applicable to hydrophobic drugs but fails to predict hydrophilic molecule absorption. Even with hydrophobic drugs, variability is high yet minimized with internal standards. The paracellular route and active transport seem to correlate with higher variability and *in vivo–in vitro* lack of correlation (Larregieu and Benet, 2013).

Regardless of the *in vitro–ex vivo* model, most of them do not promote predigestion of samples. One cannot estimate the effect of gastrointestinal fluids upon NPs without this assessment. Even nondegradable polystyrene NPs (unmodified, aminated, or carboxylated) promoted different *ex vivo* permeation profiles with predigestion, showing its relevance for *in vivo* prediction (Westerhout et al., 2017).

Drug/NP *in vivo* absorption can be estimated by plasma detection if metabolism does not influence their integrity. *In vivo* pharmacokinetics focuses on blood sampling and drug quantification at several time points, generally with rats, rabbits, or humans. The most common parameters include the amount of drug detected over time (area under the curve [AUC]),

TABLE 1 | Pharmacokinetic parameters and evaluation strategies for oral/buccal medicines.

	In vivo[a]	Drug predictors	NP predictors	*In vitro* assays/*ex vivo* assays
Absorption	T max, AUC, C_{max}	Solubility, lipophilicity (log P), molecular weight, number of hydrogen bond donor groups (Lipinski et al., 2001), log D, polar surface area and pKa (Berben et al., 2018)[b]	Charge, size, bioadhesiveness, lipophilicity, surface modification (Griffin et al., 2016)	Parallel artificial membrane permeation assay (PAMPA) and derivatives (Berben et al., 2018), cell based assays (mainly Caco-2), USP dissolution methods/derivatives[c], permeation through mucosal tissue (pig, human)
Distribution	Volume of drug distribution at steady state, tissue- plasma partition coefficients	logP, pKa	Targeting ligands	Plasma protein binding assay, *ex vivo* tissue distribution
Metabolism	Metabolites in blood, urine, feces	ligand for liver enzymes, [d]lipophilicity	Targeting ligands, size, charge, lipophilicity, surface modification (Griffin et al., 2016)	Metabolic activity of hepatocytes, cytochrome P450 (CYP) inhibition assay, liver and intestinal microsome stability
Excretion	Drug in urine, feces	Molecular weight, lipophilicity, pKa	Size	Plasma protein binding

[a]In vivo models include generally mice, rat, rabbit, dog, or monkey species. Monkeys are considered more reliable than other animal species to infer human pharmacokinetic profiles (Furukawa et al., 2014). [b]Drugs that are substrates for biological transporters do not present predictive permeability with only these parameters. [c]USP dissolution methods vary depending on the dosage form. They can be predictive for drug with dissolution rate-limited absorption, but complex release kinetics and NP environmental changes may increase in vivo correlation failure. [d]To check ligand properties, the most common method is molecular docking (Meng et al., 2011).

the highest drug level detected (C_{max}), and the time the latter happened (t_{max}). On the other hand, NPs are seldom classified based on plasma levels. Nanoparticle tracking relies mainly on marked particles with fluorescent dyes to observe biodistribution in tissues. An important reminder is that plasma levels do not discriminate buccal from gastric or intestinal absorption.

NP-IN-MATRIX DDSS

The following items present a discussion of all articles we could find with *in vivo* pharmacokinetic data of NP-in-matrix DDSs. The NP type directed subdivisions based on their main constituent. Exact values and formulation details are presented in **Table 2**.

Polymeric NPs

Polymers vary on their degradation, polarity, source, and chain size properties (Hallan et al., 2016). Polymeric based NPs present scalable manufacturing methods and capability to load a wide range of drug types (Crucho and Barros, 2017). The most common natural polymers for NPs are chitosan, sodium alginate, dextran, gelatin, and albumin. These hydrophilic proteins and carbohydrates degrade in physiological conditions, besides their biocompatibility, which helps to avoid side effects (Boateng and Areago, 2014; Madkhali et al., 2019; Bronze-Uhle et al., 2017; Kim et al., 2001). Alginate and chitosan still exhibit bioadhesive nature, which increases NP efficacy for mucosal delivery (Boateng and Areago, 2014). In turn, albumin discharges drugs *via* desorption without significant burst effects (Jiang and Stenzel, 2016). We have not found any pharmacokinetics data for NP-in-matrix systems based on gelatin or chitosan NPs; however, several studies discussed in this article address these excipients as matrix components.

Concerning alginate NPs, Garhy et al. loaded carvedilol in these carriers and further incorporated this system in buccoadhesive gels. The *in vitro* release assay showed burst behavior for all 12 different NP formulations. However, NP-in-gel formulations (FG1 and FG2) indicated that the gelling agent delayed carvedilol release, which diminished burst. FG1 gel contained hydroxypropyl methylcellulose (HPMC), whereas le FG2 presented the same HPMC concentration and sodium carboxymethylcellulose. Rabbits treated with FG2 formulation showed a two-fold increase in relative bioavailability compared to the market product. The increase in bioavailability occurred probably due to NP enhancement in drug solubility and the buccal bypass of the first-pass effect (Garhy et al., 2018).

Albumin properties were tested in exenatide-loaded bovine serum albumin/dextran NPs; the peptide was adsorbed to the carrier protein and released in a sustained manner due to dextran crosslinkings. This loaded NP was incorporated in gastroresistant microparticles of Eudragit L/HPMC. The incorporation led to macromolecule protection and decreased release rates of the peptide cargo. Consequently, pharmacokinetic data showed that NP-in-matrix resulted in a high relative oral bioavailability of 77% compared to a subcutaneous injection of the commercial equivalent medicine (Soudry-Kochavi et al., 2015).

Among the synthetic polymers, the aliphatic polyesters and their copolymers are the most used for drug delivery because of their biodegradability and biocompatibility. One of the most popular is the poly(lactic acid), often combined with glycolide to form the hydrophobic copolymer poly(lactic-co-glycolic acid) (PLGA) (Washington et al., 2017); PLGA exhibit high stability in biological fluids and long clinical experience; it was the only synthetic polymer to compose a nanostructure part of an NP-in-matrix dosage form with pharmacokinetic data. All the drugs entrapped into these studied systems are considered poorly water-soluble drugs.

Three different studies reported buccal films as matrices for PLGA NPs. The incorporated drugs were acyclovir (Al-Dhubiab et al., 2015), selegiline (Al-Dhubiab, 2016a) and zolpidem (Al-Dhubiab, 2016b). *In vitro* studies showed that film formulations prolonged drug liberation in a composition-dependent mode. The results of *ex vivo* studies with rabbit buccal mucosa showed that these nanospheres can permeate the tissue. *In vivo* results confirmed the predictions, whereas male rabbits demonstrated an increased drug bioavailability with the NP-in-film strategy. After incorporating NPs in polymeric films, the bioadhesive properties increased the residence time in oral cavity. It was also observed that C_{max}, AUC, and t_{max} improved with the use of combined systems when compared to controls (oral drug solutions, results in **Table 2**).

The PLGA NP improvements may come as well from a micro matrix strategy. Nassar et al. (Nassar et al., 2011) used docetaxel-loaded PLGA nanocapsules in entero-coated microparticles. The microcarrier released NPs that penetrated the enterocytes of rats, bypassed permeability-glycoprotein pump, and apparently circumvented gut metabolism of the drug. An oral administration of NP-in-matrix resulted in higher bioavailability than intravenous solution of the free drug (commercial formulation, 276%) and its NP formulation (400%). A subsequent study with minipigs confirmed the pattern obtained with rats; the superiority of NP-in-matrix over NPs was attributed to lymphatic transportation that changed drug biodistribution (Attili-Qadri et al., 2013).

Lipidic NPs

Lipid NPs are well-established DDSs due to their high biocompatibility, biodegradability, low toxicity, and applicability to various administration routes (Chime and Onyishi, 2013; Wissing et al., 2004; Shastri, 2017; Teixeira et al., 2017; Puri et al., 2009). The main lipid NPs reported are liposomes, solid lipid nanoparticles (SLNs), nanostructured lipid carriers, and nanoemulsions. The hydrophobic cores enhance drug solubility and protect it from the environment; the surfactant layer separates particles by steric or electrical hindrance. The exception is the liposome vesicle form, which allows loading of hydrophobic and hydrophilic drug molecules into its outer layer or aqueous core, respectively (Karamanidou et al., 2016). Among the cited particles, only NLC did not present *in vivo* data, probably because it is the most recent development among this group.

Lipidic NPs may deform under mechanical stress, such as tableting; they can also undergo lipid phase transitions upon heating, such as for film casting. Therefore, Hazzah et al. incorporated curcumin SLN in freeze-dried polymeric sponges

TABLE 2 | Pharmacokinetic data for NP-in-matrix systems.

References	Matrix type	Matrix excipients	NP-Type	NP excipients	Drug	Pharmacokinetics
(Al-Dhubiab et al., 2015)	Film	HPMC K15 + Carbopol 974P + Eudragit® RL 100 + ethyl cellulose + PEG 200	Polymeric (nanospheres)	PLGA	Acyclovir	• Model: male white rabbits. • Administration: NP-in-buccal film (1 cm^2) was wetted and applied to the buccal mucosa for 4 h; control animals received oral drug solution (1 mg dose, 1 mL). • Data for control (oral solution): C_{max} = 91.61 (ng/mL); t_{max} = 2 h; AUC_{∞} = 395.21 ng·h/mL. • Data for buccal combined system (A3): C_{max} = 306.04 (ng/mL); t_{max} = 6 h; AUC_{∞} = 3116.21 ng·h/mL.
(Nekkanti et al., 2009)**	Tablet	Mannitol	Nanocrystal	HPMC	Cardesan	• Model: male Wistar rats. •Administration: oral suspensions of spray dried drug microparticles or drug nanoparticles at a 10 mg/kg dose. • Data for drug microparticles: C_{max} = 0.16 ± 0.10 µg/mL; t_{max} = 1.81 ± 1,13 h; AUC_{∞} = 0.31 ± 0.07 ng·h/mL; • Data for drug nanoparticles: C_{max} = 0.09 ± 0.03 µg/mL t_{max} = 1.06 ± 0.38 h AUC_{∞} = 0.78 ± 0.22 µg·h/mL.
(Rana and Murthy 2013)	Patch (triple layer patch)	HPMC + carbopol + ethyl cellulose	Nanocrystals	PVA	Carvedilol	• Model: rabbits • Administration: NP-in-film (combined system) in a 250 µg/kg dose and oral tablet (control) in a 1 mg/kg dose. • Data for control: C_{max} = 48.73 ± 14.1 ng/mL; t_{max} = 2 h; AUC_{∞} = 1813.70 ± 42.53 ng·h/mL. • Data for combined system: C_{max} = 356.91 ± 29.5 ng/mL; t_{max} = 4 h; AUC_{∞} = 4154.37 ± 80.22 ng·h/mL.
(Garhy et al., 2018)	Gel	Sodium carboxymethyl cellulose + hydroxypropyl methylcellulose K4M	Polymeric (nanospheres)	Sodium alginate + Eudragit® RS100	Carvedilol	• Model: male New Zealand rabbits. • Administration: NP-in-buccal gel (3.125 mg of drug) was applied to the mucosa; control animals received equivalent oral dose of commercial tablet. • Data for FG1 (4% HPMC K4M): C_{max} = 102.27 ng/mL t_{max} = 1h $AUC0\text{-}\infty$ = 639.38 ng·h/mL Relative bioavailability = 130.3% increase compared to the market product

(Continued)

TABLE 2 | Continued

References	Matrix type	Matrix excipients	NP-Type	NP excipients	Drug	Pharmacokinetics
						• Data for FG2 (4% HPMC K4M + 2% sodium carboxymethylcellulose): C_{max} = 187.41 ng/mL t_{max} = 1h AUC0-∞ = 830.59 ng·h/mL Relative bioavailability = 130.3% increase compared to the market product • Data for control (commercial tablet): t_{max} = 1.5 h Exact values for C_{max} and AUC are not available.
(Rao et al., 2015)	Lipidic (microparticles)	Labrasol®	Inorganic nanoparticles	Silica	Cinnarizine	• Model: male Sprague-Dawley rats • Administration: one of four formulations at 10 mg/kg *via* oral gavage (unformulated cinnarizine; silica–lipid hybrid (SLH); pluronic-functionalized silica–lipid hybrid (PLU-SLH); NP-in-microparticle structure and PLU&SLH physical mixture). • Unformulated cinnarizine: C_{max} = 262 ± 41 ng/mL; t_{max} = 0.6 ± 0.1 h; AUC_{∞} = 656 ± 64 ng·h/mL • SLH: C_{max} = 258 ± 23ng/mL; t_{max} = 1.0 ± 0.0h; AUC_{∞} = 859 ± 133 ng·h/mL • PLU-SLH: C_{max} = 427 ± 5 ng/mL; t_{max} = 1.3 ± 0.3h; AUC0-α = 1400± 135 ng·h/mL • PLU&SHL: C_{max} = 326 ± 39ng/mL; t_{max} = 1.1 ± 0.3h; AUC_{∞} = 971 ± 161 ng·h/mL
(Lv et al., 2015)	Film	Carboxymethyl chitosan (CCS)	Micelle	Phospholipid and bile salts	Cucurbitacin B (Cu B)	• Model: healthy male rabbits. •Administration: films applied to buccal mucosa. CCS-films containing Cu B loaded phospholipid–sodium deoxycholate–mixed micelles (PL-SDC-MMs), conventional CCS (C-CCS) films and the conventional tablet (Hulusupian), 1 mg/kg. The tablet was administered as oral suspension. • Data for micelles-in-CCS films: C_{max} = 2.04 ± 0.50 (μg/mL); t_{max} = 5.03 ± 0.34 h; AUC0–36 = 46.43 ± 5.11 (μg·h/mL). • Data for CCS films: C_{max} = 0.52 ± 0.37 (μg/mL); t_{max} ~7.96 ± 0.97 h AUC0–36 = 4.44 ± 1.21 (μg·h/mL). • Data for Cu B marked tablet: C_{max} = 3.08 ± 0.52 (μg/mL); t_{max} = 3.01 ± 0.82 h; AUC0–36 = 17.23 ± 3.43 (μg·h/mL).

(Continued)

TABLE 2 | Continued

References	Matrix type	Matrix excipients	NP-Type	NP excipients	Drug	Pharmacokinetics
(Lv et al., 2014)	Fast-dissolving oral films (FDOFs)	Pullulan and PEG 400	Micelle	Phospholipid (PL) and bile salts (sodium deoxycholate (SDC))	Cucurbitacin B (Cu B)	• Model: male Wistar rats. • Administration: Cu B-PL/SDC-MMs, the FDOFs containing Cu B-PL/SDC-MMs, and the Cu B suspension, all corresponding to a dose of 2 mg/kg. • Data for Cu B suspension: C_{max} = 3.23 ± 0.64 (μg/mL); t_{max} = 3.01 ± 0.44 h; AUC(0–24) = 17.13 ± 3.54 (μg·h/mL). • Data for Cu B-PL/SDC-MMs: C_{max} = 7.18 ± 1.08 (μg/mL); t_{max} = 0.69 ± 0.32 h; AUC(0–24) = 42.25 ± 5.91 (μg·h/mL). • Data for Cu B-PL/SDC-MMs-in-FDOFs: C_{max} = 7.82 ± 1.21 (μg/mL); t_{max} = 0.67 ± 0.28 h; AUC(0–24) = 45.11 ± 6.13 (μg·h/mL).
(Augustine et al., 2018)*	Microparticle	Alginate + chitosan	Nanosuspension	Alginate	Darunavir/ritonavir	• Model: albine Sprague-Dawley rats. • Administration: 25 mg/kg dose of daruvanir + ritovanir. Groups: unformulated drug, the nanonized drug and the NP-in-microparticle loaded drug (NiMDS). • Data for the unformulated drug: C_{max} = 0.14 μg/mL; t_{max} = 2.63 h; AUC_{last} = 1.17 μg·h/mL; • Data for nanonized drug: C_{max} = 0.11 μg/mL; t_{max} = 1.75 h; AUC_{last} = 1.35 μg·h/mL; • Data for NiMDS: C_{max} = 0.38 μg/mL; t_{max} = 2.75 h; AUC_{last} = 2.67 μg·h/mL.
(Kevadiya et al., 2018)	Oral strip films (OSFs)	HPMC	Nanocrystals	SDS and HPMC	Fenofibrate (FNB)	• Model: New Zealand white rabbits. • Administration: orally/buccal dose equivalent of 30 mg/kg of FNB. Groups: marketed formulation (oral suspension); pristine FNB (suspension); OSFs (5.28 mg/cm^2 of FNB-NC-D). • Tricor: C_{max} = 23.1 ± 8.8μg/mL; t_{max} = 8.0 ± 3.0 h; AUC_{∞} = 654.6 ± 251 μg·h/mL. • FNB: C_{max} = 16.8 ± 12.2 μg/mL; t_{max} = 8.0 ± 5.8h; AUC_{∞} = 514.8 ± 374 μg·h/mL. • FNB-NC-D: C_{max} = 37.6 ± 10.6μg/mL; t_{max} = 6.0 ± 1.7h; AUC_{∞} = 931.2 ± 263 μg·h/mL.

(Continued)

TABLE 2 | Continued

References	Matrix type	Matrix excipients	NP-Type	NP excipients	Drug	Pharmacokinetics
(Ahmed et al., 2018)**	Lyophilized tablet (LT)	HPMC, mannitol, silica, Avicel, and plasdone XL	Self-nanoemulsion (SNE)	Anise oil; Tween 80; cosurfactant (methanol; ethanol; propanol; butanol)	Finasteride (FSD)	• Model: healthy male volunteers. • Administration: group I: FSD-SNELTs; group II: FSD-LTs; group III: FSD-marketed tablets (Proscar®), containing 5 mg of FSD. • Data for FSD-SNELTs: C_{max} = 44.635 ± 3.259 (ng/mL); t_{max} = 1.5 ± 0.289 h; AUC_{last} = 721.662 ± 55.085 (ng·h/mL). • Data for FSD-LTs: C_{max} = 37.794 ± 1.405 (ng/mL); t_{max} = 2 ± 0 h; AUC_{last} = 444.08 ± 37.283 (ng·h/mL). • Data for marketed tablets: C_{max} = 29.150 ± 4.798 (ng/mL); t_{max} = 3 ± 1 h; AUC_{last} = 487.639 ± 42.989 (ng·h/mL).
(Imperiale et al., 2015)*	Polymeric (microspheres)	Alginate + chitosan coated or not with Eudragit	Nanocrystal	Not mentioned	Indinavir	• Model: mongrel dogs. • Administration: a single dose of 10 mg/kg of: indinavir (IDV) free base, pure IDV nanoparticles and NP-in-microparticle delivery system (NiMDSs); all encapsulated within gastro-resistant capsules. • IDV base: C_{max} = 0.34 µg/mL; t_{max} = 1.10 h; AUC_{∞} = 0.83 µg·h/mL; • IDV nanoparticles: C_{max} = 1.41 µg/mL; t_{max} = 2.00 h; AUC_{∞} = 18.16 µg·h/mL; • NiMDSs: C_{max} = 0.50 µg/mL; t_{max} = 1.80 h; AUC_{∞} = 39.23 µg·h/mL.
(Nidhi et al., 2016)	Patch (transmucosal patch [TP])	Hydroxypropyl cellulose-LF (HPC-LF)	Lipidic (SLN)	Glyceryl palmitostearate + glyceryl monostearate	Lignocaine (Lig) + diclofenac diethylamine (DDEA)	• Model: white New Zealand male rabbits. • Administration: group 1: TP (0.5×0.5 cm) containing lignocaine base (LB) (0.872 mg/kg) and DDEA (1.6248 mg/kg) placed over the anterior mandibular gingiva for 12 hours. Group 2 (control): marketed Lig HCl gel (1.008 mg/kg) over the anterior mandibular gingiva and marketed diclofenac (Dic) sodium administered orally as 1.4 mg/kg. In both groups, the dose maintained was 0.872 mg/kg of Lig and 1.3033 mg/kg of Dic. • Data for TP: - Gingival crevicular fluid (GCF): C_{max} = 0.4428 ± 0.28 (µg/mL) (Lig) and 4.6213 ± 0.21 (µg/mL) (Dic); t_{max} = 0.25 h (Lig) and 2 h (Dic); AUC_{∞} = 1.6396 ± 1.02 µg·h/mL (Lig) and 808.835 ± 3.25 µg·h/mL (Dic). - Plasma: C_{max} = 0.3259 ± 0.03 (µg/mL) (Lig) and 0.1910 ± 0.02 (µg/mL) (Dic); t_{max} = 1 h (Lig) and 2 h (Dic); AUC_{∞} = 5.6502 ± 0.72 µg·h/mL (Lig) and 4.1754 ± 0.38 µg·h/mL (Dic).

(Continued)

TABLE 2 | Continued

References	Matrix type	Matrix excipients	NP-Type	NP excipients	Drug	Pharmacokinetics
						• Data for control: - Gingival crevicular fluid (GCF): C_{max} = 0.0499 ± 0.02 (μg/mL) (Lig) and 1.6495 ± 0.05 (μg/mL) (Dic); t_{max} = 0.5 h (Lig) and 2 h (Dic); AUC_{∞} = 0.1024 ± 0.31 μg·h/mL (Lig) and 8.6204 ± 0.22 μg·h/mL (Dic). - Plasma: C_{max} = 0.1645 ± 0.01 (μg/mL) (Lig) and 1.4181 ± 0.15 (μg/mL) (Dic); t_{max} = 0.5 h (Lig) and 2 h (Dic); AUC_{∞} = 0.6568 ± 0.01 μg·h/mL (Lig) and 4.6808 ± 0.26 μg·h/mL (Dic).
(Guo et al., 2015)**	Tablet	Not mentioned	Nanocrystals	Pluronic F68, HPMC K4M, HPMC E5, PVP K30	Rebamipide (REB)	• Model: male Sprague-Dawley rats • The test preparation rebamipide nanocrystal tablets (REB-NTs) were compared with that of a reference formulation of Mucosta® tablets (REB-MTs). Dose = 10 mg/kg. • REB-Nts: C_{max} = 543.4 ± 150.5 ng/mL; t_{max} = 1.67 ± 0.41 h; AUC_{∞} = 2622.3 ± 462.8 ng·min/mL. • REB-Mts: C_{max} = 281.5 ± 66.1 ng/mL; t_{max} = 1.08 ± 1.34 h; AUC_{∞} = 1187.4 ± 411.8 ng·min/mL.
(Salem et al., 2018)**	Tablet	Nano-silica, microcrystalline cellulose and croscarmellose sodium	Self-nanoemulsion	Surfactants (Tween 80 and Cremophore RH 40), oils (oleic acid, labrafac, labrafil) and cosurfactant (propylene glycol)	Rosuvastatin	• The study was performed in healthy male volunteers. • Administration: SNE-tablet and Crestor®; the tablets were administered orally at a dose of 10 mg each. • Data for Crestor®: C_{max} = 23 885 (ng/mL); t_{max} = 3 h; AUC_{last} = 264 210 (ng·h/mL). • Data for SNE tablet: C_{max} = 66 521 (ng/mL); t_{max} = 2 h; AUC_{last} = 648 219 (ng·h/mL).
(Al-Dhubiab, 2016a)	Buccal Film	HPMC K15 + Carbopol 971P + Eudragit® RS 100 + ethyl cellulose + PEG 400	Polymeric (nanospheres)	PLGA/PVA	Selegiline	• Model: male white rabbits. • Administration: NP-in-buccal film (1 cm^2) was wetted and applied to the buccal mucosa for 4 h; control animals received oral drug solution (1 mg dose, 1 mL). • Data for control (oral drug solution): C_{max} = 264.28 (ng/mL); t_{max} = 1 h; AUC_{∞} = 877.07 ng·h/mL. • Data for buccal film (F3): C_{max} = 426.58 (ng/mL); t_{max} = 4 h; AUC_{∞} = 2935.65 ng·h/mL.

(Continued)

TABLE 2 | Continued

References	Matrix type	Matrix excipients	NP-Type	NP excipients	Drug	Pharmacokinetics
(El-Say et al., 2017)**	Lyophilized tablet (LT)	Porous fumed silica, lactose, and microcrystalline cellulose (Avicel)	Self-nanoemulsion (SNE)	Labrasol, and Transcutol	Vitamin K	• Model: male human volunteers. •Administration: subjects were classified into 3 groups (6 per each). Group I: vitamin K-in-SNELTs; group II: commercial tablet; group III: injected drug ampoule intramuscularly. All groups = 10 mg. • Data for vit K-in-SNELTs: C_{max} = 1572.37 ± 120.2 (ng/mL); t_{max} = 2.5 ± 0.0 h; AUC_{last} = 7283.34 ± 85.4 (ng·h/mL). • Data for commercial tablet: C_{max} = 1054.97 ± 91.04 (ng/mL); t_{max} = 3.0 ± 0.0 h; AUC_{last} = 4379.59 ± 202.3 (ng·h/mL). • Data for intramuscular drug ampoule: C_{max} = 1868.28 ± 89.2 (ng/mL); t_{max} = 2.0 ± 0.0h; AUC_{last} = 8379.76 ± 1434.7 (ng·h/mL).
(Al-Dhubiab, 2016b)	Film	HPMC K100 + Eudragit® RL 100 + Carbopol 974P	Polymeric (nanospheres)	PLGA	Zolpidem	• Model: male white rabbits. • Administration: NP-in-buccal film (1 cm^2) was wetted and applied to the buccal mucosa for 4 h; control animals received oral drug solution (1 mg dose, 1 mL). • Data for control (oral drug solution): C_{max} = 32.34 (ng/mL); t_{max} = 1 h; AUC_{∞} = 136.06 ng·h/mL. • Data for buccal film (Z4): C_{max} = 52.54 (ng/mL); t_{max} = 1.5 h; AUC_{∞} = 236.00 ng·h/mL.
(Tong et al., 2018)**	Tablets	Anhydrous dibasic calcium phosphate (Fujicalin®)	Self-nanoemulsion (SNE)	Soybean lecithin and glycocholic acid (surfactant) and Transcutol HP (cosurfactant)	Vitamin K1 (VK1)	• Model: beagle dogs. •Administration: six healthy beagle dogs randomly divided into two groups (SNE-L tablets and conventional VK1 tablets), receiving a single 10 mg oral dose. • Data for combined system: C_{max} = 575.46 ± 84.27 (ng/mL); t_{max} = 1.67 ± 0.58 h; AUC_{∞} = 1716.33 ± 264.20 (ng·h/mL). • Data for control (commercial tablet): C_{max} = 249.23 ± 79.05 (ng/mL); t_{max} = 2.0 ± 1.0 h; AUC_{∞} = 866.14 ± 215.45 (ng·h/mL).
(Attili-Qadri et al., 2013)	Microparticle	Eudragit L + HPMC	Polymeric (nanocapsule)	Glyceryl tributyrate + oleoyl polyoxylglycerides + PLGA	Docetaxel	• Model: minipigs. • Administration: oral dose of Taxotere (commercial) and combined system (1.25 mg/kg).

(Continued)

TABLE 2 | Continued

References	Matrix type	Matrix excipients	NP-Type	NP excipients	Drug	Pharmacokinetics
						• Data for control (oral solution of commercial drug): C_{max} = 97.6 (ng/mL); AUC_{∞} = 797.7 ng·h/mL. • Data for combined system: C_{max} = 817.9 (ng/mL); AUC_{∞} = 7,923.1 ng·h/mL.
(Nassar et al., 2011)*	Microparticle	Eudragit L + HPMC	Polymeric (nanocapsule)	Glyceryl tributyrate + oleoyl polyoxylglycerides + PLGA	Docetaxel	• Model: Sprague-Dawley male rats • Administration: intravenous dose of drug-loaded NPs and oral dose of combined system (5mg/kg). • Data for drug-loaded NPs: AUC = 1,441.9 ng·h/mL. • Data for oral combined system: AUC = 5,754.5 ng·h/mL
(Soudry-Kochavi et al., 2015)**	Microparticle	Eudragit L + HPMC	Polymeric (nanosphere)	BSA + dextran + sodium trimetaphosphate	Exenatide	• Model: Sprague-Dawley male rats. • Administration: drug solution and commercial drug (Byetta™) were administered subcutaneously (SC)(65µg/kg). Combined systems DX-50 and DX-150 were administered orally (by gavage) (165 µg/kg). • Data for control (SC commercial drug): C_{max} = 1.22 µg/mL t_{max} = 1.33 h AUC = 31.01 h·µg·10^{-2}/mL. • Data for control (SC drug solution): C_{max} = 1.06 µg/mL t_{max} = 0.83 h AUC = 26.37 h·µg·10^{-2}/mL. • Data for oral combined system DX-50 (50 mg dextran): C_{max} = 2.09 µg/mL t_{max} = 1.33 h AUC = 59.45 h·µg·10^{-2}/mL. • Data for oral combined system DX-150 (150 mg dextran): C_{max} = 1.80 µg/mL t_{max} = 1.00 h AUC = 36.00 h·µg·10^{-2}/mL.

NP, nanoparticle; AUC, area under the curve that describe drug concentration over time, measured in plasma; C_{max}, the maximum drug concentration measured in plasma; t_{max}, the time taken to reach the maximum drug concentration; PVA, polyvinyl alcohol; PLGA, poly(lactic-co-glycolic acid); HPMC, hydroxypropyl methylcellulose; PEG, polyethylene glycol; SDS, sodium dodecyl sulfate; PVP, polyvinylpyrrolidone; BSA, bovine serum albumin.

**Studies comparing pharmacokinetic data for NP-in-matrix and free NPs.*

***NP-in-matrix systems for oral delivery.*

to avoid the cited issues. Human studies showed that curcumin SLN-in-polycarbophil sponge has higher C_{max}, t_{max}, and AUC than the SLN-in-HPMC sponge (**Table 2**). In accordance, polycarbophil formulation adhered to the mucosa for a longer time (15 h, compared to 4 h) and presented higher matrix porosity and homogeneous distribution of SLNs. The decreased porosity of HPMC sponges diminished swelling and consequent interaction with mucin. Also, SLNs remained onto the surface of HPMC sponges, lowering its adhesion property to the oral mucosa and releasing the NPs faster than polycarbophil. Although pure NPs were not tested *in vivo*, *in vitro* release showed that NP-in-sponge eliminated the burst effect of the nanodispersions, which improves prediction of therapy outcomes and avoids possible plasma peaks (Hazzah et al., 2015).

Ahmed et al. also used freeze-dried polymeric matrix (gelatin "tablets," no compression step) to load lipidic self-nanoemulsions (SNEs) of finasteride. Different from the mucoadhesive sponges, the freeze-dried tablets melt on the mouth upon contact with saliva. These macrocarriers aim as fast release as possible for buccal and gastrointestinal absorption. Both formulated tablets (with or without SNE) presented in human higher C_{max} and shorter t_{max} of the drug than the marketed tablets. Likewise, AUC and Mean Residence Time (MRT) indicated superiority of NP-in-tablet system. The improved drug bioavailability may enhance the therapeutic effects (Ahmed et al., 2018).

A variety of this technique decreased the low bioavailability of oral vitamin K. The SNE was loaded on porous silica carriers and later incorporated in lyophilized tablets. SNE-in-lyophilized tablets increased absorption rate and extent of vitamin K in humans compared to marketed tablets. Even better, the NP-in-matrix system presented AUC similar to the commercial intramuscular injection (El-Say et al., 2017). Powdered SNE loaded with vitamin K_1 was also incorporated into regular tablets, but with different vitamin loadings. Because SNEs form nanoparticles upon contact with gastrointestinal fluid, NP deformation was not a concern. Beagle dogs administered with SNE-in-tablet showed a 2.3-fold increase in vitamin K_1 C_{max} and 1.98-fold in AUC (Tong et al., 2018). The increment in bioavailability probably happened due to higher surface area and consequent higher drug dissolution rate in the gastrointestinal tract (Gong et al., 2016).

SNE-in-tablet was also applied to rosuvastatin delivery, increasing solubility and bypassing hepatic first-pass metabolism. Male humans taking SNE-in-tablet had rosuvastatin AUC increased 2.45 times and C_{max} increased 2.78 times compared with the intake of commercial rosuvastatin tablets. Similarly, t_{max} decreased with drug administration in SNE tablet, highlighting its benefits (Salem et al., 2018).

The latter lipid NP-in-matrix with published *in vivo* pharmacokinetics is the phospholipid-bile salts-mixed micelles. Cucurbitacin B was loaded in these micelles to address its water insolubility, toxicity, and gastrointestinal side effects. The use of fast-dissolving oral films of pullulan as a matrix maintained the *in vivo* absorption properties like micelles and promoted a significant increase in the oral bioavailability of cucurbitacin B in Wistar rats (highest values of C_{max} and AUC, lowest t_{max}), when compared to the free suspension drug. Also, the matrix did not interfere with Cu B-micelles original structure (Lv et al., 2014). These micelles in carboxymethyl chitosan buccal film rendered a mucoadhesive formulation, which released the drug for a longer period. It resulted in 2.69-fold increase in bioavailability in rabbits when compared to marketed tablets and 10.46 times the film formulation without NP. The team reported that buccal mucosa barrier probably explains higher C_{max} and lower t_{max} of oral tablets; high AUC from film formulations may be owed to the presence of permeation enhancers in it and the nanosized drug, ensuring the increase in the amount of drug penetration into the blood (Lv et al., 2015). It would be interesting to compare the influence of the different matrices in cucurbitacin B kinetics, but the animal models differ in species, drug dose, and period of evaluation.

Inorganic NPs

Inorganic nanoparticles are flexible carriers that allow surface modification, drug targeting, and modified drug release. This group includes silica, clay, and metals as excipients arranged in nanoparticles, nanotubes, or nanorods/nanoparticles, respectively (Kerdsakundee et al., 2017; Rao et al., 2011; Zhang et al., 2018). The silica-based ones were the only inorganic NP-in-matrix compositions tested *in vivo* for oral administration. Although biocompatible and with a well-defined/modifiable structure, they do not adhere to mucosa and are good candidates for matrix incorporation (Slowing et al., 2008).

To improve the oral delivery of the poorly soluble drug cinnarizine, an antihistamine and calcium-channel blocker, Rao S. et al. developed a pluronic functionalized silica–lipid hybrid microparticle. Pluronic acts as a polymeric precipitation inhibitor, avoiding recrystallization of cinnarizine dissolution; the silica–lipid hybrid microparticle improved drug partition by producing a hydrophobic microenvironment. Bioavailability was compared between the cinnarizine loaded functionalized silica-lipid hybrid system, unformulated cinnarizine and a cinnarizine loaded nonfunctionalized silica-lipid system; the in vivo design included a single dose of 10 mg/kg of each formulation *via* oral gavage. The study resulted in more than 2.1-fold improvement in the AUC and 1.6-fold improvement in C_{max} of cinnarizine of the functionalized NP-in-microparticle structure in comparison to the unformulated one and a 1.6-fold improvement in both AUC and C_{max} in comparison with the nonfunctionalized formulation, resulting in an overall improved bioavailability of cinnarizine (Rao et al., 2015).

Drug-Based NPs

Poor solubility, low bioavailability, and short stability *in vivo* are limiting problems in the development and delivery of new active ingredients (Liu et al., 2012). To overcome these issues, one can entrap the drug in a nanocarrier or reduce its particles to obtain a nanosized range, such as nanocrystals. Compared to NPs, drug-based particles offer higher drug loading (nearly 100%) with generally less excipients and uniform/stable physical nature (Liu et al., 2012).

Accordingly, indinavir nanonization increased absorption (from 0.83 to 18.16 μg·h/mL) and t_{max} (from 1.10 to 2.50 h) of the free base drug after administration of a single oral dose in mongrel dogs; however, NP-in-microparticle alginate/chitosan particles performed much better than pure nanocrystals (AUC of 39.23 μg·h/mL and $t_{½}$ value of 76.3 h). This represented an increase of the oral bioavailability and the apparent $t_{½}$ of 47 and 95 times, compared to the free drug. The increment in release time may improve HIV treatment, which demands long-term therapy and frequent dosing (Imperiale et al., 2015). Likewise, darunavir and ritonavir benefited from an NP-in-microparticle oral delivery system for nanocrystals. The difference was that NP-in-microparticle increased the oral bioavailability of the combined drugs by 2.3-fold compared with the NP only and the free drug. In this case, nanonization alone was not able to increase absorption (Augustine et al., 2018).

Nanocrystals vehicled in tablets and buccal films allow easier self-administration, increased dosage precision, and superior performance. Rebamipide presents only 10% of oral bioavailability in humans due to poor solubility, which is the reason Guo and coworkers formulated an NP-in-tablet version of the medicine. Drug nanocrystals were stabilized with HPMC and polyvinylpyrrolidone before tablet incorporation. The relative oral bioavailability of REB nanocrystal tablets was 256.8% in rats (reference Mucosta® tablets) (Guo et al., 2015). Nekkanti's group also used HPMC-stabilized nanocrystals for candesartan cilexetil delivery, further incorporated in mannitol-based tablets. This prodrug belongs to the low solubility/long-term therapy group, such as rebamipide. *In vivo* studies confirmed dosage form benefits: Wistar rats presented 2.51-fold increase in AUC, a 1.77-fold increase in C_{max}, and a decreased t_{max} (1.81–1.06 h) compared to the free prodrug (Nekkanti et al., 2009).

Rana and Murthy developed a three-layer buccal film: a mucoadhesive layer, a layer containing nanosuspension of carvedilol nanocrystals and a backing membrane. The structure aimed to prevent the first-pass metabolism, raising drug bioavailability. C_{max} of the buccal patch was 7.3 times higher than that of the oral tablet, and t_{max} exhibited by the patch was 4 h in comparison to 2 h for oral tablet. The NP in microparticle structured buccal patch has been designed as a novel platform for potential buccal delivery of drugs having high first-pass metabolism (Rana and Murthy, 2013).

Another application of nanosized drugs is the development of better suitable dosage forms of existing drugs to attend the patient needs. Kevadiya et al. developed an oral strip-film containing nanocrystals of the cholesterol-reducing agent fenofibrate, a very low solubility prodrug, aiming to create a fast disintegrating solid dosage form ideal for emergency administration and for patients with swallowing difficulties. New Zealand white rabbits were divided in three groups: the first received the oral commercial formulation Tricor in suspension form; the second received the suspension of fenofibrate nanocrystals (pristine FNB) and the third received the oral striped-films containing fenofibrate nanocrystals (OSF). Pharmacokinetics data showed a higher C_{max} and lower t_{max} of OSF when compared to the marketed Tricor formulation and pristine FNB. The AUC was also higher for OSF formulation (931.26 μg·h/mL) compared to Tricor (654.6 ± 251 μg·h/mL) and pristine FNB (514.8 ± 374 μg·h/mL); and the t_{max} (h) of OSFs was found to be 2 h earlier than the t_{max} of Tricor and pristine FNB (Kevadiya et al., 2018).

CONCLUSION

Because most of the articles we gathered date from this decade, NP-in-matrix approach still has a long way for exploitation. In our findings, most matrices belong to the polymeric group, based on classical excipients in the market, like HPMC. However, they vary from buccal to oral delivery, with rapid or slow degradation to offer an immediate or modified release. The use of an external matrix to incorporate nanoparticles brought several advantages to formulations. This type of system reduced burst effect, avoided NP degradation in gastrointestinal tract, increased residence time in the mouth, modulated t_{max}, and bypassed first-pass metabolism (buccal forms and some oral forms). Thus, the systemic bioavailability of the tested drugs was successfully enhanced.

Buccal release belongs to the trending strategies for drugs, so we expect an increase in pharmacokinetic studies concerning NP-in-matrix buccal delivery. Nanoparticle types will probably expand too, as the actual group is mainly PLGA, nanocrystals, and some lipid particles. In summary, we believe this article compiled several evidences and possible pitfalls of this strategy, which will help future developments on the field.

AUTHOR CONTRIBUTIONS

RC: synthetic polymeric NP-in-matrix research and writing. DG— inorganic NP-in-matrix research and writing. VB-d-A: lipidic NP-in-matrix research and writing. JC: tables, figures and conclusion. LO-N: review design, introduction and pharmacokinetics writing, scientific revision.

FUNDING

FAPESP 14/14457-5 - article charges funding CAPES 001 - scholarships for graduate students (RF, DG, VB-d-A, JC). This study was financed by the Coordenação de Aperfeiçoamento de Pessoal de Nível Superior - Brasil (CAPES) - Finance Code 001 and FAPESP project 2019/08281-5 and 2019/19696-1.

REFERENCES

Ahmed, T. A., El-Say, K. M., Hosny, K. M., and Aljaeid, B. M. (2018). Development of optimized self-nanoemulsifying lyophilized tablets (SNELTs) to improve finasteride clinical pharmacokinetic behavior. *Drug Dev. Ind. Pharm.* 44 (4), 652–615. doi: 10.1080/03639045.2017.1405977

Al-Dhubiab, B. E., Nair, A. B., Kumria, R., Attimarad, M., and Harsha, S. (2015). Formulation and evaluation of nano based drug delivery system for the buccal delivery of acyclovir. *Colloids and Surfaces. B. Biointerfaces* 136, 878–884. doi: 10.1016/j.colsurfb.2015.10.045

Al-Dhubiab, B. E. (2016a). Development and evaluation of buccal films impregnated with selegiline-loaded nanospheres. *Drug Delivery* 23 (7), 2154–2162. doi: 10.3109/10717544.2014.948644

Al-Dhubiab, B. E. (2016b). *In vitro* and *in vivo* evaluation of nano-based films for buccal delivery of zolpidem. *Braz. Oral Res.* 30 (1), e126. doi: 10.1590/1807-3107bor-2016.vol30.0126

Attili-Qadri, S., Karra, N., Nemirovski, A., Schwob, O., Talmon, Y., Nassar, T., et al. (2013). Oral delivery system prolongs blood circulation of docetaxel nanocapsules *via* lymphatic absorption. *Proc.Nat. Acad. Sci.* 110 (43), 17498–17503. doi: 10.1073/pnas.1313839110

Augustine, R., Ashkenazi, D. L., Arzi, R. S., Zlobin, V., Shofti, R., and Sosnik, A. (2018). Nanoparticle-in-microparticle oral drug delivery system of a clinically relevant darunavir/ritonavir antiretroviral combination. *Acta Biomater.* 74, 344–359. doi: 10.1016/j.actbio.2018.04.045

Barua, S., Kim, H., Jo, K., Seo, C. W., Park, T. J., Lee, K. B., et al. (2016). Drug delivery techniques for buccal route: formulation strategies and recent advances in dosage form design. *J. Pharm. Invest.* 46 (7), 593–6135. doi: 10.1007/s40005-016-0281-9

Berben, P., Bauer-Brandl, A., Brandl, M., Faller, B., Flaten, G. E., Jacobsen, A. C., et al. (2018). Drug permeability profiling using cell-free permeation tools: overview and applications. *Eur. J. Pharmaceut. Sci.: Off. J. Eur. Fed. Pharmaceut. Sci.* 119, 219–233. doi: 10.1016/j.ejps.2018.04.016

Bernkop-Schnürch, A., Weithaler, A., Albrecht, K., and Greimel, A. (2006). Thiomers: preparation and *in vitro* evaluation of a mucoadhesive nanoparticulate drug delivery system. *Int. J. Pharm.* 317 (1), 76–81. doi: 10.1016/j.ijpharm.2006.02.044

Boateng, J. S., and Areago, D. (2014). Composite sodium alginate and chitosan based wafers for buccal delivery of macromolecules. *Austin J. Anal. Pharmaceut. Chem.* 1, 1–7.

Bronze-Uhle, E. S., Costa, B. C., Ximenes, V. F., and Lisboa-Filho, P. N. (2017). Synthetic nanoparticles of bovine serum albumin with entrapped salicylic acid. *Nanotechnol. Sci. Appl.* 10, 11–21. doi: 10.2147/NSA.S117018

Chime, S. A., and Onyishi, I. V. (2013). Lipid-based drug delivery systems (LDDS): recent advances and applications of lipids in drug delivery. *Afr. J. Pharm. Pharmacol.* 7 (48), 3034–3595. doi: 10.5897/AJPPX2013.0004

Crucho, C. I. C., and Barros, M. T. (2017). Polymeric nanoparticles: a study on the preparation variables and characterization methods. *Mater. Sci. Eng. C. Mater. Biol. Appl.* 80, 771–784. doi: 10.1016/j.msec.2017.06.004

El-Say, K. M., Ahmed, T. A., Ahmed, O. A. A., Hosny, K. M., and Abd-Allah, F. I. (2017). Self-nanoemulsifying lyophilized tablets for flash oral transmucosal delivery of vitamin K: development and clinical evaluation. *J. Pharm. Sci.* 106 (9), 2447–2565. doi: 10.1016/j.xphs.2017.01.001

Furukawa, T., Naritomi, Y., Tetsuka, K., Nakamori, F., Moriguchi, H., Yamano, K., et al. (2014). Species differences in intestinal glucuronidation activities between humans, rats, dogs and monkeys. *Xenobiotica* 44 (3), 205–165. doi: 10.3109/00498254.2013.828362

Garhy, D. M. A., Ismail, S., Ibrahim, H. K., and Ghorab, M. M. (2018). Buccoadhesive gel of carvedilol nanoparticles for enhanced dissolution and bioavailability. *J. Drug Delivery Sci. Technol.* 47, 151–158. doi: 10.1016/j.jddst.2018.07.009

Gong, W., Wang, Y., Sun, L., Yang, J., Shan, L., Yang, M., et al. (2016). Development of itraconazole liquisolid compact: effect of polyvinylpyrrolidone on the dissolution properties. *Curr. Drug Delivery* 13 (3), 452–615. doi: 10.2174/1567201813666160216144323

Griffin, B. T., Guo, J., Presas, E., Donovan, M. D., Alonso, M. J., and O'Driscoll, C. M. (2016). Pharmacokinetic, pharmacodynamic and biodistribution following oral administration of nanocarriers containing peptide and protein drugs. *Adv. Drug Delivery Rev. Oral Delivery Pept.* 106, 367–380. doi: 10.1016/j.addr.2016.06.006

Guo, Y., Wang, Y., and Xu, L. (2015). Enhanced bioavailability of rebamipide nanocrystal tablets: formulation and *in vitro/in vivo* evaluation. *Asian J. Pharmaceut. Sci.* 10 (3), 223–229. doi: 10.1016/j.ajps.2014.09.006

Hallan, S. S., Kaur, P., Kaur, V., Mishra, N., and Vaidya, B. (2016). Lipid polymer hybrid as emerging tool in nanocarriers for oral drug delivery. *Artif. Cells Nanomed. Biotechnol.* 44 (1), 334–495. doi: 10.3109/21691401.2014.951721

Hazzah, H. A., Farid, R. M., Nasra, M. M. A., El-Massik, M. A., and Abdallah, O. Y. (2015). Lyophilized sponges loaded with curcumin solid lipid nanoparticles for buccal delivery: development and characterization. *Int. J. Pharm.* 492 (1–2), 248–257. doi: 10.1016/j.ijpharm.2015.06.022

Imperiale, J. C., Nejamkin, P., del Sole, M. J., Lanusse, C. E., and Sosnik, A. (2015). Novel protease inhibitor-loaded nanoparticle-in-microparticle delivery system leads to a dramatic improvement of the oral pharmacokinetics in dogs. *Biomaterials* 37, 383–394. doi: 10.1016/j.biomaterials.2014.10.026

Imperiale, J. C., and Sosnik, A. (2013). Nanoparticle-in-microparticle delivery systems (NiMDS): production, administration routes and clinical potential. *Text.* 3 (1), 22–38. doi: 10.1166/jbt.2013.1064

Jiang, Y., and Stenzel, M. (2016). Drug delivery vehicles based on albumin-polymer conjugates. *Macromol. Biosci.* 16 (6), 791–8025. doi: 10.1002/mabi.201500453

Kalepu, S., and Nekkanti, V. (2015). Insoluble drug delivery strategies: review of recent advances and business prospects. *Acta Pharm. Sin. B.* 5 (5), 442–535. doi: 10.1016/j.apsb.2015.07.003

Kamaly, N., Yameen, B., Wu, J., and Farokhzad, O. C. (2016). Degradable controlled-release polymers and polymeric nanoparticles: mechanisms of controlling drug release. *Chem. Rev.* 116 (4), 2602–2635. doi: 10.1021/acs.chemrev.5b00346

Karamanidou, T., Bourganis, V., Kammona, O., and Kiparissides, C. (2016). Lipid-based nanocarriers for the oral administration of biopharmaceutics. *Nanomed. (London, Engl.)* 11 (22), 3009–3255. doi: 10.2217/nnm-2016-0265

Kerdsakundee, N., Li, W., Martins, J. P., Liu, Z., Zhang, F., Kemell, M., et al. (2017). Multifunctional nanotube-mucoadhesive poly(methyl vinyl ether-co-maleic acid) @hydroxypropyl methylcellulose acetate succinate composite for site-specific oral drug delivery. *Adv. Healthcare Mater.* 6 (20), 1700629. doi: 10.1002/ adhm.201700629.

Kevadiya, B. D., Barvaliya, M., Zhang, L., Anovadiya, A., Brahmbhatt, H., Paul, P., et al. (2018). Fenofibrate nanocrystals embedded in oral strip-films for bioavailability enhancement. *Bioeng. (Basel, Switzerland)* 5 (1), 16. doi: 10.3390/bioengineering5010016

Kim, I. S., Jeong, Y. I., Kim, D. H., Lee, Y. H., and Kim, S. H. (2001). Albumin release from biodegradable hydrogels composed of dextran and poly(ethylene glycol) macromer. *Arch. Pharmacal Res.* 24 (1), 69–735. doi: 10.1007/BF02976496

Larregieu, C. A., and Benet, L. Z. (2013). Drug discovery and regulatory considerations for improving *in silico* and *in vitro* predictions that use Caco-2 as a surrogate for human intestinal permeability measurements. *AAPS J.* 15 (2), 483–497. doi: 10.1208/s12248-013-9456-8

Lipinski, C. A., Lombardo, F., Dominy, B. W. E., and Feeney, P. J. (2001). "Experimental and computational approaches to estimate solubility and permeability in drug discovery and development settings1PII of original article: S0169-409X(96)00423-1. The article was originally published in Advanced Drug Delivery Reviews 23 (1997) 3–25.1". *Adv. Drug Delivery Rev.*, Special issue dedicated to Dr. Eric Tomlinson, Advanced drug delivery reviews, a selection of the most highly cited articles, 1991–1998, 46 (1), 3–26. doi: 10.1016/S0169-409X(00)00129-0

Liu, Y., Xie, P., Zhang, D., and Zhang, Q. (2012). A mini review of nanosuspensions development. *J. Drug Targeting* 20 (3), 209–235. doi: 10.3109/1061186X.2011.645161

Meng, X. Y., Zhang, H. X., Mezei, M., and Cui, M. (2011). Molecular docking: a powerful approach for structure-based drug discovery. Curr. comput. Aided Drug Des. 7(2), 146–157.

Moore, T. L., Rodriguez-Lorenzo, L., Hirsch, V., Balog, S., Urban, D., Jud, C., et al. (2015). Nanoparticle colloidal stability in cell culture media and impact on cellular interactions. *Chem. Soc. Rev.* 44 (17), 6287–6305. doi: 10.1039/C4CS00487F

Lv, Q., Li, X., Shen, B., Dai, L., Xu, H., Shen, C., et al. (2014). A solid phospholipid-bile salts-mixed micelles based on the fast dissolving oral films to improve the oral bioavailability of poorly water-soluble drugs. *J. Nanopart. Res.* 16 (6), 24555. doi: 10.1007/s11051-014-2455-6

Lv, Q., Shen, C., Li, X., Shen, B., Yu, C., Xu, P., et al. (2015). Mucoadhesive buccal films containing phospholipid-bile salts-mixed micelles as an effective carrier for cucurbitacin B delivery. *Drug Delivery* 22 (3), 351–585. doi: 10.3109/10717544.2013.876459

Madkhali, O., Mekhail, G., and Wettig, S. D. (2019). Modified gelatin nanoparticles for gene delivery. *Int. J. Pharm.* 554, 224–234. doi: 10.1016/j.ijpharm.2018.11.001

Nassar, T., Attili-Qadri, S., Harush-Frenkel, O., Farber, S., Lecht, S., Lazarovici, P., et al. (2011). High plasma levels and effective lymphatic uptake of docetaxel in an orally available nanotransporter formulation. *Cancer Res.* 71 (8), 3018–3285. doi: 10.1158/0008-5472.CAN-10-3118

Nekkanti, V., Pillai, R., Venkateshwarlu, V., and Harisudhan, T. (2009). Development and characterization of solid oral dosage form incorporating candesartan nanoparticles. *Pharm. Dev. Technol.* 14 (3), 290–985. doi: 10.1080/10837450802585278

Nidhi, M., Patro, M. N., Kusumvalli, S., and Kusumdevi, V. (2016). Development of transmucosal patch loaded with anesthetic and analgesic for dental procedures and *in vivo* evaluation. *Int. J. Nanomed.* 11, 2901–2920. doi: 10.2147/IJN.S94658

Puri, A., Loomis, K., Smith, B., Lee, J.-H., Yavlovich, A., Heldman, E., et al. (2009). Lipid-based nanoparticles as pharmaceutical drug carriers: from concepts to clinic. *Critical Rev. Ther. Drug Carrier Syst.* 26 (6), 523–805. doi: 10.1615/CritRevTherDrugCarrierSyst.v26.i6.10

Rana, P., and Murthy, R. S. R. (2013). Formulation and evaluation of mucoadhesive buccal films impregnated with carvedilol nanosuspension: a potential approach for delivery of drugs having high first-pass metabolism". *Drug Delivery* 20 (5), 224–355. doi: 10.3109/10717544.2013.779331

Rao, S., Richter, K., Nguyen, T.-H., Boyd, B. J., Porter, C. J. H., Tan, A., et al. (2015). Pluronic-functionalized silica–lipid hybrid microparticles: improving the oral delivery of poorly water-soluble weak bases. *Mol. Pharm.* 12 (12), 4424–4335. doi: 10.1021/acs.molpharmaceut.5b00622

Rao, S., Song, Y., Peddie, F., and Evans, A. M. (2011). Particle size reduction to the nanometer range: a promising approach to improve buccal absorption of poorly water-soluble drugs. *Int. J. Nanomed.* 6, 1245–1251. doi: 10.2147/IJN.S19151

Salem, H. F., Kharshoum, R. M., Halawa, A. K. A., and Naguib, D. M. (2018). Preparation and optimization of tablets containing a self-nano-emulsifying drug delivery system loaded with rosuvastatin. *J. Liposome Res.* 28 (2), 149–605. doi: 10.1080/08982104.2017.1295990

Shastri, D. H. (2017). Effective delivery routes and strategies for solid lipid nanoparticles (SLN) and nanostructured lipid carriers (NLC). *Curr. Pharm. Des.* 23 (43), 6592–6601. doi: 10.2174/1381612823666171122111132

Slowing, I. I., Vivero-Escoto, J. L., Wu, C.-W., and Lin, V. S. Y. (2008). Mesoporous silica nanoparticles as controlled release drug delivery and gene transfection carriers. *Adv. Drug Delivery Rev. Inorg. Nanopart. Drug Delivery* 60 (11), 1278–1288. doi: 10.1016/j.addr.2008.03.012

Soudry-Kochavi, L., Naraykin, N., Nassar, T., and Benita, S. (2015). Improved oral absorption of exenatide using an original nanoencapsulation and microencapsulation approach. *J. Controlled Release: Off. J. Controlled Release Soc.* 217, 202–210. doi: 10.1016/j.jconrel.2015.09.012

Teixeira, M. C., Carbone, C., and Souto, E. B. (2017). Beyond liposomes: recent advances on lipid based nanostructures for poorly soluble/poorly permeable drug delivery. *Prog. Lipid Res.* 68, 1–11. doi: 10.1016/j.plipres.2017.07.001

Tong, Y., Wang, Y., Yang, M., Yang, J., Chen, L., Chu, X., et al. (2018). Systematic development of self-nanoemulsifying liquisolid tablets to improve the dissolution and oral bioavailability of an oily drug, vitamin K1. *Pharmaceutics* 10 (3), 96. doi: 10.3390/pharmaceutics10030096

Washington, K. E., Kularatne, R. N., Karmegam, V., Biewer, M. C., and Stefan, M. C. (2017). Recent advances in aliphatic polyesters for drug delivery applications. Wiley Interdiscip. *Rev. Nanomed. Nanobiotechnol.* 9 (4), e1446. doi: 10.1002/wnan.1446.

Westerhout J., Bellmann S., van Ee R., Havenaar R., Leeman W., et al. (2017). Prediction of Oral Absorption of Nanoparticles from Biorelevant Matrices Using a Combination of Physiologically Relevant In Vitro and Ex Vivo Models. *J. Food Chem. Nanotechnol.* 3 (4), 111–119. doi: 10.17756/jfcn.2017-046.

Wissing, S. A., Kayser, O., and Müller, R. H. (2004). Solid lipid nanoparticles for parenteral drug delivery. *Adv. Drug Delivery Rev. Adv. Lipid-Based Drug Solubilization Targeting* 56 (9), 1257–1272. doi: 10.1016/j.addr.2003.12.002

Zhang, H., Zhu, Y., Qu, L., Wu, H., Kong, H., Yang, Z., et al. (2018). Gold nanorods conjugated porous silicon nanoparticles encapsulated in calcium alginate nano hydrogels using microemulsion templates. *Nano Lett.* 18 (2), 1448–1453. doi: 10.1021/acs.nanolett.7b05210

22

Robotic Therapy: Cost, Accuracy and Times — New Challenges in the Neonatal Intensive Care Unit

*Ilaria Amodeo [1,2], Nicola Pesenti [3], Genny Raffaeli [1,2], Gabriele Sorrentino [1], Alessia Zorz [1], Silvia Traina [1], Silvia Magnani [1], Maria Teresa Russo [1], Salvatore Muscolo [1], Laura Plevani [1], Fabio Mosca [1,2] and Giacomo Cavallaro [1]**

[1] Neonatal Intensive Care Unit, Fondazione IRCCS Ca' Granda Ospedale Maggiore Policlinico, Milan, Italy, [2] Department of Clinical Sciences and Community Health, University of Milan, Milan, Italy, [3] Department of Statistics and Quantitative Methods, Division of Biostatistics, Epidemiology and Public Health, University of Milano-Bicocca, Milan, Italy

***Correspondence:**
Giacomo Cavallaro
giacomo.cavallaro@policlinico.mi.it

Background: The medication process in the Neonatal Intensive Care Unit (NICU), can be challenging in terms of costs, time, and the risk of errors. Newborns, especially if born preterm, are more vulnerable to medication errors than adults. Recently, robotic medication compounding has reportedly improved the safety and efficiency of the therapeutic process. In this study, we analyze the advantages of using the I.V. Station® system in our NICU, compared to the manual preparation of injectable drugs in terms of accuracy, cost, and time.

Method: An *in vitro* experimental controlled study was conducted to analyze 10 injectable powdered or liquid drugs. Accuracy was calculated within a 5% difference of the bottle weight during different stages of preparation (reconstitution, dilution, and final product). The overall cost of manual and automated preparations were calculated and compared. Descriptive statistics for each step of the process are presented as mean ± standard deviation or median (range).

Results: The median error observed during reconstitution, dilution, and final therapy of the drugs prepared by the I.V. Station® ranged within ±5% accuracy, with narrower ranges of error compared to those prepared manually. With increasing preparations, the I.V. Station® consumed less materials, reduced costs, decreased preparation time, and optimized the medication process, unlike the manual method. In the 10 drugs analyzed, the time saved from using the I.V. Station® ranged from 16 s for acyclovir to 2 h 57 min for teicoplanin, and cost savings varied from 8% for ampicillin to 66% for teicoplanin. These advantages are also capable of continually improving as the total amount of final product increases.

Conclusions: The I.V. Station® improved the therapeutic process in our NICU. The benefits included increased precision in drug preparation, improved safety, lowered cost, and saved time. These advantages are particularly important in areas such as the NICU, where the I.V. Station® could improve the delivery of the high complexity of care and a large amount of intravenous therapy typically required. In addition, these benefits may lead to the reduction in medication errors and improve patient and family care; however, additional studies will be required to confirm this hypothesis.

Keywords: robotic therapy, newborn, safety therapy, patient safety, robotic cost, time, accuracy

INTRODUCTION

A significant number of intravenous medications are administered in the Neonatal Intensive Care Unit (NICU) daily, and harmful medication errors are more likely to occur there compared to adult settings (Kaushal et al., 2001). Newborns are particularly vulnerable to medication errors, based on the peculiarity of the developmental pharmacotherapy (Kearns et al., 2003; Chedoe et al., 2007). Prescriptions are expressed per kilogram of body weight and require accurate calculation and multiple dilutions when administered to preterm low-birth-weight infants. Drug pharmacokinetics and pharmacodynamics change dynamically based on evolving systems and organs maturation (Tayman et al., 2011; Allegaert et al., 2013; Allegaert et al., 2014; Allegaert and Van Den Anker, 2014). The resulting patient-specific variability to drug exposure may threaten drug safety, particularly for compounds with a narrow therapeutic range (Samra et al., 2011). Lastly, most of the drugs prescribed are still off-label for neonates (Conroy et al., 1999).

Given the complexity of all these issues, the medication process can be challenging in terms of cost, time, and risk of errors, particularly for preterm newborns (Conroy et al., 1999; Chappell and Newman, 2004; Kugelman et al., 2008). In order to optimize the therapeutic process, many technologic solutions have been introduced in clinical practice in recent years, such as the use of a computerized physician order entry system (CPOE), bar-coded identification, and smart-infusion pumps (Myers et al., 1998; Bates, 2007; Vardi et al., 2007). Recently, robotic medication compounding has demonstrated an improvement in the safety and efficiency of the therapeutic process in different settings. Robotic devices have been shown to be useful in the preparation of chemotherapies, adjuvant medications, and cytotoxic drugs for adult patients (Seger et al., 2012; Nam et al., 2016; Iwamoto et al., 2017; Unluturk et al., 2018; Geersing et al., 2019). In all cases, the robot was handled by the hospital pharmacists. To date, there are no reports of robotic applications in the neonatal setting.

The I.V. Station® is an automated compounding robot that prepares ready-to-administer sterile medications through a fully-automated process (Omnicell, inc. www.omnicell.com). This technology has been specifically developed for the automated individualized preparation and distribution of injectable drugs ready for use, including drugs requiring multiple dilutions (either powdered or in solution). Several studies have already demonstrated that the use of the I.V. Station® reduces the rate of preparation errors and the waste of injectable drugs (Flynn et al., 1997). In this study, we compare the advantages obtained from the robot-assisted preparation of injectable drugs by the I.V. Station®, to the manual preparation in terms of accuracy, costs, and time in our NICU.

MATERIALS AND METHODS

Study Design

This study was conducted in the NICU of Fondazione IRCCS Ca' Granda Ospedale Maggiore Policlinico in Milan in 2016 for 2 months after the introduction of the I.V. Station® technology. We performed an *in vitro* experimental controlled study to analyze the accuracy, cost, and preparation time of medication with robot-assistance compared to manual preparation.

The analysis included 10 injectable drugs that were either powdered or liquid. For each drug, 10 manual preparations and 10 automated preparations were compared, for a total of 200 samples (100 manual and 100 automated). Prescriptions have been made considering a hypothetical newborn patient of 1000 g of body weight. Dosages were prescribed based on the pediatric and neonatal therapeutic dosage handbook (Taketomo et al., 2018). The updated annual consumption of each drug calculated from January to December 2018 in listed in **Table 1**.

Samples intended for *in vitro* analyses were not utilized for clinical purposes. Since patients were not directly involved in the study, our investigation did not require ethical approval.

Accuracy

Accuracy was calculated as <5% difference in the bottle weight during different stages of preparation (reconstitution, dilution, and final preparation) for both the manual and automated processes. This value reflects the accuracy of the concentration of the drug at the end of each step.

Automated-Preparation

Using the I.V. Station®, drugs were prepared and multiple controls were performed at different steps, specifically:

- *Reconstitution check*: for the powdered drugs (Acyclovir, Ampicillin, Ampicillin + Sulbactam, Amoxicillin + Clavulanic

TABLE 1 | Drugs, composition, therapeutic dose, and number of annual prescriptions.

Drug	*Composition*	*Therapeutic dose*	*Administrations/year*
Acyclovir	powder	20 mg/kg 3 times a day for 14-21 days	33
Ampicillin	powder	50 mg/kg 3 times a day for 7 days	6585
Ampicillin+Sulbactam	powder	50 mg/kg 2 times/day for 7 days	842
Amoxicillin+Clavulanic Acid	powder	50 mg/kg 2 times/day for 7 days	3010
Dobutamine	liquid	5 mcg/kg/min	243
Fluconazole	liquid	3 mg/kg every 72 hours (prophylaxis)	505
Metronidazole	liquid	7,5 mg/kg every 12-24 hours for 14 days	1136
Paracetamol	liquid	10 mg/kg every 4-8 hours	2623
Teicoplanin	powder	8 mg/kg every 24 hours	139
Vancomycin	powder	10 mg/kg every 24-72 hours for 7-21 days	6452

Acid, Teicoplanin, Vancomycin), the I.V. Station® maintained accuracy within a range of ±5% by assessing the weight of the solvent injected.
- *Dilution check*: for drugs requiring dilution (Acyclovir, Ampicillin, Ampicillin + Sulbactam, Amoxicillin + Clavulanic Acid, Dobutamine, Teicoplanin, Vancomycin), the I.V. Station® maintained accuracy within a range of ±5% by assessing the weight of the drug injected.
- *Final check*: for all preparations, the I.V. Station® maintained accuracy within a range of ±5% by assessing the weight of the final product.

Manual Preparation

Drugs were prepared by 6 nurses with at least 5 years of experience working in our NICU. No specific training was conducted before starting the study since we considered a minimum of 5 years NICU expertise sufficient for the purpose of the study.

The following formula was applied as we were aware of the density of each drug:

$$\bullet Accuracy\% = (measured\ weight - ideal\ weight) / (ideal\ weight) \times 100$$

Multiple controls were performed at different steps, specifically:

- *Reconstitution check*: for powdered drugs (Acyclovir, Ampicillin, Ampicillin + Sulbactam, Amoxicillin + Clavulanic Acid, Teicoplanin, Vancomycin), the nurse maintained accuracy within a range of ±5% by assessing the weight of the solvent injected.
- *Dilution check*: for drugs requiring dilution (Acyclovir, Ampicillin, Ampicillin + Sulbactam, Amoxicillin + Clavulanic Acid, Dobutamine, Teicoplanin, Vancomycin) the nurse maintained accuracy within a range of ±5% by assessing the weight of the drug injected.
- *Final check*: for all preparations, the nurse maintained accuracy within a range of ±5% by assessing the weight of the final product.

Costs

We calculated and compared the overall cost of the manual vs. automated drug preparation, considering a detailed list of items including bottles, syringes, needles, caps, solvents, gloves, sterile gauze, and stoppers. For manual preparations, costs were calculated based on a single dose of medication. For the IV Station®, since dilution takes place once, a higher number of vials are often needed to obtain the desired concentration of the stock solution, from which the IV Station® obtains the different doses of medication, but also has a larger amount of final product available. Hence, the costs included all the materials used to obtain the stock solution; however, multiple administrations can be obtained.

The costs of electricity, machine maintenance, days of detention due to possible damage or machine failure over the 2 month observation period were not considered.

Preparation Time

For each manual preparation, we considered the time required to walk to the laminar flow hood at nurse's station, prepare a single dose of each drug, prime the intravenous line, and return to the patient to begin drug administration. For automated compounds, we considered the time required to walk to the I.V. Station®, withdraw all the drugs already prepared by the robot, return to the laminar flow hood to complete the preparation and priming of the intravenous line, and return to the patient to begin drug administration.

Statistical Analysis

Descriptive statistics for each step of the process are presented as mean ± standard deviation or median (range) for both the I.V. Station® and manual preparations. The cost of each drug preparation is fixed, as a result of calculations based on the value of the drug itself and the overall material required. Therefore, a statistical comparison between the cost of the I.V. Station® and manual preparation cannot be conducted due to the absence of variability in the estimates. One-way ANOVA was used to compare time savings between the drugs for single preparations. Time differences between the I.V. Station® and manual preparations are reported. Statistical analysis is not informative when studying differences between the I.V. Station® and manual accuracy because all values lay in the range of ±5%.

Estimates of costs/savings and preparation times are presented using a heatmap plot. Boxplots are used to show the distribution of time for each drug analyzed. Statistical analyses were performed using R version 3.5.3 (R Foundation for Statistical Computing, Vienna, Austria).

RESULTS

Accuracy

The data concerning the accuracy of manual and robotic preparations are depicted in **Table 2**. For the I.V. Station® preparations, the median error observed during reconstitution, dilution, and final therapy ranged within ±5% accuracy. Narrow ranges of error were observed, and they were always included in the ±5% interval.

In the case of manual preparations, the median error lied in the range of ±5% accuracy, with the exception of the Ampicillin + Sulbactam, in which a median error 6.3% was observed during the dilution check. Moreover, higher variability and wider ranges of error were observed, which sometimes exceeded the ±5% limits. Indeed, in 5% of all manual preparations, the accuracy was outside the admitted interval between the range of ±5% (**Table 2**). A graphical representation of the accuracy in reconstitution, dilution, and final product for manual and robotic preparations is depicted in **Figures 1A–C**.

Cost and Savings

The costs related to manual and automatic drug preparations and the number of vials needed to be prepared for a single dose of medication are listed in **Table 3**. A projection of the expected costs savings with the I.V. Station® compared to manual drug

TABLE 2 | The accuracy of manual and robotic preparations.

		Reconstitution		Dilution		Final Therapy	
Drug	**Type**	**Median Error%**	**Range%**	**Median Error%**	**Range%**	**Median Error%**	**Range%**
Acyclovir	IV	2.6	2.0; 3.8	-0,5	-1.2; 0.8	3.1	2.1; 4.0
	M	-0.3	-2.9; 2.5	-1.8	-5.5; -0.4	-1.7	-3.1; -0.5
Amoxicillin + Clavulanic Acid	IV	2.5	-0.4; 2.8	0.6	0.1; 1.9	0.3	-0.5; 1.4
	M	-0.2	-3.5; 1.5	4.0	1.0; 5.3	-1.1	-2.3; 0.1
Ampicillin	IV	2.1	1.4; 2.6	-1.4	-3.6; 1.3	3.1	2.1; 4.0
	M	-0.2	-7.7; 6.9	3.9	0.2; 4.3	2.2	-1.4; 5.3
Ampicillin + Sulbactam	IV	2.8	2.0; 3.2	-0.5	-2.8; 1.0	-0.4	-1.1; 0.9
	M	0.0	-3.6; 3.6	6.3	5.0; 7.1	1.4	-0.4; 3.5
Teicoplanin	IV	1.2	-2.4; 1.8	-1.3	-2.1; 0.8	1.0	-1.5; 4.0
	M	0.0	-2.7; 1.2	-2.4	-3.6; -1.0	0.8	-0.4; 1.5
Vancomycin	IV	0.9	-5.0; 1.8	-0.4	-4.1; 1.3	1.0	-4.7; 3.7
	M	-0.8	-4.4; 1.0	1.2	0.1; 3.4	1.8	-0.9; 2.9
Dobutamine	IV			2.5	-1.0; 3.7	-0.2	-3.1; 1.8
	M			-3.5	-4.4; -2.8	-2.1	-3.1; -1.6
Fluconazole	IV					-1.0	-3.6; 0.9
	M					2.2	-1.6; 2.8
Metronidazole	IV					-0.7	-4.6; 1.7
	M					3.2	-0.6; 5.0
Paracetamol	IV					0.4	-2.0; 3.3
	M					4.1	-1.8; 6.2

IV, I.V.Station®; M, manual.

preparation is displayed in **Figure 2**. For each drug, the number of drug preparations needed to amortize the robotic preparation is shown. In our study, when a low number of preparations was required, the robotic process was more expensive than the manual one (red boxes). As the number of preparations increased, the I.V. Station® optimized the materials consumed and cost, and eventually equaled the cost of manual preparation (white boxes) or became even less expensive (green boxes). As shown in the heatmap, if a single preparation was considered, the manual method was more cost-effective in four out of 10 cases. However, with the 10 drug preparations analyzed, the I.V. Station® led to substantial savings for all the cases considered. The expected savings ranged from 8% for ampicillin to 66% for teicoplanin and may continue to rise as the total amount of final product increased.

Preparation Time

The time needed to prepare each drug separately is shown in **Figure 3**. In almost all cases, the time required to prepare a single manual dose was less than 4 min and ranged from 1 min 17 s for paracetamol to 3 min 18 s for Amoxicillin + Clavulanic Acid. The only exception was with teicoplanin, in which a single preparation took up to 18 min 43 s. In this case, the relevant difference was due to the difficulty associated with manual reconstitution and dilution of the powdered drug.

The median time required for a single I.V. Station® preparation was 2 min 59 s. This was in line with a majority of the manual results, although it was higher compared to paracetamol, fluconazole, and metronidazole (p-value < 0.001) and lower than amoxicillin + clavulanic acid (p-value = 0.007) and teicoplanin (p-value < 0.001).

Figure 4 shows a projection of the expected time-savings associated with the I.V. Station® compared to manual preparation. For each drug, the number of administrations required to amortize the I.V. Station® preparation times are depicted. In our study, when a low number of doses were required, the I.V. Station® was more time-consuming than the manual method (red boxes) in some instances. For example, if we required a single preparation, the I.V. Station® was more expensive than the manual method in half of the cases analyzed. As the number of preparations increased, the I.V. Station® led to a progressive optimization of the preparation process (green boxes). The I.V. Station® led to substantial time-savings in all the cases analyzed. The time saved ranged from 16 s for acyclovir to 2 h and 57 min for teicoplanin and may continue to rise even as the total number of medications prepared increase.

DISCUSSION

Medication errors are defined as any preventable event that can lead to inappropriate medication use or patient harm. Errors can occur at any stage in the medication-use process (prescribing, transcribing, dispensing, administering, monitoring) (Aronson, 2009). The therapeutic process includes several stages; each of which are potentially at risk for medication errors (Aronson, 2009). Infants who require more intensive levels of care are at a higher risk for medication errors and potentially fatal errors are three times more likely to occur in the NICU than in adult wards (Kaushal et al., 2001). Prescribing and drug administration challenges place newborns at risk of 10-fold and up to 100-fold potentially fatal dosing errors (Chappell and Newman, 2004; Taheri et al., 2013).

Preterm babies require a more intensive level of care and more complex therapy, which exposes them to a higher risk of

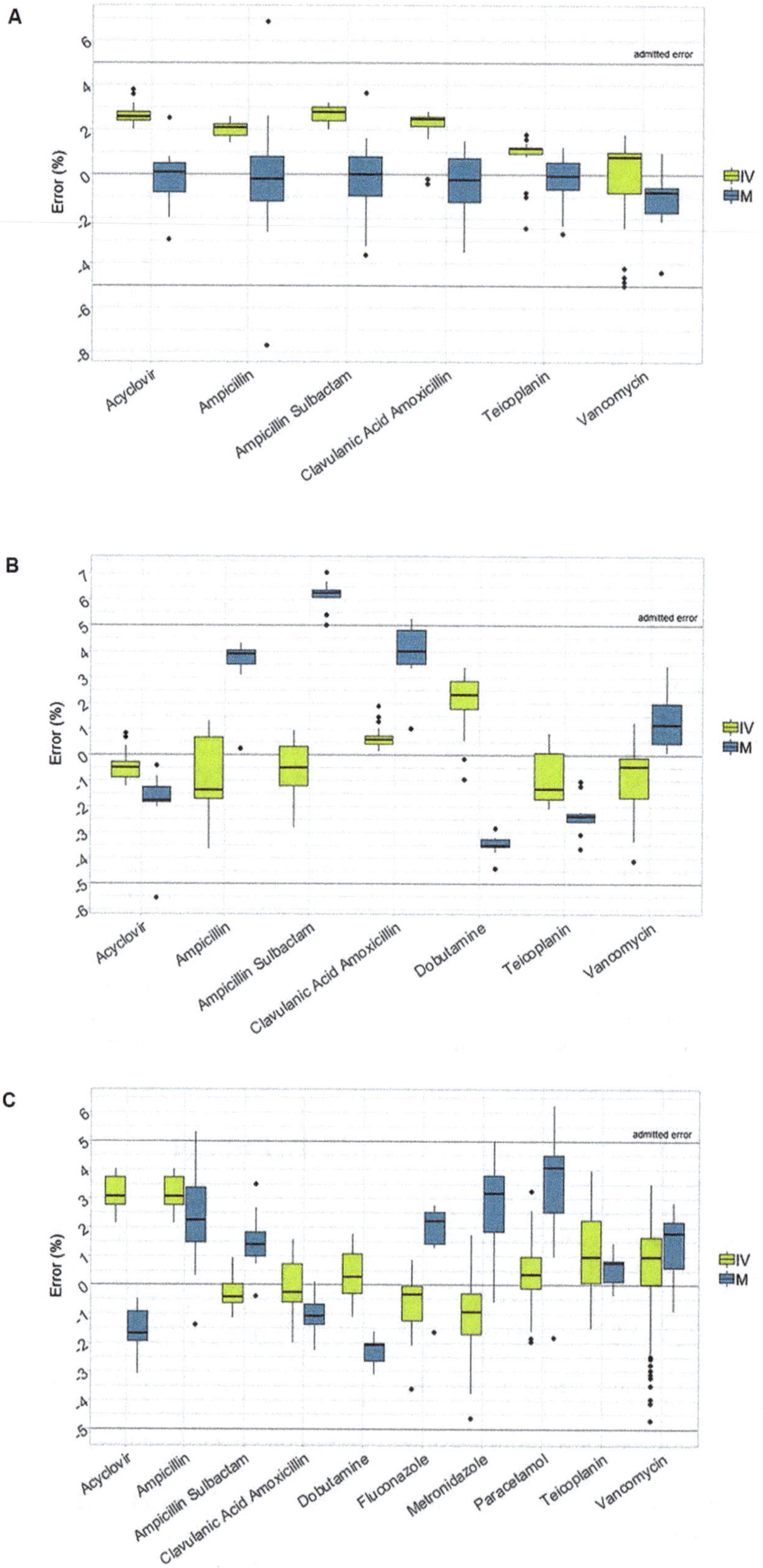

FIGURE 1 | Box-plot of accuracy in reconstitution, dilution and final product between I.V. Station® and manual preparations (IVS: I.V. Station®; M: manual). **(A)**: Accuracy in reconstitution. **(B)**: Accuracy in dilution. **(C)**: Accuracy of the final drug.

TABLE 3 | Costs of the single vial, number of vials and relative cost for the preparation of a single dose of medication (IV Station® and manual).

	IV Station										Manual									
	Acyclovir	**Ampicillin**	**Amoxicillin + Clavulanic Acid**	**Ampicillin + Sulbactam**	**Dobutamine**	**Fluconazole**	**Metronidazole**	**Paracetamol**	**Teicoplanin**	**Vancomycin**	**Acyclovir**	**Ampicillin**	**Amoxicillin + Clavulanic Acid**	**Ampicillin + Sulbactam**	**Dobutamine**	**Fluconazole**	**Metronidazole**	**Paracetamol**	**Teicoplanin**	**Vancomycin**
Single vial cost (€)	7.70	4.08	2,42	6.80	4.69	0.50	0.29	0.60	41.60	1.04	7.70	4.08	2.42	6.80	4.69	0.50	0.29	0.60	41.60	1.04
Number of vials (n)	2	5	2	5	1	1	1	1	2	1	1	1	1	1	1	1	1	1	1	1
Total cost of the drug (€)	15.40	20.40	4.84	34.00	4.69	0.50	0.29	0.60	83.20	1.04	7.70	4.08	2.42	6.80	4.69	0.50	0.29	0.60	41.60	1.04
Vial drug content (mg)	250	1000	1200	1000	250	100	500	1000	200	500	250	1000	1200	1000	250	100	500	1000	200	500
Vial drug volume (mL)	0	0	0	0	20	50	100	100	0	0	0	0	0	0	20	50	100	100	0	0
Mean drug doses pro Kg (mg/Kg/dosis)	20	50	50	50	5	3	7.5	10	8	10	20	50	50	50	5	3	7.5	10	8	10
Volume of Drug Reconstitution (mL)	5	5	5	5	0	0	0	0	5	5	10	20	20	20	30	0	0	0	20	100
Final dilution volume (mL)	108	120	108	120	109	50	100	100	108	104	50	20	20	20	50	50	100	100	20	100
Final drug concentration (mg/ml)	3.7037	33.3333	14.8148	33.3333	1.0321	2	5	10	2.9630	3.8462	5	50	60	50	5	2	5	10	10	5
Administration volume (mL)	5.4	1.5	3,4	1.5	7.0	1.5	1.5	1.0	2.7	2.6	4.0	1.0	1.0	1.0		1.5	1.5	1.0	0.8	2.0
Drug stability (h)	24	12	1	12	48	48	48	48	48	48	ns	ns	ns	ns	ns	ns	ns	ns	ns	ns
Number of possible administrations (n)	20	80	32	80	16	33	67	100	40	40	1	1	1	1	1	1	1	1	1	1
Num. admin. amortize costs (n)	2	3	2	4	2	1	2	2	2	2	1	1	1	1	1	1	1	1	1	1

h, hours; mg, milligrams; mL, milliliters; n, numbers; ns, not store. Doses of amoxicillin + clavulanate and ampicillin + sulbactam are referred to as amoxicillin and ampicillin alone.

iatrogenic events. Thus, the incidence of medication errors that occur during the care of extremely preterm newborns is reported to be quite high near 57%, compared to 3% when caring for full-term infants (Kugelman et al., 2008). In this patient category, adequate drug dosing requires serial dilutions and manipulation of the solutions, thus increasing the odds of an incorrect dose, concentration, and contamination of the final solution (Kugelman et al., 2008). As previously demonstrated in the literature, manually-prepared drugs in the ICU setting frequently show significant deviations from the target concentration, while automated-prepared drugs show less variability (Allen et al., 1995; Parshuram et al., 2003; Wheeler et al., 2008; Dehmel et al., 2011; Seger et al., 2012). This wide variability can lead to harmful consequences, such as adverse reactions due to overdosing or loss of efficacy due to underdosing (Kugelman et al., 2008). In a recent study, Iwamoto et al. demonstrated that the robotic preparation of antineoplastic drugs using APOTECA-chemo had higher accuracy and a lower absolute dose error compared to manual preparation. The risk of overdose significantly reduced, resulting in safer cancer treatment (Iwamoto et al., 2017). Geersing et al. also demonstrated that APOTECA-chemo preparations were microbiologically safe (Geersing et al., 2019).

Our data confirm that the I.V. Station® can reduce variability and thus improve accuracy at any step of the medication process (**Table 2**, **Figure 1**). Although manual method results in a tolerable median error, it shows wider variability among different preparations, with some dropping outside of the ±5% admitted interval. As recently reported in the literature, ward-based manually prepared solutions can deviate in concentration conformity more often than machine-made solutions (Kugelman et al., 2008). As can be expected in any operator-dependent process, the accuracy of the final therapy could not be guaranteed, without the possibility to identify and discard those preparations which do not respect the desired concentration. A centralized, automated preparation of standardized solutions has already been proposed as an effective means to reduce preparation error in everyday practice (Kugelman et al., 2008).

Unlike manual preparations, the I.V. Station® is set to automatically discard preparations that do not respect the predetermined range of accuracy. Hence, our data are consistent with this hypothesis. For this reason, the margin of error observed with the I.V. Station® never dropped outside the ±5% accuracy interval in any of the steps analyzed (reconstitution, dilution, final product). Therefore, the I.V. Station® may guarantee a high level of concentration conformity, and thus increased drug safety. Moreover, when combined with other strategies (i.e., electronic medical record, computerized order entry, and bar-code system) robotic technology is expected to reduce the risk of prescription and administration errors, improving safety and workflow efficiency (Dehmel et al., 2011).

Robotic preparation appears to be safer not only for the patient but also for the staff. Seger et al. observed a significant reduction in potentially harmful staff events after the

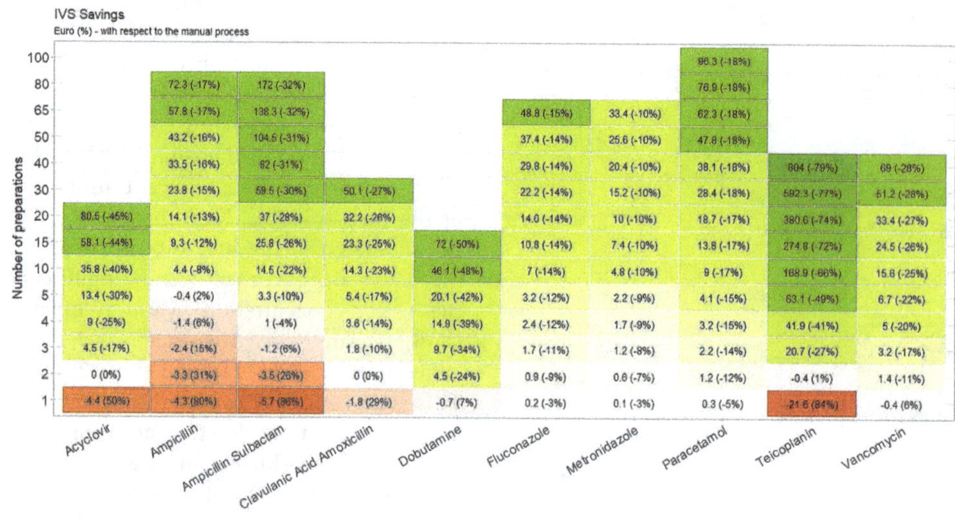

FIGURE 2 | Estimated cost savings. The robotic preparations result more expensive than the manual one in the red boxes. As the amount of preparations increases, I.V. Station® leads to an optimization of materials consumption and costs, becoming equal to manual preparation (white boxes) or even less expensive (green boxes).

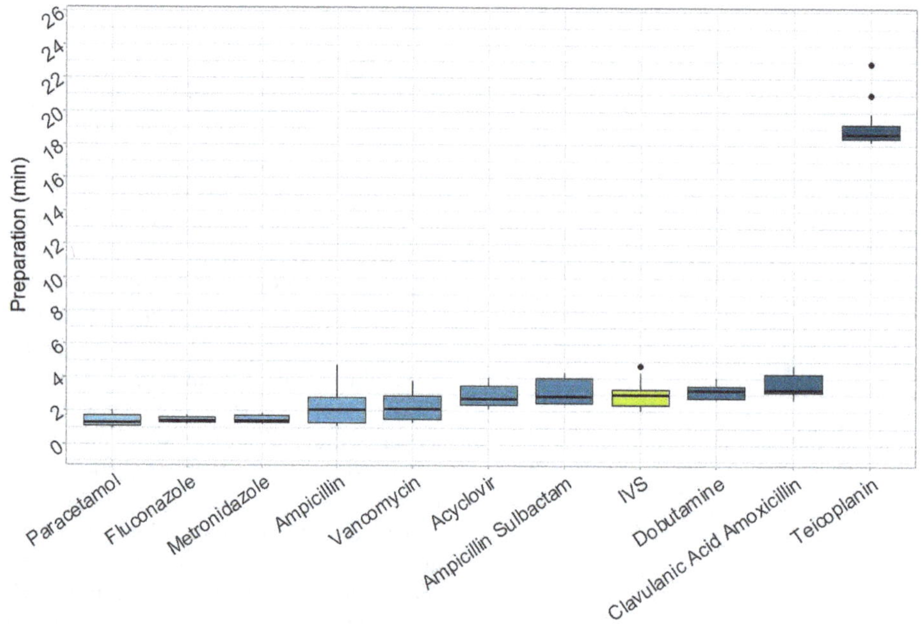

FIGURE 3 | Times for preparations. Time needed for the preparation of each drug separately (IVS: I.V. Station®).

introduction of robotic preparation of an antineoplastic drug (Seger et al., 2012). Although we did not evaluate staff events in relation to the therapeutic process, we could speculate that advantages similar to those reported by Seger et al. would occur in our NICU, where work-related risk is high. Robotic technology offers the opportunity not only for safer but also for a more cost-effective medication process. Moreover, Seger et al. found out that by introducing robotic preparation of an antineoplastic drug and adjuvant medications, they considerably reduced ancillary costs associated with several components. The savings accounted for 60% of the overall cost, and when annualized for the number of antineoplastics prepared in a year, they would have saved \$115,500 in material costs (Seger et al., 2012).

Our data confirm that robotic technology reduces the cost administering most drugs, especially when multiple preparations are needed. Benefits are expected to be even more remarkable when considering the huge number of medications prescribed in

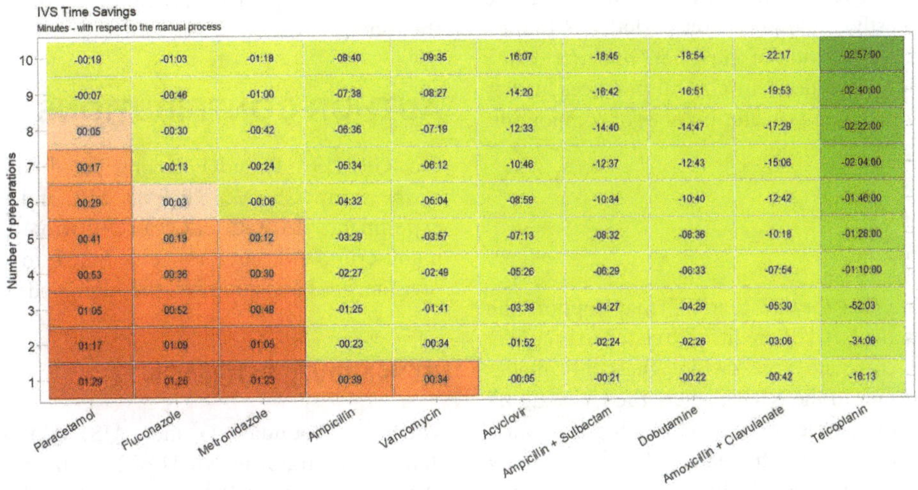

FIGURE 4 | Estimated time savings. I.V. Station® expected time-saving compared to manual preparation. With a low number of doses, I.V. Station® could result in more time-consuming than the manual method (red boxes). With the increase of preparations, I.V. Station® leads to a progressive optimization of the preparation process (green boxes).

the NICU, since the more preparations of the same drug that are required within short period, the greater are the advantage, as the robot may use the same vial.

As shown in **Figure 2**, if the number of doses prepared through the I.V. Station® is low, the material consumption is high in a first step but could be subsequently amortized by an increase in the number of preparations. The greater is the number of patients requiring the same therapy in a given period, the more remarkable the advantage. Therefore, the I.V. Station® leads to greater savings in the long run, provided that the final product is consumed within the time frame in which the diluted solution remains stable.

Hence, the robotic process could be further optimized by consistently using the I.V. Station®, to expand production to other departments of the same hospital or other NICUs in the territory, building a distribution network with centralized production. Furthermore, automated-preparation of medications allow nurses to save time during the therapeutic process. Although manual preparation is rapid for some drugs (i.e., paracetamol, which is ready for use), some drugs require multiple dilutions and a significant amount of time to be prepared (i.e., teicoplanin) (**Figure 3**).

The I.V. Station® prepares multiple drugs in a sequence that can be withdrawn at once (**Figure 4**), thus inducing relevant time savings compared to manual preparation. For liquid drugs that are ready to be used (as paracetamol), the advantage commences when the number of doses to be prepared is more than nine. In analyzing the other compounds, savings begin with a lower number of preparations and is highest with teicoplanin, as robotic process saves a great deal of time from the first administration. With costs savings, the more intravenous therapy required, the greater the advantage in terms of procedural efficiency. The saved "drug preparation time" can, therefore, be used for the direct care of the neonate. While the robot is working, the nurse could remain at the patient's bedside to better assist the baby wherever necessary, engage and educate the family, in an effort to provide the best care possible. As a result, the bond between the newborn and parents can be strongly enhanced. All these positive effects are not currently quantifiable but could represent a strong point in favor of smart robotics in the NICU setting.

Our study has some limitations. We analyzed a small number of injectable drugs, which only represents a small proportion of the intravenous therapy administered in the NICU. However, we have included the compounds that are the most commonly prescribed by neonatologists. Our analysis did not include costs concerning electricity, machine maintenance, or days of detention due to possible damage or failure of the robot. However, in 2018, the inactivity rate of the I.V. Station® was almost negligible (2.5% = 9.2/365 days), with a minimum time lag of 4.8 min up to 2.5 days of the stop. Seger et al. found some mechanical or software failure events associated with robotic preparations, which did not have harmful consequences on the patients but affected workflow efficiency and wasting of some medication (Seger et al., 2012). These are important limitations of robotic technology. The impact of ancillary costs, robot, or software failure, must be further characterized, and strategies for avoiding waste need to be implemented. Another limitation is that analysis of the microbiological safety of robotic compounds was not analyzed in this study. However, a preliminary microbiological analysis confirming the bacteriological safety was performed in 2013 before the implementation of the robot in our Unit. Based on the standard operating procedures of the I.V. Station®, the sterility of drug preparations is guaranteed for 24 h.

Based on our on-site microbiological surveillance, we have extended the sterility for liquid preparations for up to 72 h. Over 1 year, we analyzed microbiological cultures taken both from pharmaceutical preparations and the surface of the robot (daily during the first month, then weekly for three months and monthly for the rest of the year), which turned out to be negative (unpublished data). Lastly, the observation period was limited to 2 months after the introduction of the robot. To better define the advantages of the I.V. Station® in clinical practice, further analysis must be conducted on a greater number of compounds, and during a more extended period.

CONCLUSIONS

Our data demonstrate that the I.V. Station® may support the therapeutic process in the NICU. Benefits are related to accuracy in drug preparation, cost, and time-saving. These advantages are particularly important in the NICU, where the I.V. Station® could facilitate the high complexity of care, nursing workload, and the significant amount of intravenous therapy typically administered. Robotics may positively impact the patients and their families, by allocating the human resources (i.e., nurses' time and effort) to neonatal care. A possible reduction in medication errors due to the introduction of automated procedures is also possible: however, additional studies are required to confirm this hypothesis. Efforts should be directed at drugs that are not currently available in vials, in order to extend the number of pharmaceutical drugs that can be prepared by the robot.

AUTHOR CONTRIBUTIONS

GC, GR, GS, LP, and FM contributed conception and design of the study. GS, AZ, ST, SMa, MR, and SMu performed the experiments. IA, GC, GR, and NP wrote the first draft of the manuscript. All authors contributed to manuscript critical revision, read and approved the submitted version.

ACKNOWLEDGMENTS

Vodafone Foundation and AISTMAROnlus bought and donated the robot to NICU of Fondazione IRCCS Ca' Granda Ospedale Maggiore Policlinico (Milan). Vodafone Foundation and AISTMAROnlus were not involved in the study design, collection, analysis, interpretation of data, the writing of this article or the decision to submit it for publication. The authors would like to thank all the healthcare providers involved in the Neonatal Intensive Care Unit of the Fondazione IRCCS Ca' Granda Ospedale Maggiore Policlinico.

REFERENCES

Allegaert, K., and Van Den Anker, J. N. (2014). Clinical pharmacology in neonates: small size, huge variability. *Neonatology* 105, 344–349. doi: 10.1159/000360648

Allegaert, K., Naulaers, G., Vanhaesebrouck, S., and Anderson, B. J. (2013). The paracetamol concentration-effect relation in neonates. *Pediatr. Anesth.* 23, 45–50. doi: 10.1111/pan.12076

Allegaert, K., Van De Velde, M., and Van Den Anker, J. (2014). Neonatal clinical pharmacology. *Pediatr. Anesth.* 24, 30–38. doi: 10.1111/pan.12176

Allen, E. M., Boerum, D. H. V., Olsen, A. F., and Dean, J. M. (1995). Difference between the measured and ordered dose of catecholamine infusions. *Ann. Pharmacother.* 29, 1095–1100. doi: 10.1177/106002809502901104

Aronson, J. K. (2009). Medication errors: definitions and classification. *Br. J. Clin. Pharmacol.* 67, 599–604. doi: 10.1111/j.1365-2125.2009.03415.x

Bates, D. W. (2007). Preventing medication errors: a summary. *Am. J. Health-Syst. Pharm.* 64, S3–S9. doi: 10.2146/ajhp070190

Chappell, K., and Newman, C. (2004). Potential tenfold drug overdoses on a neonatal unit. *Arch. Dis. In Childhood-Fetal Neonatal. Edition* 89, F483–F484. doi: 10.1136/adc.2003.041608

Chedoe, I., Molendijk, H. A., Dittrich, S. T., Jansman, F. G., Harting, J. W., Brouwers, J. R., et al. (2007). Incidence and nature of medication errors in neonatal intensive care with strategies to improve safety. *Drug Saf.* 30, 503–513. doi: 10.2165/00002018-200730060-00004

Conroy, S., Mcintyre, J., and Choonara, I. (1999). Unlicensed and off label drug use in neonates. *Arch. Dis. In Childhood-Fetal Neonatal. Edition* 80, F142–F145. doi: 10.1136/fn.80.2.F142

Dehmel, C., Braune, S. A., Kreymann, G., Baehr, M., Langebrake, C., Hilgarth, H., et al. (2011). Do centrally pre-prepared solutions achieve more reliable drug concentrations than solutions prepared on the ward? *Intens. Care Med.* 37, 1311–1316. doi: 10.1007/s00134-011-2230-4

Flynn, E. A., Pearson, R. E., and Barker, K. N. (1997). Observational study of accuracy in compounding iv admixtures at five hospitals. *Am. J. Health-Syst. Pharm.* 54, 904–912. doi: 10.1093/ajhp/54.8.904

Geersing, T. H., Franssen, E. G. F., Pilesi, F., and Crul, M. (2019). Microbiological performance of a robotic system for aseptic compounding of cytostatic drugs. *Eur. J. Pharmaceut. Sci.* 15, 130:181–185. doi: 10.1016/j.ejps.2019.01.034

Iwamoto, T., Morikawa, T., Hioki, M., Sudo, H., Paolucci, D., and Okuda, M. (2017). Performance evaluation of the compounding robot, APOTECAchemo, for injectable anticancer drugs in a Japanese hospital. *J. Pharmaceut. Health Care Sci.* 243, 12. doi: 10.1186/s40780-017-0081-z

Kaushal, R., Bates, D. W., Landrigan, C., Mckenna, K. J., Clapp, M. D., Federico, F., et al. (2001). Medication errors and adverse drug events in pediatric inpatients. *Jama* 285, 2114–2120. doi: 10.1001/jama.285.16.2114

Kearns, G. L., Abdel-Rahman, S. M., Alander, S. W., Blowey, D. L., Leeder, J. S., and Kauffman, R. E. (2003). Developmental pharmacology-drug disposition, action, and therapy in infants and children. *New Engl. J. Med.* 349, 1157–1167. doi: 10.1056/NEJMra035092

Kugelman, A., Inbar-Sanado, E., Shinwell, E. S., Makhoul, I. R., Leshem, M., Zangen, S., et al. (2008). Iatrogenesis in neonatal intensive care units: observational and interventional, prospective, multicenter study. *Pediatrics* 122, 550–555. doi: 10.1542/peds.2007-2729

Myers, T. F., Venable, H. H., and Hansen, J. A. (1998). Computer-enhanced neonatology practice evolution in an academic medical center. NICU Clinical Effectiveness Task Force. *J. Perinatol.: Off. J. California Perinatal Assoc.* 18, S38–S44.

Nam, G. J., Joo, K., Young, J. K., Yun, K., Yeoun-Jae, A. S., Jung, K., et al. (2016). Development of Dual-Arm Anticancer Drug Compounding Robot and Preparation System with Adaptability and High-Speed. *J. Int. Soc. Simulation Surg.* 3, 64–68. doi: 10.18204/JISSiS.2016.3.2.064

Parshuram, C. S., Ng, G. Y., Ho, T. K., Klein, J., Moore, A. M., Bohn, D., et al. (2003). Discrepancies between ordered and delivered concentrations of opiate infusions in critical care. *Crit. Care Med.* 31, 2483–2487. doi: 10.1097/01.CCM.0000089638.83803.B2

Samra, H. A., Mcgrath, J. M., and Rollins, W. (2011). Patient safety in the NICU: a comprehensive review. *J. Perinatal Neonatal Nurs.* 25, 123–132. doi: 10.1097/JPN.0b013e31821693b2

Seger, A. C., Churchill, W. W., Keohane, C. A., Belisle, C. D., Wong, S. T., Sylvester, K. W., et al. (2012). Impact of robotic antineoplastic preparation on safety, workflow, and costs. *J. Oncol. Pract.* 8, 344–349. doi: 10.1200/JOP.2012.000600

Taheri, E., Nourian, M., Rasouli, M., and Kavousi, A. (2013). The study of type and amount of medication errors in neonatal intensive care units and neonatal units. *Iran J. Crit. Care Nurs.* 6 (1), 21–28.

Taketomo, C. K., Hodding J. H., and Kraus D. M. (2018). *Lexicomp pediatric & neonatal dosage handbook: with international trade names index: a global resource for clinicians treating pediatric and neonatal patients.* Hudson, Ohio: Wolters Kluwer. 24th Ed.

Tayman, C., Rayyan, M., and Allegaert, K. (2011). Neonatal pharmacology: extensive interindividual variability despite limited size. *J. Pediatr. Pharmacol. Ther.* 16, 170–184. doi: 10.5863/1551-6776-16.3.170

Unluturk, M. S., Tamer, O., and Utku, S. (2018). A robotic system to prepare IV solutions. *Int. J. Med. Inf.* 119, 61–69. doi: 10.1016/j.ijmedinf.2018.09.011

Vardi, A., Efrati, O., Levin, I., Matok, I., Rubinstein, M., Paret, G., et al. (2007). Prevention of potential errors in resuscitation medications orders by means of a computerized physician order entry in paediatric critical care. *Resuscitation* 73, 400–406. doi: 10.1016/j.resuscitation.2006.10.016

Wheeler, D. W., Degnan, B. A., Sehmi, J. S., Burnstein, R. M., Menon, D. K., and Gupta, A. K. (2008). Variability in the concentrations of intravenous drug infusions prepared in a critical care unit. *Intens. Care Med.* 34, 1441–1447. doi: 10.1007/s00134-008-1113-9

Permissions

All chapters in this book were first published by Frontiers; hereby published with permission under the Creative Commons Attribution License or equivalent. Every chapter published in this book has been scrutinized by our experts. Their significance has been extensively debated. The topics covered herein carry significant findings which will fuel the growth of the discipline. They may even be implemented as practical applications or may be referred to as a beginning point for another development.

The contributors of this book come from diverse backgrounds, making this book a truly international effort. This book will bring forth new frontiers with its revolutionizing research information and detailed analysis of the nascent developments around the world.

We would like to thank all the contributing authors for lending their expertise to make the book truly unique. They have played a crucial role in the development of this book. Without their invaluable contributions this book wouldn't have been possible. They have made vital efforts to compile up to date information on the varied aspects of this subject to make this book a valuable addition to the collection of many professionals and students.

This book was conceptualized with the vision of imparting up-to-date information and advanced data in this field. To ensure the same, a matchless editorial board was set up. Every individual on the board went through rigorous rounds of assessment to prove their worth. After which they invested a large part of their time researching and compiling the most relevant data for our readers.

The editorial board has been involved in producing this book since its inception. They have spent rigorous hours researching and exploring the diverse topics which have resulted in the successful publishing of this book. They have passed on their knowledge of decades through this book. To expedite this challenging task, the publisher supported the team at every step. A small team of assistant editors was also appointed to further simplify the editing procedure and attain best results for the readers.

Apart from the editorial board, the designing team has also invested a significant amount of their time in understanding the subject and creating the most relevant covers. They scrutinized every image to scout for the most suitable representation of the subject and create an appropriate cover for the book.

The publishing team has been an ardent support to the editorial, designing and production team. Their endless efforts to recruit the best for this project, has resulted in the accomplishment of this book. They are a veteran in the field of academics and their pool of knowledge is as vast as their experience in printing. Their expertise and guidance has proved useful at every step. Their uncompromising quality standards have made this book an exceptional effort. Their encouragement from time to time has been an inspiration for everyone.

The publisher and the editorial board hope that this book will prove to be a valuable piece of knowledge for researchers, students, practitioners and scholars across the globe.

List of Contributors

Gareth Baynam
Genetic Services of Western Australia, Department of Health, Government of Western Australia, Perth, WA, Australia
Western Australian Register of Developmental Anomalies, Perth, WA, Australia
Office of Population Health Genomics, Public Health Division, Department of Health, Government of Western Australia, Perth, WA, Australia
School of Paediatrics and Child Health, University of Western Australia, Perth, WA, Australia
Institute for Immunology and Infectious Diseases, Murdoch University, Perth, WA, Australia
Telethon Kids Institute, Perth, WA, Australia
Spatial Sciences, Department of Science and Engineering, Curtin University, Perth, WA, Australia

Alicia Bauskis, Caroline E. Walker and Caron M. Molster
Office of Population Health Genomics, Public Health Division, Department of Health, Government of Western Australia, Perth, WA, Australia

Nicholas Pachter
Genetic Services of Western Australia, Department of Health, Government of Western Australia, Perth, WA, Australia
School of Paediatrics and Child Health, University of Western Australia, Perth, WA, Australia
School of Pathology and Laboratory Medicine, University of Western Australia, Perth, WA, Australia

Lyn Schofield
Genetic Services of Western Australia, Department of Health, Government of Western Australia, Perth, WA, Australia
Centre for Comparative Genomics, Murdoch University, Perth, WA, Australia

Hedwig Verhoef
Cooperative Research Centre for Spatial Information, Perth, WA, Australia

Richard L. Palmer, Stefanie Kung, Petra Helmholz and Michael Ridout
School of Spatial Sciences, Curtin University, Perth, WA, Australia

Anne Hawkins
Genetic Services of Western Australia, Department of Health, Government of Western Australia, Perth, WA, Australia

Jack Goldblatt
Genetic Services of Western Australia, Department of Health, Government of Western Australia, Perth, WA, Australia
School of Paediatrics and Child Health, University of Western Australia, Perth, WA, Australia

Tarun S. Weeramanthri
Public Health Division, Department of Health, Government of Western Australia, Perth, WA, Australia

Hugh J. S. Dawkins
Office of Population Health Genomics, Public Health Division, Department of Health, Government of Western Australia, Perth, WA, Australia
School of Pathology and Laboratory Medicine, University of Western Australia, Perth, WA, Australia
Centre for Comparative Genomics, Murdoch University, Perth, WA, Australia
Centre for Population Health Research, Curtin Health Innovation Research Institute, Curtin University of Technology, Perth, WA, Australia

Weiduo Hou, Chenyi Ye, Weixu Li, Xiang Gao, Rongxin He, Qiang Zheng and Wei Zhang
Department of Orthopedics, Second Affiliated Hospital, School of Medicine, Zhejiang University, Hangzhou, China
Research institute of Orthopaedics, Zhejiang University, Hangzhou, China

Mo Chen
Department of Rheumatology, Second Affiliated Hospital, School of Medicine, Zhejiang University, Hangzhou, China

David B. Preen and Lakkhina Troeung
Centre for Health Services Research, School of Population and Global Health, The University of Western Australia, Perth, WA, Australia

Iris Lansdorp-Vogelaar
Department of Public Health, Erasmus University Medical Centre, Rotterdam, Netherlands

Hooi C. Ee
Department of Gastroenterology, Sir Charles Gairdner Hospital, Nedlands, WA, Australia

Cameron Platell
Colorectal Cancer Research Unit, The University of Western Australia, Perth, WA, Australia

Dayna R. Cenin
Centre for Health Services Research, School of Population and Global Health, The University of Western Australia, Perth, WA, Australia
Department of Public Health, Erasmus University Medical Centre, Rotterdam, Netherlands

Max Bulsara
Centre for Health Services Research, School of Population and Global Health, The University of Western Australia, Perth, WA, Australia
Institute for Health Research, University of Notre Dame, Fremantle, WA, Australia

Peter O'Leary
Faculty of Health Sciences, Curtin University, Perth, WA, Australia

Orenzio Soler
School of Pharmacy, Health Science Institute, Federal University of Pará, Belém, Brazil

Jorge Otávio Maia Barreto
Fiocruz School of Government, Fiocruz Brasília, Osvaldo Cruz Foundation, Brasília, Brazil

M Sanni Ali
Faculty of Epidemiology and Population Health, Department of Non-communicable Disease Epidemiology, London School of Hygiene and Tropical Medicine, London, United Kingdom
Nuffield Department of Orthopaedics, Rheumatology and Musculoskeletal Sciences (NDORMS), Center for Statistics in Medicine (CSM), University of Oxford, Oxford, United Kingdom
Centre for Data and Knowledge Integration for Health (CIDACS), Instituto Gonçalo Muniz, Fundação Osvaldo Cruz, Salvador, Brazil

Maria Yury Ichihara and Mauricio L. Barreto
Centre for Data and Knowledge Integration for Health (CIDACS), Instituto Gonçalo Muniz, Fundação Osvaldo Cruz, Salvador, Brazil
Institute of Public Health, Federal University of Bahia (UFBA), Salvador, Brazil

Luciane Cruz Lopes
University of Sorocaba–UNISO, São Paulo, Brazil
Pharmaceutical Sciences Graduate Program, University of Sorocaba (UNISO), Sorocaba, Brazil

George C.G. Barbosa, Robespierre Pita, Roberto Perez Carreiro, Dandara Ramos, Nivea Bispo and Bethania de Araujo Almeida
Centre for Data and Knowledge Integration for Health (CIDACS), Instituto Gonçalo Muniz, Fundação Osvaldo Cruz, Salvador, Brazil

Djanilson Barbosa dos Santos
Centro de Ciências da Saúde, Federal University of Recôncavo of Bahia (UFRB), Salvador, Brazil

Fabiana Raynal and Vania Canuto
Department of Management and Incorporation of Health Technology, Ministry of Health (DGITS/MS), Brasília, Brazil

Rosemeire L. Fiaccone
Centre for Data and Knowledge Integration for Health (CIDACS), Instituto Gonçalo Muniz, Fundação Osvaldo Cruz, Salvador, Brazil
Institute of Public Health, Federal University of Bahia (UFBA), Salvador, Brazil
Department of Statistics, Federal University of Bahia (UFBA), Salvador, Brazil

Marcos E. Barreto
Centre for Data and Knowledge Integration for Health (CIDACS), Instituto Gonçalo Muniz, Fundação Osvaldo Cruz, Salvador, Brazil
Department of Computing, Federal University of Bahia (UFBA), Salvador, Brazil
Institute of Health Informatics, University College London, London, United Kingdom

Liam Smeeth
Faculty of Epidemiology and Population Health, Department of Non-communicable Disease Epidemiology, London School of Hygiene and Tropical Medicine, London, United Kingdom
Centre for Data and Knowledge Integration for Health (CIDACS), Instituto Gonçalo Muniz, Fundação Osvaldo Cruz, Salvador, Brazil

Jasleen K. Jolly
Nuffield Laboratory of Ophthalmology, Nuffield Department of Clinical Neurosciences, University of Oxford, Oxford, United Kingdom
Wellcome Integrative Neuroimaging Centre, Nuffield Department of Clinical Neurosciences, University of Oxford, Oxford, United Kingdom
Oxford Eye Hospital, Oxford University Hospitals NHS Foundation Trust, Oxford, United Kingdom

Holly Bridge
Wellcome Integrative Neuroimaging Centre, Nuffield Department of Clinical Neurosciences, University of Oxford, Oxford, United Kingdom

Robert E. MacLaren
Nuffield Laboratory of Ophthalmology, Nuffield Department of Clinical Neurosciences, University of Oxford, Oxford, United Kingdom
Oxford Eye Hospital, Oxford University Hospitals NHS Foundation Trust, Oxford, United Kingdom

Jianguo Xiao, Tony Spicer, Grace Yajuan Yun, Changying Shao, Andrew Robertson and Tarun Stephen Weeramanthri
Public Health Division, Department of Health, Government of Western Australia, Perth, WA, Australia

Le Jian
Public Health Division, Department of Health, Government of Western Australia, Perth, WA, Australia
School of Public Health, Curtin University, Perth, WA, Australia

John Nairn
Australian Bureau of Meteorology, Adelaide, SA, Australia

Robert J. B. Fawcett
Australian Bureau of Meteorology, Melbourne, VIC, Australia

Adriana Muñoz-Talavera and María Cristina Islas-Carbajal
Department of Physiology, Institute of Experimental and Clinical Therapeutics, University Center for Health Sciences, University of Guadalajara, Guadalajara, Mexico

Miguel Ángel Gómez-Lim and Alberto Cristian López-Calleja
Department of Genetic Engineering, Center for Research and Advanced Studies of the National Polytechnic Institute, Irapuato, Mexico

Luis A. Salazar-Olivo
Division of Molecular Biology, Institute for Scientific and Technological Research of San Luis Potosí, San Luis Potosí, Mexico

Jörg Reinders
Scientific Support Unit Analytical Chemistry, Leibniz Research Centre for Working Environment and Human Factors, Dortmund, Germany

Katharina Lim
Institute of Functional Genomics, University of Regensburg, Regensburg, Germany

Abraham Escobedo-Moratilla
CONACYT-Consortium for Research, Innovation, and Development of the Drylands (CIIDZA), IPICYT, San Luis Potosí, Mexico

Ana Rosa Rincón-Sánchez
Institute of Molecular Biology and Gene Therapy, Department of Molecular Biology and Genomic, University Center for Health Sciences, University of Guadalajara, Guadalajara, Mexico

Richard P. Mann
School of Mathematics, University of Leeds, Leeds, UK

Faisal Mushtaq, Gabriel Mata-Cervantes, Tom Pike, Richard M. Wilkie and Mark Mon-Williams
Faculty of Medicine and Health, University of Leeds, Leeds, UK

Alan D. White
Faculty of Medicine and Health, University of Leeds, Leeds, UK
Big Data and Analytics Unit, Institute of Global Health Innovation, Imperial College London, London, UK

Dalton Coker
Big Data and Analytics Unit, Institute of Global Health Innovation, Imperial College London, London, UK

Stuart Murdoch, Tim Hiles, Clare Smith, David Berridge and Suzanne Hinchliffe
Leeds Teaching Hospitals NHS Trust, Leeds, UK

Geoff Hall, Stephen Smye and J. Peter A. Lodge
Faculty of Medicine and Health, University of Leeds, Leeds, UK
Leeds Teaching Hospitals NHS Trust, Leeds, UK

Chhabi Lal Ranabhat
Policy Research Institute, Kathmandu, Nepal
Institute for Poverty Alleviation and International Development, Yonsei University, Wonju, South Korea
Manmohan Memorial Institute of Health Science, Kathmandu, Nepal,
Department of Gerontology, Pai Chai University, Daejeon, South Korea

Chun-Bae Kim
Institute for Poverty Alleviation and International Development, Yonsei University, Wonju, South Korea
Department of Preventive Medicine, Yonsei University Wonju College of Medicine, Wonju, South Korea

Myung Bae Park
Department of Gerontology, Pai Chai University, Daejeon, South Korea

Mihajlo (Michael) Jakovljevic
Department of Global Health Economics and Policy, University of Kragujevac, Kragujevac, Serbia
Division of Health Economics, Lund University, Lund, Sweden

Anthony S. Gunnell
Exercise Medicine Research Institute, Edith Cowan University, Joondalup, WA, Australia
School of Population Health, University of Western Australia, Nedlands, WA, Australia

Sarah Joyce and Stephania Tomlin
Public Health and Clinical Services Division, Western Australian Department of Health, East Perth, WA, Australia

Dennis R. Taaffe
Exercise Medicine Research Institute, Edith Cowan University, Joondalup, WA, Australia
School of Medical and Health Sciences, Edith Cowan University, Joondalup, WA, Australia
School of Human Movement and Nutrition Sciences, The University of Queensland, St. Lucia, QLD, Australia

Prue Cormie
Institute for Health and Ageing, Australian Catholic University, Melbourne, VIC, Australia

Robert U. Newton
Exercise Medicine Research Institute, Edith Cowan University, Joondalup, WA, Australia
School of Medical and Health Sciences, Edith Cowan University, Joondalup, WA, Australia
University of Queensland Centre for Clinical Research, The University of Queensland, Brisbane, QLD, Australia

David Joseph
Exercise Medicine Research Institute, Edith Cowan University, Joondalup, WA, Australia
Department of Radiation Oncology, Sir Charles Gairdner Hospital, Nedlands, WA, Australia
Faculty of Medicine, University of Western Australia, Nedlands, WA, Australia

Nigel Spry
Exercise Medicine Research Institute, Edith Cowan University, Joondalup, WA, Australia
Faculty of Medicine, University of Western Australia, Nedlands, WA, Australia
Genesis Cancer Care, Joondalup, WA, Australia

Kristjana Einarsdóttir
Centre of Public Health Sciences and Unit for Nutrition Research, School of Health Sciences, University of Iceland, Reykjavik, Iceland

Daniel A. Galvão
Exercise Medicine Research Institute, Edith Cowan University, Joondalup, WA, Australia
School of Medical and Health Sciences, Edith Cowan University, Joondalup, WA, Australia

Bruna Cipriano Almeida Barros
Hematology Graduate Program, Federal University of São Paulo (UNIFESP), São Paulo, Brazil

Mayara Costa de Camargo, Izabela Fulone, Marcus Tolentino Silva, Miriam Sanches do Nascimento Silveira, Iara Alves de Camargo, Silvio Barberato-Filho and Fernando de Sá Del Fiol
Pharmaceutical Sciences Graduate Program, University of Sorocaba (UNISO), Sorocaba, Brazil

Angela Acosta
ISAGS, South American Institute of Government in Health, UNASUR, Rio de Janeiro, Brazil
RAM Group, National University of Colombia, Bogotá, Colombia

Egdda Patricia Vanegas
ISAGS, South American Institute of Government in Health, UNASUR, Rio de Janeiro, Brazil
SEPRO Research Group, National University of Colombia, Bogotá, Colombia

Joan Rovira
ISAGS, South American Institute of Government in Health, UNASUR, Rio de Janeiro, Brazil
Andalusian School of Public Health, Granada, Spain

Brian Godman
ISAGS, South American Institute of Government in Health, UNASUR, Rio de Janeiro, Brazil
Strathclyde Institute of Pharmacy and Biomedical Sciences, University of Strathclyde, Glasgow, United Kingdom
Division of Clinical Pharmacology, Karolinska Institute, Karolinska University Hospital Huddinge, Stockholm, Sweden
School of Pharmacy, Sefako Makgatho Health Sciences University, Garankuwa, South Africa

Tomasz Bochenek
ISAGS, South American Institute of Government in Health, UNASUR, Rio de Janeiro, Brazil
Department of Drug Management, Faculty of Health Sciences, Jagiellonian University Medical College, Krakow, Poland

Timothy J. J. Inglis and Nadia Urosevic
The Marshall Centre for Infectious Diseases Training and Research, School of Biomedical Sciences, University of Western Australia, Perth, WA, Australia
Department of Microbiology, PathWest Laboratory Medicine WA, Queen Elizabeth II Medical Centre, Nedlands, WA, Australia

Joseph O. Fadare
Department of Pharmacology and Therapeutics, Ekiti State University College of Medicine, Ado-Ekiti, Nigeria

Abimbola Margaret Obimakinde
Family Medicine Unit, Department of Community Medicine, College of Medicine, University of Ibadan, Ibadan, Nigeria
Family Medicine Department, University College Hospital, Ibadan, Nigeria

Okezie O. Enwere
Department of Medicine, Imo State University, Orlu, Nigeria

Olufemi O. Desalu
Department of Medicine, College of Health Sciences, University of Ilorin, Ilorin, Nigeria

Raphael Olasoji Ibidapo
Department of Medicine, Ekiti State University Teaching Hospital, Ado-Ekiti, Nigeria

Jennifer Girschik and Laura Jean Miller
Public Health Division, Department of Health Western Australia, Perth, WA, Australia

Tony Addiscott
Health Consumers Council, Perth, WA, Australia

Mike Daube
Faculty of Health Sciences, Curtin University, Perth, WA, Australia

Paul Katris
Western Australian Clinical Oncology Group, Perth, WA, Australia

David Ransom
Cancer and Palliative Care Network, Department of Health Western Australia, Perth, WA, Australia

Terry Slevin
Cancer Council Western Australia, Perth, WA, Australia

Tim Threlfall
Western Australian Cancer Registry, Department of Health Western Australia, Perth, WA, Australia

Flávia Campos Barcelos and Mario Jorge Sobreira da Silva
Brazilian National Cancer Institute (INCA), Rio de Janeiro, Brazil

Guacira Corrêa de Matos and Elisangela da Costa Lima
Faculty of Pharmacy, Federal University of Rio de Janeiro, Rio de Janeiro, Brazil

Fabrício Alves Barbosa da Silva
Oswaldo Cruz Foundation (Fiocruz), Rio de Janeiro, Brazil

Marleen E. Jansen
Section Community Genetics, Department of Clinical Genetics, Amsterdam Public Health Research Institute, Amsterdam, Netherlands
Institute for Public Health Genomics, School for Oncology and Developmental Biology (GROW), Faculty of Health, Medicine, and Life Sciences, Maastricht University, Maastricht, Netherlands

Karla J. Lister
Screening Policy Section, Office of Population Health Genomics, Department of Health, Government of Western Australia, Perth, WA, Australia

Henk J. van Kranen
Institute for Public Health Genomics, School for Oncology and Developmental Biology (GROW), Faculty of Health, Medicine, and Life Sciences, Maastricht University, Maastricht, Netherlands
Center for Nutrition, Prevention and Health Services, National Institute for Public Health and the Environment, Bilthoven, Netherlands

Martina C. Cornel
Section Community Genetics, Department of Clinical Genetics, Amsterdam Public Health Research Institute, Amsterdam, Netherlands

Isa Brito Félix, Anabela Mendes and Adriana Henriques
Unidade de Investigação e Desenvolvimento em Enfermagem (UI&DE), Lisbon Nursing School, Lisbon, Portugal

Mara Pereira Guerreiro
Unidade de Investigação e Desenvolvimento em Enfermagem (UI&DE), Lisbon Nursing School, Lisbon, Portugal
Centro de Investigação Interdisciplinar Egas Moniz (CiiEM), Instituto Universitário Egas Moniz, Monte de Caparica, Portugal

Afonso Cavaco
iMed. ULisboa, Faculty of Pharmacy, University of Lisbon, Lisbon, Portugal

Ana Paula Cláudio, João Balsa and Maria Beatriz Carmo
Biosystems & Integrative Sciences Institute (BioISI), Faculty of Sciences, University of Lisbon, Lisbon, Portugal

Nuno Pimenta
Sport Sciences School of Rio Maior, Polytechnic Institute of Santarém, Santarém, Portugal

John P. Newnham and Scott W. White
School of Women's and Infants' Health, The University of Western Australia, Crawley, WA, Australia

Matthew W. Kemp, Catherine A. Arrese, Roger J. Hart and Jeffrey A. Keelan
School of Women's and Infants' Health, The University of Western Australia, Crawley, WA, Australia

Renata Carvalho Feitosa, Danilo Costa Geraldes and Juliana Souza Ribeiro Costa
Laboratory of Pharmaceutical Technology (Latef), Faculty of Pharmaceutical Sciences, State University of Campinas, Campinas, Brazil
Institute of Biology, State University of Campinas, Campinas, Brazil

Viviane Lucia Beraldo-de-Araújo and Laura Oliveira-Nascimento
Laboratory of Pharmaceutical Technology (Latef), Faculty of Pharmaceutical Sciences, State University of Campinas, Campinas, Brazil

Ilaria Amodeo, Fabio Mosca and Genny Raffaeli
Neonatal Intensive Care Unit, Fondazione IRCCS Ca' Granda Ospedale Maggiore Policlinico, Milan, Italy
Department of Clinical Sciences and Community Health, University of Milan, Milan, Italy

Nicola Pesenti
Department of Statistics and Quantitative Methods, Division of Biostatistics, Epidemiology and Public Health, University of Milano-Bicocca, Milan, Italy

Gabriele Sorrentino, Alessia Zorz, Silvia Traina, Silvia Magnani, Maria Teresa Russo, Salvatore Muscolo, Laura Plevani and Giacomo Cavallaro
Neonatal Intensive Care Unit, Fondazione IRCCS Ca' Granda Ospedale Maggiore Policlinico, Milan, Italy
Department of Clinical Sciences and Community Health, University of Milan, Milan, Italy

Index

www.ingramcontent.com/pod-product-compliance
Lightning Source LLC
LaVergne TN
LVHW082136200926
848484LV00008B/2059